Moghissi's
Essentials of Thoracic and Cardiac Surgery

Second Edition

EDITED BY

K. MOGHISSI

J.A.C. THORPE

F. CIULLI

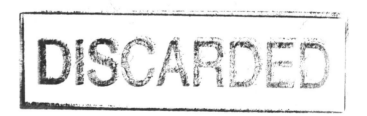
2003

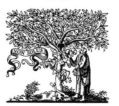

ELSEVIER

AMSTERDAM – BOSTON – LONDON – NEW YORK – OXFORD – PARIS
SAN DIEGO – SAN FRANCISCO – SINGAPORE – SYDNEY – TOKYO

ELSEVIER SCIENCE B.V.
Sara Burgerhartstraat 25
P.O. Box 211, 1000 AE Amsterdam, The Netherlands

First edition: Heinemann Medical 1986
Second edition: Elsevier Science B.V. 2003

Library of Congress Cataloging-in-Publication Data

Moghissi's essentials of thoracic and cardiac surgery / edited by Keyvan Moghissi, James
 A.C. Thorpe, Franco Ciulli.–2nd ed.
     p.; cm.
   Rev. ed. of: Essentials of thoracic and cardiac surgery / Keyvan Moghissi. 1986.
   Includes bibliographical references and index.
   ISBN 0-444-82975-X (alk. paper)
   1. Heart--Surgery. 2. Chest--Surgery. I. Title: Essentials of thoracic and cardiac
 surgery. II. Moghissi, K. (Keyvan) III. Thorpe, James A.C. IV. Ciulli, Franco. V.
 Moghissi, K. (Keyvan). Essentials of thoracic and cardiac surgery.
   [DNLM: 1. Thoracic Surgical Procedures–methods. WF 980 M696 2003]
 RD598.M553 2003
 617.4'12--dc21

                                                    2002192851

British Library Cataloguing in Publication Data

Moghissi's essentials of thoracic and cardiac surgery. –
  2nd ed.
  1. Chest – Surgery 2. Heart - -Surgery
  I. Moghissi, K. (Keyvan) II. Thorpe, J.A.C. III. Ciulli, F.
  IV. Essentials of thoracic and cardiac surgery
  617.5'4

  ISBN 044482975X

ISBN: 0-444-82975-X

⊗ The paper used in this publication meets the requirements of ANSI/NISO Z39.48-1992 (Permanence of Paper).
Printed in The Netherlands.

List of Contributors

Gianni D. Angelini, *MD, FRCS*, Professor of Cardiac Surgery, Bristol Heart Institute, University of Bristol, UK

Raimondo Ascione, *MD*, Senior Lecturer in Cardiothoracic Surgery, Bristol Heart Institute, University of Bristol, UK

Gerard R. Avery, *BMedSci, BM BS, MSc, FRCR*, Consultant Radiologist, Hull and East Yorkshire Hospitals, Hull, UK

Robert S. Bonser, *FRCP, FRCS, FESC*, Consultant Cardiothoracic Surgeon, Cardiothoracic Surgical Unit, Queen Elizabeth Hospital, Edgbaston, Birmingham, UK

Philip A. Boreham, *MBBS, MRCP*, Consultant Cardiologist, Frenchay Hospital, Bristol, UK

Linda Boruta, *BA (Hons) Psychol, Grad Assoc Phys, MCSP*, Senior Physiotherapist, Cardiac Rehabilitation and Cardiopulmonary Transplantation Unit, Northern General Hospital, Sheffield, UK

Franco Ciulli, *MD*, Consultant Cardiothoracic Surgeon, Clinical Director of Cardiothoracic Services, Bristol Royal Infirmary and Honorary Senior Lecturer, University of Bristol, UK

Graham J. Cooper, *MBChB, MD, FRCS*, Consultant Cardiothoracic Surgeon, Northern General Hospital, Sheffield, UK

Georges Decker, *MD*, Department of Thoracic and Esophageal Surgery, University Hospital, Gasthuisberg, Belgium

Kate Dixon, *BA (Hons)*, Director and General Manager, Yorkshire Laser Centre, Goole and District Hospital, Goole, UK

Pierre Fuentes, *MD*, Professor and Chief of Thoracic Surgery Department, Hôpital Sainte Marguerite, 13274 Marseille, France

Sunit Ghosh, *BSc, MBBS, FRCA*, Consultant Cardiothoracic Anaesthetist, Department of Anaesthesia, Papworth Hospital, Cambridge, UK

Iftikhar Ul Haq, *MD, MBChB, MRCP, MBA*, Consultant Cardiologist, Royal Victoria Infirmary, Newcastle, UK

Jürg Hamacher, *MD*, Department of Thoracic Surgery, University Hospital, Zurich, Switzerland

Deborah Harrington, *MBChB, MRCS*, Cardiothoracic Surgical Unit, Queen Elizabeth Hospital, Edgbaston, Birmingham, UK

Hans A. Huysmans, *MD, PhD*, Professor of Cardiac Surgery and Director of The European Board of Thoracic and Cardiovascular Surgeons, Oegstgeest, The Netherlands

Antoon Lerut, *MD*, Professor and Head of Department, Thoracic and Esophageal Surgery, University Hospital, Gasthuisberg, Belgium

Keith McNeill, Consultant Respiratory and Transplant Physician, Transplant Unit, Papworth Hospital, Cambridge, UK

Alan J. Mearns, *MBChB, FRCS*, Consultant Cardiothoracic Surgeon, Bradford Royal Infirmary, Bradford, UK

Keyvan Moghissi, *BSc, MD, Dip Med Specialist en Chirurgie, Genève, FRCS, FETCS,* Membre Associé Academie Chirurgie, Paris. Consultant Cardiothoracic Surgeon and Clinical Director, Yorkshire Laser Centre, Goole and District Hospital, UK. Emeritus Honorary Professor, Department of Applied Physics (Laser), University of Hull, UK

Anil Mulpur, *FRCS,* Consultant Cardiothoracic Surgeon, Leeds General Infirmary, Leeds, UK

Daniel Nikzas, *MD,* Assistant Consultant, Second Surgical Department, Konstantopoulio General Hospital, Nea Ionia, Athens, Greece

Daniel J. Penny, *MD, MRCP,* Consultant in Cardiac Intensive Care, Cardiothoracic Unit, Great Ormond Street Hospital for Children NHS Trust, London, UK

Claudia Paoloni, *MD,* Department of Anaesthesia, Papworth Hospital, Cambridge, UK

Karen Pearson, *RGN, Ad Dip Couns,* Specialist Nurse, Cardiac Rehabilitation and Cardiopulmonary Transplantation Unit, Northern General Hospital, Sheffield, UK

David A.C. Sharpe, *MBChB, FRCS,* Consultant Cardiothoracic Surgeon, Blackpool Victoria Hospital, Blackpool, UK

Freyja–Maria Smolle–Juettner, *MD, PhD,* Professor, Thoracic and Hyperbaric Surgery, General and University Hospital, Burgfriedweg 8, A-8010 Graz, Austria

Uz Stammberger, *MD,* Department of Thoracic Surgery, University Hospital, Zurich, Switzerland

Mark R. Stringer, *BSc, PhD,* Senior Research Fellow, Department of Medical Physics, University of Leeds, UK

Pascal Thomas, *MD, FECTS,* Professor, Thoracic Surgery Department, Hôpital Sainte Marguerite, 13274 Marseille, France

J. Andrew C. Thorpe, *MBChB, FRCS, FETCS,* Consultant Cardiothoracic Surgeon, Leeds General Infirmary and Honorary Senior Lecturer, Leeds University, Leeds, UK

Victor T. Tsang, *MD, MS, MSc, FRCS,* Consultant Cardiothoracic Surgeon, Cardiothoracic Unit, Great Ormond Street Hospital for Children NHS Trust, London, UK

Malcolm J. Underwood, *MBChB, MD, FRCS,* Consultant Cardiothoracic Surgeon, Senior Lecturer in Cardiac Surgery, Bristol Heart Institute, Bristol Royal Infirmary, UK

William S. Walker, *MA, FRCS, FRCSE,* Consultant Cardiothoracic Surgeon, The Royal Infirmary of Edinburgh, Edinburgh, Scotland, UK

Walter Weder, *MD,* Professor and Head of Department, Department of Thoracic Surgery, University Hospital, Zurich, Switzerland

Nigel M. Wheeldon, *MD, MBChB, FRCP, FESC,* Consultant Cardiologist, Department of Cardiology, South Yorkshire Cardiothoracic Centre, Northern General Hospital, Sheffield, UK

Peter Wilde, *BSc, BMBCh, MRCP, FRCR,* Consultant Cardiac Radiologist, Bristol Royal Infirmary, UK

Mark Yeatman, *BSc (Hons), FRCS,* Specialist Registrar, Bristol Royal Infirmary, UK

Foreword

This second edition of Moghissi's *Essentials of Thoracic and Cardiac Surgery* represents a major contribution to the rapidly changing and growing field of cardiothoracic surgery. It is a systematic, profound collection of knowledge and techniques, brought up to date by Keyvan Moghissi and his co-editors, Andrew Thorpe and Franco Ciulli, ably assisted by an illustrious group of international experts.

According to Prof Moghissi himself, the book addresses primarily the surgeon in training, not only acquainting him or her with major advances in the field, but also providing a solid foundation of basic knowledge of thoracic surgery, like surgical anatomy, diagnostics and technical approaches. But it is not only the trainee who should be studying this book: an established cardiothoracic surgeon will find here a wealth of new knowledge, critically assembled and commented upon by leading European experts and by the editors themselves.

This book nicely complements a series of recent similar works about cardiac surgery, and will give all cardiothoracic surgeons a solid basis upon which they can formulate their own opinions and search for strategies in complex thoracic problems. All new techniques, such as VATS, lung volume reduction surgery and lasers, receive profound, critical attention; so the book can be truly considered as a repository of present knowledge in the field of cardiothoracic surgery. It should become an essential part of every department's library and a companion of trainees and established cardiothoracic surgeons.

Marko Turina, *MD*
Chairman, Department of Surgery
Director, Clinic for Cardiovascular Surgery
University Hospital
Zurich, Switzerland

Foreword

This book is the ideal text for the modern generation of trainee cardiothoracic surgeons and candidates for speciality examinations, particularly the European examination in General Thoracic Surgery. Thoracic surgeons are expected to have experience in general cardiac surgery and knowledge in all the many aspects of thoracic surgery; that is the emphasis in this book.

Thoracic surgery became established in the first half of the 20th century. It was the era of infective lung disease, and surgeons took on the management of empyema, bronchiectasis and tuberculosis in the days before antibiotics. Thoracic surgery emerged from the generality of surgery and developed as a speciality partly for the simple geographical reason that these surgeons worked in hospitals that were perforce specialised sanatoria, often situated out of town, for the care of those with lung disease. This new and challenging area of surgery demanded dedication and close collaboration with a new range of skills in anaesthesia. Thoracic surgeons operated nearer and nearer to the heart, successfully closing the persistent ductus arteriosus and relieving coarctation and then reaching inside the heart to open stenosed mitral and then pulmonary valves. The pioneer surgeons for these operations were Gross, Tubbs, Crafoord, Bailey, Harken, Brock and Holmes-Sellors. Holmes-Sellors wrote the foreword to the first edition (1986) of Moghissi's *Essentials of Thoracic and Cardiac Surgery* and was my predecessor at Middlesex Hospital in London.

These were of course thoracic surgeons, for heart surgery had not yet been invented. Heart surgery grew from these beginnings in the second half of the 20th century, latterly driven by the increasing volume of cases in the epidemic of coronary artery disease in the developed world. It naturally fell to the thoracic units to develop and to take on this work. The non-cardiac work, or what is now often called "general" thoracic surgery, has developed and changed, too, and will of course continue to do so: that is the nature of surgical practice.

Specialisation has been an essential feature of surgery but the way in which specialists have emerged has varied from place to place and time to time. Much thoracic surgery is performed by surgeons who trained in cardiothoracic surgery and continue to operate in both areas. Some have come from general visceral surgery and have specialised in work above the diaphragm. This diversity has great advantages for the speciality. The thoracic surgeon works with pulmonologists and oncologists in the great variety of diseases that affect the chest. This is recognized in the requirements for training in Europe and in the nature of the European Board examinations. This second edition takes into account these new developments carrying us forward into the 21st century.

Keyvan Moghissi has helped in developing the harmonisation of the speciality in Europe as a founding father of the European Association for Cardiothoracic Surgery, serving as its president in 1987 just after the first edition of this book was published.

He is a great European. His MD was gained at the University of Geneva where he trained in surgery. On coming to Britain he became a Fellow of the Royal College of Surgeons specialising in Cardiothoracic Surgery and spending his professional life largely in Yorkshire. He is the Thoracic Editor of the European Journal of Cardiothoracic Surgery.

That he is a great teacher and didactic writer can be seen from this book. He has recruited other authors but the lion's share is from the hands of Professor Moghissi himself.

Tom Treasure, *MD MS FRCS*
Professor of Cardiothoracic Surgery
Consultant Thoracic Surgeon
Guy's and St Thomas's Hospitals
London, UK

Section IV. Topics in Thoracic Surgery

Section V. Topics in Cardiac Surgery

The Lung and Pleura

K. Moghissi, J.A.C. Thorpe and F. Ciulli (Eds.)
Moghissi's Essentials of Thoracic and Cardiac Surgery
© 2003 Elsevier Science B.V. All rights reserved

CHAPTER I.1

Surgical anatomy of the chest

K. Moghissi

1. Introduction

Many textbooks of anatomy refer to the bony skeleton of the chest as "the thoracic cage". This is an excellent description as it highlights some of the characteristics of the bony framework of the chest which are important to the surgeon. Particularly, it reflects the fact that the chest is made up of bars of bone, the ribs, interspersed with soft tissue, which thus provides an easy access to the interior of the chest. This arrangement also combines mobility with firmness which is a functional requirement of the thorax.

The architectural design of the thorax consists of two vertical pillars: one anterior, the sternum; the other posterior, the vertebral column. These two are held in position by obliquely slanting ribs. The anterior pillar (sternum) is shorter in length than the posterior pillar (vertebral column). This discrepancy between the length of the two pillars has two consequences: firstly the direction of ribs from vertebral column to sternum is oblique and not horizontal; secondly the lowest five ribs cannot directly articulate with the sternum. Three of these, namely ribs 8–10, join the 7th costal cartilage to make the costal margin. The last two ribs, 11 and 12, have no attachment anteriorly and are known as floating ribs. The incomplete bony wall of the chest so constructed (Fig. 1) is completed by intercostals overlaid by other muscles which, for the most part, cover the chest and also provide a firm attachment for the shoulder girdle. The thoracic cage is open at its base into the abdomen but the diaphragm closes the opening and thus separates the thoracic from the abdominal cavity. The apex of the chest is the root of the neck and a membrane, Sibson's fascia, separates the thoracic cavity from the neck.

1.1. Thoracic Vertebral Column

This forms the posterior pillar of the thoracic cage and consists of 12 thoracic vertebrae and their intervertebral discs. The column so constructed may be likened to a string of threaded beads which, when pulled together, becomes strong but has mobility.

1.2. Sternum

The sternum is 10–15 cm long and forms the anterior pillar of the thoracic cage. It consists of three parts: the manubrium, body and xiphoid process. Since the sternum is shorter than the thoracic vertebral column, it follows that the lower five ribs cannot join directly to the sternum (false ribs). The junction of the manubrium to the body forms a visible and palpable ridge known as the angle of Louis. The manubrium provides a facet on each side for articulation with the clavicles. The sternoclavicular joints are greatly strengthened by interclavicular ligaments which follow the contour of the suprasternal notch. These joints are firm but allow free movement of the clavicles on the sternum, protecting them from dislocation in cases of trauma, though the clavicle tends to fracture. However, if the ligaments of these joints are torn by trauma, anterior dislocation of the clavicle occurs without harm to the posteriorly placed great vessels.

The following anatomical landmarks are of practical importance:

The superior margin of the manubrium is level with the lower border of the body of the 2nd thoracic vertebra; the distance between the two is about 5 cm.

The angle of Louis is level with the lower border of the body of the 4th thoracic vertebra. Lateral to the angle of Louis there are articular facets (one

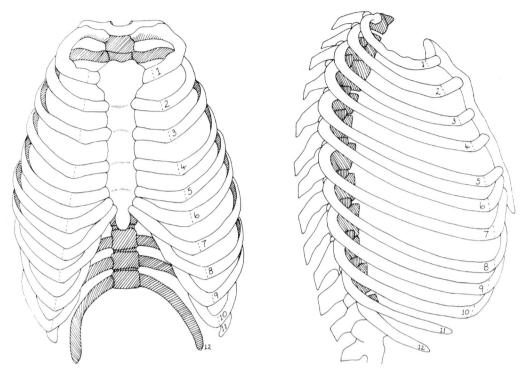

Fig. 1. Thoracic cage, front and lateral view.

on each side) for the 2nd costal cartilages. This allows accurate identification of intercostal spaces anteriorly, as laterally and just below it lies the second intercostal space.

An imaginary horizontal line drawn between the angle of Louis and the 4th thoracic vertebra is a dividing line between the superior and inferior mediastinum. On this line is found:

– The division of the trachea into two main bronchi.
– The arch of the aorta, which commences behind the right lateral end of the angle of Louis and terminates on the left aspect of the body of the 5th thoracic vertebra.
– The azygos vein which enters the superior vena cava.

The body of the sternum provides articular facets for the costal cartilages of all true ribs (3rd–7th). The xiphoid process joins the body of the sternum level with discs between the 9th and 10th thoracic vertebrae.

1.3. Ribs and Intercostal Spaces

Twelve pairs of ribs form the bony bars of the thoracic cage and the protective shield of the chest cavity. Seven pairs are true ribs whose costal carti-

lages attach directly to the sternum. The remaining five pairs are false ribs, of which the upper three (8, 9 and 10) have their cartilages attached to the one above to make the costal margin. The last two pairs of ribs (11 and 12) are floating ribs and have no anterior attachment.

Between the ribs are the 11 intercostal spaces, the first of which is situated between the 1st and 2nd rib and the last between the 11th and 12th ribs. Intercostal spaces are occupied by external and internal intercostal muscles. These are essentially two sheets of muscle. The external intercostal muscle fibres extend from the lower border of the upper rib to the upper border of the rib below. Their fibres are directed obliquely downwards and forward (in the same direction as the external oblique muscles). The internal intercostal muscles extend from the upper margin of the costal groove of the rib above to the upper border of the rib below. Their fibres are directed obliquely downwards and backwards. This 'X' arrangement of fibres of the two sets of intercostal muscles is an important factor contributing to the elasticity of the chest wall as a whole. In between the two sets of intercostal muscles are intercostal vessels and nerves, with the vein, artery and nerve (mnemonic: VAN) situated from above downwards.

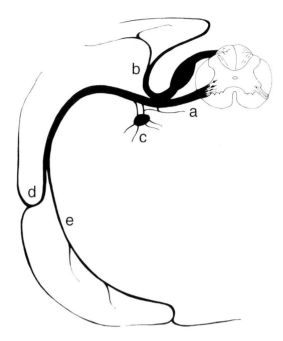

Fig. 2. Intercostal nerve: (a) anterior primary ramus, (b) posterior primary ramus, (c) sympathetic ganglion, (d) lateral cutaneous branch, (e) continuation of anterior primary ramus (intercostals nerve).

Posteriorly the intercostal vessels are protected in the subcostal groove in the inferior border of the ribs but anteriorly the vessels are not protected by the ribs but are exposed. This point should be borne in mind in aspiration of the chest. The vessels are not likely to be injured when an aspirating needle is introduced into the chest above the superior border of a rib.

1.3.1. Intercostal Nerves

An intercostal nerve is a mixed nerve (Fig. 2) , and is the anterior primary ramus of a thoracic spinal nerve. On emerging from the vertebral foramen a spinal nerve divides into a posterior and an anterior branch (posterior and anterior primary rami). The posterior branch (posterior primary ramus) itself divides into medial and lateral branches which are concerned with the extensor muscles of the vertebral column and the skin overlying them. The cutaneous branch of the posterior division supplies skin over a wider area from the posterior mid-line almost to the posterior axillary line.

The anterior division (anterior primary ramus) is the *intercostal nerve*.

There are 11 intercostal nerves; the anterior primary ramus of the 12th thoracic spinal nerve is the subcostal nerve. Intercostal nerves have the following branches:

- *Communicans branches* (two in number). One is a white ramus communicans which goes to a ganglion of the sympathetic trunk, and the other a grey ramus communicans which is a branch which the ramus receives from a sympathetic ganglion.
- *Collateral branch.* Concerned with the supply of intercostal muscles, parietal pleura and the periosteum of the rib.
- *Lateral cutaneous branch.* Pierces the intercostal and other overlying muscles to supply a wide area of the skin of the chest wall from the axilla to the mid line anteriorly, as well as the skin of the abdominal wall.
- *Anterior cutaneous branch.* Pierces the intercostal space anteriorly to supply the skin over the front of the chest and the abdomen.

Through the greater part of their course intercostal nerves lie between the intercostal muscles (in company with the artery and vein). The upper six intercostal nerves end near the sternum as the anterior cutaneous nerves. The lower six intercostal nerves leave the thorax, passing between the internal oblique and the transversus abdominis muscles and end by piercing the rectus muscle to supply the skin of the abdominal wall. The lateral cutaneous branch of the 2nd intercostal nerve is the intercostobrachial nerve which supplies the skin of the upper and back part of the arm.

Knowledge of the intercostal nerves and their distribution explains some of the extrathoracic pains which can originate from the chest and some of the extrathoracic lesions which can manifest as pain in the chest.

2. Muscles of the chest

Ribs, intercostal muscles and their neurovascular content are overlaid externally by two layers of muscles. The deeper layer consists of serratus anterior, anterolaterally, and the rhomboids (major and minor) posteriorly. These muscles are then covered by a larger superficial group which consists of pectoralis major and minor anteriorly and trapezius and latissimus dorsi posteriorly.

Knowledge of the anatomical arrangement and topography of the chest wall musculature have important practical relevance to surgical access to the thoracic cavity and to a number of other operative procedures. It is therefore useful to recall the anatomical characteristics of some of these muscles.

2.1. Trapezius

This large muscle covers the upper part of the posterior aspect of the neck and chest. Its fibres arise from an elongated line which extends from the occipital bone to the ligamentum nuchae and spinous process of all the thoracic vertebrae including the supra spinous ligament. From these origins the muscle fibres are directed towards the posterior border of the clavicle to be attached to the lateral one third of that bone and in continuation to the acromion and the upper border of the spine of the scapula. The lower fibres of the muscle form the upper side of a triangle known as the triangle of auscultation whose lower side is formed by the upper border of the latissimus dorsi muscle. The nerve to the muscle is derived from the accessory nerve (C_3, C_4) which enters its deep surface together with its vessels.

2.2. Latissimus Dorsi

This muscle has also a wide origin from:
- Spine and supra spinous ligaments of the lower six thoracic vertebrae under cover of the trapezius.
- Lumbar fascia and spines of lumbar vertebrae.
- Outer lip of the posterior part of crest of the ilium.
- Lower four ribs.
- Angle of scapula.

The muscle fibres converge forwards around the lateral wall of the thorax and are inserted into the floor of the bicipital inter tubercular groove of the humerous. The innervation of the muscle is from the posterior cord of the brachial plexus (C_6, C_7, C_8 roots) which enters the anterior border of the muscle. The upper border of the muscle, on emergence from under the trapezium, forms the lower side of the triangle of auscultation.

2.3. Serratus anterior

This muscle is covered partially by lattissimus dorsi. It originates from the outer surfaces of the upper eight ribs and is attached to the costal surface of the medial border of the scapula from the superior and including the inferior angle. The muscle is innervated by the long thoracic nerve.

2.4. Pectoralis major

The anterior wall of the chest is, to a large extent, covered by the pectoralis major. This muscle arises from three distinct heads:

- Clavicular head originates from the medial half of the anterior aspect of the clavicle.
- Steno-costal head arises from the anterior surface of the sternum and adjacent six costal cartilages.
- Abdominal head takes its origin from the upper part of the aponeurosis of the external oblique muscle.

The muscle fibres from these heads are directed towards the humerous where they are inserted to the greater tubercle and the lateral lip of the bicipital (inter-tubercular) groove.

2.5. Pectoralis minor

The muscle takes origin from the anterior aspect of the 2nd to 4th rib near the costal cartilages. The fibres form a small triangular muscle which is inserted to the coracoid process of the scapular.

The nerve to the pectoralis muscles from the medial and lateral pectoral nerves (for pectoralis major) and medial pectoral nerve (pectoralis minor) are branches of the medial and lateral cords of the brachial plexus respectively.

3. Skin and subcutaneous nerves of the thorax

The thoracic cage and its muscles are covered by the fascia, subcutaneous fat and skin. The skin of the thorax is thinner in front than behind. Lines of cleavage of the skin run horizontally around the chest. Incisions made along these lines heal more quickly and with a better cosmetic result than incisions made across the lines of cleavage. This is taken into account in thoracotomy, particularly when the cosmetic element is of importance. However, in certain situations, such as drainage of a chronic empyema requiring rib resection and a permanent or long-term opening for drainage, a vertical incision (across the lines of cleavage) is clearly preferable.

The skin of the chest is supplied segmentally by the 2nd–12th thoracic spinal nerves which also innervate the skin of the abdominal wall. A strip of skin posteriorly is supplied by the posterior primary rami of these spinal nerves. The rest of the skin anterolaterally and posterolaterally is supplied by branches of the anterior primary rami (intercostal nerves).

4. Thoracic cavity and pleural space

The external contour of the thorax is oval. The anterior bulge of the vertebral column makes the

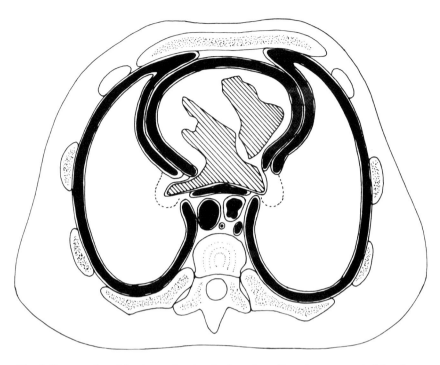

Fig. 3. Trans-section of the thorax showing the thoracic cavity and arrangement of the pleura.

transverse section of the interior of the thoracic cavity kidney shaped. The thoracic cavity is divided into three compartments (Fig. 3). The two lateral compartments accommodate the lungs. The middle, the mediastinum, contains the heart and the great vessels, the trachea and its bifurcation, the oesophagus, thymus gland, lymphatics and nerves. The thoracic cavity is lined by the pleura which covers it like wallpaper. This is the parietal pleura. It then reflects to cover the lungs as the visceral pleura.

The pleura is a serous membrane which forms independent closed sacs on each side of the chest. Like the hemithorax itself the pleura is in the shape of a truncated cone. The medial aspect of the pleural sac into which the lung is projected becomes inseparably attached to the lung itself. This is the visceral pleura. The parietal pleura covers the inner surface of the thoracic cavity. The original sac, now between the parietal and visceral pleura, becomes the pleural space. At the apex of the thorax the parietal pleura strengthens Sibson's fascia. At the base it drapes the diaphragm forming the diaphragmatic pleura. Medially, the parietal pleura lines the mediastinum as the mediastinal pleura. At the root of the lung the mediastinal pleura covers the structures of the root. It then continues as the visceral pleura to drape the lung. It is important to note that normally the parietal

pleura can be stripped off the chest wall with ease and can then be seen as a glistening membrane.

Such separation of visceral pleura from the lung is not possible as it is attended by damage to the pulmonary parenchyma. The visceral pleura covering the lungs falls short of the parietal pleura covering the chest wall in all areas. In some areas however, the space is wider, forming pleural recesses.

The surface marking of the parietal and visceral pleura is important (Fig. 4). The parietal pleura covers the costal surfaces of the thorax. At the apex of the chest it projects some 2.5 cm above the medial third of the clavicle. It then turns anteromedially towards the sternoclavicular joint where it continues as the mediastinal pleura and meets its opposite number at the level of the 2nd costal cartilage. From that level to the 4th costal cartilages the two mediastinal pleurae descend together at the back of the sternum. At the level of the 4th costal cartilage the mediastinal pleurae diverge. The right continues vertically and the left turns laterally towards the apex of the heart thus leaving part of the pericardium bare of pleura. Near the 6th costal cartilage the mediastinal pleura diverges further by turning laterally to reach the mid-clavicular line and mid-axillary line at about the 8th and 10th ribs, respectively. From the mid-axillary line the pleura passes horizontally to reach the

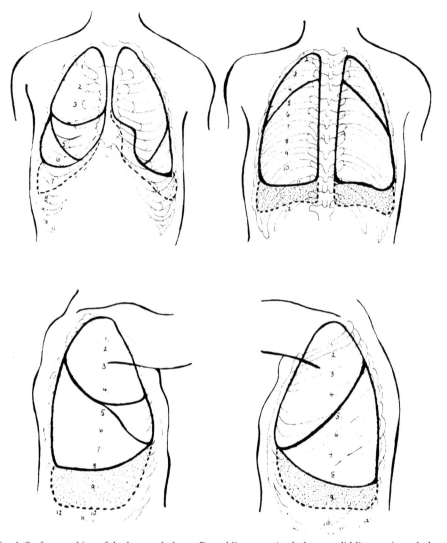

Fig. 4. Surface marking of the lung and pleura. Dotted line = parietal pleura; solid line = visceral pleura.

thoracic vertebrae 1–2 cm below the 12th ribs. In the process of turning laterally the pleura covers the upper surface of the diaphragm. The lung covered by the visceral pleura closely follows the parietal pleura at the apex and on the costal walls. Inferiorly however, it falls short of the pleura so that at the mid clavicular line it is at the level of the 6th rib and at the mid-axillary line it is level with the 8th rib. It then passes posteriorly at the level of the 8th rib.

The oblique fissure of the lung is almost in line with the 6th rib. On the right side, the anterior part of the horizontal fissure is level with the 4th costal cartilage and the line of fissure passes horizontally towards the oblique fissure approximately under the 6th rib.

5. Surgical anatomy of the lungs and bronchopulmonary segments

5.1. Gross anatomical description

The gross anatomical description accords two lobes for the left lung (upper and lower lobes) and three lobes for the right lung (upper, middle and lower lobes) which can be identified by fissures that are visible clefts between the lobes lined by the visceral pleura.

The left lung has a single fissure, the oblique fissure, which divides the upper from the lower lobe. The right lung has an oblique fissure which, like that of the left lung, divides the lung into an upper

Table 1

Bronchopulmonary segments

Right lung	Left lung
Upper lobe	*Upper*
Segment 1. Apical	Segment 1. Apical posterior
Segment 2. Posterior	Segment 2.
Segment 3. Anterior	Segment 3. Anterior
Middle lobe	*Lingula*
Segment 4. Lateral	Segment 4. Superior
Segment 5. Medial	Segment 5. Inferior
Lower lobe	*Lower lobe*
Segment 6. Apical	Segment 6. Apical
(dorsal lobe)	(dorsal lobe)
Segment 7. Medial basal	Segment 7. Medial basal
(cardiac)	(absent)
Segment 8. Anterior basal	Segment 8. Anterior basal
Segment 9. Lateral basal	Segment 9. Lateral basal
Segment 10. Posterior basal	Segment 10. Posterior basal

Each segment of the lung receives a segmental branch of the bronchus bearing the name and the number of the pulmonary segment which it enters (see Fig. 5a in this chapter.)

and lower portion. In addition, a horizontal fissure divides the upper portion into upper and middle lobes. The lower portion of the right lung below the oblique fissure is the lower lobe.

Each lung has a lateral or costal surface which is convex and adapted to the configuration of the chest wall, an apex that projects behind the medial third of the clavicle into the neck, a base, which is concave, resting on the diaphragm and the medial surface which flanks the mediastinal structures, notably the pericardium. All surfaces of the lung present the impression of the intrathoracic structure against which they lie. The mediastinal surface is of particular importance as it contains the hilum, the area into which the bronchi, vessels and lymphatics pass to form the root of the lung. The hilum (or hilus) is surrounded by the pleura which covers the structure of the root forming a large cuff. Below the root the pleura is reflected down from the hilum to form the pulmonary ligament. From the surgical point of view the anatomical unit of the lung is the bronchopulmonary segment. It is this portion of the lung which receives a branch of the bronchus (the segmental bronchus), a branch of the pulmonary artery and one or more branches of the pulmonary vein. A bronchopulmonary segment can be dissected and resected.

Because the lobes of the lungs are lined and separated by visceral pleura covering the "fissure",

a lobectomy results in minimal air leaks from the alveoli. Segmentectomy (segmental resection) will cause a certain amount of air to leak because the boundaries of pulmonary segments are not lined, nor are they demarcated by the visceral pleura.

In both lungs the segmental branches of the pulmonary artery to the posterior segment of the upper lobe, the middle lobe (or the lingula on the left side) and the lower lobe emerge from the main trunk after turning into the oblique fissure. This is of practical surgical importance since dissection of the fissure and division of the visceral pleural opening exposes the sheath of the artery overlaid by lymph nodes. This arrangement facilitates the dissection, ligation and division of the segmental arteries in pulmonary resection. Each lung has ten segments which are named and numbered as shown in Table 1 and Fig. 5a.

5.2. Bronchial Tree

Two aspects of the bronchial tree (Fig. 5b) are important to the surgeon:
- Anatomical.
- Endoscopic.

5.2.1. Anatomical aspect
This defines the main bronchi and their distribution to the lobes, segments and sub-segments of the lung. The bronchi (right and left) commence at the bifurcation of the trachea and are directed to the hilum of the right and left lung, respectively. The bifurcation is indicated in the interior of the trachea by a ridge, the carina, situated in the middle of the lower trachea in between the two bronchial openings.

The right main bronchus gives off:

The upper lobe bronchus which subdivides into three branches, namely the apical (1), posterior (2), and the anterior (3) segmental bronchi.

The right middle lobe bronchus which in turn subdivides into the lateral (4), and the medial (5) segmental bronchi.

The right lower lobe bronchus which subdivides into the apical (6), medial (7), anterior (8), lateral (9), and posterior (10) segmental bronchi.

The left main bronchus gives off:

The main stem bronchus for the upper lobe and the lingula. This branch immediately divides into the left upper lobe bronchus for the upper lobe of the lung proper. This in turn divides into the apical (1), posterior (2), and anterior (3) segmental bronchi. The apical and posterior segmental bronchi usually emerge as

(a)

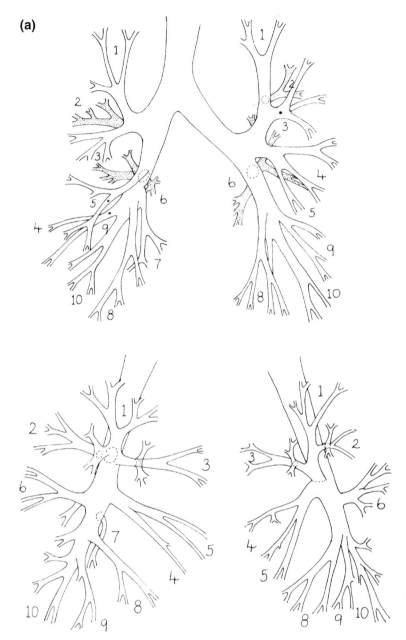

Fig. 5. (a) Bronchopulmonary segments.

one branch i.e. the apical–posterior bronchus, which then subdivides. The lingular bronchus which divides into two branches, the superior lingular (4), and inferior lingular (5) segmental bronchi.

N.B. The numbers in parentheses correspond to the standard "universal" numbering of the bronchi.

The left lower lobe bronchus divides, like the right lower lobe bronchus, into five segmental branches, namely: the apical (6), medial basal (7), anterior basal (8), lateral basal (9), posterior basal and (10) segmental bronchi.

The medial basal segmental bronchus on the left side is often small or non-existent. This is due to the absence of the medial basal pulmonary segment itself because of the projection of the heart into the left chest.

5.2.2. Endoscopic aspect (bronchoscopy)
The bronchoscopic appearance of the bronchial tree (Fig. 5c) is as follows.

The carina is seen as a ridge, separating the orifices of the right and left main bronchi.

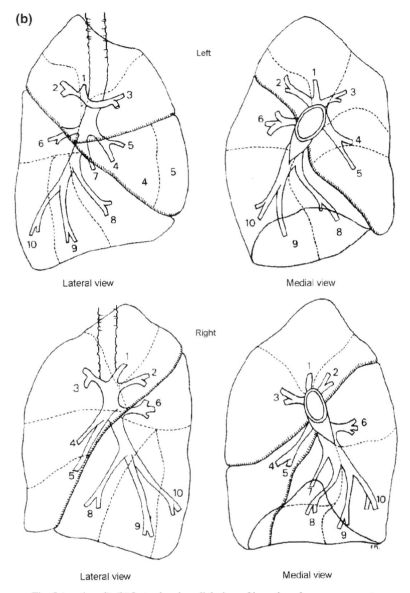

Fig. 5 (continued). (b) Lateral and medial view of bronchopulmonary segments.

At the right lateral aspect of the right main bronchus, level with the carina, is the orifice of the right upper lobe bronchus. With a rigid bronchoscope, the orifice alone is usually seen without its segmental divisions. When a telescopic view is obtained using either the right-angle telescope or the flexible fibreoptic bronchoscope the orifice is seen to contain three subsidiary orifices. These are the apical, posterior and anterior segmental orifices. When the bronchoscope is introduced into the right main bronchus below the right upper lobe opening for a distance of 1.5–2 cm the following bronchial segmental orifices are seen:

- Anteriorly at about 12 o'clock there is the middle lobe orifice.
- Almost opposite posteriorly at 6 o'clock is the apical segmental orifice of the lower lobe.
- Just below these two orifices are seen the openings of the segmental bronchi for the basal segments of the lower lobe, viz: the anterior, posterior medial and the lateral segmental bronchial openings.

On the left of the carina the opening of the left main bronchus is seen leading to the bronchial lumen, which is directed downwards and laterally making an angle of about 60 degrees with the mid-

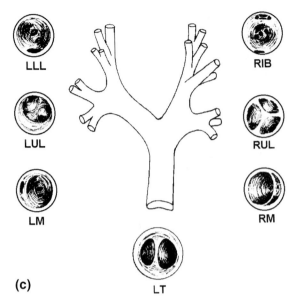

(c)

Fig. 5 (continued). (c) Endoscopic aspect of the bronchial tree: LT = lower trachea, RM and LM = right and left main bronchi, RUL and LUL = right and left upper lobe orifices, RIB = right intermediate bronchus (towards the lower lobe), LLL = left lower lobe bronchial orifice.

line of the carina. 2–2.5 cm below the carina on the lateral wall of the main bronchus the common opening of the left upper lobe and that of the lingular segments is seen. The former emerges almost at a right angle, whereas the latter is directed more obliquely downwards. Normally, with a rigid bronchoscope

placed within the left main bronchus, only the common orifice of the upper lobe is seen. The division of the upper lobe bronchus into two main branches (upper lobe proper, and lingula) becomes visible using a right-angle telescope or a flexible fibreoptic bronchoscope. When the latter instrument is directed within the opening of the main stem of the upper lobe bronchus the two divisions are easily seen. The opening of the left upper lobe bronchus proper is seen to divide into a further two or, at times, three segmental bronchi which are the apical–posterior segmental and the anterior segmental bronchi.

As has been noted, the apical and posterior segmental bronchi of the left upper lobe arise as a single stem dividing into two, unlike the right upper lobe where they arise individually.

The lingular segmental bronchus forms the lower division of the common left upper lobe opening. Its orifice is seen below the opening of the bronchus for the upper lobe proper. It soon divides into its two branches, the superior and inferior segmental bronchi of the lingula. Less than 0.5 cm below the stem of the left upper lobe opening, the orifice of the main lower lobe bronchus is seen. Its lumen is directed downwards and more medially than that of the upper lobe in continuation with the left main bronchus. The openings of the segmental bronchi to the left lobe are seen with the apical segmental orifice situated posteriorly at 6 o'clock or at the floor of the bronchus when viewed with the patient in a supine position.

K. Moghissi, J.A.C. Thorpe and F. Ciulli (Eds.)
Moghissi's Essentials of Thoracic and Cardiac Surgery

Clinical manifestations and diagnostic methods

K. Moghissi and J.A.C. Thorpe

1. Clinical manifestations of lung disease

1.1. Introduction

Despite the availability of a wide range of investigatory methods the value of clinical history and examination in the diagnosis of respiratory disease must not be underestimated. It should be appreciated that in the vast majority of cases patients initially consult their doctors because of symptoms. Symptoms and signs are useful guides in the initiation of investigations relevant to the case.

1.2. Cough

This is the commonest symptom of respiratory disease. The cough reflex is a protective mechanism to clear the respiratory tract. It is both the result of an irritant and protection against the damaging effects of abnormal materials in the airway. A cough may be productive (associated with sputum) or dry. In thoracic surgical patients cough is usually productive and should not be stopped or suppressed by means of medication, except in patients with widespread neoplasia who are to be sedated in the terminal phase of their disease, when all efforts should be made to make their ending peaceful.

It must not be forgotten that:
- Cough is frequently associated with upper respiratory tract infection.
- Irritation from ear, nose and throat can stimulate the cough reflex.
- Even in the absence of other symptoms, a patient with a persistent cough for over 2–3 weeks should have further investigations and most importantly a chest radiograph.
- Paroxysmal cough, when prolonged, can produce syncope because of raised intracranial pressure and hypoxia.

1.3. Sputum

Excessive normal or abnormal secretions in the respiratory tract constitute sputum which can be of a variety of colours and consistencies. The normal amount of respiratory tract mucus secreted, estimated at between 50–100 ml/day is cleared insensibly by ciliary action of the mucous membrane without development of cough. However, in circumstances such as inflammatory conditions or when the amount of secretion is increased, clearance is carried out by means of cough. In thoracic surgery it is important to note:
- Volume of sputum/day, which must be collected and measured.
- Character of sputum for which a descriptive classification may be adopted such as *mucoid, yellow/green purulent, black* (containing black particles of atmospheric or cigarette smoke) and *bloodstained* (haemoptysis).

1.4. Haemoptysis

This can take the form of heavily bloodstained sputum, rusty coloured secretions, frank and fresh bleeding with cough, or dark bloodstained fluid emitted during coughing. The latter is particularly important in post-pulmonary resection cases. All patients with haemoptysis should be investigated further. It must be emphasised that a normal chest radiograph in such patients may conceal a tumour in the trachea or bronchi which has not caused sufficient impression on the bronchial lumen to cause atelectasis which would be shown radiologically.

Chest radiography and bronchoscopy is mandatory in patients with haemoptysis, particularly in those with no previous symptoms.

Table 1

Showing the grades of Dyspnoea

Grade I	Normal
Grade II	The individual can walk with a normal person of his/her own age, sex and build on the level but cannot do so on hills or stairs
Grade III	The individual can walk a long distance at his/her own pace but cannot keep pace with a normal person
Grade IV	The individual can walk about 100 yards but develops dyspnoea after that distance
Grade V	Dyspnoea develops even after a few steps, or in carrying out washing or dressing

1.5. Dyspnoea

This is a subjective sensation which denotes abnormal awareness of breathing. However, the term is used to describe difficulty in breathing, shortness of breath and painful breathing.

Dyspnoea may be classified as:
- *Exertional dyspnoea* which may or may not be due to pulmonary disease
- *Dyspnoea at rest.*

1.5.1. Grades of dyspnoea
To evaluate the severity of dyspnoea various grading systems have been suggested; the most frequently employed is shown on Table 1.

The Medical Research Council's Committee on Chronic Bronchitis (1965) suggests a useful questionnaire given to patients for self assessment of dyspnoea as follows:
I. Are you breathless when hurrying on level ground or walking up a slight hill?
II. Or when walking with people of your own age on level ground?
III. Do you stop for breath when walking at your own pace on level ground?

A negative answer to the first question means no dyspnoea. A positive answer to the first question signifies dyspnoea whose severity is assessed by a positive answer to the second or third questions. It should be noted that subjective evaluation of grading of dyspnoea does not necessarily correlate with the pulmonary function found on objective testing.

1.6. Wheeze

This is a hissing noise which is heard often on expiration, usually on auscultation and sometimes without the help of a stethoscope. It denotes obstruction to the flow of air. A bronchial lumen narrowed from whatever cause produces wheeze. A localised wheeze caused by plugs of thick mucus secretions may disappear on coughing but bronchial narrowing caused by organic lesions such as neoplasms will remain even after coughing. Development of localised wheeze in patients with no previous history of chest disease or bronchitis must be investigated further.

1.7. Stridor

This is a characteristic snoring type of noise which accompanies the inspiratory phase of breathing and is usually associated with obstructive lesions of trachea or larynx. In children and infants the sudden onset of stridor suggests inhalation of a foreign body. Such cases must be investigated urgently. In adults stridor is usually associated with tracheal obstruction.

1.8. Chest pain

Chest pain is a symptom which is present in many respiratory and other conditions affecting intrathoracic viscera. It can also originate from outside the thorax. It should be remembered that the visceral pleura does not contain sensory pain nerve endings but the parietal pleura is extremely sensitive to pain. Pain which is associated with chest wall or respiratory disease needs to be distinguished from cardiac and oesophageal pain. Typical pleuritic pain is worse on breathing or coughing. Intercostal pain of fibrositis or costochondritis can be localised by the patient and the site is tender on palpation. Thoracic pain may be referred to other areas, notably the abdomen.

1.8.1. Pleuritic pain
The pleura can frequently be involved in pulmonary diseases such as pneumonia, tuberculosis and malignancies. Such pain is not diffuse and tends to be distributed along the intercostal segmental distribution. The pain is exacerbated by chest movement such as breathing or coughing.

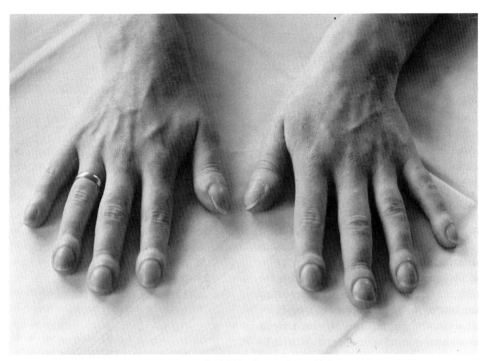

Fig. 1. Gross finger nail clubbing in a patient with lung cancer.

1.8.2. Intercostal neuritis

This type of pain is similar to that of pleuritic pain but more superficial and not related so much to respiratory movement.

1.9. Clubbing of finger nails

Finger nail clubbing (Fig. 1) is frequently associated with chronic pulmonary conditions particularly with lung cancer and is present in 30% of patients with bronchogenic carcinoma.

The mechanism of the production of clubbing is not certain and none of the theories which are advanced to explain its development explain its association with such a range of diseases.

1.10. Hypertrophic Pulmonary Osteo-arthropathy (HPOA)

This condition consists of painful arthropathies of ankles, wrists, knees and less commonly fingers and other joints. Radiologically the bones, notably those of forearms, wrists and the lower legs, are widened with cortical reaction. In 80% of cases HPOA is caused by bronchial carcinoma and in only 5% is intrathoracic suppuration the cause. The pathogenesis of the condition is uncertain. It is interesting that both clubbing and pulmonary arthropathy are reversible. Removal of the tumour is followed by the gradual return of the nails and finger clubbing to their original normal shape. There is almost immediate relief of pain in the bones and joints after operation.

1.11. Cyanosis

Cyanosis is defined as a bluish discoloration of the conjunctiva, mucous membrane and skin. When severe, it can be readily detected clinically. In its mild form it may be difficult to diagnose cyanosis, particularly in patients with dark pigmented skin.[1]

Cyanosis is due to an abnormally high level of reduced haemoglobin compared with oxyhaemoglobin in the blood circulating in the minute vessels. It becomes manifest when there is a minimum of 5 g of reduced haemoglobin in every 100 ml of blood. As each gram of haemoglobin takes up 1.34 ml of oxygen when fully saturated, 5 g will take up

---

[1] The normal colour of the skin is dependant on pigmentation, which in turn is governed by the amount and distribution of the pigment melanin in the melanoblasts (the pigment cells of the skin) and the basal cells of the epidermis. The melanoblasts manufacture the pigment and then pass it on to the basal cells.

$5 \times 1.34 = 6.7$ ml of oxygen per 100 ml of blood, which is the minimum amount of oxygen deficiency necessary to produce cyanosis. Fully saturated blood contains $15 \times 1.34 =$ approximately 20 ml of oxygen per 100 ml. This has to fall to 13.3 ml of oxygen per 100 ml ($20–6.7 = 13.3$ corresponding to oxygen saturation of 85%) before cyanosis develops. It must be noted that the tissue extraction of oxygen is not uniform; the blood circulating through the skin in some circumstances may be so desaturated as to cause cyanosis. This phenomenon may be entirely local due to the disturbance of skin circulation. The cyanosis in such cases is peripheral.

Peripheral cyanosis can also occur through local stagnation of blood, as in peripheral vascular failure and venous obstruction. Peripheral cyanosis may be accompanied by low cardiac output, in which case the extremities are both cold and blue, but other signs of low cardiac output will also be present. In cases of peripheral cyanosis the mucosa of the tongue remains pink. Inspection of the tongue is, therefore, a better index of central cyanosis and reflects generalised oxygen desaturation of the circulating haemoglobin. It occurs in respiratory system diseases when the blood, after its passage through the lung, remains desaturated. It also occurs when there is a substantial shunting of blood from the right to left heart or is caused by gross perfusion/ventilation mismatching. The magnitude of the shunt to cause cyanosis is about one-third of cardiac output.

It must be emphasised that:
- As central cyanosis is dependent on oxygen desaturation of haemoglobin, anaemia is not a contributing factor in cyanosis, but in polycythaemic patients a smaller drop in saturation will produce cyanosis.
- In haemoglobinopathies, e.g. methaemoglobinaemia, where the chemical combination of oxygen is interfered with, central cyanosis can be produced
- In pulmonary collapse, when the lung is perfused but not ventilated, the situation is similar to that of right to left shunting (i.e. pulmonary to systemic shunting). Cyanosis will therefore develop depending on:
  - the magnitude (extent) of the collapse,
  - the extent of the perfusion through the collapsed lung.

Both of the above accentuate ventilation/perfusion mismatching.

2. Diagnostic methods in pulmonary diseases

The purpose of investigatory method is:
- To help in the establishment of diagnosis.
- To ascertain the patient's suitability for a particular treatment (e.g. surgery)
- To reveal related or unrelated associated pathological conditions.
- Prognosis.

Specific diagnostic procedures in respiratory disease are:

2-1 Sputum examination
2-2 Skin hypersensitivity tests
2-3 Bronchoscopy
2-4 Diagnostic thoracoscopy
2-5 Biopsies
2-6 Respiratory function tests.

2.1. Sputum examination

The volume and macroscopic appearance of expectorations are an important diagnostic guide in some respiratory diseases. The spot diagnosis of lung abscess or bronchopleural fistula following pulmonary surgery may be made with accuracy by the large offensive purulent expectorations of the former and the bloodstained water secretion of the latter. More detailed study of the cytology and the microbiology of sputum provides valuable diagnostic information. Sputum for laboratory examination should be fresh and unspoiled by food debris.

2.1.1. Cytology for malignant cells
The objective of cytological examination is to identify a cell population in a sample of sputum, bronchial secretion or pleural fluid. The examination is of great importance in the search for abnormal and malignant cells which are shed in the respiratory tract and/or pleural fluids. The principle is based on the fact that cells from neoplastic tissues are shed more readily and are recognisable by their anomalies. The accuracy with which the diagnosis is made depends on the experience of the examiner as well as on the type and location of tumour.

2.1.2. Microbiological studies
Direct smear examination. This is a valuable test for the identification of organisms in respiratory diseases and is a standard test for the diagnosis of tuberculosis from sputum or other material suspected of containing tubercle bacilli. In addition, asbestos

bodies and *Entamoeba histolytica* may be identified by this method.

Culture. This is mandatory in respiratory disease. Some indication of the possible diagnosis should be given to the bacteriologist in order to culture the sputum in the most appropriate culture medium. It is also essential in the pre-operative investigation of patients undergoing surgery and in the post-operative phase particularly when antibiotic policy has to be decided.

2.1.3. Other sputum examinations
A variety of other tests may be carried out for a specific purpose such as identification of asbestos bodies.

2.2. Skin hypersensitivity tests

2.2.1. Tuberculin testing
The test is based on the delayed type hypersensitivity reaction displayed by the sensitive individual when challenged with the tubercle bacillus antigens. One of several methods can be used to elicit hypersensitivity reaction; these are:

Mantoux test. This is carried out by intradermal injection of tuberculin contained in 0.1 ml solution. The injection is made on the anterior surface of the forearm. The test is assessed 48–72 hours later. When positive, the skin shows inflammation and induration of at least 10 mm in diameter and 1 mm in thickness. Coloration is not significant but the diameter of induration is taken into account when interpreting the test.

Heaf multiple puncture test. This is carried out with a special instrument consisting of six pointed needles on a plate. The tuberculin fluid is placed on the skin with the instrument set over it. The catch is then released allowing the needles to inject the fluid into the skin to a depth of 2 mm (the depth of the needles can be adjusted to 1 mm for children). The result is read between 3 and 6 days later. The reaction is gauged in three or four grades. Grade I shows at least four separate papules. In Grade II the papules are fused to form a ring. In Grade III the ring is filled in the centre and there is, in addition, induration spreading outwards. An additional grade, Grade IV, is described when there is necrosis.

Tine test. This is also a multiple puncture test which is carried out by disposable units. Each unit has four

teeth or tines, 2 mm in length which are mounted on a disc. These are dipped into old tuberculin and then sterilised. The tines are pressed onto the anterior aspect of the skin of the forearm forming four punctures which introduce the tuberculin into the skin. The results is read 48–72 hours after. An induration of 2 mm or more in diameter is taken as a positive result.

2.2.2. Interpretation of tuberculin tests
A positive reaction gives support to the diagnosis of active tuberculosis or that the patient has had tuberculosis at some time in the past but is still immune.

A negative reaction indicates that the patient under investigation is not suffering from tuberculosis. The Heaf test is less accurate but convenient for out-patients. Grade III reaction supports the diagnosis of active tuberculosis but in the presence of positive Grade I and II reactions, this diagnosis is less likely.

2.3. Bronchoscopy

Bronchoscopy is an important method of investigation and in conjunction with radiology is the most helpful diagnostic procedure with regard to bronchopulmonary neoplasm.

Although bronchoscopy implies visual inspection and examination of the bronchial tree, it has two main purposes:

2.3.1. Diagnosis of bronchopulmonary lesion
Even in the presence of a normal chest radiograph, patients suffering from persistent bronchopulmonary symptoms, particularly haemoptysis, should have a screening bronchoscopy. A lesion may be in its early development or tracheal lesions may be present in a patient with normal chest radiograph. Failure to carry out bronchoscopy in patients with haemoptysis and normal chest radiograph may have serious consequences (see section 2 in chapter II.1). In addition to visual examination of the bronchial tree, bronchoscopy is useful in the assessment of operability in cases of lung cancer and for the design of the intended operative procedure. For this reason many, including the author, believe that such bronchoscopies should be carried out by the thoracic surgeon who intends to undertake operation, even when the histological diagnosis is established by previous bronchoscopy. Besides visual examination diagnostic bronchoscopy is useful for:

(a) Obtaining samples of bronchial secretions for:

(i) Identification of pathogenic micro-organisms and sensitivity to anti-microbial chemotherapy.

(ii) Cytological examination, notably identification of malignant cells.

(b) Recovery of biopsy material for histological examination.

2.3.2. Therapeutic Bronchoscopy purposes include:

(a) Bronchoscopy for removal of a foreign body lodged within the airway (see chapter I.6).

(b) Clearing the bronchial tree of normal or abnormal secretions. This is particularly relevant to sputum retention following surgery and also after traumatic injuries of the chest.

(c) Bronchial lavage using normal saline or suitable aqueous antiseptic solution in patients with bronchiectasis particularly those whose secretions contain either antibiotic resistant microbial or fungal organism and/or in the condition of alveolar pulmonary proteinosis.

2.3.3. Contraindications for bronchoscopy

In experienced hands there are no contraindications for bronchoscopy. Caution must be exercised when the rigid instrument is used in the following categories of patient:

- Patients with deformity of the spine. These patients can present the risk of spinal cord compression during hyperextension of the neck.

- Patients with severe superior vena caval obstruction. In some of these patients even slight trauma

can cause profuse bleeding. In addition there may be considerable oedema of the upper respiratory tract which intensifies the respiratory embarrassment of such patients. The addition of bronchoscopy trauma to such respiratory airways can cause considerable mechanical obstruction.

- In patients with high obstructive tracheal lesions. Some of these patients can bleed easily, resulting in complete respiratory tract obstruction.

- Patients with aneurysm of the ascending aorta or aortic arch in whom there is a definite risk of rupture of aneurysm.

- In very ill patients with severe cardio-respiratory failure. The necessity of bronchoscopic examination must be weighed against the risks involved. In such patients the use of a rigid instrument under topical/surface anaesthesia has the advantage that ventilation and aspiration, if and when required, can be provided more easily than with the use of the fibreoptic instrument.

2.3.4. Bronchoscopy — procedure

Bronchoscopy can be carried out using either a rigid or flexible fibreoptic bronchoscope.

Instruments.

- Rigid bronchoscope (Fig. 2)
  This is essentially a light-carrying tube with a connecting cable to a light source. This instrument permits direct viewing of the interior of the larynx, trachea and main and segmental bronchi. A complete range of rigid bronchoscopes includes adult,

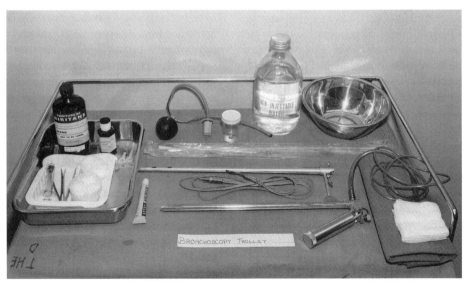

Fig. 2. Rigid bronchoscopy trolley, showing also instrument with battery operated light source.

Table 2

Specifications of rigid bronchoscopes (G.U. Manufacturing Company)

	Outside diameter (mm)	Inside diameter (mm)	Length (cm)
Adult	11.0	10.0	40
Adult small	10.0	9.0	40
Adolescent	9.0	8.0	40
Adolescent small	8.0	7.0	40
Child	8.0	7.0	30
Infant	6.0	5.4	27.5
Suckling	4.8	4.1	27.5
Suckling short	4.3	3.7	18
Lower bronchus	7.0	6.4	45
Adult aspirating	8.5	7.5	40
Child aspirating	7.5	6.5	30

male and female, adolescent, child, infant and suckling (Table 2). There are direct and angled telescopes which allow magnification and visualisation of those bronchial openings which are not in direct line of the bronchoscopic field of vision. Accessories include straight and angled bronchial biopsy punches and foreign body extractors of different sizes.

• Flexible fibreoptic bronchoscope (Fig. 3)

The flexible fibreoptic bronchoscope is made of light-transmitting flexible fibres. This instrument provides a telescopic view of the bronchial tree. Because of its flexibility it can negotiate the different angles at which the bronchial orifices emerge from the main bronchi and can therefore enter the main lobar and even segmental openings to provide an excellent view. The flexible fibreoptic bronchoscope accommodates both suction and separate biopsy probe side channels. The bronchial brush can also be directed through the biopsy channel if required. The accessories of the bronchoscope include a side viewing teaching arm to allow simultaneous examination by two individuals and a camera for photography of the bronchial tree. Most units also use video equipment comprising camera, monitor and video recorder.

The two bronchoscopes (rigid and flexible) have some individual characteristics which are shown in Table 3.

Bronchoscopy procedure (Fig. 4). Bronchoscopy can be carried out under general or topical anaesthesia. In diagnostic bronchoscopy, carried out generally by the respiratory physician, the fibreoptic instrument is usually used with the patient receiving topical anaesthesia. Surgeons prefer to carry out bronchoscopy under general anaesthesia using the rigid instrument and, if necessary, introduce the fibreoptic bronchoscope into the rigid one for detailed examination of the segmental bronchi. Interventional bronchoscopy is best carried out using the rigid instrument with the patient under general anaesthesia.

Prior to bronchoscopy the procedure should be fully explained to the patient. It is particularly important to explain the steps of operation when this is done under topical anaesthesia.

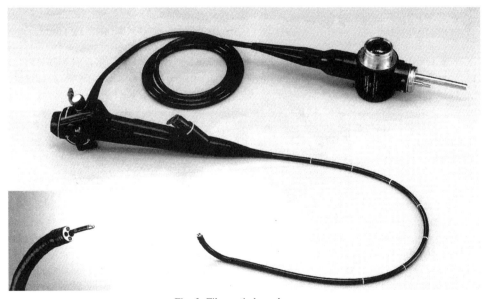

Fig. 3. Fibreoptic bronchoscope.

Table 3

Comparison of bronchoscopes

	Rigid instrument	Fibreoptic (flexible) instrument
Viewing	Direct	Indirect
Field of vision	Good for main and lobar bronchi	Good for main, lobar and segmental bronchi.
Biopsy forceps	Good $\geq$ 5 mm × 4 mm	Small $\leq$ 2 mm × 2 mm
Interventional Bronchoscopy	Good to very good	Poor
(a) Control of bleeding	(a) good	(a) not good
(b) Suction (emergency)	(b) very good	(b) not good
(c) Diathermy/laser	(c) good	(c) good
(d) Ventilation	(d) good	(d) not so good
(e) FB [a] extraction	(e) good	(e) not good (?impossible)
Anaesthesia	General usually	Topical usually
	Topical possible	General possible

[a] Foreign body.

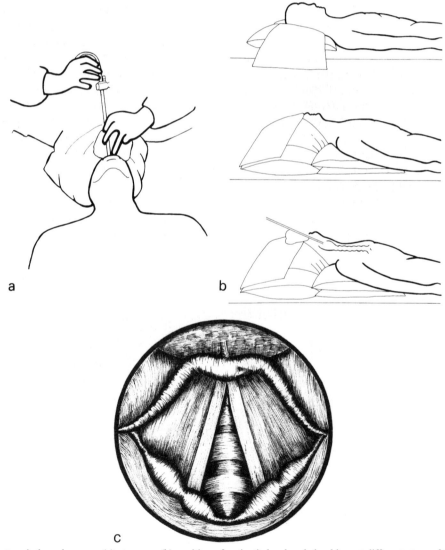

Fig. 4. Different steps in bronchoscopy. (a) step one, (b) position of patient's head and shoulders at different steps of the procedure, (c) bronchoscopic view of the laryngopharynx and vocal cords from above downwards, back of the tongue, tip of the epiglottis and vocal cords, view of the trachea through the aperture, aryepiglottic folds and pharyngeal wall.

Oxygenation during the procedure must be maintained. All modern rigid instruments have a ventilating side venturi which can be connected to a ventilating source usually with positive pressure mechanism. Ventilation/oxygenation can be undertaken by a variety of techniques such as:

- Apnoea and intermittent ventilation: using a bronchoscope fitted with an eyepiece which closes the top of the instrument during ventilation.
- Sanders Injector: this is a device which injects oxygen with a high positive pressure into the venturi port of the bronchoscope.
- High frequency positive pressure ventilation: oxygenation is maintained by high frequency positive pressure introduction of oxygen through the bronchoscope.

Patient ECG and oxygen saturation are monitored throughout the procedure, the latter by using a pulse oximeter.

When bronchoscopy is performed under general anaesthesia using the flexible instrument the latter may be passed through the rigid bronchoscope which is first placed into the trachea. This then can receive a supply of oxygen by injector fitted to the side of the rigid instrument. Alternatively, a wide endotracheal tube is inserted and the flexible instrument is passed through it. In this case oxygen is supplied through the side of a connector opening. When bronchoscopy is carried out under local anaesthesia, the patient can breathe normally.

Technique of rigid bronchoscopy:

The patient is positioned on his back with his head slightly flexed over a pillow:

Step 1 A square surgical towel is placed under the head. When the patient is anaesthetised this will cover his head and eyes leaving the nose and mouth uncovered (Fig. 4a).

Step 2 The patient's upper lip and teeth are protected by a small swab. The bronchoscope is lightly lubricated using sterile gel and is introduced through the mouth and into the trachea by lifting the epiglottis forward with the beak of the instrument thus bringing the vocal cords into view (Fig. 4a, b and c).

Some operators introduce the bronchoscope through the right side of the mouth. In the author's opinion it is preferable to introduce the bronchoscope centrally through the mouth. This has a recognisable midline structure, the uvula. Next, locate the upper border of the epiglottis (seen like a crescent moon rising over a mountain), then go behind to lift it

forwards. In neonates, bronchoscopy may be particularly difficult, necessitating the use of a laryngoscope to view the opening of the glottis.

Step 3 The instrument is then rotated 90 degrees to allow its oval opening to be easily admitted into the inverted V-shaped aperture of the larynx between the vocal cords.

Step 4 The instrument is gently pushed forwards into the trachea. The pillow under the head is moved down and placed under the shoulders to raise them slightly, so extending the head. This movement should take place gently so that the instrument in the upper trachea does not inflict trauma.

On introducing the instrument, the larynx and the trachea are examined. Particular attention is paid to the carina indicating the division of the trachea into the main bronchi.

Step 5 The bronchscope is now introduced further into each of the main bronchi by turning the patient's head to the opposite side.

In each main bronchus the upper lobe orifice and its component segments, followed by the lower lobe and its segments, are examined. A complete bronchoscopy consists of examination of:

- Larynx and vocal cords
- Trachea
- Carina
- Right bronchial tree:
  Right upper lobe bronchus and its three segmental orifices
  Right intermediate bronchus
  Right middle lobe bronchus opening
  Right lower lobe bronchus with its segmental orifices
- Left bronchial tree:
  Left main bronchus
  Left upper lobe and its components
  (a) Left upper lobe bronchus proper and its three (often only two) segmental orifices
  (b) Lingular bronchus and its segmental openings
  Left lower lobe bronchus and its segmental orifice

Technique of flexible fibreoptic bronchoscopy:

In many instances this technique is carried out under topical anaesthesia (see below). Lubrication of the instrument with lignocaine gel provides additional assistance. The instrument is introduced into the trachea either through the nose or mouth. The former approach is more advantageous as the internal meatus of the nose and the nasopharynx are in a direct line with the laryngopharynx, and therefore it is easier to pass the instrument into the trachea. When the fibroscope is passed through the mouth it can be introduced directly or through the rigid bronchoscope, which is then placed first into the trachea. Alternatively, the fibroscope can be introduced into the endotracheal tube which is placed first into the trachea. The two latter techniques are particularly suitable for patients receiving general anaesthesia.

The systematic examination of the bronchial trees on either side is undertaken in the same manner as for the rigid bronchoscope (see previous page).

2.3.5. Bronchoscopy in special circumstances
In some cases the bronchoscopy technique may have to be altered according to special circumstances. Post-operative bronchoscopy and bronchial aspiration may need to be carried out in the intensive therapy unit and/or in-ward with the patient in bed. It is preferable for such bronchoscopies to be performed by the surgical team using the rigid instrument under topical anaesthesia.

2.3.6. Topical (local) anaesthesia for bronchoscopy
The patient is given sedation, a small dose of Diazepam (2.5–5 mg) or Midazolam intravenously, and the tongue and throat are sprayed with 4% lignocaine to produce surface anaesthesia. Alternatively, 2–3 ml of 4% lignocaine is injected into the lumen of the trachea, through the cicothyroid membrane. Care is taken to inject the local anaesthetic into the lumen and not onto the wall of the trachea. For this, the patient's neck is extended, the prominence of the thyroid cartilage is palpated and followed down to reach the cricothyroid membrane. A 5 ml syringe with a no. 1 needle is prepared containing 3 ml of 4% lignocaine. The skin over the cricothyroid membrane is cleaned with an antiseptic solution. The needle is then introduced through the membrane into the trachea for aspiration of air, confirming that the needle is positioned in the lumen and not in the wall. The injection is then given rapidly and the needle withdrawn. The injection provokes a bout of coughing which splashes the topical anaesthesia around the trachea and larynx. Patients should be warned about this and the operator must withdraw the needle quickly after the injection to prevent injury.

2.3.7. Complications of bronchoscopy
Complications of bronchoscopy are rare but they can be serious. The following complications are important:

Haemorrhage. This is usually caused by a punch biopsy which is taken too deeply. The complication is more prevalent when the rigid instrument with its larger biopsy punch is used. Suction, packing by ribbon gauze, topical application of pledglet soaked with 1/100.000 solution of adrenalin, YAG laser application, introduction of a double lumen tube and emergency thoracotomy are the therapeutic possibilities to be considered, depending on the circumstances. These measures are easier to undertake when within the operating theatre campus with the surgeon and the anaesthetist at hand. Usually the bleeding subsides. Exceptionally, in patients with necrotic tumour in a main stem bronchus, a small amount of bleeding can cause embarrassing hypoxea.

Perforation of the trachea, bronchus or bronchiole. This can occur in uncooperative patients under topical, or local, anaesthesia or by biopsy punch. These may cause surgical subcutaneous or mediastinal emphysema. This is a rare complication associated with bronchoscopy with the use of the rigid instrument.

Pneumothorax. This may be caused by forcible jet oxygenation during bronchoscopy under general anaesthesia especially in children, using a rigid bronchoscope. It may also occur 'spontaneously' during bronchoscopy using the fibreoptic instrument particularly in an anxious or uncooperative patient and those with emphysematous lung or bullae.

Laryngeal/subglottic oedema. May complicate bronchoscopy in children and infants.

Bronchospasm. May occur in some patients, particularly asthmatics.

Cardiac dysthymic complication. In elderly and in the presence of hypoxia, a variety of abnormal rhythms may occur.

Trauma to teeth. This complication can be avoided if the bronchoscope is not allowed to press on the teeth by using the method as indicated.

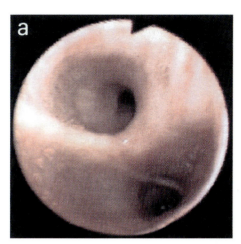 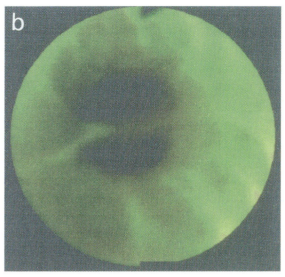

Fig. 5. Fluorescence bronchoscopy: normal image, (a) white light, (b) fluorescence.

2.3.8. Fluorescence Bronchoscopy

Introduction. About 50% of lung cancer, especially squamous cell carcinoma, develops centrally in the bronchi and can be diagnosed bronchoscopically using conventional white light. However the diagnostic yield, even in experienced hands, depends largely on the stage of cancer. The localisation of early lung cancers at carcinoma in situ stage or with subtle mucosal changes is extremely difficult, if not impossible. Radiology is also unhelpful. Even experienced bronchoscopists fail to diagnose carcinoma in situ in over 70% of cases when conventional bronchoscopy is used (Woolner et al., 1984).

Specificity and sensitivity of bronchoscopic detection can be improved using diagnostic fluorescence imaging. There are principally two methods of fluorescence bronchoscopy:

Photodynamic/Drug enhancement methods: The principle of this method is that using a photosensitising drug which selectively accumulates in cancer tissue, the discriminative power of fluorescence imaging can be enhanced. Low dose Photofrin and 5 Amino Levulinic Acid (5-ALA) have been used for this purpose. 5-ALA in particular can be absorbed topically. Absorption leads to accumulation of protoporphyrin IX in malignant and pre-malignant tissue which fluoresces when exposed to light of 390–420 nm wavelength.

Autofluorescence method: This method relies on excitation of 'chromophores' in bronchial submucosa by specific light which fluoresces. Biochemical and structural changes of surface epithelium of bronchial mucosa results in alteration (reduction) of the fluorescence intensity. It therefore follows that mucosal excitation by a light of a specific wavelength results in the differential fluorescence being imaged. Also an optimal light wavelength can achieve the greatest (optimal) discrimination between normal and abnormal mucosa. Early in 1990 the British Columbia Cancer Agency, in collaboration with Xillix Technologies Corporation, Canada, developed a light induced fluorescence endoscope (LIFE) which is now commercially available. (See Fig. 5 and Fig. 6).

The LIFE lung system allows an over two-fold increase in the detection rate of severe dysplasia and carcinoma in situ compared with white light bronchoscopy. Other systems are also being developed. However, the results from trials are awaited.

2.4. Diagnostic Thoracoscopy

In 1910 a Swedish physician, Jacobaeus, developed a cystoscope to examine serous cavities. In the 1950s thoracoscopy was used for the diagnosis of pleural disease. Up until recent developments of Video Assisted Thoracic Surgery (VATS), thoracoscopy was used largely by European physicians and some surgeons essentially for diagnosis of intra-thoracic conditions. VATS and the gamut of its uses are described in a separate chapter in this book (see chapter IV.1). At this juncture, for the purpose of completeness, it should be remembered that thoracoscopy maintains its position and indications for the diagnosis of:

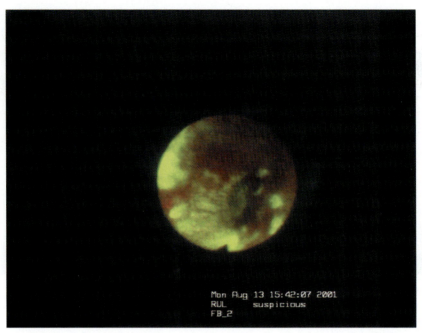

Mon Aug 13 15:42:07 2001
RUL   suspicious
FB_2

Fig. 6. Fluorescence bronchoscopy: dyplastic charges showing as red/brown areas.

- Pleural effusion (malignant/benign)
- Diffuse lung disease
- Localised lung lesions
- Mediastinal tumours
- Others

2.5. Biopsies

In many respiratory diseases the histological diagnosis is, ultimately, of paramount importance. Tissue samples may be obtained by:
- Bronchial biopsy.
- Lymph node biopsy: Supraclavicular nodes, when palpable, and the scalene group of nodes (palpable or not) may be biopsied for histological diagnosis (see below).
- Mediastinal node biopsies can be obtained via mediastinoscopy or by mediastinotomy (see chapter II.3).
- Lung biopsy: This is particularly relevant to widespread parenchymal disease of the lung. The biopsy material can be obtained by needle usually under CT or ultrasonic guidance, by thoracoscopic technique and via open mini thoracotomy.
- Pleural biopsy: The biopsy of parietal pleura can provide invaluable information about the diagnosis of pleural effusion. Biopsy material may be obtained by several means.

2.5.1. Scalene node biopsy

Scalene nodes are part of the inferior group of deep cervical lymph nodes which are found around the jugular vein and extend from behind the sternomastoid muscles into the posterior triangle of the neck to appear as supraclavicular glands. These nodes are included in a pad of fat, the areolar tissues, situated over the scalenus anterior muscle in the root of the neck. They have special significance in the diagnosis of pulmonary diseases.

The scalene node biopsy is of value in a variety of pulmonary and mediastinal disorders but its greatest value is in sarcoidosis, tuberculosis and diffuse pulmonary diseases, including undifferentiated types of carcinoma

The right scalene nodes are concerned with the whole of the right lung and the lower lobe of the left lung. Therefore, when there is no palpable gland it is more relevant to excise nodes from the right side except when the left upper lobe is diseased. When there is a palpable node, biopsy is taken from that side.

The operation. Scalene node biopsy operations may be carried out under general or local anaesthesia. The former is particularly indicated if the procedure is carried out following bronchoscopy or other examination for which general anaesthesia is required.

The patient is placed in a supine position with a

pillow under the shoulders and the head turned to the opposite side. An incision is made 2 cm above and parallel to the upper border of the clavicle from the anterior border of the trapezius, to the clavicular head of the sternomastoid muscle. When the skin and platysma are incised, the edge of the sternomastoid becomes visible. This is retracted anteromedially and the dissection carried out further with blunt ended scissors and forceps. The pad of fat, containing multiple small glands, can be seen behind and medial to the internal jugular vein. Notice laterally the brachial plexus and posteriorly the scalenus anterior muscle covered by its fascia, with the phrenic nerve beneath the fascia. The pad of fat with the glands is lifted upwards and out of the wound using a pair of tissue forceps (e.g. Babcock forceps); the pad of fat is then clamped at its base by 1 or 2 artery forceps (Spencer Wells), and excised. When there is a definitely enlarged or pathological gland this is excised without the pad of fat. The wound is then closed.

2.6. Respiratory function tests

2.6.1. Assessment of pulmonary function in thoracic surgery

The aim of this chapter is to familiarise the reader with the basics of pulmonary physiology and the application of pulmonary function tests commonly used. For a deeper insight refer to the key references.

In 1846, John Hutchison, a surgeon, invented the spirometer and coined the term "Vital Capacity". Since that time there have been many reported tests for pulmonary assessment from Sniders match blowing test (inability to blow out a match at 7 to 8 cm) to sophisticated analysis of lung volumes in a whole body plethysmograph and invasive pulmonary artery pressure measurements. This chapter hopefully provides a practical approach to preoperative respiratory assessment.

During the initial patient encounter, a careful history and examination are vitally important. Simple spirometry, estimation of carbon monoxide transfer factor and blood gas analysis are essential in the majority of patients undergoing thoracic surgery. More sophisticated tests, e.g. exercise testing, six-minute walk test and assessment of oxygen utilisation, VO_2 max., may provide useful information in patients with borderline spirometry. No one test can give an accurate picture of respiratory function and all these investigations must be related to the planned operation and assessed in conjunction with the CT scan and ventilation perfusion scan.

2.6.2. Mechanics of ventilation and lung volumes

To allow adequate gas exchange at the alveolar capillary membrane, sufficient ventilation of the alveolated region of the lung (the so-called respiratory zone) must occur. Contraction of the diaphragm and the action of intercostal muscles, which raise the ribs increasing the cross sectional area, cause volume increase of the thorax on inspiration. Accessory muscles, e.g. sternomastoid, are called into action in a severe case of dyspnoea or stridor.

The volume of fresh gas entering the respiratory zone each minute is 5250 ml/min (effective tidal volume — 350 ml × 15 — respiratory rate). Inspired air flows to the terminal bronchioles and thereafter the velocity of airflow becomes less. It is important to be aware that there are normally regional variations in ventilation. Using Xenon-133 gas it has been shown that the lower regions of the lung ventilate better than the upper zones. In the lateral position the dependent lung is best ventilated. Volume change per unit of pressure is known as compliance. Elasticity therefore, is the reciprocal of compliance. Compliance is decreased with age and also by emphysema.

Flow volume curves are particular useful to assess inspiratory and expiratory effort and can be used to calculate the work of breathing (Table 4).

Diffusion of gas takes place in the respiratory zone, which has a volume of 2.5 to 3 litres. Figure 7 describes simple spirometric lung volumes.

- *Tidal volume.* This is the volume of air inspired or expired in each resting breath. In adults this is

Table 4

Parameters measured in pulmonary function testing (example of a patient's test results)

	Pred.	Meas.	% Pred.
Lung volumes			
Vital capacity (l)	5.39	4.96	92
Total lung capacity – box (l)	6.98	6.57	94
Total lung capacity – SB (l)	6.98	6.25	90
FRC (PL)	3.25	2.83	87
Residual volume (l)	1.63	1.62	99
Lung mechanics			
FEV_1 litres	4.35	4.01	92
FVC litres	5.15	4.81	93
FEV_1/FVC %	83	83	
sGaw 1/kPa s^{-1}	>0.85	2.63	
FEF 25–75% l/min	303	236	78
Diffusing capacity			
DLCO mmol/kPa min^{-1}	11.9	9.8	83
DLCO/VA DLCO/l	1.70	1.58	93
Exp. CO ppm			

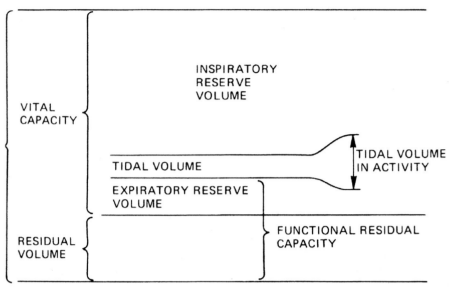

Fig. 7. Simple spirometic lung volumes.

approximately 500 ml of which 150 ml is incorporated in the 'dead space' created by the trachea and large airways where gas exchange does not take place. Effective tidal volume is therefore 350 ml.

• Vital capacity is the summation of inspiratory reserve and expiratory reserve volume. Gas that remains in the lung after maximal expiration is the 'residual volume'.

The volume of gas in the lung after a normal expiration is the 'functional residual capacity'. The residual volume and functional residual volume cannot be measured by spirometry but can be measured by a helium gas dilution method or by using a whole body plethysmograph (West, 1995).

Airway resistance in normal lungs is low due to the elasticity and compliance of the lung together with the surface tension lowering effects of surfactant. Surfactant contains the phospholipid-di-palmitoyl phosphatidyl choline (DPCC) which is an important component. This is produced from fatty acids in Type 11 cells lining the alveolus. Lack of this in the newborn causes respiratory distress. The viscosity and density of the gases inspired will also contribute to resistance. Resistance can be calculated from Ohm's Law:

$$\text{Resistance} = \frac{\text{Pressure drop}}{\text{Rate of flow}}$$

$$\text{or} \quad \text{Resistance (percent)} = \frac{\text{FEV}_1}{\text{VC}} \times 100$$

Accurate measurements of resistance are best performed in a whole body plethysmogaph.

Chest wall deformity, kyphoscoliosis, phrenic nerve paralysis, myaesthenia and many other conditions affecting the musculoskeletal system of the chest wall can all adversely affect gas transfer and impair ventilation.

2.6.3. Diffusion

This is the passive transfer of gases across the alveolar-capillary membrane. Fick's Law states that the rate of transfer of a gas through a sheet of tissue is proportional to the tissue area and the difference in gas partial pressure between the two sides, and inversely proportional to the tissue thickness. The rate of transfer depends on the solubility and molecular weight of the gas. The blood-gas barrier in the lung is enormous (50 to 100 square meters) and the thickness is only 0.3 microns, which makes an ideal barrier for diffusion to take place. CO_2 diffuses about 20 times more rapidly than O_2 as it has a much higher solubility. Diffusion capacity of the lung can be measured using carbon monoxide, which has a high affinity for the haemoglobin molecule. In the 'single breath method' a single inspiration of a dilute mixture of carbon monoxide is made and the rate of disappearance of carbon monoxide from the alveolar gas during a 10 second breath hold is calculated. This is usually performed by analysing inspired and expired concentrations with an infrared analyser. Helium can be added to the inspired gas to give a measurement of lung volume by dilution. Diffusion capacity is a useful investigation. This can be elevated or reduced depending on the disease process.

2.6.4. Perfusion

In health, the cardiac output of the left heart equals that of the right heart. The right ventricular and pulmonary artery pressures are ten times lower than the systemic arterial blood pressure. Mean pressure in the main pulmonary artery is about 15 mmHg. Alveolar vessels are exposed to alveolar pressure and larger vessels outside the lung substance are exposed to intrapleural pressure. Resistance therefore determines the pulmonary flow.

$$\text{Vascular resistance} = \frac{\text{Input pressure outpressure}}{\text{Blood pressure}}$$

The pressure drop from the pulmonary artery to left atrium is about 10 mmHg. If the pulmonary blood flow is 6 l/min then the pulmonary arterial resistance is 10/6, which is about 1.7 mmHg/l/min. The pulmonary bed is a vascular bed and is very compliant with any increase in pulmonary vascular pressure; closed capillaries open up (recruitment) and distension of vessels also occurs. Lung volume is another important determinant of pulmonary vascular resistance. If the lung is collapsed the resistance is increased. If alveolar pressure rises the capillaries will be squashed and the resistance will increase.

2.6.5. Measurement of pulmonary blood flow

The volume of blood flowing through the lungs each minute can be calculated using the Fick principle:

$$\text{Blood flow} = \frac{\text{Oxygen uptake (ml/min)}}{\text{(Arterial-venous) oxygen difference (ml/l)}}$$

This can be measured by a dye dilution technique or by nuclear scanning techniques. From radioactive xenon studies in the upright human lung there is a linear decrease in perfusion from base to apex and this distribution is affected by posture and exercise. In mild exercise both upper and lower perfusion increase. Ventilated non-perfused lung is called the 'alveolar dead space'. Perfused and non-ventilated lung equates with 'physiological dead space'.

The pulmonary vasculature responds rapidly to hypoxia. If the alveolar PO_2 drops, hypoxic vasoconstriction occurs due to contraction of smooth muscle in the walls of small arterioles. The precise mechanism for this response is unknown but is likely mediated by humoral factors, e.g. histamine, catecholamines and prostaglandins. Nitric oxide is an endothelium derived relaxing factor and may be important in vessel wall relaxation. Acid base balance and autonomic regulation are considered important.

Ventilation/perfusion nuclear scans are invaluable in the assessment of patients with pulmonary embolism, where respiratory function is borderline prior to surgery and in the assessment of patients for volume reduction surgery in emphysema.

2.6.6. Control of Breathing

To meet the metabolic demands of the body the process of respiration is finely controlled to allow efficient oxygenation, elimination of carbon dioxide and maintenance of blood pH (Fig. 8). The central control resides in the brain with autonomic control residing in the brain stem and voluntary control in the cerebrum.

Brain stem control of breathing originates in neurons located within the pons and medulla, which are organised into separate groups called the respiratory centres. There are three separate areas named the pneumotaxic centre, the apneustic centre and the medullary centre, which is divided into an expiratory centre and a gasping centre. The medullary centre is located in the reticular formation of the medulla and consists of dorsal neurones involved with inspiration and a ventral group involved with expiration.

The system of sensors is complex and consists of chemoreceptors in the medulla as well as in the carotid and aortic bodies, which respond to changes in pH, and in CO_2 and PO_2. Other mechanoreceptors are sited in the lungs and chest wall.

2.6.7. Disorders of ventilation

Spirometry is one of the most universally applied tests of pulmonary function but it is important to realise that normal values have a range and are based on age, sex and height. Certain ethnic groups may have lower values. Disorders can be obstructive or restrictive (Table 5).

Peak flow is an alternative test to spirometry and gives a snapshot of flow. It can be readily assessed at home or by the bedside using a small hand held recorder, which are now electronic giving a digital readout.

2.6.8. Clinical Application of pulmonary function tests

Pulmonary function tests are useful for both the physician and surgeon in diagnosis, evaluation of the progress of disease and its response to treatment, e.g. steroid response. They are of particular use to the surgeon in planning surgery as well as judging the amount of pulmonary parenchyma to resect. Predictive postoperative pulmonary function can be calculated from the preoperative spirometry and CT

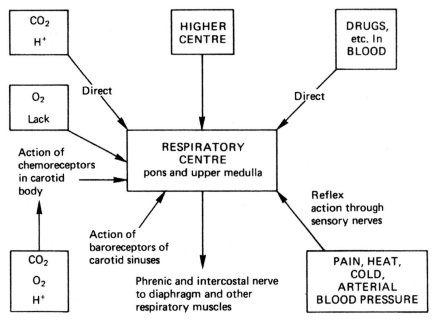

Fig. 8. Respiratory centre and control of breathing.

Table 5

Disorders of ventilation

Common obstructive ventilatory disorders	Uncommon obstructive ventilatory disorders	Common restrictive ventilatory disorders
Asthma	Bronchiolitis obliterans	Idiopathic fibrosing alveolitis
Asthma bronchitis	Eosinophilic granuloma	Interstitial pneumonitis and fibrosis
Chronic obstructive bronchitis	Lymphangiomyomatosis	Disseminated granulomatosis e.g TB
Chronic obstructive pulmonary disease (COPD)	Sarcoidosis (advanced disease)	Sarcoidosis
Cystic fibrosis		Thoracic deformities
Emphysema		Congestive heart failure

scan where the number of pulmonary segments to be resected can be calculated.

$$\text{Postoperative FEV}_1 = \text{Preoperative FEV}_1$$
$$\times \%\text{function in the remaining lung.}$$

The most important tests preoperatively are spirometry, flow-volume loop, diffusing capacity (dlCO), ventilation/perfusion scan and blood gas analysis. PO_2, PCO_2 and pH are easily measured from arterial blood samples with a blood/gas electrode. Hypoxaemia may be caused by altitude, hypoventilation, ventilation/perfusion defects or anatomic shunts. The interpretation of pulmonary function has to be taken into account with the clinical scenario and few pulmonary function tests have a clear-cut relationship to post operative risk and outcome. A good FEV_1 appears to be the most important in predicting outcome of lung resection. Guidelines and protocols for pulmonary function in thoracic surgical patients have been published by the British Thoracic Society (1998). Recommendations that advise no pulmonary resection in patients with an FEV_1 of less than 1.0 litre can be misleading. For instance in patients with heterogenous emphysema with an associated carcinoma a successful result can be obtained from surgical resection in the presence of poor respiratory function. In essence, volume reduction surgery is being performed which may even improve function. Borderline cases such as this should be discussed with a thoracic surgeon in the setting of a multidisciplinary team. Pulmonary function tests, despite their sophistication, have not replaced the experienced clinician.

References and further reading

The British Thoracic Society. BTS Recommendations to respiratory physicians for organising the care of patients with lung cancer. Thorax 1998; 53(Suppl 1): S1–S8.

The Committee on the Aetiology of Chronic Bronchitis. Definition and classification of chronic bronchitis for clinical and epidemiological purposes. A report to the Medical Research Council. Lancet 1965; 1(7389): 775–779.

Griffith Pearson F, et al. Thoracic Surgery. New York, Churchill Livingstone, 1993.

Jacobaeus HC. Über die Möglichkeit die Zystoscopie bei untersuchung seroser Hohlungen Anzuwended. Munch Med Wschr 1910; 57: 2090–2092.

West JB. Respiratory physiology, the essentials (5th ed.). Baltimore: Williams A. Wilkins, 1995.

Woolner LB, Fontana RS, Cortese DA, et al. Roentgenographically occult lung cancer. Pathologic findings and frequency of multiplicity during a ten year period. Mayo Clinic Proc 1984; 59: 453–466.

K. Moghissi, J.A.C. Thorpe and F. Ciulli (Eds.)
Moghissi's Essentials of Thoracic and Cardiac Surgery
© 2003 Elsevier Science B.V. All rights reserved

CHAPTER I.3

Thoracic imaging

G. Avery

In this chapter a brief description is given of the radiological and scintigraphic techniques available for imaging of the chest with the main emphasis on chest radiography.

1. Chest radiography

This is the first step in the radiological investigation of respiratory disease. It is important that the Thoracic Surgeon has understanding of technique and film interpretation. The following areas will be addressed:
1-1 Acquisition Techniques
1-2 Film interpretation
1-3 Description
1-4 Normal appearance

1.1. Acquisition techniques

The Postero Anterior (PA) chest radiograph is taken with the patient erect, not rotated, the arms positioned to project the scapulae free of the lungs and at suspended full inspiratory effort.

There are two different techniques, which depend on the kilovoltage of the X-ray tube.
- Low kilovoltage, 60–80 kVp (peak kilovoltage), tube/film distance at 6 feet.
- High kilovoltage, 145 kVp, tube/film distance 10 feet, 6 inch patient/film air gap

The higher kVp technique allows better visualisation of the lung that is partially obscured by the heart and mediastinum, although there is reduced visualisation of parenchymal calcification and ribs.

On a plain chest radiograph (Fig. 1a), in addition to PA view, the patient position can be altered to allow assessment of different areas:
- Lateral View: Allowing assessment of areas poorly

visualised on the PA film, this view helps localisation of lesions (Fig. 1b).
- Oblique: Mainly used for the assessment of pleural or rib and chest wall lesions.
- Lordotic: Allows assessment of the lung apices by projecting the clavicles and first ribs away from the lungs.
- Lateral Decubitus: This can demonstrate small amounts of pleural fluid on the dependent side
- Antero Posterior (AP) view: Can be useful to assess whether opacities are intrapulmonary or within a rib.
- Expiratory film: Can detect a small pneumothorax and air trapping; this is useful in detection of foreign body inhalation.

In thoracic surgical emergency and post-operative cases, portable X-ray apparatus is brought to the patient's bed. The portable examination is usually inferior to a departmental film for several reasons:
- The AP projection with a small tube/film distance causes magnification of the heart and mediastinal outlines making theses areas difficult to assess and obscuring areas of lung.
- The patient positioning, often semi-erect or supine can make pleural effusions difficult to recognise.
- A poor inspiration can mimic parenchymal opacification and give apparent cardiomegaly.

Conventional film is gradually being replaced by digital radiography. Digital detectors have a wider range of sensitivity than film/screen combinations allowing improved image contrast. It is also possible to manipulate the digital image, which can provide additional information. Digital systems are essential for the development of Picture Archiving and Communications Systems (PACS) which allow the electronic transfer of radiographs both within and between hospitals.

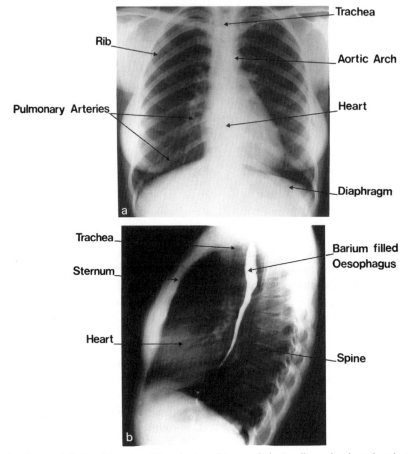

Fig. 1. (a) normal chest radiograph – PA projection; (b) normal chest radiograph – lateral projection.

1.2. Film interpretation

Mental discipline is required to look at a film systematically in order to interpret it correctly. The commonest error in interpretation is to not see an abnormality that is present on the film. The chest radiograph should be examined systematically, starting with the patient details and the date of the examination.

The next step is to assess the technique: projection, radiographic exposure, inspiratory effort and patient positioning. Patient rotation can be checked by assessing the symmetry of the medial ends of the clavicles to the spinous process of the vertebral body at the same level. If there is rotation then the hemithorax closer to the film will be of increased density compared to the contralateral hemithorax.

It is then important to examine the following areas, the order in which this is done is not important but should be consistent.

- Lungs (Parenchyma)
- Hila of the lungs
- Mediastinum
- Heart
- Diaphragm
- Pleura/ribs/chest wall
- Abdomen, parts which are visible on the chest film

There are three areas that should be consciously reviewed as lung lesions can be partially obscured by superimposed structures.

- The apices, in particular behind the confluence of the clavicle and first rib.
- The retrocardiac lung which is partially obscured by the heart.
- The posterior costophrenic angles which are difficult to see due to the overlying diaphragm.

When assessing a chest radiograph it is important to look both for abnormal opacities and the loss of normally visible structures.

It is important to appreciate that as the X-ray beam passes through the chest, it is attenuated. The magnitude of this is dependent upon the density of the tissues encountered. The denser the tissue, the more energy absorbed. There are only four densities which can be clearly differentiated on the chest radiograph: calcium, soft tissue, fat and air.

Structures are visualised because their margins represent interfaces between two different densities: air/soft tissue at the diaphragm, mediastinum and heart; bone/soft tissue for the ribs and vertebrae: fat/soft tissue in the chest wall. Where two structures of the same density abut each other it is not possible to differentiate their margins, for example vascular structures within the mediastinum. When interpreting a radiograph it must be appreciated that fluid is of soft tissue density, this is demonstrated by the appearance of the pulmonary vessels at the hila and within the lung.

Felson and Felson (1950) introduced the "silhouette sign" which is the loss of a normal interface between two structures of differing radiographic density. In the chest this is usually due to the replacement of air by soft tissue. This is an important sign and can be seen in the loss of the right heart border with middle lobe consolidation (Fig. 2) or the loss of a hemidiaphragmatic outline with lower lobe consolidation and pleural fluid.

It is also useful to assess the thickness of normally seen structures, e.g. the right paratracheal stripe, which is visible on a PA film, is usually 2–3 mm thick; an increase in this is evidence of mediastinal disease, often lymphadenopathy.

1.3. Description

It is important that the person interpreting the radiograph can accurately describe the findings to a colleague who has not seen the X-ray, the descriptive terms used must therefore be understandable to all. The thoracic surgeon should be totally "au fait" with some of the commonly used terminology. The Fleischner Society published a glossary of chest radiology terms in 1984.

Several of the terms used are given below.

- *Atelactasis*: Less than normal inflation of all or a portion of lung with corresponding diminution of volume. Qualifiers may be used to indicate severity, mechanism or distribution.

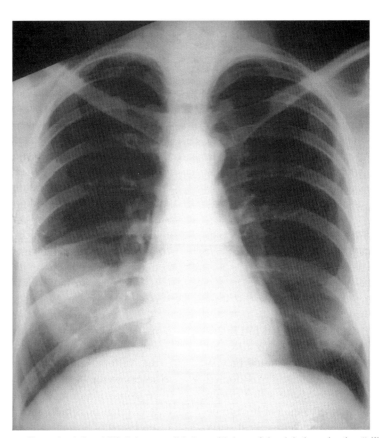

Fig. 2. PA chest radiograph: right middle lobe consolidation with loss of the right heart border: "silhouette sign".

- *Cavity*: A gas containing space within the lung surrounded by a wall whose thickness is greater than 1 mm and usually irregular in contour.
- *Coin Lesion*: A sharply defined circular opacity within the lung suggestive of the appearance of a coin and usually representing a spherical or nodular lesion.
- *Collapse*: A state in which lung tissue has undergone complete atelectasis. Mainly used in respect to lobar disease.
- *Consolidation*: An essentially homogenous opacity of the lung characterised by little or no loss of volume, by effacement of pulmonary blood vessels and sometimes by the presence of an air bronchogram.
- *Lucency*: The shadow of an absorber that attenuates the primary X-ray beam less effectively than do surrounding absorbers. Hence on an X-ray any circumscribed area that appears more nearly black than its surroundings.
- *Opacity*: The shadow of an absorber that attenuates the primary X-ray beam more effectively than do surrounding absorbers. Hence on an X-ray any circumscribed area that appears more nearly white than its surroundings
- *Reticulonodular*: A collection of innumerable small, linear and nodular opacities that together produce a composite appearance resembling a net with small superimposed nodules. Usually indicates predominant abnormality in the pulmonary interstitium.
- *Septal Line(s)*: A straight linear opacity 1.5–2 cm in length and 1–2 mm in width usually situated at the lung base and oriented at right angles to the pleural surface with which it is in contact.
  Other terms that are commonly used include:
- *Ill-defined opacity*: an irregular opacity that has indistinct margins.
- *Patch*: often used to describe ill-defined areas e.g. patchy consolidation

1.4. Normal appearance

- PA Projection (Fig. 1a)
  If the radiograph is taken at suspended full inspiration the anterior ends of the upper six ribs and the posterior aspect of the10th ribs should be visible through the lungs. The diaphragm is domed with the apex at least 1.5 cm above a line drawn from the costophrenic angle to the cardiophrenic angle. The right hemidiaphragm is usually slightly higher than the left -approximately 1.5 cm, however in 9% of normal people they are the same height or the left slightly higher (Felson, 1973).
  The pulmonary markings are mainly produced by vessels and bronchial walls. The pulmonary arteries, bronchial arteries, bronchi and lymphatics run closely together and fan out from the hila. They gradually reduce in size and are visible up to 1–2 cm from the visceral pleura. The pulmonary veins are usually lateral to the arteries in the upper lobes and run horizontally in the lower lobes allowing them to be distinguished from the arteries.
  It is useful to assess the bronchus and artery for the upper lobe anterior segments; these are often seen end on and are usually similar in size. If the artery is greater than 1.5 times the size of the bronchus it is considered to be enlarged.
  The hila outlines are predominately vascular in origin with normal lymph nodes and bronchial walls having a minor role. The lower lobe pulmonary arteries should measure between 9 to16 mm prior to their segmental division.
  The mediastinal outline on the right is formed superiorly to inferiorly by the superior vena cava, the ascending aorta which becomes more prominent with age, the right atrium and a short segment of the inferior vena cava; formation on the left is by the aortic knuckle, the pulmonary artery, the left atrial appendage and the left ventricle. Fat pads may partially obscure the cardiophrenic angles.
  Heart size is usually assessed by the cardiothoracic ratio (CTR). The cardiac diameter is the sum of the maximal displacement of the right heart border from the midline and the maximal displacement of the left heart border from the midline. The thoracic diameter is measured from internal to internal borders of the ribs. A ratio of up to 50% is considered normal.
- Lateral projection (Fig. 1b)
  This allows assessment of areas poorly seen on the PA film, e.g. the anterior mediastinum and the posterior costophrenic angles, localisation of lesions seen on the PA film and a different view of structures already seen, e.g. the hila.
  There should be a radiolucent space retrosternally; this is lost with lesions in the anterior mediastinum. Similarly, the apparent density of the vertebral bodies should decrease from the apices to the bases. In the presence of lower lobe consolidation or mass lesion this is also lost.
  It is often possible to localise lesions from their alteration of normal silhouettes on the PA film but the lateral view is a very helpful adjuvant. It is

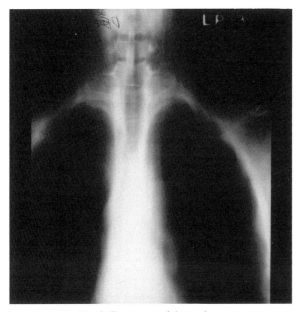

Fig. 3. Tomogram of the trachea.

also useful to confirm the presence of suspected abnormalities seen on the PA view.

The hila overlie each other on the lateral film but is possible to differentiate them due to their difference in height. The upper lobe bronchi can be seen end-on and the posterior walls of both the trachea and right bronchus intermedius demonstrated.

1.5. Tomography

Within the chest this technique (Fig. 3) has mainly been superseded by computed tomography (CT) and magnetic resonance imaging (MRI), however it is a useful procedure and is essential in intravenous urography. It is a method of imaging a particular layer (depth) within the patient whilst blurring out detail from all other layers. This may be said to be sectioned or "sliced" radiography. The X-ray tube and film move in opposite directions either linked by a rod or electronically, the alterable fulcrum point of which provides the level for the tomogram.

In the chest, the method can be useful for assessing tracheal disease, in particular benign strictures but MRI is preferable for malignant disease due to the better visualisation of adjacent structures.

2. Computed tomography (CT) (Figs. 4a–e and 5)

Considerable advances have occurred in CT with the advent of spiral/helical CT. All CT scanners require a rotating X-ray tube producing a narrow fan-beam of X-rays that pass through the transverse plane of the patient to detectors opposite. This data is then reconstructed to produce the image.

Older scanners work on a step and shoot principle; the tube rotates 360° to produce one image then stops, the table moves a set distance then stops and the scan is repeated. In spiral CT there is continuous rotation of the tube and continuous table movement allowing acquisition of volume data sets, several of which may be obtained during one patient examination

The advantages of spiral CT include shorter scan times and single breath hold scans allowing flexible post processing including multiplanar reconstructions, 3D reconstructions and virtual endoscopy. This has become accepted as the standard CT mode.

Each reconstructed axial slice is made up of pixels, usually a 512×512 matrix. Each pixel has an attenuation value, measured in Houndsfield Units (HU) determined by its radiographic density. The density range is from $-1,000$ HU (air) to $1,000$ HU (bone) with water having a density of 0HU. It is possible to view each image centered at any desired attenuation value (window level) with any desired range (window width). This allows assessment of lung, soft tissue and bone from the same data set.

There are multiple different acquisition protocols available for thoracic CT and techniques vary dependent upon the clinical situation. In general an iodine based intravenous contrast medium is required to assess the mediastinum and hila (Fig. 6a and b). Without contrast there is little difference in attenuation values between vessels and adjacent structures, e.g. lymph nodes. Iodine causes increased absorption of the X-ray beam and a consequent increase in the attenuation value so that vascular structures appear brighter or "enhanced" allowing their differentiation from adjacent soft tissues. The slice thickness can vary from 2 to 10 mm with thinner slices being useful where partial voluming may be a problem, e.g. the aorto-pulmonary window or with the complex anatomy of the hila.

The resolution of CT can be assessed in two projections, it is maximal in the transverse section where it is dependent upon the field of view, pixel size and reconstruction algorithm. In the through-plane or Z-axis in spiral CT the resolution is dependent upon slice width, pitch of acquisition and reconstruction algorithm. The maximal resolution is in high resolution CT (HRCT) in which 1 mm thick slices are obtained and where structures measuring 0.1 to 0.2 mm can be visualised, e.g. interlobular septa.

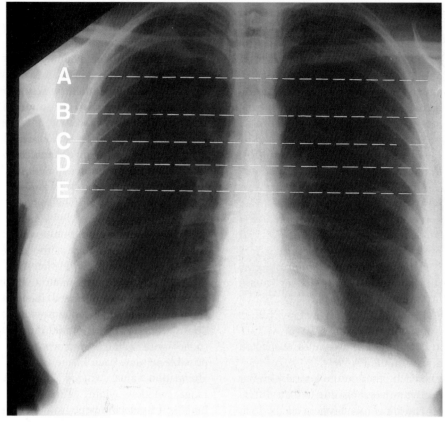

Fig. 4. Axial 8mm thick CT images of a normal mediastinum with intravenous contrast. Scout view showing level of axial images (see right for corresponding axial images A through E).

CT is the method of choice for the staging/pre-operative assessment of lung cancer. In this situation the liver and adrenals should be scanned routinely and delayed scans may be helpful in the characterising lesions in these organs. (Szolar et al., 1998).

CT can be used to assess pulmonary nodules, mediastinal masses, persisting pulmonary consolidation/collapse, aortic disease and, more recently, pulmonary emboli (Remy-Jardin et al., 1995).

High resolution CT (HRCT) refers to a specific technique for the assessment of interstitial lung disease or bronchiectasis. 1 to 2 mm thick slices are obtained at intervals of 1 to 2 cm through the lung. Initially performed on suspended deep inspiration, expiratory or prone scans may also be required to assess air trapping and the posterior lung bases.

Spiral CT allows excellent multiplanar reconstruction giving better spatial awareness of pathology. Virtual bronchoscopic techniques may in the future augment conventional bronchoscopy.

The disadvantages of CT include:

- The ability to only scan in axial sections compared to MRI although spiral CT now allows excellent reconstructions.
- High radiation dose. In 1992 CT represented 2% of examinations yet contributed 20% of effective patient dose (Document of NRPB, 1992). Since then, changes in technology have reduced the dose per examination but an increased number of studies are performed.
- Possible complications from intravenous contrast, these include local extravasation and allergic reactions, which can range from urticaria to anaphylaxis.

3. Nuclear medicine

The principle of nuclear medicine is the provision of functional rather than anatomical information. Many different agents can be used, which are labelled with a gamma ray emitting radionuclide and then injected, inhaled or ingested by the patient. These agents act as tracers of physiological function, e.g. pulmonary

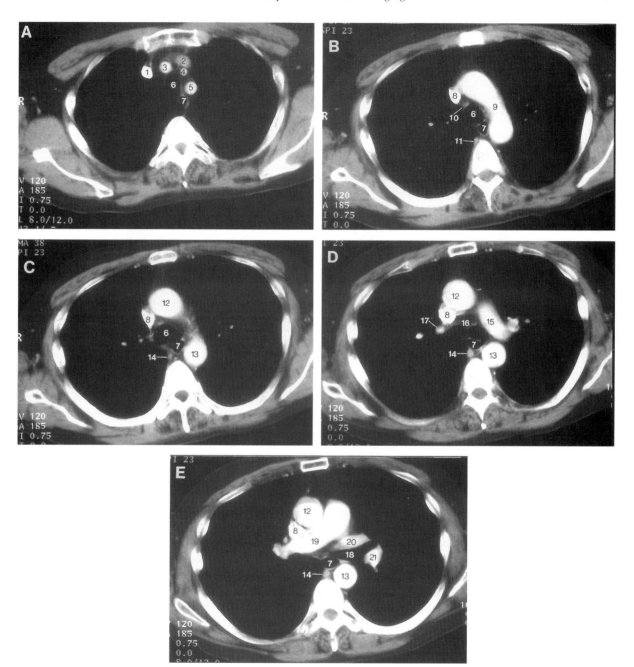

Fig. 4 (continued). 1. Right Innominate Vein, 2. Left Innominate Vein, 3. Innominate Artery, 4. Left Carotid Artery, 5. Left subclavian Vein, 6. Trachea, 7. Oesophagus, 8. Superior Vena Cava, 9. Aortic Arch, 10. Lymph node, 11. Superior Right Intercostal Vein, 12. Ascending Aorta, 13. Descending Aorta, 14. Azygous vein, 15. Left Main Pulmonary Artery, 16. Tracheal bifurcation, 17. Right Upper Lobe Artery, 18. Left Main Bronchus, 19. Right Main Pulmonary Artery, 20. Left Superior Pulmonary Vein, 21. Left Interlobar Artery.

perfusion or ventilation, with the emitted gamma rays being detected by a gamma camera.

The gamma camera consists of a sodium iodide crystal in which incident gamma rays produce a light scintillation. These are detected by a series of photomultiplier tubes. The spatial resolution is 6–12 mm at a distance of 10 cm from the camera.

The mainstay of pulmonary nuclear medicine is the ventilation/perfusion scan (Fig. 7a and b). The perfusion study is performed by an intravenous injection of ^{99m}Technetium (Tc) labelled macroaggregated albumin. Up to 500,00 particles are injected which will obstruct approximately 0.1% of the vascular bed. Images are then taken in 6 to 8 different projections.

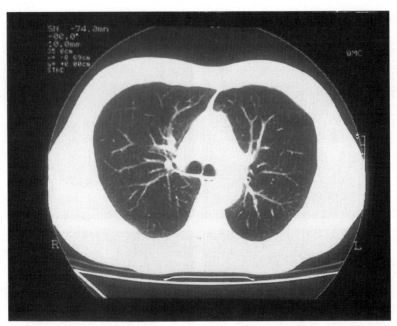

Fig. 5. Axial 10 mm thick CT image on lung windows at the level of the tracheal bifurcation showing normal parenchymal appearance.

There are several different agents available for ventilation imaging, either gaseous or particle aerosols.

There are two gaseous agents. [133]Xenon is commonly used. It has the advantages of being easily available and allowing assessment of the wash in, equilibrium and wash out of the tracer although only from one projection, usually posterior which is performed prior to the perfusion study. [81m]Krypton has the advantage of allowing multiple views to be acquired in conjunction with the perfusion study. However, it has a half life of only 13 seconds and is produced via a cyclotron making it difficult to obtain in many hospitals.

The radioaerosol usually used is Diethylene triamine pentaacetic acid (DTPA) labelled with [99m]Tc. This is readily available and multiple views can be obtained although central deposition of the tracer can be a problem in patients with chronic obstructive pulmonary disease.

The applications of ventilation/perfusion scanning include:
- Pulmonary embolism — Multiple, large, wedge-shaped pleural based perfusion defects with normal ventilation is the classical appearance of pulmonary emboli. Unfortunately most studies do not show this pattern and therefore diagnostic criteria have been proposed for their interpretation, e.g. PIOPED criteria (Gottschalk et al., 1993).
- Pre-operative assessment of lung function — This is mandatory for a patient with borderline lung function requiring a pneumonectomy. Important ventilation and perfusion defects in the residual (healthy) lung or good, matched ventilation and perfusion in the lung to be resected would constitute a contraindication since the quality of life after pneumonectomy would be compromised.
- Assessment of chronic obstructive pulmonary disease (COPD) and bullous emphysema — Matched ventilation and perfusion defects are demonstrated often with a patchy distribution within the lungs.

Radionuclide bone scanning can play an important role in the assessment of lung cancer, in the evaluation of bone pain and the search for distant metastases.

There are many other agents which may be useful, e.g. if a retrosternal thyroid is suspected [123]Iodine can be used to confirm functioning thyroid tissue and is preferred to ^{99m}Tc-pertechnetate due to its higher target to background ratio. Ectopic parathyroid adenomas within the mediastinum may be detected using ^{99m}Tc-sestamibi.

Positron emission tomography (PET) scanning with [18]Fluoro-deoxy glucose ([18]FDG) may become an important imaging agent due to its ability to differentiate between benign and malignant disease of the lungs and pleura due to variations in glucose transport and utilisation which leads to high uptake in malignant tissue (Bury et al., 1997). The ability to perform whole body imaging may be useful in pre-

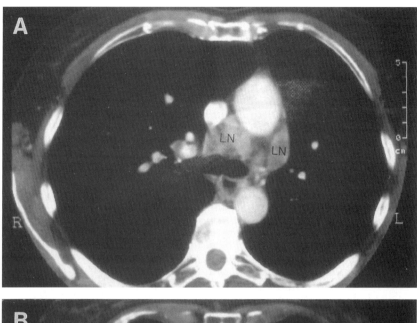

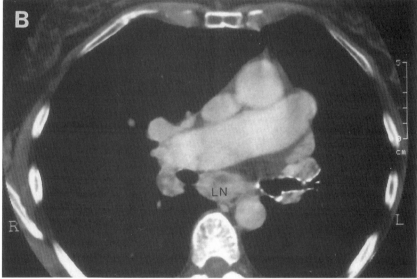

Fig. 6. Axial 8 mm CT images with intravenous contrast showing mediastinal lymphadenopathy (LN): (a) precarinal and aortopulmonary window lymphadenopathy, (b) subcarinal lymphadenopathy.

operative staging of lung cancer allowing detection of distant metastases, although the normally high brain activity limits detection of cerebral metastases. Gamma cameras are now available that can perform PET scanning; however, [18]FDG is produced in a cyclotron and has a half life of 118 minutes, which are limiting factors to its use.

4. Ultrasound

Images are produced due to the reflection of the ultrasound beam as it passes through the body. This occurs when it attempts to cross a boundary between two tissues of different acoustic impedance. In extreme mismatches of impedance, complete reflection occurs with an "acoustic shadow" distally, this happens at interfaces between soft tissue/bone and soft tissue/air and is the limiting factor for the use of ultrasound in the chest.

There are however specific areas where ultrasound is a valuable investigation:

Localisation of pleural fluid — assessment of site, volume, loculation and differentiation of fluid from pleural thickening (Fig. 8).

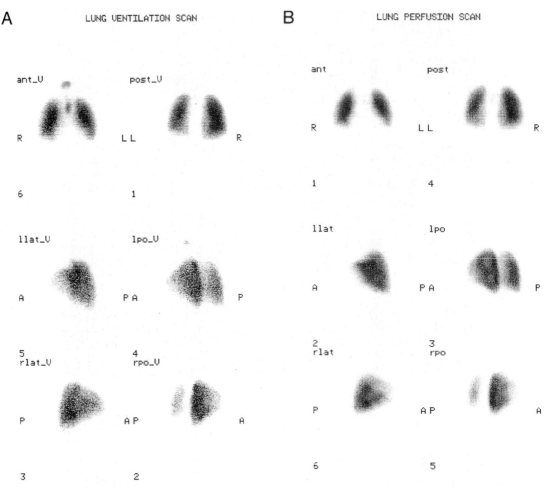

Fig. 7. Normal radioisotope ventilation and perfusion images: (a) ventilation study using ^{99m}Tc-DTPA aerosol, (b) perfusion study using ^{99m}Tc-MAA, performed after the ventilation study, residual ventilation activity is noted in the mouth and oesophagus.

Assessment of pleural tumour or pulmonary disease abutting the chest wall; it can be very effective in assessing chest wall invasion.

Differentiation of solid and cystic masses.

Ultrasound guided intervention — aspiration, biopsy or drainage procedures.

5. Magnetic resonance imaging (MRI)

This technique, MRI (Fig. 9a and b), utilises a strong magnetic field and radiofrequency pulses to obtain signals from hydrogen nuclei within the tissues. There are many different pulse sequences that can be used to obtain images, the two basic sequences are T_1 and T_2 weighted.

T_1 weighted images show water and fluid as dark. On T_2 weighted images these areas appear bright so that tissue with a high water content, e.g. inflamma-tory or malignant tissue, shows as high signal areas on the T_2 sequence.

MRI contrast agents, e.g. Gadolinium-DTPA, act by enhancing the signal from water molecules particularly on T_1 sequences causing enhanced signal from tissue with a high water content.

STIR sequences suppress the signal from normal fat tissue allowing better assessment of disease processes extending through fat planes or into fat.

The strengths of MRI include: the lack of ionising radiation, ability to image in any plane, characterisation of soft tissues and the assessment of vascular structures without intravenous contrast.

Acquisition times of 3 to 7 minutes per sequence can give problems with breathing or cardiac motion artifacts. ECG gating can be used to reduce cardiac motion but respiratory gating would significantly increase the acquisition time and is not routinely

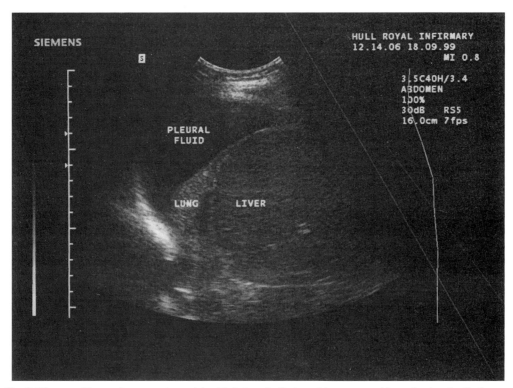

Fig. 8. Ultrasound image demonstrating a right-sided pleural effusion with non-aerated lung abutting the diaphragm.

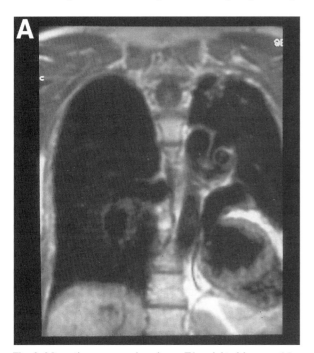

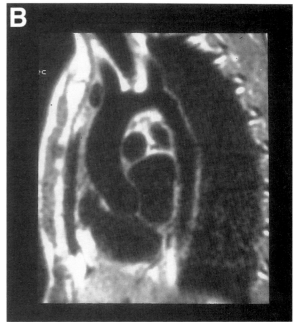

Fig. 9. Magnetic resonance imaging – T1-weighted images: (a) coronal image through the aortic arch and descending aorta, (b)sagittal image through the aorta. *(Images courtesy of Dr. A. Nicholson, Hull Royal Infirmary.)*

used. Usually several sequences are obtained in each study with combinations of axial, coronal and sagittal scans and a variety of different sequences.

The visualisation of parenchymal disease is poorer than in CT, in part due to the respiratory motion. <1 cm nodules are better seen on CT and the morpholog-

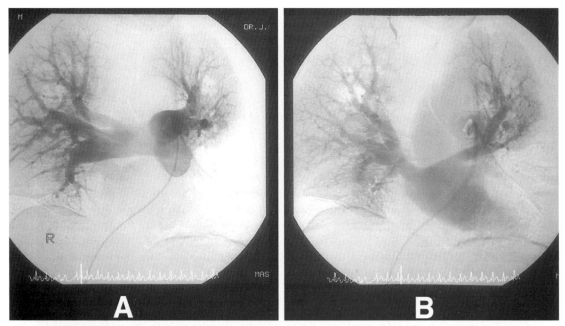

Fig. 10. Digital subtraction pulmonary angiography (normal): (a) pulmonary arteries, (b) pulmonary veins and left atrium.

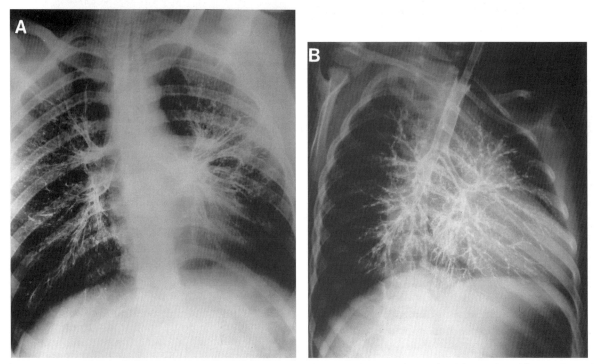

Fig. 11. Normal bronchography: (a) PA radiograph demonstrating major bronchi in both lungs, (b) right anterior oblique radiograph demonstrating major bronchi in both lungs.

ical characterisation of larger nodules, e.g. the presence of calcification or spiculation, is superior on CT (Bittner and Felix, 1998).

Contraindications include cardiac pacemakers, metallic foreign bodies and ferromagnetic surgical implants although all cardiac valve replacements except the Starr-Edwards are unaffected (Hartnell et al., 1997).

The uses of MRI within the thorax include: vascular — cardiac and great vessels, e.g. aortic dissection, the assessment of superior sulcus invasion, staging of oesophageal tumours, the characterisation of mediastinal masses and chest wall disease.

The spatial resolution of CT and MRI is similar in the mediastinum and the choice between the two techniques is often dependent upon availability/access as well as the information required by the examination.

6. Angiography

Angiography (Fig. 10a and 10b) is study of the vasculature by catheterisation of the vessels and injection of intravascular iodinated contrast media. The use of digital subtraction allows visualisation of the vessels without the overlying structures. Interventional vascular radiology has an important role in thoracic radiology.

Excluding the heart, there are several areas where angiography has a major role:

Pulmonary Arteries: Angiography remains the gold standard for the diagnosis of pulmonary emboli although there is inter-observer variation in the interpretation of the images. It is also used for the diagnosis of pulmonary arteriovenous malformations and pulmonary artery aneurysms; these can be treated by embolization, usually with coils.

Bronchial Arteries: Catheterisation is usually in response to severe life-threatening haemoptysis in patients with chronic inflammatory lung disease with the aim of embolising the responsible vessel. It may be necessary to assess intercostal or internal mammary arteries as these can occasionally be implicated.

Aorta: Although MRI and CT can demonstrate certain pathologies such as dissection and trauma, aortography remains an important investigation. Aortic coarctation can be managed by balloon dilatation and the aberrant systemic arteries to sequestrated lung segments demonstrated.

Superior Vena Cava: The imaging of superior vena cava obstruction is important as intraluminal stenting allows immediate relief of symptoms. Imaging is also valuable in patients requiring surgical reconstruction.

Inferior Vena Cava: The placement of intraluminal filters has become an essential procedure in the management of severe pulmonary embolism.

7. Bronchography

Developments and advances in CT have reduced the indications of bronchography (Figs. 11a and 11b) to such an extent that the procedure is regarded by many as "a thing of the past." For the diagnosis of bronchiectasis high resolution CT has become the procedure of choice. Nevertheless, to the thoracic surgeon, bronchography is more than the mere diagnosis of diseased bronchi and peribronchial parenchyma, which is presented on CT images. The surgeon needs visualisation of the precise anatomical configuration of segmental bronchi in their whole length, which is not afforded by the CT image. It is also important to the assessment of the distribution of normal and abnormal bronchi outlined.

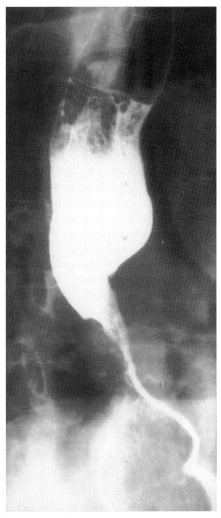

Fig. 12. Barium swallow demonstrating an oesophageal carcinoma. *(Image courtesy of Dr. A.D. Taylor, Hull Royal Infirmary)*

In bronchography a contrast medium is introduced into the lumen of the lower trachea. By changing the position of the patient on the X-ray table, the contrast will flow and fill the bronchial tree. To avoid overlapping images of the bronchial tree radiographs are taken from different angles; a minimum of PA, right lateral and left oblique views are needed. In cases of selected bronchography contrast is introduced via a catheter positioned in the lobar or segmental bronchus.

7.1. Techniques

Bronchoscopic: a catheter passed via either a rigid or fibreoptic bronchoscope through which is injected contrast into the trachea, main or lobar bronchi (see bronchoscopy: section 2.3 in chapter I.2).

Percutaneous trans-tracheal injection: A wide bore short needle or catheter is passed through the cricothyroid membrane. The larynx and trachea should be well-anaesthetised beforehand (for technique, see section 2.3.6 in chapter I.2).

Nasotracheal fine tube intubation: Following topical anaesthesia of the nasolarngopharynx, a fine nasogastric catheter is passed via the nose into the trachea. It is important to ensure the catheter lies well above the carina before introduction of the dye. This can be checked by X-ray.

The important points in achieving success, irrespective of the technique used, is for patients with copious sputum to have extensive physiotherapy, postural drainage and/or even bronchoscopic clearing of the bronchial tree prior to bronchography.

After bronchography the patient should be given physiotherapy and encouraged to cough and expectorate in order to clear the bronchi of excess sputum and the contrast. In some cases bronchoscopy (rigid) and bronchial aspiration/clearing of the airway may be necessary.

8. Oesophageal investigation

Plain chest and neck radiography can demonstrate presence of an opaque foreign body retained in the oesophagus. It is important to have a lateral view X-ray film to avoid the cardiac and mediastinal structures obscuring the foreign body.

The Barium swallow is the commonest examination; this can be used to assess either morphology or motility (Fig. 12).

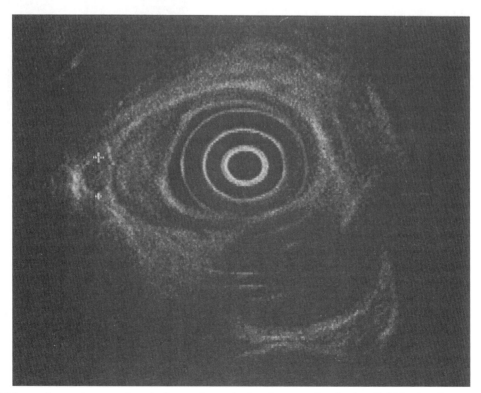

Fig. 13. Axial image from a transoesophageal ultrasound examination demonstrating focal wall thickening due to an oesophageal carcinoma with an adjacent lymph node marked by the calipers. *(Image courtesy of Dr. A.D. Taylor, Hull Royal Infirmary)*

If oesophageal motility is to be assessed this requires a video recording of the patient swallowing both liquid barium and a solid bolus with the oropharynx examined in both PA and lateral projections. It is also important to assess motility with the patient both erect and lying on the screening table, often prone.

In looking for morphological abnormalities both an effervescent agent releasing carbon dioxide and a smooth muscle relaxant, e.g. Hyoscine butylbromide, are often used.

In some circumstances water-soluble contrast media is employed for swallow studies. This does not give the same mucosal detail as Barium but is the contrast of choice for investigating oesophageal perforations, leaks or post surgical anastamotic integrity.

Oesophageal carcinomas can be staged by both CT and MRI for assessment of local spread and distant metastatic disease with similar results. Although liver and paraaortic nodular metastases are well-demonstrated, the depth of tumour penetration of the wall and the presence of adjacent nodes are poorly visualised.

Endoluminal ultrasound (Fig. 13) can be also be used for the local staging. This has the resolution to accurately assess depth of penetration and infiltration into adjacent structures although it tends to overestimate local nodal involvement (Rankin and Mason, 1992).

Radioisotope studies of the oesophagus are mainly concerned with motility. Using a combination of ^{99m}Tc and ^{111}Indium it is possible to study liquid and solid motility simultaneously. The presence of ectopic gastric mucosa in a Barrett's oesophagus can be detected with ^{99m}Tc pertechnetate.

References and further reading

Bittner RC, Felix R. Magnetic resonance (MR) imaging of the chest: state of the art. Eur Respir J 1998; 11: 1392–1404.

Bury Th, Paulus P, Dowlatti A, Corhay JL, Rigo P, Radermecker MF. Evaluation of pleural diseases with FDG-PET imaging: preliminary report. Thorax 1997; 52: 187–189.

Documents of the NRPB 3; 4: 1-16. National Radiological Protection Board, Oxon UK, Chilton, Didcot, 1992.

Felson B. Chest Roentgenology. Philadelphia, WB Saunders, 1973.

Felson B, Felson H. Localization of intrathoracic lesions by means of the postero-anterior roentgenogram. The silhouette sign. Radiology 1950; 55: 363–374.

The Fleischner Society. Glossary of terms for thoracic radiology: Recommendations of the nomenclature committee of the Fleischner Society. Am J Roentgenol 1984; 143: 509.

Gottschalk A, Sostman HD, Coleman RE et al. Ventilation-perfusion scintigraphy in the PIOPED study Part II. Evaluation of the scintigraphic criteria and interpretations. J Nucl Med 1993; 34: 1119–1126.

Hartnell CG, Spence L, Hughes LA, Cohen MC, Saouef R, Buff B. Safety of MR imaging in patients who have retained metallic materials after cardiac surgery. Am J Roentgenol 1997; 168: 1157–1159.

Rankin S, Mason R. Review: Staging of oesophageal carcinoma. Clin Radiol 1992; 46: 373–377.

Remy-Jardin M, Remy J, Petyt L, Duhamel A, Marchandise X. Diagnosis of acute pulmonary embolism with spiral CT: comparison with pulmonary angiography and scintigraphy. Radiology 1995; 197: 303.

Szolar DH, Kammerhuber FH. Adrenal adenomas and nonadenomas: assessment of washout at delayed contrast-enhanced CT. Radiology 1998; 207: 369–375.

K. Moghissi, J.A.C. Thorpe and F. Ciulli (Eds.)
Moghissi's Essentials of Thoracic and Cardiac Surgery
© 2003 Elsevier Science B.V. All rights reserved

CHAPTER I.4

Thoracic incisions — surgical access to thoracic operations

K. Moghissi

This chapter is devoted to thoracic incisions and surgical access to the chest, which constitutes the key to surgical exposure.

The technical aspects of incisions and approaches to the standard and commonly practised cardiothoracic operations are given in some detail. Modification and variation of the standard are accommodated as far as possible.

1. General principles of surgical incision and access to the thoracic cavity

Intrathoracic organs may be surgically approached anteriorly, antero-laterally, postero-laterally and posteriorly. The thoracotomy incision is planned according to the operative requirement and the topography of the organ which is the surgical target within the thorax. There are, however, some general principles which apply to all thoracotomies.

- The skin incision is usually made along skin creases and following the line of a rib.
- Incisions for exposure of the anterior mediastinum are usually carried over the sternum with transverse or vertical sternotomy if a wider exposure is needed.
- The chest wall muscles are incised or split in layers.
- Posteriorly the trapezius and latissimus dorsi are divided in continuation. Between the two, the triangle of auscultation is bare of muscles and is covered only by fascia. Incision through this fascia exposes the rhomboids and indicates the direction of the underlying ribs.
- The serratus anterior should be cut nearer to its costal digitation rather than near to the scapula.
- Excision of a rib, once a common practice is, as a rule, unnecessary.

- The chest is usually entered through an intercostal space, by incising and stripping the costal periosteum together with the intercostal muscles from the upper border of a rib, thus gaining access to the thoracic cavity. This is done using the rougine (periosteum elevator) and proceeding from the posterior to the anterior end of the upper border of the rib.
- A wider space may be created by incising the posterior end of the rib using a costotome or, alternatively, dislocating the costo-transverse joint with the use of a Semb raspatory.
- In anterior thoracotomy the perichondrium is stripped and the costal cartilages may be incised in order to provide a wider space.
- In all cases, a self-retaining rib spreader is inserted between two adjacent ribs and the space widened as required for surgical manoeuvres within the chest.
- Before closure and repair of thoracotomy wounds, the chest is usually drained using a tube connected to an underwater sealed drainage system.

2. Standard posterolateral thoracotomy technique

This is the most frequently used thoracotomy and is the standard approach for pulmonary surgery (Fig. 1).

- Posterolateral thoracotomy is usually carried out with the patient in the lateral position. Very occasionally, postero-lateral thoracotomy is carried out with the patient placed in a prone position.
- For lateral position thoracotomy the hemithorax to be entered is placed uppermost. To obtain a good lateral position, the spine should be parallel to the longitudinal axis of the operating table. To

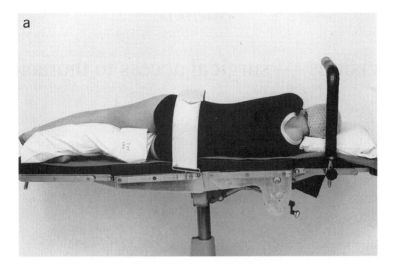

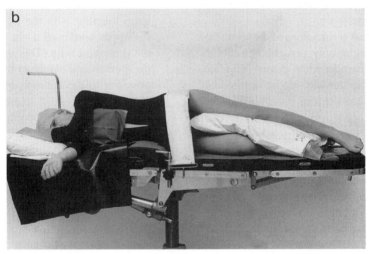

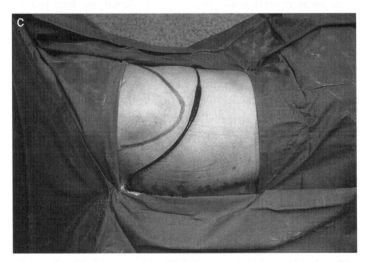

Fig. 1. The position of the patient on the table for postero-lateral left thoracotomy: (a) posterior view, (b) anterior view of the same, (c) shows the towelling of the patient for postero-lateral thoracotomy (right). Angle of the scapula is outlined and the incision is made.

facilitate surgical manipulation and manoeuvres the patient's back is placed near to the edge of the operating table. Belts, sandbags and supports are used to obtain firm fixation of the patient to the table and prevent movement during the operation. Armrests and boards are used as necessary to position the upper limbs and facilitate the running of i.v. infusions. Anaesthetic screens are helpful and assist the anaesthetist's manipulations during operation without transgressing into the operative field.

- ECG electrodes and central venous catheter are placed out of the surgical field.
- Bony prominences are protected.
- The uppermost leg is extended and the lower leg flexed beneath it to about 90°. A pillow is placed between the legs protecting the bony prominence of knees. The diathermy pad is then placed and fixed around the uppermost leg.

2.1. Skin preparation and drapes

A wide area of the skin, including the wall of the hemithorax on the thoracotomy side and the upper quadrant of the abdomen below the costal margin, is cleaned with a disinfectant solution. Four square surgical drapes[1], two larger and two smaller, are placed to border a rectangular area surrounding the area for the thoracotomy wound. One large drape covers the whole lower part of the body to overlap the table on all sides except for its upper edge which is placed horizontally across the lower chest below the incision, taking into account that an area below the incision and above the drape is required for the insertion of the intercostal drainage tubes. The second large drape covers the upper parts of the patient, overlapping the table on all sides except for its lower border, and is placed obliquely across the upper part of the scapula above the site of the incision, from the upper thoracic vertebra to the sternum. The higher the thoracotomy the higher the lower border of this drape must be placed. The two smaller drapes are laid one posteriorly in the line of the spine, the other parallel to the long axis of the sternum, thus exposing the full length of the middle ribs and, in particular, those under and adjacent to the line of incision. Each of the smaller drapes overlaps the larger ones and are fixed to them and

then to the skin by towel clips. Often, two additional drapes are required to stretch between the anaesthetic screen and a drip stand to screen off the table and its surroundings.

2.2. Incision and entry to the chest

Incision (Fig. 2) is made parallel to the line of the obliquity of the ribs starting in front, lateral to the sternocostal junction running backwards 3 to 4 cm below the angle of the scapula, then upwards between the vertebral border of the scapula and the spine for a variable distance, according to the selected thoracotomy site, but not higher than the upper border of the scapula. Many surgeons make extensive use of the electrosurgical unit. The skin incision is made with a scalpel but the flat muscles of the chest are divided by cutting diathermy. The vessels are picked up using a fine tooth forceps, electrocoagulated and then divided. Using this technique very few blood vessels require ligating. After division of the chest wall muscles in layers, the ribs and intercostal muscular planes are reached. Ribs are counted by introducing a hand under the scapula and identifying the horizontal border of the first rib. The required rib is selected and the periosteum near its upper border is incised. A rougine (periosteum elevator) is next used to raise the periosteum and the intercostal muscular attachments of the upper border of the rib, starting from the posterior end of the rib and sliding the rougine forwards towards the costal cartilage. The pleura is incised first by a scalpel and then by a pair of scissors. Following this, the rib spreader (chest spreader) is introduced and the intercostal space between the two ribs opened wide.

2.2.1. Note about electrosurgery
Some European thoracic surgeons have been hesitant about electrosurgery fearing greater tissue necrosis following its use. There is however no evidence to support this.

Electrosurgery is employed for:
(a) Electrocoagulating small blood vessels.
(b) Cutting and coagulating at the same time using blended current.
(c) Controlling ooze type of superficial bleeding (e.g. chest wall, etc.) using a ball shaped blunt applicator.

---

[1] In many countries, disposable drapes are made for a specific operation.

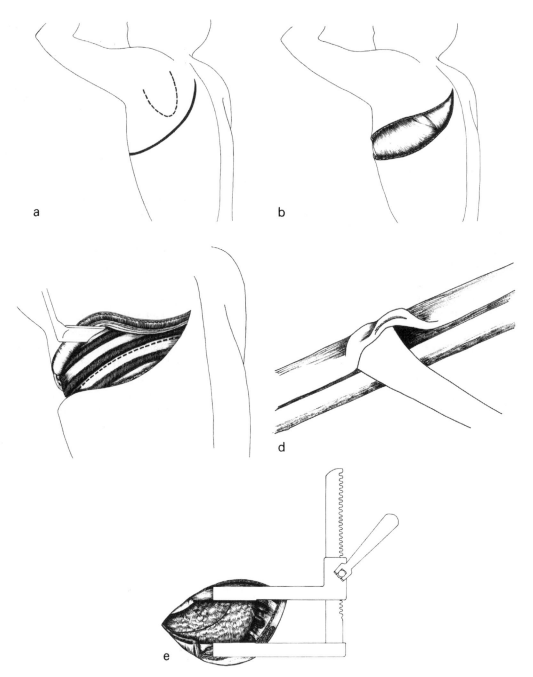

Fig. 2. Diagram showing the steps of postero-lateral thoracotomy (left): (a) position of the patient and the incision, (b) incision has been made and superficial layers of chest muscles are shown, (c) the intercostal layer is reached and the periosteum of the rib is incised, (d) periosteum is elevated using the rougine, (e) the pleural space is entered and the chest spreader inserted.

3. Thoracotomy — prone position (Overholt and Sellors-Brown position)

Prone position thoracotomy was used in the past for patients with copious bronchial secretions. This approach has been largely superseded by the advent of double lumen tube intubation. Nevertheless, the position is useful for children and when double lumen tubes are not available or cannot be placed.

The patient is placed on the table lying flat and face down (Fig. 3). The upper part of the thorax and the pelvis are lifted off the table by pads and padded

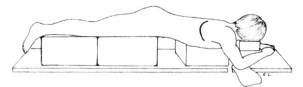

Fig. 3. Prone position thoracotomy.

rests, so that the upper abdomen and the lower chest (diaphragmatic area) are away from the table. Slight Trendelenburg tilt is made and the head is turned to one side. On the thoracotomy side the arm hangs down but with no pressure on the axilla. The essence of this position is that the lungs and trachea are placed higher than the mouth, allowing free passage of secretion from the lungs into a large endotracheal tube which can be aspirated by the anaesthetist. This position prevents the spill over of bronchial secretion from the diseased into the healthy side which may occur during thoracotomy in the lateral position when a double lumen airway tube is not used. Surgical towelling does not differ from thoracotomy in the lateral position. Drapes are placed in such a manner as to allow the fullest possible incision and to allow for placement of drainage tubes.

3.1. Closure (repair) of Postero-lateral thoracotomy wound

3.1.1. General principles
Before proceeding to the thoracotomy closure, one or more drains are inserted through a lower intercostal space into the pleural cavity and connected to an underwater sealed drainage system. Closure of the thoracotomy wound requires layer by layer stitching. Five anatomical planes can be recognised and should be stitched.

- Intercostal layers, including the parietal pleura: This means the stitching of the pleura, intercostal muscles and the periosteum above the thoracotomy opening with the intercostal muscles of the space below. A rib approximator (Fig. 4) is usually required to facilitate repair of this layer. In practice, one limb of the instrument is inserted into the intercostal space above the thoracotomy and the other limb inserted into the next but one intercostal space below the thoracotomy. By approximating the two limbs of the instrument, the soft tissue of the intercostal spaces adjacent to the thoracotomy is raised and will cover the rib adjacent to the thoracotomy. This can then be stitched together.

  Closure of the intercostal layer has to be airtight. This can be achieved using continuous run-

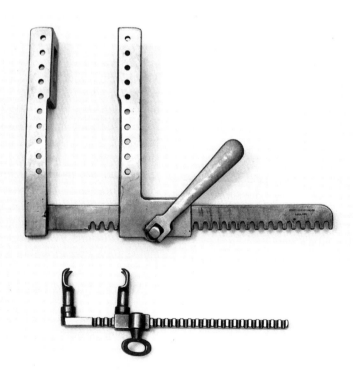

Fig. 4. Showing rib spreader above and Sellors' combined rib approximator and spreader below.

ning stitching, non or slow absorbable (No. 2/0). Sometimes it becomes necessary to apply additional interrupted stitches or pericostals to embrace the ribs above and below the thoracotomy.

- Deep muscular layer: The divided border of each of the individual muscles (serratus anterior and the rhomboids) are approximated using continuous stitches.
- Superficial muscular layer. The muscles in this layer consist of trapezius and latissimus dorsi in the posterolateral and pectoralis muscles in anterior and antero-lateral thoracotomies. The divided components of each muscle should be carefully approximated.
- Subcutaneous layer: This often requires a separate closure but can occasionally be included in the skin sutures.
- Skin closure: Skin suture can be effected in several ways, depending on the experience and the preference of the surgeon. This may be a continuous running, mattress stitches or subcuticular stitching. Alternatively clips may be used.

4. Antero-lateral thoracotomy

This thoracotomy approach (Fig. 5) is not particularly convenient for accessing all segments of the lung but it is useful in a variety of operations on the heart and oesophagus. On the left side it provides exposure to pericardium and the apex of the heart.

4.1. Position

The patient is placed supine on the operating table and the operative side is elevated about 30 degrees or more. To achieve this, padded sandbags are placed behind the buttock and back preventing the pelvis falling back. The upper shoulder is rotated backwards for about 30 degrees and the elbow is flexed. The position is secured by tapes, table-rests and supports.

- Arrangement of surgical drapes is similar to lateral position thoracotomy with some modification. Six towels are required. Two large towels are placed above and below the site of the incision. Al-

lowance is made for the site of the drainage tubes which should be included in the exposed area. Two smaller towels are laid anteriorly and posteriorly respectively, each placed well beyond the anterior and posterior extremities of the planned incision and fixed to the larger towels and the skin by towel clips. The anterior towel is fixed beyond the opposite sternal border making the mid-sternal line visible. Finally, the remaining two towels are placed from the anaesthetic screen to expand supero-laterally on each side (the wings).

4.2. Incision and entry to the thorax

A sub-mammary incision is made from the lateral border of the sternum anteriorily, extending for a variable length posteriorly and laterally along the line of the rib curve. In this position the pectoralis major and sometimes the pectoralis minor, according to the level of the incision, are divided anteriorly. The division of latissimus dorsi should be avoided. The serratus anterior fibres should be divided near to their insertion. The incision is then taken down to the intercostal space. When the incision extends beyond the costo-chondral junction, the periochondrium is elevated in continuation with the periosteum of the rib. To obtain a wider exposure, the chondro-sternal joint may be disarticulated; the internal mammary vessels may require stitching and dividing.

4.3. Closure of antero-lateral thoracotomy

This does not differ in principle from other thoracotomy closures. However, the intercostal space between the bony part of the ribs is easier to approximate and to stitch than the space between cartilages. In effect, the further forward the thoracotomy incision extends, the less soft tissue is available in the space and the more difficult a completely airtight closure becomes. Additional pericostal stitches (see previous page), and at times a linear incision through one of the adjacent cartilages with a scalpel, facilitate the closure. The muscles, subcutaneous tissues and skin are then closed in layers.

5. Anterior thoracotomy

In anterior thoracotomy (Fig. 6), the patient is placed in a supine position and surgical drapes laid in a manner to expose a square area of the upper abdomen above the umbilicus and the whole of hemithorax below the clavicle. Inclusion of the angle of Louis and

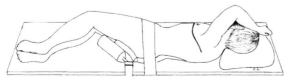

Fig. 5. Antero-lateral thoracotomy.

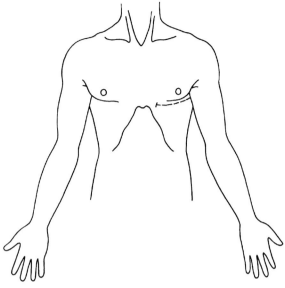

Fig. 6. Anterior thoracotomy.

the 2nd costal cartilage in the exposed area facilitates the identification of ribs and the accurate position of the incision.

5.1. Incision

A sub-mammary incision is made along the rib, starting from the lateral border of the sternum and extending laterally for a variable distance. The underlying muscles are divided. In emergency situations the intercostal muscles and the pleura are incised directly, otherwise the periosteum is elevated from the upper border of the rib together with the intercostal muscles. In either case, a chest spreader is introduced and the opening widened by winding up the retractor. Closure of an anterior thoracotomy wound is similar to that of antero–lateral thoracotomy.

5.2. Anterior Thoracotomy with trans-sternal extension

When further exposure of the mediastinum becomes necessary, the transverse section of the sternum is carried out in continuation with the anterior end of the incision. The transverse section of the sternum can be performed by using the Lebsche sternum chisel (sternum splitter) or Gigli's saw. To split the sternum with Gigli's instrument, long (Robert's type) artery forceps are passed behind the sternum from the side of the thoracotomy to puncture the corresponding opposite intercostal space lateral to the

sternal border. The chain of Gigli's saw is then picked up by the instrument and drawn under the sternum. The periosteum of the sternum is incised, the two ends of the Gigli's saw are hooked with the two hands and sawing can proceed. During the sawing an assistant places an instrument, such as Robert's artery forceps, over the anterior surface of the sternum so as to prevent the chain of the Gigli's saw projecting upwards when the bone is divided.

It is important to secure the internal mammary vessels or protect them. Closure of the transverse section of the sternum is achieved by approximating the divided edges of the sternum using two wire stitches.

6. Median sternotomy

This approach (Fig. 7) is most commonly used for all types of open-heart surgical operation. It is also a choice incision for access to anterior mediastinal tumour and for thymectomy. In combination with other incisions it provides a wide exposure for exploration and for operations in the root of the neck and some difficult cases of Morgagni type hernia.

6.1. Incision and entry to thorax

The patient is placed in supine position. A vertical midline incision is made extending from the suprasternal notch to a point midway between the

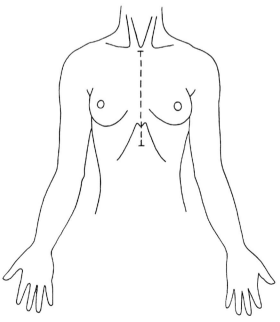

Fig. 7. Median sternotomy.

xiphoid process and the umbilicus. Below the skin, subcutaneous tissue, pectoralis major fascia (and sometimes muscle fibres) and periosteum are incised with diathermy. The sternum is next divided using an electric saw (with a substernal protection guard). The sternal section is made from the suprasternal notch downwards or from below upwards. In the latter case it is necessary to free the xiphoid process and incise it in the middle with a pair of strong scissors. This is done in order to place the guard under the bone and engage the blade in the xiphoid incision. It is important to be aware of the one or two veins around the xiphoid which can cause bleeding. For incising the bone from above downwards a space is created just above the sternal notch and the index finger is passed behind the sternum. The substernal guard of the saw is then placed substernally and the bone is incised. Subsidiaries to jugular veins, sometimes forming a venous plexus, need to be identified and coagulated. Whilst sternal division is proceeding, the lungs are hyperventilated to avoid accidental opening of the mediastinal pleura.

Once the sternum is divided the strong inter-clavicular ligament, situated just above suprasternal notch, requires division with scissors. The upper part of the linea alba also needs incising to allow wide separation of the two components of the sternum.

Note that the oscillating compressed air-saw, Leb-sche's sternum chisel or Gigli's saw can be used as an alternative to the electric saw. The principle of Gigli's saw is to pass the chain under the sternum, snug to the bone, with one end emerging through the suprasternal notch and the other below the xiphoid which is incised with a pair of strong scissors. The handles (hooks) are attached and sawing carried out. Strong forceps (e.g. Roberts artery forceps) are held by an assistant against the bone to prevent the chain springing up when the bone is divided. When Lebsche's chisel is used to divide the sternum, its guard is placed under the manubrium through the suprasternal notch and the instrument is held with an upwards pull. The mallet is then used to strike the chisel which then cuts the bone with each strike.

In all cases, whilst sternal sawing is undertaken, positive pressure ventilation is momentarily stopped in order to prevent unnecessary mediastinal pleural injury and unplanned entry to the pleural cavity.

Following the sternotomy, small periosteal and bony (trabecular) bleedings are diathermied. Bone wax may also be used for the same purpose and sealing of raw edges. The sternal retractor is applied to widen the incision and acquire exposure.

6.2. Closure of median sternotomy wound

On completion of the operation, the mediastinal/pericardial drains, if any, are led out through a stab incision placed below and lateral to the incision. All drains are connected to an underwater sealed system. Approximation of the two divided edges of the sternum is achieved usually with five heavy stainless steel wires or strong absorbable sutures. The wire may be placed through the bone or at the extreme anterior end of the intercostal spaces, i.e. around the sternum. Care should be taken to avoid injury to internal mammary vessels. The wires are crossed and twisted bringing the sternal edges together. The excess length of each wire is cut and the twisted portion is buried in the bone. Attention should be paid not to entrap drains in the sternal edges or the wires. The periosteum together with fascia and the linea alba, the subcutaneous tissue and the skin are closed in sequence. The skin is closed with subcuticular stitches or otherwise as desired.

7. Trans-sternal bilateral thoracotomy (Syn clamshell thoracotomy/transverse sternotomy)

In the early days of open heart surgery bilateral transverse thoracotomy and sternotomy was the standard route of access to the heart. This was replaced by a vertical incision with median sternotomy which is more convenient and less painful (Fig. 8). The "clamshell" incision is currently used for bilateral lung transplantation, some cases of bilateral pulmonary metastatectomies and when simultaneous bilateral pleural space access is required. A variant of bilateral thoracotomy and transverse sternotomy is to proceed with anterior bilateral thoracotomies without sternotomy.

7.1. Incision and entry to the chest

The patient is placed in supine position on the operating table, with both arms abducted on support boards. A bilateral submammary incision is made from one mid-axillary line to follow the curvature of the 4th and/or 5th ribs and in continuation, transversely over the sternum. The incision is carried down to reach the intercostal spaces bilaterally. It is necessary to incise the fascia over the pectoralis major and to divide digitations of serratus anterior to reach intercostal spaces and muscles. These muscles and endothoracic fascia are divided next to reach the pleura. Positive pressure ventilation is

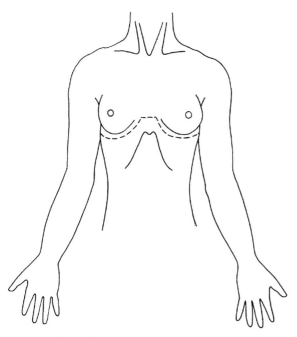

Fig. 8. Trans-sternal bilateral thoracotomy.

best discontinued in order to incise the pleura without the risk of injuring the underlying lung. The internal mammary vessels are identified and tied securely or stitched and then divided. The sternum is now divided transversally using Gigli's saw, Lebsche chisel or electric saw (see sections 5 and 6 above, transverse and median sternotomy). Bleeding from pericostal vessels is coagulated and bone wax used in addition.

7.2. Closure

Closure of the wound is carried out as per anterior and antero-lateral thoracotomy with approximation of sternal "moities" by two wire sutures.

8. Thoraco-laparotomies

A number of surgical procedures require access both to the thoracic and abdominal cavities and there are essentially two methods to achieve this (see chapter III.17).

8.1. Thoraco-phreno-laparotomy

The patient is placed in the lateral or oblique position as per postero-lateral or antero-lateral position (see Fig. 1 in this chapter). The whole of the hemi-thorax and the upper abdomen is cleaned and draped as for

thoracotomy but with the drapes placed to provide upper abdominal access.

8.1.1. Incision and exposure

The thoracic part of the incision follows the line of an appropriate rib selected for the target organ. The abdominal portion of the incision continues from the anterior end of the thoracic incision over the costal margin obliquely towards the umbilicus. Deepening of the incision exposes the fascia and digitation of serratus anterior and latissimus dorsi and in continuation the aponeurosis of external oblique and the rectus sheath. The external oblique is divided in the direction of its fibres. The rectus sheath and the muscle will need to be divided, when a wide exposure is required. The incision is carried down to open up the peritoneum. The costal margin is divided and a small piece of cartilaginous arch is excised. The diaphragm is now incised peripherally and circumfrentially 3 to 4 cm away from its attachment to the rib for a variable distance from the costal margin backwards.

The decision as to whether to include the oesophageal hiatus in this incision depends on the type of disease and the target organ. As a rule, malignancies at that level will require excision of the peripheral tissue and reconstruction. Therefore, the diaphragmatic incision will include the hiatus. Bleeding is controlled by electrocoagulation or stitching as necessary. The anchoring of the cut edges of the diaphragm by stitches to the intercostal and ribs bordering the wound facilitate manipulation in addition to tidying up the field.

8.1.2. Closure of the wound consists of:
- Closure of the diaphragm in two layers using non-absorbable sutures. We prefer one layer of interrupted horizontal mattress and a second layer of continuous running stitches. The hiatus requires reconstruction.
- Costal margin is repaired. Excision of a piece of cartilage helps alignment and overriding the repair requires two non-absorbable stitches or branded wire.
- Closure of the abdominal cavity: It is important to totally eliminate gaps at the anterior end of the diaphragm between the thoracic and abdominal cavities. An easy way to achieve this is to carry backwards the end of the continuous stitching from the upper part of the peritoneal (and fascia) closure to include the anterior end of the diaphragm, anchoring it on the way to the under surface of the costal margin.

- The chest is closed in layers as per thoracotomy.
- The abdominal wall is repaired as per routine in standard fashion. Note: attention should be paid to ensure that no gaps are left between the abdomen and thorax which might become the route for herniation.
- All drains in the abdomen and chest should be connected to an underwater sealed system.

8.1.3. Variations of thoraco-phreno-laparotomy incision as described above

- The abdominal incision may be paramedian in continuation with the thoracotomy incision.
- Incision and section of costal margin may be omitted, using thoraco-phreno-laparotomy without disruption of costal margin.

8.2. Thoraco-laparotomy (thoraco-phrenotomy) without abdominal incision

This is an extended postero-lateral or antero-lateral thoracotomy to which is added division of the hemi-diaphragm as described above. The incision is ideal for operations involving lower chest and upper abdomen. More specifically, we find this approach an excellent route of access for reconstructive processes of the oesophagus with the use of stomach, jejunum, or colon, after oesophagectomy.

9. Miscellaneous and other thoracic incisions and accesses

Under this heading are grouped together other incisions which are used to access the chest. Some of these are extensions or modifications of the aforementioned incisions which have proved to be invaluable in accessing difficult operations.

9.1. Extended antero-lateral Thoracotomy (Hemi-clamshell – Trap door incision)

This approach (Fig. 9) provides access to the superior mediastinum and structures of the root of the neck. It is also a convenient approach to access the great vessels of the root of the neck and thoracic outlet tumours. The patient is placed more favourably in supine position and the arm on the operating side is abducted.

The incision has three components:
(a) Cervical which can be oblique along the anterior border of the sterno-mastoid 4 to 5 cm above the suprasternal notch. Alternatively, this part of the

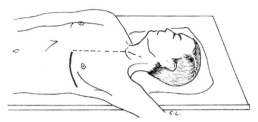

Fig. 9. Extended antero-lateral thoracotomy (hemi-clamshell)

incision can be more horizontal above the clavicle for 4 to 5 cm lateral to the sterno-clavicular joint.
(b) Sternal which is a midline incision over the manubrium and the upper part of the body of the sternum to 2nd or 3rd costal cartilage.
(c) The anterior thoracotomy component is a curved incision following the line of the 3rd rib anteriorly towards the anterior axillary line.

The three components of this composite incision are carried down; platysma and deep cervical fascia are incised and the sterno-mastoid muscle can be divided if necessary. The sternum is divided in the mid-line using the Lebsche chisel or an electric saw. Internal mammary vessels need securing. Anterior thoracotomy necessitates division of the pectoralis major fascia and muscle and some fibres of pectoralis minor. This approach provides a flap which, like a trap door, can be lifted upwards and laterally to expose structures in the root of the neck and superior mediastinum.

9.2. Modifications of antero-lateral thoracotomy (Anterior-cervico — Thoracic)

In order to obtain a good exposure in cases of pancoast tumours, Dartevelle and colleagues (1994) proposed access through an L shaped incision which provides an anterior trans-cervical approach. The vertical limb of the incision follows the anterior border of sterno-mastoid to sterno-clavicular joint. The horizontal part of the incision turns laterally under the medial half of the inferior border of the clavicle. This part of the bone is excised and the sternal attachment of sterno mastoid detached providing access to the root of the neck.

9.3. Abdomino-mediastinal incision

This is a convenient approach to the inferior part of the anterior mediastinum and upper abdomen. It is extremely useful in the repair of complicated

Morgagni's hernia and/or some oesophageal bypass operations. The patient is placed in a supine position on the operating table. A midline incision is made over the lower one third of the sternum and in continuity over the upper abdomen. The skin incision is carried down to achieve median laparotomy. The lower sternum is then divided in the mid line using an electric saw or Lebsche chisel. A small sternal retractor (e.g. small Tudor-Edwards or child Finochietto or similar) is placed and the two sides of the sternotomy are separated. This usually provides a good exposure. If a wider space is needed, the skin incision over the sternum is undercut and a small transverse incision of the sternum on one or both sides is made. After completion of the operation the abdomen is closed and the sternum is repaired using two wire stitches.

9.4. Subxiphoid access

Access through the subxiphoid is a convenient approach to the inferior part of the anterior mediastinum and to the pericardium or left ventricle. An incision is made over the xiphoid process and vertically downwards towards the umbilicus for 6 to 8 cm. The incision is deepened to divide the fascia and the upper part of the linea alba. The xiphoid is lifted or excised. The lower 3 to 4 cm of the sternum may be divided. Pericardial and sternal attachments to the diaphragm are divided. The inferior pericardium space is exposed by lifting of the sternum by an assistant using one or two suitable retractors (Langenbecks type).

10. Limited and muscle sparing thoracotomies

10.1. Introduction

In standard thoracotomies, large muscles of the chest wall and shoulder girdle are divided resulting in pain and slow post-operative mobilisation. In patients with borderline pulmonary function, the combination of pain, lack of movement and use of high dose analgesics may result in pulmonary collapse. In addition, in many cases of intrathoracic intervention, a wide exposure may not be necessary. Therefore, increasingly, limited and muscle sparing thoracotomies are used. These thoracotomies have been practised since the 1970s for simple procedures such as pleurectomy, wedge resection of the lung and local excision of tumours. More recently, particularly since the advent of thoracoscopic surgery,

there has been a new impetus to expand the range of operations through muscle sparing thoracotomies.

The basic principle of these thoracotomies is to gain access to the thoracic cavity through intercostal spaces which are not covered by large chest wall muscles. Appraisal of the anatomical arrangement of the chest wall and its muscular covering indicates two such zones:

- A postero-lateral triangular area known as the triangle of auscultation is situated below the inferior angle of the scapula, between the lower border of the trapezius and the upper border of the latissimus dorsi muscle. The space is covered by fascia overlying the ribs and intercostal muscle.
- Sub axillary space: This is the area between the upwards rising postero lateral border of the pectoralis major anteriorly and the anterior border of the latissimus dorsi muscle. The floor is covered by digitation of serratus anterior. Incision over this area together with detachment or division of some of the fibres of serratus anterior provides easy access to the chest.

Taking these anatomical arrangements into account, the following muscle sparing thoracotomies are currently in use:

10.1.1. Limited/postero-lateral (para scapular) thoracotomy

With the patient in a lateral thoracotomy position and the arm extended forward, skin incision is made over the triangle of auscultation (see section 10.1 above). The incision is carried along the medial border of the scapula and is extended downwards and forward for 8 to 10 cm below the inferior angle of the scapula. The fascia covering the floor of the triangle is opened to expose a portion of ribs 5–7 and their intercostal spaces. Elevation of the angle of scapula by an assistant helps this exposure. The trapezius and the latissimus muscles are retracted posterio-medially and anterior inferiorly respectively in order to gain better intra thoracic exposure. Entry to the chest is made through the 5th or 6th intercostal space as in standard postero-lateral thoracotomy. The closure is carried out in layers.

10.1.2. Axillary and sub-axillary thoracotomies

The patient is placed either in a lateral decubitus or oblique position. The arm is at 90 degrees abduction. In either case there are options for:

(a) Oblique incision (Fig. 10a)
(b) Horizontal incision
(c) Vertical incision (Fig. 10b)

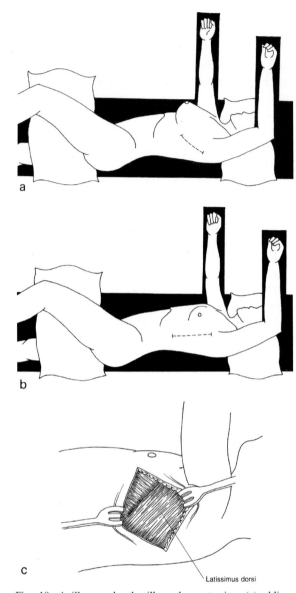

Fig. 10. Axillary and subaxillary thoracotomies: (a) oblique incision, (b) vertical incision, (c) exposure of muscles in axillary incision.

In all cases, the incision is made in such a way as to avoid the posterior border of the pectoralis major and the anterior border of the latissimus dorsi (Fig. 10c). The latter muscle is retracted posteriorly and the digitations of the serratus are divided anteriorly in order to reach ribs and intercostal muscles.

10.2. Indications for muscle sparing thoracotomies

- Limited lung resection
- Pleurectomy
- Exploratory thoracotomy with the possibility of extending the incision allowing better access to the posterior mediastinum and nodal dissection for broncho-plastic procedures.
- Pericardial drainage
- As a 'utility incision' in conjunction with video-assisted thoracoscopic surgery (VATS).

The axillary thoracotomy, particularly with vertical incision, offers a better choice of intercostal space for pleurectomy or local excision of anteriorly placed tumours.

For many pulmonary excisions the author prefers limited muscle sparing postero-lateral incision and thoracotomy through the triangle of auscultation which permits extension to standard postero-lateral thoracotomy if a wider exposure becomes necessary. For pleurectomy and anterior mediastinal operation, preference is given to the axillary and sub-axillary approach.

10.3. Advantages/disadvantages of muscle sparing thoracotomies

10.3.1. Advantages of muscle sparing thoracotomies
- Reduction of post-operative pain
- Reduction of post-operative complications incidence (e.g. pulmonary collapse)
- Reduction of morbidity rate

10.3.2. Disadvantages of muscle sparing thoracotomies
- Limitation of exposure
- Limitation for extensive lymph node excision in cancer surgery
- Difficulty of undertaking complicated surgery such as broncho-vascular plastic operations
- Difficulty in dealing speedily with major vascular accidental haemorrhage in complicated dissections
- Difficulty in identifying sources of bleeding on re-opening the wound in cases of early post-operative clot retention and haemothorax.

Some of these disadvantages may be eliminated by combining such incisions and accesses with video-thoracoscopic surgery.

References and further reading

Baeza OR, Foster ED. Vertical axillary thoracotomy: a functional and cosmetically appealing incision. Ann Thorac Surg 1976; 22: 287–288.
Bethencourt DM, Holmes EC. Muscle-sparing posterolateral tho-

racotomy. Ann Thorac Surg 1988; 45: 337–339.

Casha AR, Yang L, Kay PH, et al. A biomechanical study of median sternotomy closure technique. Eur J Cardiothorac Surg 1999; 15: 365–369.

Dartvelle PG, Chapelier AR, Machiarini P, et al. Anterior trans thoracic approach for radical resection of lung tumours invading the thoracic inlet. J Thorac Cardiovasc Surg 1994; 108: 389–392.

Ginsberg RJ. Alternative (muscle-sparing) incision in thoracic surgery. Ann Thorac Surg 1993; 53: 752–754.

Hazelrigg SR, Landreneau RL, Boley TM, et al. The effect of muscle-sparing versus standard postero-lateral thoracotomy on pulmonary function, muscle strength and post operative pain. J Thorac Cardiovasc Surg 1991; 101: 394–401.

Kittle CF. Which way in? The thoracotomy incision. Ann Thorac Surg 1988; 45: 234.

Kraus DH, Huo J, Burt M. Surgical access to tumours of the cervicothoracic junction. Head Neck 1995; 17: 131–136.

Lardinois D, Sippel M, Gugger M. Morbidity and validity of the hemi-clamshell approach for thoracic surgery. Eur J Cardiothorac Surg 1999; 16: 194–199.

Macchiarini P, Ladurie FL, Cerrina J, et al. Clamshell or sternotomy for double lung or heart-lung transplantation. Eur J Cardiothorac Surg 1999; 15: 333–339.

Mitchell R L. The lateral limited thoracotomy incision: standard for pulmonary operation. J Thorac Cardiovasc Surg 1990; 99: 590–596.

Moghissi K. Median sternotomy wound disruption. J R Coll Surg Edinb 1977; 22: 156–157.

Ponn RB, Ferneini A, Diagnostino RS, et al. Comparison of later pulmonary function after postero-lateral and muscle-sparing thoracotomy. Ann Thorac Surg 1992; 53: 670–674.

Rothenberg SR, Pokorny WJ. Experience with a total muscle-sparing approach for thoracotomies in neonate, infant and children. J Paediat Surg 1992; 27: 1157–1160.

Stoney WS, Alford WC, Burrus GR, et al. Median sternotomy dehiscence. Ann Thorac Surg 1978; 26: 421–426.

CHAPTER I.5

Congenital abnormalities of the lung

K. Moghissi

1. Introduction

Congenital abnormalities of the lung originate from developmental anomalies of the primitive foregut and its derivatives. In about the 4th week of intrauterine life, a groove develops in the ventral aspect of the foregut. At five to six weeks an out-pouching or diverticulum appears from the pharyngeal part of the foregut lined by endodermal epithelium and invested by mesenchyme. At this time the respiratory part of the primitive foregut and the oesophagus share a common tube. Separation begins to occur by ingrowth of lateral mesenchymal septa. The diverticulum grows, elongates, divides and subdivides to form one tube and then a succession of tubes giving rise to a bronchial tree and lung buds.

Subsequent subdivision takes place and the air sacs are formed. Differentiation of the epithelium of the air sacs occurs during the 24th week. At the 28th week some cells (referred to as type II) are responsible for the production of surfactant. The terminal air sacs continue their budding to produce a new generation of alveoli which continues after birth, during infancy and childhood up to the age of 8 or 9 years. The blood and lymphatic channels derive from mesenchyme. The pulmonary blood vessels derive from two sources; the mesenchymal network of vessels and also the heart.

2. Congenital lobar emphysema (syn infantile lobar emphysema)

By definition this is over-inflation of the air spaces of a segment or lobe of the lung without important parenchymal destruction. The condition arises after birth and is caused by:

- Over expansion of part of the lung by air trapping due to ball-valve obstruction of the bronchus
- Weak or absent bronchial cartilage
- Bronchial obstruction by extrinsic compression.

The disease most commonly affects the upper lobe predominantly on the right side. The symptoms are generally noticed at birth or soon after in the form of respiratory distress. Dyspnoea, tachypnoea and cyanosis are the usual features. In severe cases stridor and nasal flare are also present.

Clinical examination is often inconclusive. Chest X-ray and CT of the thorax show hyper-distension of the affected part, shift of the mediastinum and herniation of the lobe. Pulmonary scintigraphy may demonstrate loss of perfusion.

Diagnostic bronchoscopy is useful to eliminate presence of a foreign body, external compression and endoluminal disease.

The list of conditions to be considered in differential diagnosis is long and collaboration between paediatric respiratory physician, radiologist and surgeon is required to achieve correct diagnosis and management.

Treatment consists of excision of the emphysematous part. Cases which result from external compression through cardiovascular anomalies are treated according to their aetiology. In severe, life-threatening cases, endotracheal intubation and urgent or emergency surgery is required. In less severe cases, comprehensive investigation including ventilation/perfusion scintigraphy should be undertaken prior to surgical intervention.

3. Bronchogenic cyst

This is a malformation in which the primitive lung bud does not pouch-out properly. The result is formation of a bronchogenic cyst or cystic duplication of the oesophagus. Bronchogenic cyst may be lined by respiratory (ciliated) columnar or squamous epithelium with presence of mucus secreting glands. Topographically, in descending order of frequency, cysts are found in the middle mediastinum, within the lung and in or at proximity of the inferior pulmonary ligament. The majority of bronchogenic cysts have no communication with the tracheobronchial tree.

The majority of patients are symptomatic and present with pain, cough, fever, dyspnoea and occasionally haemoptysis. Presentation in the newborn infant can be one of life-threatening cardio-respiratory distress. Asymptomatic cases are discovered coincidentally. Chest radiography and CT scan will characteristically show the cystic lesion. However, at times, diagnosis may be difficult. Lung abscess, hydatid cyst and a host of other lesions can project images similar to that of a bronchogenic cyst. Bronchoscopy may only show compressive signs and rarely the communication of the cyst to the bronchial tree.

Complications of bronchogenic cysts are infection, haemoptysis and rarely, malignant degeneration. Treatment consists of surgical excision of the cyst. It is important to disrupt the tracheo-bronchial communication if present. Mediastinal cysts can be removed with no pulmonary parenchymal resection. Cysts in the lung often require lobectomy.

4. Congenital cystic adenomatoid malformation (CCAM)

This condition, which was first described by Chin and Tang in 1949, consists of an overgrowth of terminal bronchioles and lack of maturation of aleveoli. The resulting abnormality presents as a cyst lined by cuboidal or pseudo-stratified columnar epithelium. The condition is often described under three types:

Type I: Large cystic space within a single lobe (about 50% of cases)
Type II: Multiple small cysts
Type III: Tumour-like mass without cysts but with adenomatoid hyperplastic bronchial structures.

The primary deficit in this malformation is generally attributed to atresia of the lobar, segmental or sub-segmental bronchi. Clinical features are related to symptoms and signs of respiratory distress generally at birth or soon after. Dyspnoea, tachypnoea and cynanosis are the usual presenting symptoms. In a small number of newborn infants, when the cyst is confined to a segment, the only symptom may be difficulty in feeding and repeated chest infections in infancy a month or more after birth. Occasionally some cases are quasi-asymptomatic and the condition is discovered in adulthood. Diagnosis is essentially made by imaging. Chest radiograph and CT scan show the cystic appearance of the lesion containing air and fluid. Mediastinal shift is, at times, also present. The pictures may mimic a diaphragmatic hernia with loops of bowel in the chest. Barium contrast study is then helpful.

With the development of prenatal diagnostic procedures, there is the possibility of identification in the foetus and intra-uterine treatment of this lesion. Post-natal treatment consists of resectional surgery with conservation of healthy parenchyma.

5. Pulmonary sequestration

Pulmonary sequestration (Fig. 1a and b) is a rare congental malformation in which a portion of lung does not communicate with the bronchial tree and is supplied by an aberrant systemic artery. The consequences of this pathological entity principally are:

(a) Repeated infection in the sequestrated part
(b) A mass of pulmonary tissue not subscribing to any function and causing complications

Two forms of pulmonary sequestration are described: intra-lobar and extra-lobar. Intra-lobar sequestration, by far the commonest, lacks independent pleural coverage and is within the normal pulmonary parenchyma. The extra-lobar variety possesses its own pleural covering and is almost an accessory lobe with abnormal bronchovascular supply.

In either form of sequestration the majority of sufferers present with recurrent pulmonary symptoms, repeated chest infection being the commonest. Pleuritic pain, haemoptysis, at times massive, and haemothorax are present in 10 to 15% of cases. In some cases tuberculous and fungal infection within the sequestrated part can supervene. The sequestration may have a fistulous communication with the upper gastro-intestinal tract with manifestation in childhood.

Diagnosis is suspected by chest radiography and confirmed by CT scan and retrograde aortography. The latter demonstrates the arterial supply which can be multiple.

The treatment is surgical resection, which is indicated in all except those cases having definite contraindication for surgical intervention. The result of operation is generally excellent.

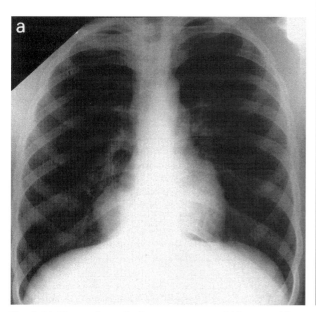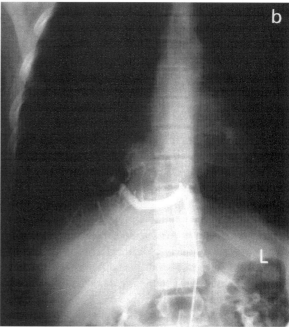

Fig. 1. (a) Chest radiograph of a young man, aged 18 years, with an opacity in the right lower lobe, which, on investigation, showed to be a sequestrated lung, (b) aortogram of the same patient clearly showing the sequestrated part of the lung supplied by the systemic artery.

6. Agenesis, aplasia and hypoplasia

These abnormalities represent a spectrum of pulmonary malformations extending from total absence of the lung in agenesis to a rudimentary functionless lung in hypoplasia. In the case of agenesis the carina, bronchi, blood vessels and pulmonary parenchyma are absent. In many such cases there are also associated cardiac abnormalities. In aplasia the main bronchus is present but pulmonary vessels and parenchyma are absent. Hypoplasia consists of malformed bronchi with poorly developed unaerated lungs. Generally, unilateral anomalies without associated cardiac deficit have a favourable outcome. Bilateral conditions or those with associated cardiac deficit do not.

7. Congenital pulmonary vascular abnormalities

7.1. Stenosis and atresia of the main pulmonary vessels

Stenosis and atresia of the main pulmonary vessels are usually associated with congenital heart disease.

7.2. Idiopathic hyperlucent lung (McLeod's syndrome)

This is often the result of chronic infection. The condition is characterised by diminished calibre of vessels.

7.3. Pulmonary arterio-venous abnormal communication

This is the commonest vascular malformation and represents a spectrum of anomalies in which there is a direct communication between the branches of pulmonary arteries and veins. The anomaly may be an arterio-venous aneurysm or microscopic communication between the network of branches of arteries and veins.

Macroscopically, the aneurysm consists of a pool of blood with a thin surrounding membrane with an afferent pulmonary branch (feeder) and efferent pulmonary vein tributaries. The malformation may present with hereditary haemorrhagic telangiectasis (Rendu–Osler syndrome) with cutaneous and mucosal spider form angioma.

The patient may be asymptomatic but the condition may be diagnosed by symptoms of dyspnoea, haemoptysis, chest pain and palpitations. Chest radiography shows an opacity and the feeder artery may be recognisable. CT scan of the thorax with contrast and pulmonary angiography are mandatory to plan therapy and to precisely indicate the anatomy of the lesion. More recently, magnetic resonance imaging with contrast has been employed to identify the lesion and the afferent-efferent vessels.

Indications for treatment are:

- Existence of symptoms
- Prevention of complications in asymptomatic patients (haemoptysis, haemothorax and/or stroke)

Surgical treatment consists of parenchyma-saving pulmonary resection (resection of a segment/lobe with enclosed lesion). Embolisation may be attempted by expert interventional radiologists. In some cases, with a large lesion, combined embolisation and resection is indicated. This is to reduce the risk of surgical operation and prevent a large mass (infarcted lung) becoming a constant source of infection when left in situ.

References and further reading

Aktogu S, Yuncu G, Halil Colar H, Buduneli T. Bronchogenic cysts: clinico-pathological presentation and treatment. Eur Respir J 1996; 9: 2017–2021.

Al-Bassam A, Al-Rebeeah A, Al-Nassar S, Al-Mobaireek K, Al-Rawaf A, Banjer H, Al-Mogari I. Congenital cystic disease of the lung in infants and children (experience with 57 cases). Eur J Pediatr Surg 1999; 9: 364–368.

Chin KY, Tang MY. Congenital adenomatoid malformation of one lobe of along with general anasarca. Arch Pathol Lab Med 1949; 48: 221–229.

Cuypers PH, De Leyn P, Cappelle L, et al. Bronchogenic cysts: a review of 20 cases. Eur J Cardiothorac Surg 1996; 10: 393–396.

Dahabreh J, Zisis C, Vassiliou M, Arnogiannaki N. Congenital cystic adenomatoid malformation in an adult presenting as lung abscess. Eur J Cardiothorac Surg 2000; 18: 720–723.

Evrard V, Ceulemans J, Coosemans W, De Baere T, De Leyn P, Deneffe G, Devlieger H, De Boeck C, Van Raemdonk D, Lerut T. Congenital parenchymatous malformations of the lung. World J Surg 1999; 23: 1123–1132.

Halkic N, Cuenoud PF, Corthesy ME, Ksontini R, Boumghar M. Pulmonary sequestration: a review of 26 cases. Eur J Cardiothorac Surg 1998; 14: 127–133.

Hellmuth D, Glerant JC, Sevestre H, Remond A, Jounieaux V. Pulmonary adenomatoid malformation presenting as unilobar cysts in an adult. Respir Med 1998; 92: 1364–1372.

Karnak I, Senocak ME, Ciftci AO, Buyukpamukca N. Congenital lobar emphysema: diagnostic and therapeutic considerations. J Pediatr Surg 1999; 34: 1347–1351.

Kravitz RM. Congenital malformations of the lung. Paed Clin N Am 1994; 4133: 453–473.

Lackner RP, Thompson AB 3rd, Rikkers LF. Galbraith TA. Cystic adenomatoid malformation involving an entire lung in a 22 year old woman. Ann Thorac Surg 1996; 61: 1827–1829.

Patel S, Meeker D, Biscotti C, et al. Presentation and management of bronchogenic cysts in the adult. Chest 1994; 106: 79–85.

St Georges R, Deslauriers J, Durancea A, et al. Clinical spectrum of bronchogenic cysts of the mediastinum and lung in the adult. Ann Thorac Surg 1991; 52: 52–56.

Stocker JT. Congenital and developmental diseases. In Dali DH, Hammar SP (eds.), Pulmonary pathology (2nd ed.). New York, Springer-Verlag. 1994; 155–190.

Thakral CL, Maji DC, Sjawani MJ. Congenital lobar emphysema: experience with 21 cases. Paediatr Surg Int 2001; 17: 88–91.

Van Roaemdonck D, De Boeck K, Devlieger H, Demedts M, et al. Pulmonary sequestration, a comparison between paediatric and adult patients. Eur J Cardiothorac Surg 2001; 19: 388–395.

Vogt-Maykopf I, Rau B, Branscheid D. Surgery for congenital malformation of the lung. Ann Radiol (Paris) 1993; 36(2): 145–160.

Watine B, Mensier E, Delecluse P, et al. Pulmonary sequestration treated by video assisted thoracoscopic resection. Eur J Cardiothorac Surg 1994; 8: 155–156.

CHAPTER I.6

Foreign bodies in the airways

K. Moghissi

Accidental inhalation and impaction of foreign bodies in the airways is not uncommon, particularly amongst children. Each thoracic unit has a collection of curious objects recovered from air passages (Fig. 1). The effect of a foreign body in the airways depends on the:

- Size of the object.
- Nature of the object, and its chemical composition.
- Patient's age.
- Anatomical site of the impaction.
- Duration of impaction.

In an infant, any object disproportionate to the diameter of the trachea can be fatal. In one case treated by the author, a plastic bead was impacted in the lower trachea of an 11 month infant, who presented with severe cyanosis and was unconscious on admission. The orifice in the centre of the bead, the only means of passage of air, had kept the infant alive until the object was extracted (with some difficulty) and the child recovered.

1. Clinical presentation and diagnosis

In an adult, the background and clinical history draw attention to the possibility of foreign body inhalation. In infants and children, clinical history may also be available to raise suspicion of the incident

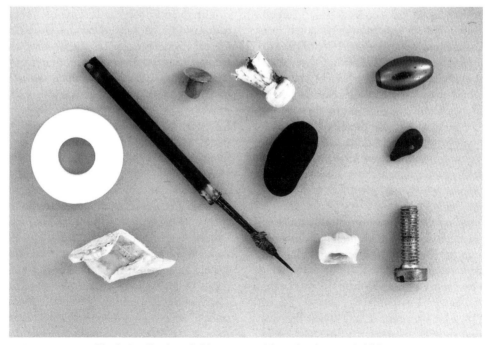

Fig. 1. A collection of objects removed from the airways of children.

though, in many instances, a clear history may not be obtained. The subject, usually a child, develops a sudden attack of cough, dyspnoea, wheeze and stridor; cyanosis may be present. If the object is small it migrates to the bronchi (usually the right) and, after some initial symptoms, purulent and haemorrhagic bronchitis develops followed by pneumonitis and lung abscess. In such a case, the clinical picture is one of pulmonary suppuration.

The diagnosis is made at an early stage by the history of events leading to the development of symptoms. If no severe symptoms present, the inhalation incident may often pass unnoticed.

In all children with a localised infection and/or an abscess on admission, the possibility of foreign body inhalation should be considered.

In the early stages (within 12 to 24 hours), auscultatory signs are wheeze or the absence of breath sounds, both indicating bronchial obstruction. Later, with the development of pneumonitis and lung abscess, clinical findings are those of pulmonary suppuration.

A chest radiograph is the most important investigation and should never be omitted when a patient presents with a history which could suggest inhalation of a foreign body. Postero-anterior and lateral views are necessary. It must be realised that even a radio opaque object may not be visible on a postero-anterior view chest radiograph because of its being overshadowed on X-ray film by mediastinal structure density, hence the necessity for a lateral view chest radiograph. It should also be noted that an object may be impacted in the pharyngo-larynx or the upper trachea. Therefore, the radiographs should include views of the neck as well as the chest. In the case of a non-radio opaque object, particularly in children, the chest radiograph should be both on inspiration and expiration. The radiological findings on plain chest radiography are variable, dependent on the size of the object and the duration of impaction and may be one of the following:

- Normal appearance with or without visible radio-opaque foreign body.
- Hyperclarity in one lobe or in one lung indicating the existence of air which has entered on inspiration through the partially obstructed bronchus but cannot get out on expiration. The area is therefore hyperexpanded compared with the rest of the lung.
- Collapse of a lobe or even a lung when the size of the inhaled object is disproportionately larger than the diameter of the bronchus (Fig. 2).

- Signs of pulmonary infiltration and consolidation, indicating inflammatory reaction created by the foreign body.

The only exception to full radiological investigation is in an extreme emergency situation due to suffocating airway obstruction. In this case there is no time and the provision of airway should be the primary concern. This was the case with the infant to which reference was made above.

2. Management

When the diagnosis is suspected and after appropriate radiological investigation, bronchoscopy should be carried out as a matter of urgency to extract the foreign body or exclude its presence in the airways. Even in the absence of radiological signs but with the history of foreign body inhalation, bronchoscopy must be carried out. Failure to remove a foreign body can result in pulmonary infection. In one case referred to us, a plastic screw had remained in the bronchial tree causing lung abscess and empyema. The X-ray in an accident and emergency department, taken days previously, was reported as 'normal'.

When the diagnosis is established the aim is to retrieve the foreign body and to prevent or treat any infective complication. Removal of a foreign body from the airways can nearly always be carried out by bronchoscopy, under general anaesthetic using a rigid bronchoscope. In the case of children, the procedure must be carried out by an experienced operator. Bronchoscopy on the neonate must be performed by an expert thoracic surgeon and an experienced anaesthetist, within a department where a range of endoscopic equipment, including various sizes of foreign body extractors, is at hand. In the case of infants, bronchoscopy may be difficult, requiring prior exposure of the larynx by a laryngoscope following which, under adequate vision, the suckling or infant bronchoscope can be introduced.

After bronchoscopic retrieval of the foreign body, thorough inspection of the bronchial tree should be carried out to ensure that there is no additional foreign body present. The author administers intravenous broad spectrum antibiotic in all cases. Further doses of an appropriate antibiotic (according to the microbiological culture of the secretions) are given only in cases of purulent bronchial secretion or pulmonary infiltration. We also lavage the bronchial tree with a solution of normal saline or an aqueous

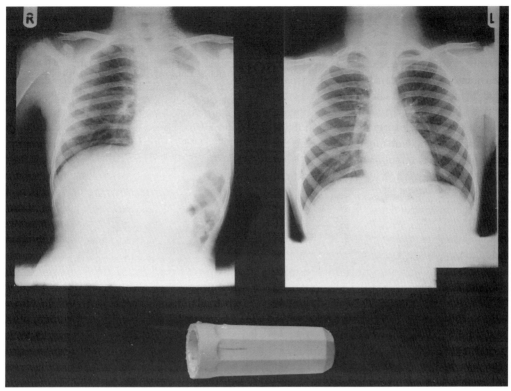

Fig. 2. Top left: almost complete collapse of the left lung by inhalation of a plastic pen cover (bottom). Top right: expanded lung following removal of object.

solution of 1/5000 dilution of chlorhexidine, after extraction of the foreign body has been undertaken. The patient is discharged from hospital 24 to 48 hours later. Small children should be watched carefully after bronchoscopy, as trauma to the larynx may cause upper airway obstruction. Some foreign bodies, especially peanuts and some sweets, may cause chemical bronchiolitis in addition to their obstructive effect. Such cases should be kept under observation after the removal of the object.

In cases presenting after a few days or when an unsuccessful attempt has been made to remove a small object from a basal segmental bronchi, the foreign body may disappear from view and/or penetrate into the lung substance. Bronchoscopy in such cases shows pus, granulation tissue and much bleeding and does not always achieve the objective. Nevertheless, bronchoscopy should be performed though the surgical extraction of the foreign body may become inevitable. In this event, through an appropriate limited thoracotomy approach (section 10 in chapter I.4), the bronchus containing the foreign body is exposed and the object is removed by bronchotomy (incising the bronchus), or by incising the pulmonary sub-

stance. The bronchus is repaired by fine interrupted stitches applied transversely and the lung tissue by appropriate absorbable sutures.

3. Complications

A retained foreign body can migrate:
(a) through the wall into the oesophagus or mediastinum
(b) downwards into terminal bronchi to disappear from the bronchoscopic field of vision into terminal bronchi to remain lodged enveloped by inflammation and granulation tissue. At times the foreign body penetrates the bronchial wall and enters the substance of the pulmonary parenchyma.

4. Pitfalls

• Clinical history and symptoms of inhaled and/or ingested foreign body can at times be confused. Bronchoscopy should be carried out soon after the diagnosis is made or suspected before inflammatory changes make the object invisible. An

experienced anaesthetist is essential, particularly
for infants and children.

- Rarely the inhaled foreign body may be multiple.
- If the foreign body is not recovered a clear note
  should be made of the incident. The primary care
  doctor and the patient should be informed.
- At least one follow up visit should be arranged
  particularly in those who at presentation have
  pulmonary parenchymal changes and when the
  foreign body has not been recovered.

References and further reading

Kreuzer A (ed.). Foreign body extraction from the airways in
  adults. In: Strausz, J Pulmonary Endoscopy and Biopsy techniques. Eur Respir Monogr 1998; 3(9): 36–48.

Oguzkaya F, Akcali Y, Kahrman C, et al. Tracheobronchial
  foreign body aspirations in childhood: a 10 year experience.
  Eur J Cardiothorac Surg 1998; 14: 388–392.

Prakash UBS, Cortese DA. Tracheo Bronchial Foreign Bodies.
  In: Prakash UBS (ed.), Bronchoscopy. Mayo Foundation,
  New York, Raven Press Ltd. 1994, pp. 253–277.

CHAPTER I.7

Chest trauma

A. Mulpur and J.A.C. Thorpe

1. Introduction

The incidence of chest trauma varies from country to country. Some 20 to 25% of traumatic deaths result from thoracic trauma and chest injuries. One third of trauma victims in automobile accidents sustain major thoracic trauma.

1.1. Classification

Thoracic trauma can be classified as in Scheme 1.

1.2. Spectrum

Thoracic trauma may involve a wide range of skeletal and/or soft tissue injuries of the chest wall and a variety of chest cavity visceral injuries. Evaluation of the patient's injuries must be systematic and comprehensive. Assessment should take account of the following possibilities:

- Chest wall injuries:
  - Rib fracture.
  - Sternal fracture.
  - Clavicular fracture.
  - Vertebral fracture.
  - Scapular fracture.
  - Soft tissue injury.
- Haemothorax.
- Pneumothorax.
- Parenchymal pulmonary injury.
- Airway injury.
- Diaphragmatic injury.
- Oesophageal injury.
- Thoracic duct injury.
- Cardiac tamponade.
- Cardiac injury.

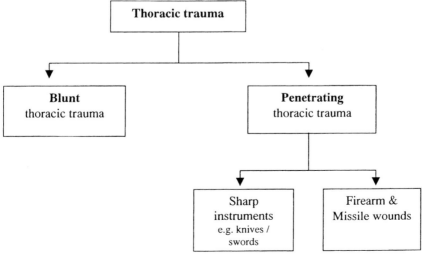

Scheme 1.

- Great vessel injury — aortic dissection.
- Sympathetic chain injury.
- Additional injuries:
  - Laceration
  - Contusion
  - Haematoma

1.3. Initial management

The trauma victim should be assessed as a whole. However, initial resuscitation methods concentrate on airway, breathing and circulation (ABC). Assessment of thoracic and extrathoracic injuries and quantification of degree of shock are vitally important. Overzealous fluid administration plays an important role in the development of adult respiratory distress syndrome (ARDS) and thus a proper fluid balance chart should be maintained. The patient should be mechanically ventilated as per the criteria listed in Table 1.

It is important to remember that trauma to the lower chest may commonly involve the liver and spleen in addition to the diaphragm.

1.3.1. Clinical evaluation

This begins with inspection of the neck veins and trachea. If the neck veins are distended, cardiac tamponade and tension pneumothorax must be considered. Contralateral tracheal deviation may mean tension pneumothorax or a massive haemothorax. Flail chest produces a paradoxical movement of the chest wall. With inspiration the chest wall moves outwards, whereas the flail segment moves inwards and vice-versa. Open and sucking wounds are obvious and must be closed with an intercostal drain insertion. Symmetry of the chest wall movement with respiratory excursion must be ascertained.

- Palpation of the chest detects tracheal deviation and subcutaneous surgical emphysema. Demonstration of fracture crepitus for sternal and rib fractures is very painful and should not be specifically elicited. Apical impulse of the heart should be noted.
- Percussion must be gentle. This reveals hyperresonance in pneumothorax and a stony dull note in haemothorax. Its value is limited in most of the trauma clinical situations.
- Auscultation can be misleading. Distant heart sounds are the hallmark of cardiac tamponade. Conducted breath sounds are commonly heard even with a collapsed lung due to haemo/pneu-

Table 1

Criteria for mechanical ventilation

Parameter	Unit	Indication	Normal range
Respiratory rate	Breaths/min	>35	10–20
Tidal volume	ml/kg	<5	5–7
Vital capacity	ml/kg	<15	65–75
Max. Insp. pressure	cm H_2O	<25	75–100
$P_a O_2$	mmHg	<60	75–110
$P_a CO_2$	mmHg	>60	35–45
$V_d : V_t$ ratio	...	>0.6	0.3
$P (A - a DO_2)$	mmHg	>350	25–65
			$(FiO_2 = 1)$

mothorax and too much reliance should not be placed on clinical findings alone.

1.4. Investigations

Plain chest X-ray is the initial investigation. Wherever possible posteroanterior (PA) films should be obtained. In trauma, chest X-rays are most often supine anteroposterior (AP) films. It is difficult to appreciate mediastinal widening and increased cardiothoracic ratio in AP film. Obliteration of costophrenic angle may not show up in this type of X-ray, even when a significant haemothorax exists. Clavicular, sternal and scapular fractures are easy to miss and must be specifically looked for in every case. Soft tissue injuries, mediastinal emphysema, widened superior mediastinum and diaphragm rupture are amongst the failures of plain X-ray to demonstrate. Supine chest radiographs can miss 50 to 60% of pneumothoraces while CT has a 100% pickup rate. Lateral and oblique decubitus films are theoretically superior in detecting haemothorax but are rarely practical in a polytrauma victim. 'Deep sulcus sign' refers to asymmetric costophrenic angles due to anterolateral location of pneumothorax in supine film.

Ultrasound scan is useful to detect haemopericardium, cardiac tamponade, intrapleural collections and associated liver and splenic trauma.

Computerised axial tomography (CAT scan) and magnetic resonance imaging (MRI) are useful in selected patients to evaluate intra-thoracic vascular injuries and subtle diaphragmatic trauma.

Video assisted thoracoscopy is useful in a small number of patients to especially evaluate diaphragmatic trauma and find the source of continued bleeding in cases of haemothorax.

Bronchoscopy, both flexible and rigid is needed to assess airway injuries.

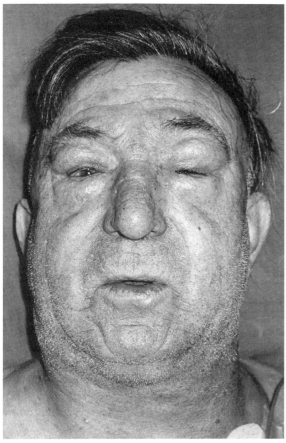

Fig. 1. Gross surgical emphysema of the face in a patient involved in a road traffic accident.

A variety of possible thoracic traumatic conditions is briefly presented here.

1.4.1. Subcutaneous and mediastinal emphysema (Fig. 1)

Injuries of the tracheobronchial tree, oesophagus and pulmonary parenchyma can result in this condition (Fig. 1). This can occur with or without a pneumothorax and extend into the neck, face, abdominal wall, extremities and genitalia and result in "Michelin Man". Subcuteaneous emphysema may result in dysphonia, which can be painful and may be severe enough to cause obstruction to venous return from the face. Primary injury should be dealt with and sometimes the underlying culprit is an improperly placed or slipped out intercostal chest drainage tube. Multiple small incisions are rarely required to allow egress of the air in very severe cases with haemodynamic compromise.

1.4.2. Sternal fracture

This occurs in 4 to 8% of thoracic trauma victims. Front seat occupants in an automobile involved in a frontal collision are typical victims. Sternal fracture is typically a transverse fracture located in the body of the sternum and is rarely displaced. It does not show up on frontal projections and lateral X-ray of the sternum should be obtained. Underlying cardiac injury should be ruled out by estimation of cardiac enzymes and cardiac ultrasound examination. Analgesia is all that is required in most cases. Sternal fracture with significant displacement must be managed with open reduction through a midline incision. Costochondral disruption resulting in a flail sternum can be managed using external or internal fixation techniques.

1.4.3. Scapular fractures

Considerable force is required to fracture the scapula and therefore multiple, severe injuries are possibly associated with this injury. These patients have a 10% mortality rate. As the scapula is well padded with muscles, there is usually little displacement. Most are managed conservatively. Internal fixation is indicated in selected cases of glenoid involvement.

1.4.4. Clavicular fractures

The clavicle may be involved in direct or indirect trauma. Neurovascular examination of the upper limb should be routinely performed. Most are closed fractures occurring in the mid-shaft of the clavicle and fragments frequently overlap. Fractures of the lateral end of the clavicle may involve the coracoclavicular ligament and result in superior displacement of the bone. The majority are treated conservatively with a broad arm sling for three weeks. Figure-of-8 bandage is difficult to maintain and is unnecessary. Open reduction is reserved for cases with skin, vascular or neurological compromise. Malunion is common but rarely causes a functional disability. Nonunion is seen in 5% of the cases and requires surgery if symptomatic, with internal fixation and bone grafting.

1.4.5. Rib fractures

First and second ribs require considerable force to fracture and, as in scapular fractures, this signifies serious impact. Careful search for associated intra- and extra-thoracic injuries must be made as 35 to 40% of thoracic trauma victims have rib fractures. Associated haemo/pneumothorax should be ruled out.

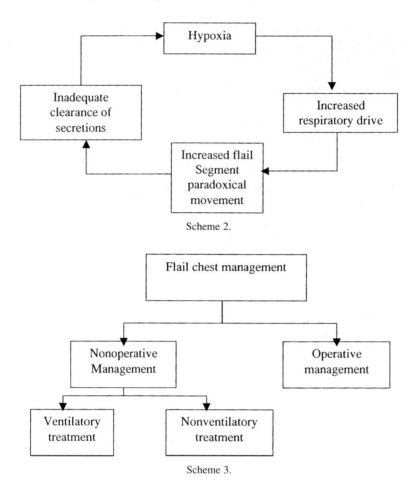

Scheme 2.

Scheme 3.

For isolated fractures of ribs, the mainstay is pain relief. A wide variety of analgesic regimen are in use. Non-steroidal anti-inflammatory drugs (NSAID), oral or parenteral narcotics especially patient controlled analgesia system (PCAS) with morphine, epidural analgesia, intercostal nerve blocks, intrapleural regional analgesia, transcutaneous electric nerve stimulation have all been used and must be tailored to the individual patient. Physiotherapy, mobilisation and deep vein thrombosis prophylaxis should be used as appropriate. Mortality rates for isolated rib fractures is 5% in children and 10–20% in adults.

1.4.6. Flail chest

Two or more ribs, with each rib fractured at more than one site, usually constitutes a flail segment. 5% of thoracic trauma victims have a flail chest. Flail chest is uncommon in children. Pathophysiology of flail chest is depicted in the following diagram. Flail segment movement can lead to ARDS, when there is an associated pulmonary contusion (Scheme 2).

Management of flail chest is controversial. There are mainly two lines of management (Scheme 3). Non-operative management consists of analgesia, incentive spirometry, physiotherapy, bronchoscopy when needed and mechanical ventilation in selected cases using the criteria listed in Table 1. Physiotherapy includes suctioning, breathing exercises, humidification of inspired air and chest percussion. Trinkle regime (Trinkle et al., 1975) for the management of flail chest consists of the following components:

(1) Restricting intravenous fluids to less than 1000 ml during resuscitation and to 50 ml/hour thereafter.
(2) Frusemide to promote urinary flow.
(3) Methylprednisolone 500 mg every six hours for 48 to 72 hours.
(4) Salt-poor albumin.
(5) Non-crystalloid replacement of blood loss.
(6) Analgesia.
(7) Nasal oxygen.
(8) Mechanical ventilation if pO_2 is below 60 mmHg on room air or below 80 mmHg on supplemental oxygen.

Internal fixation of the fractured ribs using Keith needles, bone plates and Kirschner wires is a useful technique in selected cases. Some authorities limit the use of internal fixation of ribs in a flail segment to those cases which require thoracotomy for other reasons. Others are more liberal in the operative treatment of the flail segment. Proponents of the latter argue that early and better functional recovery, evacuation of clots and therefore decreased chance of empyema and cost effectiveness are the major advantages of the operative intervention for flail chest. Multicentre, prospective randomised trials are needed to define the role of operative management of the flail chest. Mortality from flail chest is 10–15%.

1.4.7. Pulmonary contusion, haematoma and laceration of the lung

Pulmonary contusion Pulmonary contusion is sometimes associated with fractured ribs but more frequently there are no fractures. Symptoms can vary according to the extent and severity of the associated injuries. When pulmonary contusion is the sole injury the patient may have few respiratory symptoms; chest pains and dyspnoea being the commonest. Haemoptysis is absent in most cases. Clinical examination may show no abnormality or reveal a reduction in breath sounds in the affected area together with wheeze and course crepitation in the surrounding area. Fever is often present after a few days.

The chest radiograph of pulmonary contusion is characteristic. An ill-defined, patchy infiltration is often present. The radiological features of contusion appear within 24 to 48 hours of trauma. The resolution of the contusion occurs from 2 to 3 days after.

- Management
  In the absence of other thoracic injuries patients are treated by:
  - Early mobilisation and physiotherapy
  - Broad spectrum antibiotics
  - Mild analgesic
  - Repeated chest radiograph is required to check the progress

The patient is observed for a few days following which he is discharged.

Pulmonary haematoma In some instances of blunt trauma there is much intrapulmonary haemorrhage but the visceral pleura remains intact and unbroken. A fractured rib may or may not be present. Pain, dys-

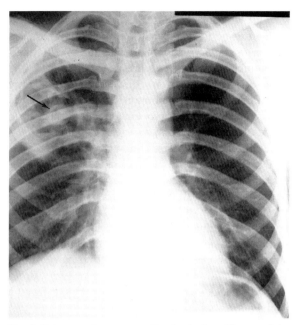

Fig. 2. Pulmonary haematoma. Opacity in the mid zone of the right lung. This remained unchanged for four weeks before disappearing.

pnoea and haemoptysis are the usual symptoms. The chest radiograph usually shows no haemopneumothorax but a homogeneous opacity. Unlike pulmonary contusion, the opacity in the case of pulmonary haematoma may persist for 3 or 4 weeks or more. In some cases, the central part of the lesion becomes necrotic and is drained through the airways (coughed up by the patient). The X-ray appearance then assumes the characteristics of a cavitating lesion which may persist for 3 to 4 weeks or more before clearing (Fig. 2)

- Management
  Patients with pulmonary haematoma should undergo bronchoscopy on account of their haemoptysis. Bronchial tear, bleeding from a major vessel and major laceration have to be excluded. Uncomplicated pulmonary haematoma is treated conservatively by:
  - Broad spectrum antibiotics
  - Physiotherapy
  - Mobilisation

When the patient's condition is stabilised, and if there are no other injuries, they may be discharged but checked every two weeks as an outpatient until complete radiological resolution of the lesion.

Laceration of the lung In contrast to perforating injuries, blunt trauma to the chest rarely causes pulmonary laceration. Whilst the cases of minor lacerations can be managed with conservative measures similar to those for pulmonary haematoma, by intercostal tube drainage of the haemopneumothorax, the cases of major laceration require early thoracotomy and repair. The most common symptoms and signs are dyspnoea, haemoptysis and shock. Although rib fractures may be present, the laceration is not due to penetration of a broken rib fragment into the lung.

Diagnosis is made by the radiological appearance aided by bronchoscopy. Chest radiograph shows haemothorax of variable size, together with a shallow (3 to 5 cm) pneumothorax. Chest radiograph taken after drainage of the haemopneumothorax indicates a slight change (unlike that observed in simple haemopneumothorax which usually shows a great improvement following drainage). Bronchoscopy will indicate seeping of blood from a segmental/lobar bronchi.

- Management

  In the first instance the haemopneumothorax is drained by an intercostal drain. When the diagnosis of laceration is made, a standard posterolateral thoracotomy is carried out using single lung ventilation. The pleural cavity is cleared of blood clots. The laceration is usually visible and the lung tissues surrounding the laceration area present with much haematoma; these need suturing with chromic catgut stitches. The air leak and bleeding points are seen much more easily when the lacerated area is cleared with normal saline solution. There are usually some bleeding vessels in the substance of the lung which require ligation. Also small bronchioles or subsegmental bronchi are seen to leak air when the lung is ventilated (the anaesthetist should be asked to ventilate the injured lung).

  The lacerated area is then cleared of the blood clot and repaired using chromic catgut sutures either as continuous horizontal mattress followed by running over-and-over stitching or as through-and-through stitching. When the lung is emphysematous, Teflon felt may be used to prevent the stitches cutting through the parenchyma. The chest is closed with an apical and a lower drain connected to an underwater sealed drainage system. Post-operative care is on similar lines to the post-operative care of thoracotomy and pulmonary resection patients.

1.4.8. Penetrating chest wall wounds

Large defects should be promptly covered with impermeable dressings and a chest tube should be inserted to aid pulmonary expansion. Operative debridement and chest wall defect closure should be undertaken after initial stabilisation of the patient. Prolene and Marlex meshes can be used in clean wounds. Polymethylmethacrylate cement with two mesh layer sandwich can be used to cover defects. Potentially infected wounds are best closed with myocutaneous flaps. Pectoralis major and latissimus dorsi are the favoured flaps.

Smaller wounds may be explored under local or general anaesthesia and treated on the merits of the wound. Exploratory thoracotomy may be needed for patients with haemodynamic instability.

1.5. Pneumothorax

Traumatic pneumothorax may be isolated pneumothorax or haemopneumothorax (Fig. 3). The following is the approach to pneumothorax (Scheme 4).

In urgent situations, a wide-bore needle is passed into the pleural cavity and a length of intravenous fluid administration set tubing is attached to the needle. The other end of the tubing is placed under a basin of water. Intercostal tube drainage is carried out in an expedite manner. Underwater seal is connected to negative suction of 20–30 mmHg. Duration of suction depends on the air leak. If there is no air leak, the suction can be switched off in 24 hours. The drain is removed after satisfactory clinicoradiological expansion of lung.

1.6. Haemothorax

Haemothorax is diagnosed by the finding of decreased respiratory movements, dull note on percussion and diminished/absent breath sounds on the side involved. It is confirmed by chest X-ray and ultrasound examination. Blunting of the costophrenic angle means at least 500 ml of blood in the pleural cavity. In major trauma, where AP film is taken, the haemothorax is not readily visible. Hazy lung field on the suspected side should raise the suspicion. Chest ultrasound and CT scans readily diagnose haemothorax.

Source of haemorrhage into the chest can be intercostal arteries, internal thoracic artery, pulmonary parenchyma, hilar vessels, aorta, pulmonary artery or one of the chambers of the heart.

Initial chest drainage >1500 ml (>20 ml/kg) or

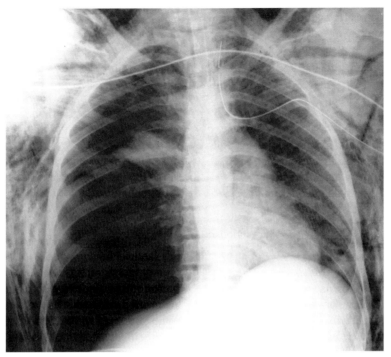

Fig. 3. Chest radiograph of a patient with traumatic pneumothorax. The left chest was drained and there was also pneumothorax of right side under some tension.

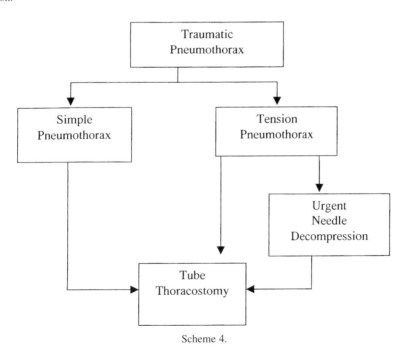

Scheme 4.

hourly bleeding in excess of 200 ml/hour (2 ml/kg/hour), for 2 to 4 hours is an indication for thoracotomy unless clotting is severely deranged. Any residual haemothorax should be aggressively treated by video assisted thoracoscopic evacuation of the clot to prevent the empyema.

1.7. Air embolism after chest trauma

This is a rare and interesting complication of chest trauma encountered in about 4% of patients. 2/3 have penetrating trauma and 1/3 have blunt trauma. Pathophysiology can be depicted as in Scheme 5.

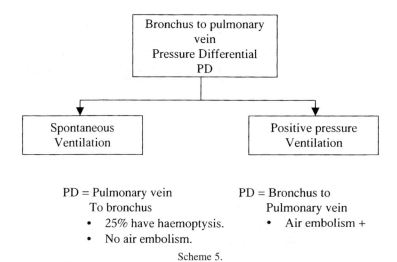

Scheme 5.

Air embolism should be suspected in any ventilated patient with chest trauma who develops focal or lateralising neurological signs or sudden haemodynamic deterioration. Frothy arterial blood gas specimen is a classic but very rare clue. Retinal arteries may show air bubbles on retinoscopy.

When diagnosed, thoracotomy should be carried out without delay and the hilum of the lung should be clamped. The patient should be kept in Trendelenburg head low position and the left ventricle should be vented. The offending lesion should be treated by lobectomy or pneumonectomy. Salvage rate from air embolism of this nature is 20% in blunt trauma group and 55% in penetrating chest injuries.

1.8. Tracheobronchial injuries

These are seen in 1% of patients with major thoracic trauma. Trachea and bronchi are implicated more commonly in penetrating injuries. Cervical tracheal injuries are more common than intrathoracic tracheobronchial injuries.

Penetrating injuries can occur anywhere but blunt tracheobronchial injuries are usually close to the carina. Chief symptoms include dyspnoea, dysphonia and haemoptysis. Subcutaneous emphysema, especially in the supraclavicular fossae and neck is a valuable clue. A major, persistent air leak and/or failure of the lung to expand, must alert the clinician to the possibility of tracheobronchial injury. Unger's 'fallen lung sign', wherein the lung collapses laterally to the chest wall is an impressive radiological sign. Bronchoscopy is the mainstay for diagnosis. CT scan of the neck and chest are also useful in selected cases.

Injuries involving <1/3 of the circumference of major airways may be managed conservatively. When surgery is indicated, exposure of the cervical trachea is through a collar incision. Tracheal injury without tissue loss or devitalisation is treated with direct suture using absorbable material. When tissue loss is significant, the wound may be converted into a tracheostomy and, wherever possible, this is brought out through a separate skin incision. A low pressure cuff endotracheal tube is left as a stent for up to seven days.

Intrathoracic trachea and carina may be approached through a partial or complete sternotomy. Main bronchial injury is dealt with through posterolateral thoracotomy. When the repair is fragile, pleural flap, intercostal muscle flap or pedicled omental flap may be used as support. In combined tracheo-oesophageal trauma, viable soft tissue interposition between them is a sound policy to prevent tracheo-oesophageal fistula.

1.9. Thoracic duct injury

This is more common in penetrating injuries. The draining fluid from the pleural cavity is milky and stains with Sudan III, which is a stain for fat. The chylothorax rarely gets infected because of bacteriostatic property of chyle.

Most cases are managed conservatively with chest drainage and total parenteral nutrition and the majority of leaks gradually subside. In a minority of cases transthoracic ligation of the thoracic duct at the diaphragmatic level is the procedure of choice. Repair of the thoracic duct and pleuroperitoneal shunt are the other methods of management.

1.10. Diaphragmatic injuries

The diaphragm may be injured in blunt and penetrating thoracic trauma. It is more common on the left side with the left to right ratio being about 3 : 1. As a result of the injury, stomach, spleen, liver, small intestine, large intestine and omentum may herniate into the pleural cavity. Respiratory distress is of variable intensity. Deviated trachea and audible bowel sounds in the chest are recognised signs. A chest X-ray may show indistinct diaphragmatic contour, elevated hemidiaphragm and air containing visceral shadow in the pleural cavity along with a blunted costophrenic angle. Ultrasound examination, fluoroscopy, CT, MRI and VATS are useful to evaluate the patient. If there is an associated abdominal injury, the repair can be carried out at laparotomy. If not, thoracotomy through the 7th or 8th space gives excellent exposure. The principle is to close the defect using non-absorbable suture. Large defects may be repaired with patch material like Goretex or bovine pericardium.

1.11. Oesophageal trauma

Oesophageal trauma can be classified in two ways: First, depending on the mode of injury (Scheme 6).

In to out injuries include those due to iatrogenic instrumentation, ingestion of a foreign body and increased intraluminal pressure. Out to in injuries include those due to stab injuries and gunshot wounds.

The second classification depends on the location of the injury (Scheme 7).

Clinical symptoms and signs of oesophageal injury may take several hours to develop fully. Dysphagia is the important, classical symptom. Pain may be in the neck, retrosternal area or in the upper back. Dysphonia and respiratory distress may also be noted. Fever, tenderness and subcutaneous emphysema in the neck are noteworthy signs.

Chest X-ray may reveal subcutaneous emphysema, pneumomediastinum and air fluid level in pleural cavity.

Contrast swallow with a water soluble agent such as gastrografin is the most useful investigation.

CT scan is of value in doubtful cases.

A carefully performed flexible oesophagoscopy has been advocated by some groups. This is especially useful in distal oesophageal injuries.

Management of oesophageal injuries is based on the three cardinal principles: drainage, nutrition and antibiotics (DNA)

Instrumental trauma tends to involve the oesoph-

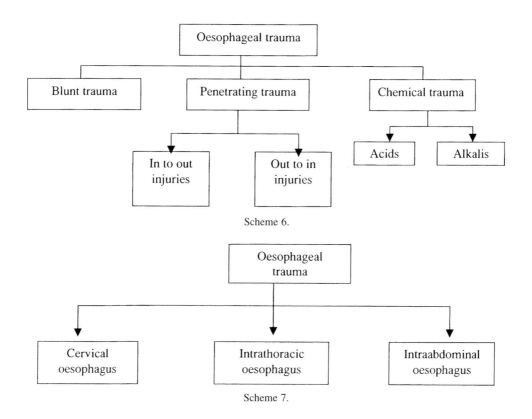

Scheme 6.

Scheme 7.

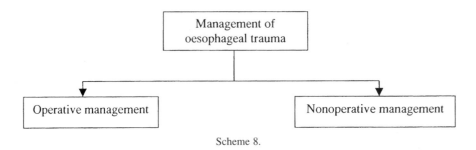

Scheme 8.

agus at the two levels of anatomical narrowing, the junction of inferior constrictor and cricopharyngeus and the oesophagogastric junction. The third area of anatomical narrowing at the level of the left main bronchus and aortic arch is rarely involved. Penetrating injuries are more common in the neck than in the intrathoracic oesophagus.

Surgical management is the preferred option (Scheme 8). The management policy in oesophageal trauma depends on the following factors: age, duration and extent of the injury, presence of obstructing lesions in the oesophagus, co-morbid factors and the general condition of the patient.

The following are the currently available surgical management options in oesophageal trauma:
(1) Primary closure
(2) Primary closure with buttress of repair.
(3) Exclusion and diversion.
(4) Esophageal resection and primary/delayed reconstruction.
(5) Abbott's T tube drainage.
(6) Intraluminal stenting.
(7) Drainage only.

Surgical approach to the cervical oesophagus is through an incision along the anterior border of left or right sternocleidomastoid muscle. The intrathoracic oesophagus is approached through a posterolateral thoracotomy in the appropriate space depending on the location and extent of the injury.

Primary closure uses 4-0 non-absorbable or slow absorbable sutures and the repair is carried out in two layers. Buttress may be using intercostal muscle flap or pedicled omental flap.

Conservative management is carried out in a small group of patients with oesophageal perforation selected using the following criteria:
(1) Perforation <24 hours.
(2) No significant intrapleural soiling.
(3) No obstructing lesion in the oesophagus.
(4) No significant sepsis.
(5) Haemodynamic stability.

(6) Contained perforation within the mediastinum
(7) Good flow of contrast into the distal segment.

2. Acute respiratory distress syndrome

ARDS is the term used to describe non-cardiogenic pulmonary dysfunction characterised by refractory hypoxia, decreased pulmonary compliance and diffuse interstitial infiltrates on the chest X-ray. Adult respiratory distress syndrome, traumatic wet lung, shock lung, Da nang lung, post perfusion lung and post pump lung are all synonymous with acute respiratory syndrome.

There are two terms which need clarification: Acute lung injury and ARDS. Acute lung injury is characterised by acute onset, PaO_2/FIO_2 200–300 mmHg regardless of the PEEP, bilateral infiltrate on CXR and pulmonary oedema. ARDS has all the criteria but the PaO_2/FIO_2 is <200 mmHg. Usage of diuretics, steroids, O_2 etc should be carried out very judiciously and is beyond the scope of this book.

2.1. Traumatic aortic rupture

10 to 25% of deaths due to automobile accidents are as a direct result of traumatic aortic rupture. It is interesting to note that the greatest tensile strength of the aorta rests in adventitia and not in intima or media. Site of the aortic injury depends on the mechanism of injury. Horizontal deceleration injuries involve the aortic isthmus in the region of ligamentum arteriosum, while vertical deceleration injuries affect the ascending aorta and the arch. It is possible to have ruptured aorta with minimal external injuries to the chest wall. Easily correctable hypovolaemic shock does not rule out the possibility of aortic rupture.

Symptoms of aortic rupture include interscapular chest pain, dyspnoea, dysphonia due to recurrent laryngeal nerve involvement, dysphagia due to oesophageal compression and paraplegia.

Signs which should alert the clinician to the possibility of traumatic aortic rupture are neck haematoma, systolic murmur over precordium and interscapular area and upper limb hypertension with lower limb hypotension — the acute coarctation syndrome. This results because of reduced flow to the lower body due to compression by haematoma. Tracheal deviation and stridor are the other infrequently encountered clinical signs.

Chest X-rays may be normal in some patients with traumatic aortic rupture. Recognised radiological findings include: mediastinal widening to 8 cm or more in AP film, indistinct aortic knuckle, aortopulmonary window obliteration, inferior and rightward displacement of left main bronchus, oesophageal and tracheal deviation to the right and left pleural effusion. Associated skeletal injuries of the first rib, sternum, clavicle and thoracic spine may be evident and give a clue to the mechanism and severity of initial injury. CT scan and MRI scan are useful in selected cases. Aortography offers definite diagnosis of traumatic aortic rupture.

Surgical treatment of traumatic aortic rupture is carried out mainly through left posterolateral thoracotomy. The "clamp and sew" technique refers to the method popularised by Crawford. Aortic occlusion time should be under 30 minutes to prevent paraplegia. Bleeding is less as no heparinisation is involved.

The second technique for repair of thoracic aortic rupture employs a Gott shunt. This refers to the usage of a heparin bonded shunt in aortoaortic or ventriculoaortic position to allow aortic perfusion distal to the distal clamp. Systemic heparinisation is avoided again and using this technique the aortic clamp time can be safely extended to 60 minutes.

The third technique of surgical treatment of traumatic aortic rupture employs cardiopulmonary bypass. This can be either partial or total cardiopulmonary bypass. In partial bypass, the femoral vein and artery can be used for cannulation, employing an oxygenator, or left atrial to femoral artery bypass can be established using just the roller pump without the oxygenator. In total bypass, right atrial or femoral vein cannula can be used for the venous return and a Y connector on arterial line can be used to perfuse head, neck, upper limbs and lower half of the body allowing the surgeon to work on the ruptured aorta. Associated intracranial injury and pulmonary injuries preclude the use of cardiopulmonary bypass as heparinisation can potentiate these injuries. Thus, the surgeon should be equipped with knowledge and

competence of all the techniques described above and should use the most appropriate technique in a given situation.

2.2. Cardiac tamponade

Cardiac tamponade is more common with penetrating cardiac trauma but can be seen following blunt cardiac trauma. Clinical features depend on the amount of blood in the pericardial cavity and the rate of accumulation of the same.

Tachycardia and hypotension associated with high central venous pressure should alert the clinician to the possibility of cardiac tamponade. Whenever the degree of circulatory collapse is out of proportion to the observed injury, cardiac tamponade must be ruled out. 'Beck's triad', is a combination of elevation of central venous pressure, indistinct heart sounds and hypotension and this triad is not always present. Kussmaul's sign refers to paradoxical elevation of venous pressure during deep inspiration and is due to impaired diastolic filling of the heart. Emergency cardiac ultrasound is the single most important investigation. Diagnostic and therapeutic pericardiocentesis should be performed only when the facility for emergency cardiac ultrasound is not available. Urgent thoracotomy or sternotomy must be arranged depending on the site of the injury.

2.3. Cardiac injuries

Cardiac injuries in thoracic trauma may be classified as in Scheme 9.

The range of possible injuries can be one or more of the following: cardiac tamponade, vena caval injuries, injuries to the cardiac chambers, aortic and pulmonary arterial injuries, coronary arterial injuries, valve injuries and septal injuries with intracardiac shunt.

A patient with cardiac trauma should be resuscitated initially as any other trauma patient with attention to airway, breathing and circulation. Inadvertent hypertension due to overzealous fluid administration should be avoided. If the radial pulse is palpable, even if the patient is hypotensive, no further attempts should be made to get the pressures to normal values as this may aggravate bleeding. This concept is referred to as "Permissive Hypotension". Emergency cardiac ultrasound is a very useful diagnostic tool in resuscitation. This enables confident and noninvasive diagnosis of cardiac tamponade, valvular injuries and intracardiac shunt. Diagnostic pericardiocentesis

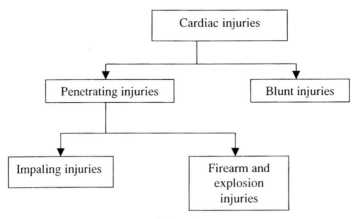

Scheme 9.

should be carried out only when the facility for cardiac ultrasound is not available. Pericardiocentesis has a limited therapeutic role in a patient waiting to get to operation theatre for emergency thoracotomy. To carry this out, a 16# or larger needle is inserted making an angle of 45 degrees from the mid-line aiming towards the right shoulder and 45 degrees away from the skin. The patient is at 45 degrees reclination. The point of entry is just to the left of the xiphoid process. ECG monitoring is helpful to avoid cardiac injury.

The surgical approach to the heart is via either left anterolateral thoracotomy or median sternotomy, depending on the site of the injury and the place where the surgery is being undertaken. Left antero-lateral thoracotomy in the 5th intercostal space can be rapidly done in the resuscitation room and must be performed by the most experienced member of the team.

Caval, aortic, pulmonary arterial and chamber injuries can be initially controlled with digital pressure and can be closed with direct or pledgeted monofilament non-absorbable sutures such as 3(0) or 4(0) polypropylene, without the aid of cardiopulmonary bypass. Associated valvular or coronary arterial injuries may require the institution of cardiopulmonary bypass. Ligation should be reserved only for the small coronary arterial branches. Otherwise, the injury should be repaired directly or using a vein patch, or coronary artery bypass grafting may have to be carried out.

Associated inter-atrial or inter-ventricular septal injury may be operated on at the same time, or at a later date, depending on the degree of left to right shunt and associated intracranial injuries. There are

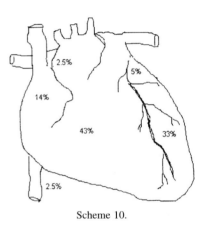

Scheme 10.

two reasons for this approach: firstly, heparinisation is avoided when an acute intracranial injury is present and secondly, small intra-cardiac shunts may disappear in the ensuing weeks and months and the patient may be followed up using serial echocardiographic evaluation and, when needed, cardiac catheterisation.

Aortic valve injuries are more common than mitral valve injuries and, depending on the extent of the injury, repair or replacement may be needed.

The regional distribution of the cardiac injuries may be depicted as in Scheme 10.

References and further reading

Moghissi K. Laceration of the lung following blunt trauma. Thorax 1971; 26: 322.

Trinkle JK, Richardson JD, Franz JL, Grover FL, Arom KV, Holmstrom FM. Management of flail chest without mechanical ventilation. Ann Thorac Surg 1975; 19: 355–363.

Bronchiectasis

K. Moghissi

1. Bronchiectasis

Bronchistasis was first described by Laennec (1819) as a suppurative condition characterised by cough, purulent sputum and haemoptysis.

2. Pathology

The macroscopic features of the condition are dominated by widely dilated bronchi. These may be described as:
- Tubular (cylindrical) with dilated bronchi but of fairly regular calibre.
- Varicose with irregular dilatation.
- Saccular (cystic) where there is bronchial dilatation distally.

The pulmonary parenchyma may contain abscesses or be consolidated and scarred. Histological changes vary according to the severity of the condition and associated pulmonary parenchymal complications. The characteristic picture is one of dilated bronchi with atrophy of the wall and epithelial changes, usually loss of cilia and variable pulmonary parenchymal changes. In the majority of cases the disease affects the lower lobes with or without, the middle lobe or lingula. The left lower lobe is the commonest site of involvement; between 45 to 60%. In approximately half of these the lingula is also involved. The right middle and lower lobe is the next combination. Less common bronchiectasis of the upper lobes is probably the sequallae of adult pulmonary tuberculosis. Bilateral distribution is not uncommon. However, it must be realised that in the past 40 years the incidence of disease has altered. Also segmental/lobar distribution is dependent on aetiological factors which are subject to geographical and temporal variations.

The pattern of bronchiectasis, as seen by bronchographic and macroscopic pathological appearances, is largely based on disruptive terminology such as cylindrical, cystic and saccular. However, there is no relationship between macroscopic appearance, clinical features and evolution of the disease. These terms have long been in use and are an established part of bronchographic interpretation.

2.1. Aetiology

Three main factors are implicated in the genesis of bronchiectasis:
- Congenital
- Obstructive
- Infective

Congenital bronchiectasis results from abnormal development of the bronchial tree. In such cases there are often other anomalies or immune deficiency syndromes. Examples of these are:
- Garner Kartagener's Syndrome Triad: bronchiectasis, dextrocardia and sinusitis, or absence of frontal sinuses
- William Campbell syndrome: bronchiectasis, abnormality or absence of cartilage.

A variety of immune deficiency conditions, such as anti alpha tripsine deficiency and hypo-gamma-glubolinaemia are also involved in promoting the development of bronchiectasis.

Bronchial occlusion: Bronchial obstruction may be from: *without* or *within*.

In cases with peribronchial lymphadenitis and lymph node enlargement bronchial stenosis can ensue. Development of bronchiectasis in children following exanthemas or primary tuberculosis are examples of extrinsic lymph node compression resulting in bronchial stenosis, infection and bronchiectasis. Such lymphadenitis, sometimes with calcification, affecting the right lower and middle lobe broncho-pulmonary lymph nodes, following tuberculosis in particular, has earned the name of *middle lobe syndrome*. In this condition proximal stenosis of the right middle lobe bronchus leads to bronchiectasis of more distal segments or divisions. Besides retention of contaminated secretion, infection directly affects the bronchial wall leading to bronchiectasis. Pneumonia in childhood or complicated measles or whooping cough have, in the past, contributed to the development of this disease. In adults, repeated staphylococcal broncho-pulmonary infection and tuberculosis are liable to be complicated by bronchiectasis.

3. Clinical features

3.1. Cough and purulent sputum are the common symptoms of bronchiectasis

The volume of expectoration is usually an indication of the severity of the disease and repeated chest infection is one of its characteristics. Affected children miss school because of periods of exacerbation characterised by fever, malaise and purulent sputum. Untreated, pneumonia and lung abscess complicate these episodes. In young adults loss of weight and daytime fatigue are present in many cases. Haemoptysis or bloodstained sputum is also frequently present in bronchiectatic patients, indicating infection. Dyspnoea and wheeze are sometimes present due to parenchymal damage or obstruction of segmental bronchi by thick secretion and/or some degree of bronchial stenosis. Auscultation of the lung in uncomplicated cases reveals a range of fine and coarse crepitations. It is worthwhile noting that persistent physical signs in an area of the chest over a period of time are strongly suggestive of bronchiectatic changes.

3.2. Diagnosis

Diagnosis of bronchiectasis is based on clinical history and examination, sputum tests and radiology. Clinical history and examination such as described above are not specific to bronchiectasis.

Sputum: The sputum is purulent in character, sometimes stained with blood and usually colonised by pathogens. Haemophilus influenzae and streptococcus pneumoniae are common inhabitants. It is not uncommon for patients to harbour gram-negative

and fungal organisms, the consequence of overzealous anti-microbial therapy.

As a rule, cytology of sputum in bronchiectasis is non-eosinophilic (except for broncho-pulmonary aspergillosis added to bronchiectasis)

Sinusitis and rhino-sinusitis are commonly associated with bronchiectasis. In any form of therapy, it is important to consider this association and to investigate the extent and severity of rhino-sinusitis, clinically and radiologically.

Radiology: On the plain chest radiograph cystic and saccular lesions, when gross, can easily be seen as air or fluid-containing lesions. Tubular (cylindrical) bronchiectasis is more difficult to discern on plain radiography unless there are areas of consolidation and fibrosis. A CT scan is an important diagnostic aid (Fig. 1). Thin section CT has a higher diagnostic sensitivity than standard thick section cuts. The calibre and thickness of the walls of bronchi can be assessed by CT but cylindrical bronchiectasis is more difficult to diagnose by CT methods. The sensitivity and specificity of CT in the diagnosis of bronchiectasis is between 66% to 84% and 82% to 92%, respectively.

Bronchography: With the decline of surgical resection and the availability of highly diagnostically accurate CT, the role of bronchography in the management of bronchiectasis has been reduced. Nevertheless, bilateral bronchography remains essential if bronchiectatic cases are to be candidates for surgical treatment. Before surgical resection, it is not only necessary to know the anatomical pattern of disease but also the anatomy of normal bronchi. This is best provided by bronchogram (Fig. 2).

4. Complications of Bronchiectasis

Prior to the antibiotic era the complications of bronchiectasis were many and varied but mostly related to sepsis and infection. At present the following complications are encountered with variable frequency:
- Pulmonary infections.
- Pleural infections.
- Brain abscess is now a rare complication but in the past was frequently a cause of death.
- Amyloidosis is now extremely rare.
- Fungal infection: whilst the recovery of fungal organisms from the long standing case is not unusual, true fungal infection remains a less common complication. Repeated antibiotic administration is largely to blame for fungal organisms replacing the usual microorganisms.

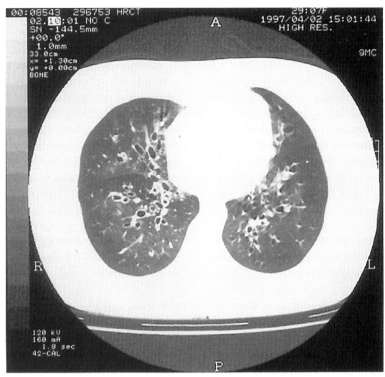

Fig. 1. CT scan of the chest showing bilateral bronchiectasis.

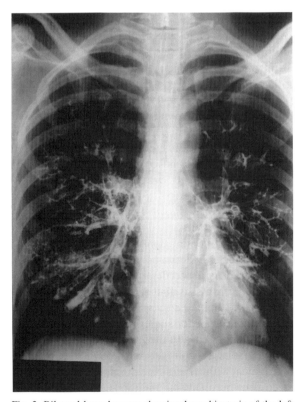

Fig. 2. Bilateral bronchogram showing bronchiectasis of the left lower lobe and basal segments of the right lower lobe.

- Sinusitis — there is a close association between sinusitis and bronchiectasis. In many severely bronchiectatic patients, sinusitis is a common occurrence. This is not really surprising since the infective complications of bronchiectasis can affect the whole of the respiratory tract.
- Haemoptysis: blood staining of the sputum, or small haemoptysis, can occur in any bronchiectatic case complicated by chest infection. This requires treatment by appropriate anti-microbial agents or bronchoscopic disinfection and therapeutic lavage followed by a course of antibiotics. In young bronchiectatic female patients, it is not unusual to have small haemoptysis or blood staining of sputum at the start of menstruation. In the absence of pulmonary endometriosis, hormone therapy (contraceptive) should be recommended if such haemoptysis becomes troublesome.
- Life threatening haemoptysis requires emergency measures which, in the case of known bronchiectasis, could involve emergency resection of the culprit segment or lobar bronchi.

5. Management of bronchiectasis

5.1. Prevention

Those cases of bronchiectasis with strong congenital or familial aetiology cannot be prevented but may be kept in check and discouraged from expansion or aggravation (see below). Amongst the known causal factors of the disease, bronchial obstruction must be considered the most important single factor. Bronchial clearance, therefore, constitutes an important preventative measure. An inhaled foreign body must not be allowed to remain in the bronchial tree in the hope of it being expectorated.

Respiratory infection, particularly in children, must be treated vigorously with appropriate antibiotic agents and physiotherapy. The progress of such infection should be monitored radiologically. When the definite diagnosis of bronchiectasis is made an equally definite management scheme should be instituted: this is described below.

5.2. Medical and conservative management

This applies to cases with:
- Widespread but scattered bronchiectasis.
- Localised bronchiectasis not suitable for surgical operation on account of general condition or inadequate respiratory function.
- Minimal symptoms and infrequent complications.

Medical management consists of: institution of self chest physiotherapy, in which patients undertake their own physiotherapy after being initiated by the professional physiotherapist. Deep breathing and postural drainage are carried out twice daily. A sample of sputum is periodically sent to the laboratory for identification of organisms and sensitivity to antibiotics

5.2.1. Medication
Expectorant: In some cases of bronchiectasis with tenacious secretions, expectorants containing mucolytic agents are helpful in reducing the viscosity of the sputum; this can then be expectorated more easily.

Bronchodilators: The bronchiectatic patient with airflow obstruction when receiving conservative treatment will benefit from the addition of bronchodilators.

Corticosteroid: Some patients, particularly those with airway hyper-responsiveness to Methacholine, appear to benefit from aerosol corticosteroid.

Mucolytic: Nebulized or inhaled mucolytics have beneficial effects in promoting more effective drainage of sputum.

Antibiotics: For some years physicians have adopted either a regular pulsed regimen or a continuous course of anti-microbial therapy. The aim has been to reduce pathogenic organisms and their effect. However, this has been responsible for antibiotic resistant organisms, reduction of patients' resistance to infection and the development of fungal organisms. Whilst, for example, a group of bronchiectatic patients with cystic fibrosis could be candidates for such long term therapies, other patients also have been subjected to such regular and/or continuous regimens with no benefit. We believe antibiotic administration should be reserved for episodes of infective complications.

5.3. Bronchial lavage

This is therapeutic bronchial lavage. The aims are:
- Bronchoscopic aspiration of thick, purulent and at times inspissated secretions which can totally block the bronchiolar (segmental and sub-segmental bronchi) lumen.
- Bronchial lavage using 500 to 1000 ml of warm (body temperature) sterile physiological saline solution. The procedure is performed under general anaesthetic using a rigid bronchoscope. 50 ml of saline solution is delivered via a syringe into the lumen of the bronchoscope. This is removed by suction and the procedure repeated 10 to 20 times. The volume aspirated is recorded and should equal within ± 20–30 ml of the volume of saline solution delivered into the bronchial tree through the bronchoscope. Lavage of the right and left bronchial tree is undertaken separately.

5.4. Surgical management

Pulmonary resection constitutes the only curative treatment for bronchiectasis. Bronchography is mandatory not only to determine the extent and distribution of the disease but also to indicate the overall extent of the unaffected segments.

The indications for surgery are:
- Localised disease limited to segments of a lobe or to a lobe as a whole.
- Patients with severe symptoms, such as cough, copious purulent sputum, repeated chest infection and/or haemoptysis.

Surgery should not be undertaken in mildly symptomatic patients because of bronchographic evidence of bronchiectasis.

- Patients with bilateral disease or those with disease affecting the whole of one lung may benefit from operation and need not be excluded if symptoms are severe provided that the pulmonary function is judged to be satisfactory for such extensive surgery. The decision may be difficult as the disease is severely disabling, yet the surgical resection may leave the individual with inadequate post-operative respiratory capacity.

The principle of surgical resection is to excise all bronchiectatic segments and to preserve healthy parenchyma. This may not be feasible in all cases. For instance, patients with gross left lower lobe bronchiectasis may have one segment in the right middle lobe with bronchiectasis; experience shows that left lower lobectomy alone will suffice. Such patients are then kept under medical surveillance.

References and further reading

Brock RC. Post-tuberculous broncho-stenosis and bronchiectasis of the middle lobe. Thorax 1950; 5: 5.

Corless JA, Warburton CJ. Surgery vs. non-surgical treatment for bronchiectasis (Cochrane review). Cochrane Database Syst Rev 2000; 4: CD002180.

Kang EY, Miller RR, Muller NL. Bronchiectasis: comparison of pre-operative thin-section CT and pathologic findings in resected specimens. Radiology 1995; 195: 649–654.

Kartagener M. Zur Pathogenese der Bronchiektasien. Mitteilung: Bronchiektasien bei Situs viscerium inversus. Beitr Klin Erforsch Tuberk Lungenkr 1933; 83: 489–501.

Laennec RTH. Traité de l'auscultation médiate ou traité des maladies du poumon et du coeur fondé principalement sur ce nouveau mode de l'exploration. Paris, J-A Brason and JS Chaude, 1819.

Mal H, Rullonn I, Mellot F, Brugiere O, Sleiman C, Menu Y, Fournier M. Immediate and long term results of bronchial artery embolization for life threatening haemoptysis. Chest 1999; 115: 996–1001.

Perry MA, Holmes Sellor T. Bronchiectasis. In: Chest Diseases. London, Butterworth, 1963; pp. 364–392.

Prieto D, Bernardo J, Matos MJ, Eugenio L, Antunes M. Surgery for bronchiectasis. Eur J Cardiothorac Surg 2001; 20(1): 19–24.

Roeslin N, Wihlm JM, Morand G. Évolution post-opératoire de 82 cas de dilatation bronchique. Poumon-Coeur 1981; 37: 203–205.

CHAPTER I.9

Lung abscess

K. Moghissi

1. Introduction

Lung abscess is a localised suppuration and necrosis within the substance of the lung. This definition embraces many unrelated and diverse conditions such as pyogenic and fungal abscesses and suppuration in necrotic tumours, all of which are characterised by cavitation and suppuration.

Prior to antibiotics, lung abscess was common and was attended by high mortality. The availability of antimicrobial agents has brought about a change in the natural history of the disease, its incidence and management. In recent years, though, there has been resurgence in the incidence of lung abscess due to an increase in the number of immuno-compromised individuals, occasioned by widespread use of immuno-suppressive drugs in conjunction with organ transplantation and also associated with HIV infection.

2. Aetiology

Lung abscess may have the following origins:

2.1. Bronchogenic

Inhalation/aspiration of a foreign body or infected material, when retained in the bronchi, can be complicated by abscess formation. This type of abscess is frequently solitary and located in the right lung, as the right main bronchus is more in line with the trachea than the left main bronchus. Lung abscess after abdominal operation and that resulting from retention of sputum have similar pathogenesis.

2.2. Hematogenous

In these the abscess follows septic emboli and infected pulmonary infarct arising from septic thrombophlebitis. An embolic abscess may be aseptic initially but become infected secondarily.

With the increased use of parenteral nutrition, occasional abscesses are encountered which arise from septic thrombophlebitis and catheter sepsis.

2.3. Post-pneumonic

A consolidated area of the lung such as that from staphylococcal pneumonia can become complicated by necrosis and suppuration with abscess formation. In infants and young children, staphylococcal pneumonia develops a characteristic lesion with cavity formation, which later becomes an air cyst (Fig. 1a and b). This type of abscess and cyst can be further complicated by an empyema or a pyopneumothorax, at times under tension (tension pyopneumothorax). Apart from staphylococcal pneumonia, Klebsiella pneumonia has a tendency towards abscess formation.

2.4. Post-traumatic

Traumatic pulmonary haematoma and laceration may be followed by localised necrosis and infection with subsequent abscess formation.

2.5. Miscellaneous

Abscess can follow bronchogenic carcinoma or hydatid cyst by super-added infection.

Three factors appear to be important in the pathogenesis of lung abscesses, namely bronchial obstruction, ischemic necrosis and infection by invading pathogenic micro-organisms of the area beyond bronchial obstruction.

Evolution of abscess is:
- Rupture of abscess:

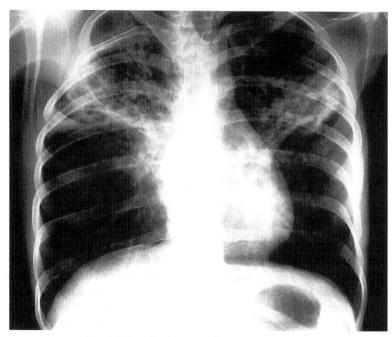

Fig. 1. Bilateral pulmonary tuberculous cavitations.

invade the tissues and create a tuberculous focus, a subpleural granuloma consisting of an accumulation of macrophages (epitheloid cells) and multi-nucleated Langhans cells, monocytes and lymphocytes. There is also caseation, a type of necrosis, at the centre of the granuloma. Associated with the granuloma is lymphadenitis (Gohn lesion). This lesion is known as a primary complex (Stage I). The primary complex usually resolves spontaneously leaving an insignificant scar and a positive tuberculin test as a reminder. In certain circumstances, such as high-risk individuals, malnourished communities and immune deficient children, the primary lesion may proceed to a fulminating generalised tuberculosis (Stage II).

Stage III disease is also known as adult tuberculosis, which is characterised by destructive cavitary tuberculosis. Apart from some of the complications of Stage I or II disease, such as abscess or concurrent empyema, the main therapeutic concern of the thoracic surgeon relates to Stage III disease (Fig. 1).

3. Clinical features and diagnosis

Pulmonary tuberculosis may present with non-specific chest symptoms; cough, dyspnoea, low grade pyrexia, fatigue, loss of weight and haemoptysis. The acute fulminant type is now rare but could mimic acute broncho-pneumonia.

3.1. Diagnosis

Clinical history and examination can be indicative of pulmonary tuberculosis. However, radiology and laboratory testing are essential to establish the diagnosis. Plain chest radiograph and CT scanning will indicate cavitation/infiltration or pleural effusion. In many cases the disease is discovered radiologically and often in the form of tuberculoma presenting as a pulmonary "coin" lesion. The recovery of mycobacterium tuberculosis from a clinical specimen is important to confirm the diagnosis.

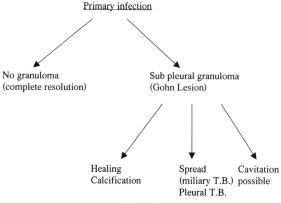

Scheme 1.

3.1.1. Clinical samples

Sputum, bronchial lavage aspirate, gastric aspirate and/or pleural fluid aspirate are dispatched to the laboratory for microbiological studies including fresh smear examination and culture. Any excised or biopsy tissue material should also be cultured as well as being examined histopathologically.

3.1.2. Immunodiagnosis

This is based on T lymphocyte recognition of *M. tuberculosis* (see tuberculin skin test). The positive test is indicative of the individual's previous exposure to *M. tuberculosis* antigens and cannot distinguish between active disease, latent infection or B.C.G. (Bacillus Calmet Guerin) vaccinated (immune) individuals. Another drawback of the test is that it fails to detect some 20% of those co-infected with human immunodeficiency virus (HIV).

3.1.3. Biopsies

Lymph node biopsy, pleural and pulmonary needle biopsies are performed to obtain samples of tissue. Thoracoscopy may be used with great advantage to obtain pleural/pulmonary tissue samples.

4. Management

4.1. Management and evolution

Since the 1950s, the availability of tuberculous chemotherapeutic agents has completely altered the management and the evolution of pulmonary tuberculosis. The commonly used drugs are Isoniazid (INAH), Rifampicin (R), Pyrazinamide (Z), Ethambutol (E), and Streptomycin (S). Different regimens are devised and recommended for different populations according to the at-risk susceptibility of that population and the prevalence of drug resistant organisms. The regimen consists of a combination of drugs, frequency of their administration and duration of treatment. The recommended regimen in the UK and many developed countries is an initial two month course of three drugs of INAH + R + Z followed by four months of INAH + R. If there is a high risk of initial Isoniozid resistance, the regimen is changed to two months of E + INAH + R + Z followed by four months of INAH + R. Detailed anti-tuberculous chemotherapy regimens and their schedules are beyond the scope of this chapter. Reference should be made to appropriate texts. It is however to be noted that anti-tuberculous chemotherapy is attended by morbidity as well as mortality.

4.2. The role of surgery

In the present state of drug therapy, the role of surgery in management of pulmonary tuberculosis is limited and can be described under the following:
- Patients with multi-drug resistance (resistance to at least two drugs) mycobacteria and persisting cavities.
- Patients with localised destroyed pulmonary parenchyma with evidence of relapsing disease.
- Patients with serious complications, notably aspergilloma or life threatening haemoptysis.
- Serious bronchial stenosis with distant non-healing cavity.
- Patients with tuberculous bronchiectasis not responding to therapy.
- Bronchopleural fistula and empyema (see chapters I.20 and I.25).

In most developed countries, some cases fall into the above categories.

The goals of surgery are:
- To eliminate the mycobacteria and to surgically excise the cavity or other pulmonary lesions which are the actual and/or potential "breeding ground".
- To achieve minimal resection with conservation of parenchyma.

These aims may be achieved by wedge/segmental resection although in some cases, the loss of parenchyma can be limited to two segments (apical and posterior segments of the upper lobes). However, lobectomy and/or even pneumonectomy may become necessary. In fact, the proportion of pneumonectomies in a recently reported series has increased to 50% or more.

4.2.1. Pre-surgical investigation and preparation

Patients who are candidates for pulmonary resection should be thoroughly investigated in order to establish suitability for surgical operation and type of operation. The pre-requisite is that all such patients will have had sufficient and appropriate anti-tuberculosis chemotherapy with a team approach to treatment involving a respiratory physician. The following are the pre-surgical requirements:
- Plain chest radiography and CT scan.
- Bronchoscopy to exclude active tuberculous bronchial lesion.
- Pulmonary function and ventilation perfusion isotope scan. With regard to the latter; the more extensive the resection considered, the more essential the V/Q scan becomes.
- Nutritional assessment is necessary in debilitated

patients; correction of severe deficiencies are important to reduce post-operative morbidity and mortality.

- Conversion to negative culture is not achievable in many drug resistant cases and is not a pre-requisite of resection. However, peri-operative drug therapy will be necessary and, usually, long term medical treatment will need to extend to many months.

5. Special note on pulmonary surgery for tuberculosis

5.1. Access

- At the present time, apart from cases which present as a peripheral pulmonary nodule (tuberculoma), which may be excised thoracoscopically, others require standard thoracotomy (postero-lateral).
- A double lumen endotracheal tube should be used to isolate the diseased lung.
- Cavitating lesions and bronchiectatic areas should be resected. Segmentectomy (apical and posterior segments of the upper lobe and/or lobar resection) can usually be achieved. Pneumonectomy should be avoided if at all possible though in a totally destroyed lung with reasonably healthy and functionally acceptable controlateral lung, particularly in the presence of multi-resistant organism, pneumonectomy may be performed.
- The author prefers hand sewing of the bronchus but staples have been used with no particular disadvantage. Effort should be made to cover the bronchial stump; pedicle (intercostal muscle) graft is used by many including the author.
- Expansion of the residual lung is important to prevent pleural space infection, though in patients with "stiff" lung this may be difficult.
- In many cases it is advantageous to mobilise the lung extra-pleurally, particularly in chronic cases and if there has been previous artificial pneumothorax.
- Candidates for operation should have received adequate chemotherapy. The adequacy of drug therapy is judged by monitoring the evolution of the disease, taking into account therapy and compliance of the patient, and may take from one to ten years or more.
- Effort should be made to achieve negative culture pre-operatively. However, this may not be achievable and does not in itself constitute contra-indication to surgery.

6. Tuberculosis and the relevance of human immunodeficiency virus (HIV) infection to surgery

HIV infection affects the course and evolution of pulmonary tuberculosis in a number of ways but mainly as follows:

- Emergence of multi-drug-resistant organisms.
- Reactivation of quiescent disease and rapid evolution of primary infection to progressive infection.
- Acute tuberculosis also accelerates the clinical progression of HIV.

Since one of the major indications of surgery in tuberculosis is related to cases with multi-drug resistance, this is an important area where thoracic surgery will have a therapeutic role. Apart from precautionary measures related to HIV infection, no alteration of indications or technique applies with respect to medical treatment.

- Medical therapy for HIV infected patients with tuberculosis is no different from those with HIV sero negative. However, the multiple drug resistant tuberculosis in HIV sero positive patients is a problem for medical treatment and it is these patients who may require surgical therapy as the medical treatment fails.

7. Complications and results of surgery for pulmonary tuberculosis

- Broncho pleural fistula (BPF) is the most important complication reaching to about 10% in multi-drug resistant cases requiring extensive surgery.
- The incidence of post resection haemothorax is also higher than for non-tuberculosis resection.
- Empyema.

The result of surgery is good in the majority of patients, even those with multi-drug resistance who do not convert to negative culture for mycobacteria. Anti-tuberculosis drugs should be continued after surgical resection.

References and further reading

Ashour M. Pneumonectomy for tuberculosis. Eur J Cardiothorac Surg 1997; 12: 209–213.

Connolly MA, Chaule P, Raniglione MC. Epidimiology of tuberculosis in Tuberculosis. In: R Wilson (ed.), European Respiratory Monograph (Vol. 2), European Respiratory Journal, Sheffield, UK, 1997; pp. 51–67.

Hudson EH, Holmes Sellors T. Pulmonary tuberculosis surgical treatment. In: Perry and Holmes Sellors (eds.), Chest Disease, London, Butterworth, 1963: pp. 309–345.

Kir A, Tahaoglu K, Okur E. Role of surgery in multi-drug-resistant tuberculosis: results of 27 cases. Eur J Cardiothorac Surg 1997; 12: 531–534.

Masden LA, Isman MD. Management of drug-resistant tuberculosis. Chest Surg Clin North Am 1994; 3: 715–721.

Moroni M, Antinuir S, Eposito R. Tuberculosis, atypical mycobacteria and human immunodeficiency virus: an overview in Tuberculosis. In: Wilson R (ed.), European Respiratory Society Monograph (Vol. 2). European Respiratory Journal, Sheffield, UK, 1997.

Ormerod LP. Chemotherapy of tuberculosis in Tuberculosis. In: Wilson R (ed.), European Respiratory Society Monograph (Vol. 2). European Respiratory Journal, Sheffield, UK, 1997.

Pomerantz M, Masden L, Goble M, et al. Surgical management of resistant mycobacterial tuberculosis and other mycobacterial pulmonary infections. Ann Thorac Surg 1991; 52: 1108–1112.

Sung SW, Kang CH, Kim YT, et al. Surgery increased the chance of cure in multi-drug-resistant pulmonary tuberculosis. Eur J Cardiothorac Surg 1999; 16(2): 187–193.

Treasure RL, Seaworth BJ. Current role of surgery in *Mycobacterium tuberculosis*. Ann Thorac Surg 1995; 59: 1406–1409.

Tuberculosis. Wilson R (ed.). European Respiratory Monograph Vol. 2, 1997, European Respiratory Society Journal Ltd, Sheffield, UK.

CHAPTER I.11

Sarcoidosis

K. Moghissi

1. Introduction

Sarcoidosis is a multi-system granulomatous disorder of unknown aetiology which commonly affects the young and which most typically presents itself as bilateral pulmonary hilar lymphadenopathy. Thoracic sarcoidosis constitutes 70% of all cases. The other organs affected by the disease are the liver, spleen, eyes and phalangeal bones.

The disease affects the lungs in a number of ways:
- sarcoid granuloma (resembling tuberculosis) eventually leading to pulmonary fibrosis;
- mediastinal lymphadenopathy;
- peri-bronchial lymphadenopathy with bronchial stenosis, pulmonary atelectasis and infection.

1.1. Presentation and clinical manifestation

The lung is the most common site for sarcoidosis. In many instances the condition is asymptomatic and is discovered in the course of chest radiography. In symptomatic patients the presentation is variable, ranging from insidious onset of malaise, fatigue and fever to more acute respiratory disease symptoms. Cough, usually without expectoration, wheeze and dyspnoea are usually present. Occasionally, thoracic sarcoid is part of a more prominent clinical manifestation of the sarcoidosis of other systems such as:
- sarcoid of the skin, which manifests itself as erythema nodosum associated with bilateral pulmonary hilar sarcoid lymphadenopathy (Lofgren's syndrome);
- in Heerfordt's syndrome (uveoparotid fever) there is uveitis, parotid gland swelling, fever and cranial nerve palsies.

2. Investigation and diagnosis

2.1. Radiology

- Plain chest radiograph shows a variety of images depending on the stage of the disease. Characteristically, hilar lymphadenopathy is the earliest change (Stage I). More advanced cases demonstrate diffuse interstitial infiltration (Stage II) with hilar lymphadenopathy (Stage III), or without.
  In further advanced cases, core infiltration, honeycombing and hilar retraction are seen.
- CT Scan shows lymphadenopathy of the mediastinum, peribronchial and perivascular node enlargement.

2.2. Bronchoscopy

Bronchoscopy may show extrinsic lobar and/or segment bronchial stenosis.

2.3. Laboratory tests

Laboratory findings are helpful in the elimination of other granulomatous conditions rather than in the diagnosis of sarcoidosis. Blood count shows no special characteristics and biochemical profile abnormalities such as hypercalcaemia and hyperglobulinaemia are non-specific.

The diagnosis is based essentially on tissue biopsy and histology. This is where the thoracic surgeon becomes involved in sarcoidosis, which is not a surgical disease.

2.4. Surgical investigatory methods

2.4.1. Lymph node biopsy
(a) Scalene node biopsy will provide the histological diagnosis in over 70% of cases.

(b) Transbronchial biopsy of lung is useful with 70–90% diagnostic yield in those with pulmonary infiltration.
(c) Mediastinoscopy and mediastinal node biopsy is almost always diagnostic in patients with mediastinal lymphadenopathy.
(d) Mediastinotomy is always diagnostic in experienced hands.
(e) Thoracoscopy (Video-Assisted Thoracoscopy) is useful not only for gland biopsy but also for lung biopsy.

2.4.2. Open lung biopsy

With the re-emergence of VATs, this method is now less favoured. Nevertheless, it is sometimes necessary to perform open lung biopsy, in which case limited thoracotomy is carried out via an appropriate route using muscle-sparing technique.

2.4.3. Biopsy of skin, visible lesion or palpable lymph node

Biopsy of skin, visible lesion or palpable lymph node can have variable yield but should be tried if easily accessible.

2.4.4. Kveim test

This is based on inoculation by the injection of sarcoid products into the skin (usually suspension of 0.1 ml of 10%) which, in patients with sarcoidosis, will induce a sarcoid nodule to develop at the site of injection. The nodule is then excised and examined under the microscope.

The advantage of the test is that in difficult cases, it may remove the necessity for a thoracotomy. However, its great disadvantage is the delay (4–6 weeks) in development of a nodule which may be excised and examined histologically showing the typical sarcoid tissue. This delay may be harmful when therapeutic measures are urgently required.

3. Pathology and evolution

The lesion in sarcoidosis is akin to tuberculous granuloma but there is no caseation and no micobacteria as in the case of tuberculosis.

The effect of sarcoid progression depends on the topography of the lymphadenopathy and the importance of pulmonary infiltration. Sarcoid granuloma of a bronchial lymph node may cause bronchial stenosis and distal bronchiectasis, pulmonary infection and scarring. Independently, pulmonary infiltrate and granuloma will eventually lead to pulmonary fibrosis.

However, not all cases of sarcoidosis progress to the final stage of scarring/fibrosis; in some cases there is spontaneous resolution of the disease.

Corticosteroid therapy in advanced symptomatic cases is helpful to relieve symptoms and will delay evolution of the disease.

4. Treatment

The aetiology of sarcoidosis is unknown and there is no specific treatment for the disease; however, medications are helpful for symptom relief and for the treatment of complications.

Treatment is warranted:

- in patients with progressive pulmonary infiltration and fibrosis (Stage II and Stage III disease) who develop symptoms;
- in those patients with hypercalcaemia;
- in patients with involvement of eye, kidney, heart or central nervous system.

The usual treatment is corticosteroidal. In severe cases a high dose of 40–60 mg (0.5–1 mg/kg b.w.) may be initiated, tapering the dose with improvement. Other medications such as Chloroquine and Cyclosporine have been tried with as yet unproven efficiency.

In end stage disease the choice is limited to transplantation.

References and further reading

Blewett CJ, Bennett WF, Miller JD, Urschel JD. Open lung biopsy as an outpatient procedure. Ann Thorac Surg 2001; 71(4): 1113–1115.

English JC 3rd, Patel PJ, Greer KE. Sarcoidosis. J Am Acad Dermatol 2001; 44(5): 725–743.

James DG. Sarcoidosis 2001. Postgrad Med J 2001; 77(905): 177–180.

Judson MA, Uflacker R. Treatment of a solitary pulmonary sarcoidosis mass by CT guided direct intralesional injection of corticosteroid. Chest 2001; 120(1): 316–317.

Luisetti M, Beretta A, Casali L. Genetic aspects in sarcoidosis. Eur Respir J 2000; 16(4): 768–780.

Shorr AF, Torrington KG, Hnatiuk OW. Endobronchial biopsy for sarcoidosis: a prospective study. Chest 2001; 120(1): 109–114.

Statement on sarcoidosis. Joint statement of the American Thoracic Society (ATS), the European Respiratory Society (ERS) and the World Association of Sarcoidosis and Other Granulomatous Disorders (WASOG) adopted by the ATS Board of Directors and by the ERS Executive Committee, February 1999. Am J Respir Crit Care Med 1999; 160: 736–755.

K. Moghissi, J.A.C. Thorpe and F. Ciulli (Eds.)
Moghissi's Essentials of Thoracic and Cardiac Surgery
© 2003 Elsevier Science B.V. All rights reserved

CHAPTER I.12

Fungal infections of the lung

K. Moghissi

1. Introduction

1.1. General characteristics

Of the variety of fungal infections, many share the following common general characteristics:
- An overall majority of fungi are soil organisms.
- The mode of infection is by inhalation and the port of entry is the respiratory system.
- In many cases, inhalation of the organism is not followed by infection, or the infection remains subclinical as evidenced by positive skin and serological tests with no clinical sign of infection.
- The presentation in some is influenza-like symptoms with no permanent pathological sequallae. In a few, systemic and pulmonary infection follows; patchy infiltration and changes akin to bronchopneumonia is the characteristic radiological finding.
- Many chronic fungal infections of the lung present with thick walled cavity or abscess.
- In some cases, when infection is unresolved, single or multiple nodular lesions persist in the lung and mimic neoplastic lesions.
- Two types of serological tests are useful for the diagnosis of fungal infection:
  - detection of antibodies against a specific fungal antigen;
  - identification of circulatory antigens. Serial serological testing is undertaken usually at 3–4 weekly intervals.

1.2. Role of the thoracic surgeon

The role of the thoracic surgeon in the management of fungal pulmonary disease is related to:
- diagnosis: when either endoscopy or biopsy is needed for identification of the organism;

- resection of lesions suspected of being malignant;
- when medical treatment cannot control the disease and/or there are complications despite active therapy.

1.3. Factors influencing treatment

In recent years two additional important groups of factors have influenced treatment: outcome and the role of surgery in fungal infections.

There has been an increase in the number of immuno-compromised patients due to:
- widespread use of immuno-suppressive agents in conjunction with organ transplantation;
- cancer chemotherapy;
- HIV infections.

These have complicated the management task. The development and availability of antifungal drugs have had a positive effect in reducing the complications of these infections.

Description in detail of fungal diseases and their characteristics is beyond the scope of this book. However, a summary of those which most frequently affect the lung is recorded in Table 1. Aspergillosis will be described separately in some detail because of its particular relevance to thoracic surgery.

2. Aspergillosis infection of the lung

2.1. Causes and types

The disease is usually caused by *Aspergillus fumigatus*, and less commonly by *Aspergillus niger* and *Aspergillus flavus*. Aspergilli are saprophytes: Aspergillosis rarely affects normal tissue or healthy individuals but tends to attack debilitated subjects and devitalised parts of the body.

Bronchopulmonary Aspergillosis is of three types:

Table 1

Fungal organisms/infections of the lung

Name	Organisms	Port of entry / Type of infection	Presentation
Actinomycosis and nocardiosis	• *Actinomyces israelii* • *Nocardia asteroid*	• Opportunistic • Endogenous (Tonsilar cryptes, carious teeth) • Aspiration of organism	• Insidious onset (cough, sputum, pain) • Haemoptysis possible
Aspergillosis	*Aspergillus fumigatus* *A. niger* *A. flavus*	• Respiratory/Inhalation • Allergic • Abscess • Aspergilloma	• Depends on type
Blastomycosis	• Dimorphic fungus • *Blastomyces dermatitidis*	• Respiratory/Inhalation • Often no infection (immuno-competent) • Sometimes systemic • Lungs • Skeletal • Skin	• Acute respiratory infection • Influenza type • Cough • Severe pain
Coccidioido–Mycocis	• Dimorphic fungus • *Coccidioides immitis*	• Respiratory/Inhalation • Often asymptomatic/few symptoms • Pulmonary • Disseminated • Meningitis	• Asymptomatic or influenza type symptoms (fever, cough, chest pain) • Skin rash possible (Erythema nodosum) • Chronic form lasting for weeks/months unless treated
Cryptococcosis (Formerly Torulosis)	• *Cryptococcus neoformans* (encapsulated yeast like in soil + avian [pigeon] excreta)	• Inhalation • Respiratory tract	• Chronic bronchopulmonary disease • Meningitis • Prevalence + in immuno-compromised
Histoplasmosis	• *Histoplasma capsulatum*	• Respiratory/Inhalation • Often none or mild symptoms similar to common cold • Systemic disease possible	• Asymptomatic • Influenza-like symptoms • Acute respiratory infection
Moniliasis (of human respiratory tract and intestine)	• *Candida albicans* yeast like organism	• Endogenous	• Distressing cough • Bronchial moniliasis • No pyrexia
Mucormycosis	• Class Zygomycetes • Order Mucorales	• Respiratory/inhalation always predisposing factors	• Fever • Cough • Severe dyspnoea • Haemoptysis
Sporotrichosis	• Dimorphic fungus • *Sporotrix schencki* (found worldwide in soil)	• Usually subcutaneous inoculation of spore • Inhalation possible • Pulmonary lesion rare: mimic TB	• Verrucous ulceration of skin and lymph node

Abbreviations: Amph B = Amphotericin B; CNS = Central nervous system; TB = Tuberculosis; CSF = Cerebrospinal fluid.

• Allergic type: *Aspergillus fumigatus* colonises the bronchial tree; bronchitis or bronchial infection with asthmatic or allergic manifestation will en-sue. Some cases progress into bronchiectasis. This type is not of surgical concern.

• Invasive or disseminated Aspergillosis with necro-

Evolution	Radiology (CXR)	Diagnosis	Treatment
• Primary pulmonary abscess and sinuses tracking to chest wall. • Secondary haematogenous dissemination – CNS • Soft tissue abscess + sinuses • Pyogenic pulmonary lesions	• Infiltration • Necrosis + cavitation	• Organism identification in sputum • Sulfur granule • Bronchoscopy + brush, biopsy, lung aspiration	• Medical • Penicillin Sulfonamide • Surgery for abscess • Drainage of empyema
• Abscess • Aspergilloma	• Typical in Aspergilloma	• Isolation + Culture	• Medical – if no complication • Surgical in bleeding Aspergilloma
• Sometimes lymphatic spread to lymph nodes • Pulmonary suppuration + cavitation	• Acute phase infective feature • Chronic cavity or mass mimicking carcinoma	• Organism culture identification • Immunological tests unreliable	• Medical • Surgery for complications • Thoracotomy for mass
• Complete healing • Small number (bronchiectasis, pulmonary abscess, pulmonary nodules) • Meningitis • Empyema	• Pneumonitis/infiltration • Pleural effusion • Cystic cavity with secondary abscess • Tumour like density • Pneumothorax • Empyema	• Organism identification in tissue • Isolation of organism in culture • Skin sensitivity • Compliment fixation	• Symptomatic • Amph B • Surgery for cavity or tumour mass • Surgery for complications
• Spontaneous remission • Pulmonary form – benign • CNS: Serious/Fatal	• Non specific • Pneumonitis • Tumour like mass	• Usually diagnosis is made after resection • Examine CSF if organism seen in sputum/resected specimen • Serology – doubtful value	• Medical • Amph B • 5-Fluoro-cytosine • Surgery for tumour like mass
• Lymphatic involvement – granuloma • Necrosis in lung (caseating granuloma)	• Patchy consolidation • Cavity • Nodular lesions • Solitary nodule (like Cancer) • Mediastinal Granulomatosis	• Direct sputum examination • Culture of organism from pathological specimen • Serology not entirely reliable	• Amph B • Surgery for complications
• Pulmonary minilosis	• Ill-defined patchy shadows	• Sputum • Mucous membrane sample examination	• Disinfections • Improve general health • No antibiotics
• Pulmonary contamination • Fatal haemoptysis	• Cavitation • Pulmonary infiltration	• Tissue sample • Histology (after staining)	• Medical – Amph B and/or surgical excision
• Mostly skin • If pulmonary it can mimic TB/histoplasmosis	• Chronic pneumonitis • Infiltration • Cavity	• Identification of organism in sputum + culture	• Medical – Potassium iodide (skin) • Amph B (pulmonary) • Surgery for complications + residual cavity

tising bronchopneumonia: This typically occurs in immuno-deficient and/or immuno-suppressed and debilitated individuals.
• Saprophytic type: aspergilloma or "fungus ball".

Most infections are caused by *A. fumigatus*. The organism can be recovered from pathological material by isolation and culture.

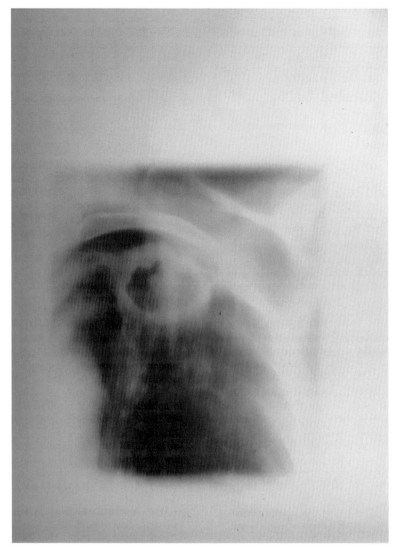

Fig. 1. Pulmonary aspergilloma in a tuberculous cavity.

2.2. Aspergilloma (Fig. 1)

The thoracic surgeon is generally concerned with aspergilloma which is caused by *A. fumigatus*, an organism found in soil and decaying vegetation. The spores of the organism are inhaled and colonise lungs already damaged by chronic lung disease and/or pre-existing cavities such as bronchogenic cysts and/or tuberculosis.

2.2.1. Presentation
In about 50% of cases, aspergillomas present as episodes of haemoptysis, which at times can be serious and life threatening. However, many patients remain asymptomatic or are discovered in the course of radiological follow-up for the progress of a treatment or during routine radiology. Evolution to systemic disease is rare and some may resolve spontaneously.

2.2.2. Radiological appearance
The radiological appearance of aspergilloma is so typical as to be diagnostic. The characteristic features are:
– A cavity with a solid tumour-like mass within it, leaving a translucent crescent halo above it, usually in the upper lobe. This image is due to the fungus ball (mycetoma) within an air-containing cavity. The fungus ball is a matted sphere of hyphae, fibrin with inflammatory cells and necrotic amorphous material.

2.3. Treatment

2.3.1. Antifungal drugs

Medical treatment using antifungal drugs such as Amphotericin B systemically is of little help in aspergillomas because the cavity containing the "ball" is poorly perfused. However, in invasive aspergillosis, common in immuno-compromised patients, intravenous administration of Amphotericin B is an effective treatment.

2.3.2. Bronchial artery embolisation

Combined with the intravenous administration of Amphotericin B, this is effective in patients with haemoptysis who are unsuitable for major resectional surgery.

2.3.3. Percutaneous cavernostomy

In elderly patients of poor physical condition in whom major surgery is contraindicated, cavernostomy may be carried out using a percutaneous method. In this method a catheter is inserted under imaging guidance and the aspergilloma cavity is first washed and then sodium iodide or Amphotericin B is instilled into it. In invasive aspergillosis, common in immuno-compromised patients, intravenous administration of Amphotericin B is an effective treatment.

2.3.4. Surgical cavernostomy

Aspergilloma is approached through standard or even limited access thoracotomy. The cavity is incised and its content is evacuated. The author sutures any bronchial opening identified by underwater (saline) testing whilst the anaesthetist inflates the lung with pressure of 30 cm of water. The wall is then obliterated by suturing the walls of the cavity together. Some surgeons leave the cavity open or apply intercostal muscle (myoplasty) over it.

2.3.5. Surgical resection

In patients with haemoptysis, surgical resection is the treatment of choice, provided that the patient is fit for such an operation. It is important to bear in mind that surgical resection for aspergilloma can, in some cases, be tedious because of dense pleural and chest wall adhesions and because of considerable fibrous scarring of the pulmonary parenchyma around the aspergilloma. There is also a high incidence of postoperative complication, particularly in thick-walled cavity aspergillomas and in those with pericavitary parenchymal Aspergillous infiltration (complex aspergilloma). Given the above scenario it is the general opinion that asymptomatic patients should not be offered surgery except for those with associated lesions.

Post resection complications. Post resection complications most commonly encountered are:
- haemothorax;
- persistent/prolonged air leak;
- poor expansion of the lung leaving residual pleural space;
- empyema;
- bronchopleural fistula;
- wound infection.

2.3.6. Results of surgical resection

Mortality from 4.5% to over 40% has been recorded (Babatasi et al., 2000; Battaglini et al., 1985; Jewkes et al., 1983; Massard et al., 1992). The present-day mortality is within 4–10% depending on the complexity of the case. All reported series highlight the high morbidity rate of 30% or more. In a series of 84 patients with aspergilloma reported by Csekeo et al. (1997), 52 patients had lobectomy, 13 had wedge resection and 6 had pneumonectomy. Of the remaining 13 patients, 12 had cavernostomy and one had exploration and lung biopsies. Peri-operative mortality and morbidity for 72 patients who had resection were 9.7% and 40% respectively.

3. Mucormycosis

Mucormycosis is a rare fungal infection which particularly affects those receiving immuno-suppression therapy, diabetics and patients with serious haematological disorders.

The pulmonary manifestations present with productive cough, dyspnoea and haemoptysis. The latter should be considered as a serious sign of a poor prognosis.

The diagnosis of mucormycosis is based on identification of characteristic hyphae by staining (hematoxylin and eosin or indigo carmine stains) at histological examination. Culture of the organism is difficult. Radiology is not pathognomonic and usually demonstrates cavitation with/without pulmonary infiltration. Treatment consists of Amphotericin B and/or surgery. Mortality is high for either treatment, often as a result of haemoptysis.

The characteristic pathological feature is penetration of the fungus through the broncho-vascular wall to cause bronchial obstruction or vascular embolism.

References and further reading

Al-Kattan K, Ashour M, Hajjar W et al. Surgery of pulmonary aspergilloma in post tuberculous vs. immuno-compromised patients. Eur J Cardiothorac Surg 2001; 20: 728–733.

Babatasi G, Massetti M, Chapelier A, Fadel E, Macchiarini P, Khayat A, Dartvelle P. Surgical treatment of pulmonary aspergilloma: current outcome. J Thorac Cardiovasc Surg 2000; 119: 906–912.

Battaglini JW, Murray GF, Keagy BA et al. Surgical management of symptomatic pulmonary Aspergilloma. Ann Thorac Surg 1985; 39: 512–516.

Chemotherapy of the pulmonary mycoses. Official statement of the American Thoracic Society. Am Rev Resp Dis 1988; 138: 1078–1081.

Chen KY, Ko SC, Hsueh PR, Luh KT, Yang PC. Pulmonary fungal infection: emphasis on microbiological spectra: patient outcome and prognostic factors. Chest 2001; 120: 177–184.

Collins DM, Dillard TA, Grathwohl KW, Giacoppe GN, Arnold BF. Bronchial mucormycosis with progressive air trapping. Mayo Clin Proc 1999; 74: 698–701.

Csekeo A, Agocs L, Egeruary M, Heilen Z. Surgery for pulmonary aspergillosis. Eur J Cardiothorac Surg 1997; 12: 876–879.

Daly R, Pairolero PC, Piehler JM et al. Pulmonary aspergilloma: results of surgical treatment. J Thorac Cardiovasc Surg 1986; 92: 981–988.

Fitzgerald EJ, Coblentz C. Fungal microabscesses in immuno-suppressed patients: CT appearances. Can Assoc Radiol J 1988; 39: 10–12.

Grover FL, Hopeman AR. Mycotic infection. In: Pearson FG, Deslauriers J, Ginsberg RJ (eds.), Thoracic Surgery. Churchill Livingstone, New York. 1995; pp 476–503.

Hay RJ. Antifungal therapy and the new Azole compounds. J Antimicrob Chemother 1991; 28: 35–46.

Israel RH, Poe RH, Greenblatt DW, Swalback WG. Differentiation of tuberculous from nontuberculous cavitary lung disease. Respiration 1985; 47: 151–157.

Jewkes J, Kay PH, Paneth M, Citron KM. Pulmonary aspergilloma: analysis of prognosis in relation to haemoptysis and survey of treatment. Thorax 1983; 38: 572–578.

Johnson PC, Sarosi GA. The endemic mycoses: surgical considerations. Semin Thorac Cardiovasc Surg 1995; 2: 95–103.

Lee FY, Mossad SB, Adal KA. Pulmonary mucormycosis: the last 30 years. Arch Intern Med 1999; 159: 1301–1309.

Lyman CA, Walsh TJ. Systemically administered antifungal agents. A review of their clinical pharmacology and therapeutic applications. Drugs 1992; 44(1): 9–35.

Magilligan DJ, Ravipati S, Zayat P et al. Massive haemoptysis control by transcatheter bronchial artery embolisation. Ann Thorac Surg 1981; 32:39.

Massard G, Roselin N, Wihlm JM et al. Pleuro-pulmonary aspergilloma: clinical spectrum and results of surgical treatment. Ann Thorac Surg 1992; 54: 1159–1164.

Moghissi K. Discussion of a paper by Csekeo A, Agocs L, Egervary M et al. Surgery for pulmonary aspergillosis. Eur J Cardiothorac Surg 1997; 12: 876–879.

Nicod LP, Pache JC, Howarth N. Fungal infections in transplant recipients. Eur Respir J 2001; 17: 133–140.

Row S, Cheadle WG. Complications of nosocomial pneumonia in the surgical patient. Am J Surg 2000; 179: 63–68.

Sarosi GA. Amphotericin B still the gold standard for antifungal therapy. Postgrad Med 1990; 88: 151–152.

Schiffman RL, Johnson TS, Weinberger SE, Weiss S St., Schwartz A. Candida lung abscess: successful treatment with Amphotericin B and 5-Flycytosine. Am Rev Resp Dis 1982; 125: 766–768.

Schwartz JR, Nagle MG, Elkins RC, Mohr JA. Mucormycosis of the trachea: an unusual cause of acute upper airway obstruction. Chest 1982; 81: 653–654.

Swanson KL, Johnson CM, Prakash UB et al. Bronchial artery embolisation: experience with 54 patients. Chest 2002; 121: 789–795.

Takaro T. Fungal infection. In: Grillo HG, Austin WC, Wilkins EW et al. (eds.), Current therapy in cardiothoracic surgery. Philadelphia: BC Decker, 1989; p. 161.

Vantrigt P. Lung infections and diffuse interstitial lung disease. In: Sabiston DC and Spencer FC (eds.), Surgery of the chest (Vol. 1). Philadelphia: WB Saunders Co, 1995; pp. 676–730.

Wong ML, Szkup P, Hopley MJ. Percutaneous embolotherapy for life-threatening haemoptysis. Chest 2002; 121: 95–102.

K. Moghissi, J.A.C. Thorpe and F. Ciulli (Eds.)
Moghissi's Essentials of Thoracic and Cardiac Surgery

CHAPTER I.13

Thoracic hydatid disease

K. Moghissi

1. Introduction

Hydatid disease is commonly caused by the cestodes *Echinococcus granulosus* and very rarely by *Echinococcus multilocularis*. The adult parasite measures 4–6 mm and comprises a head and 3 segments, each called proglottid. The last segment (pregnant proglottid) contains the eggs. In an infected animal this is the segment which, with its eggs, is discharged in the excrement. The detached eggs released from this segment are extremely resistant to physical and chemical agents. The human, in a similar way to sheep and cattle, is an intermediate host. The scheme of life cycle and infestation of human and sheep is shown in Fig. 1.

Humans acquire the disease through the alimentary tract by eating contaminated food which contain the ova. In the small intestine the ova develop into embryos which enter the portal vein to reach the capillaries of the liver and/or the lung where they lodge. Many embryos are destroyed by phagocytes but those who survive develop to the larval stage of the cestode which is in fact the hydatid cyst.

On reaching the liver the surviving embryos form cysts or migrate further to the lungs. If the embryo succeeds in passing through the pulmonary arterial capillaries to the pulmonary vein, hydatidosis in other organs could result. In the human, the distribution of the disease is about 56% in the liver, 25% in the lung and 19% in other organs.

A hydatid cyst possesses two membranes, an outer ectocyst and an inner endocyst (Fig. 2). The latter is the germinal layer which forms many sacs (brood capsules). From the inner part of the sac a head (scolex) is formed which then matures to a complete worm about 4–6 mm in length. The inner membrane of the cyst contains a clear fluid. The hydatid cyst is surrounded by an adventitious membrane formed by the host tissue reaction which is called the pericyst.

1.1. Epidemiology

In a number of countries there is a high incidence of the disease: Argentina, Chile and Uruguay in South America; Algeria and Tunisia in Africa; Turkey and Iran in Asia; the Balkans in Europe; and New Zealand and Australia. However, even in a low-risk country or in regions of a country with low incidence of the disease, hydatidosis can be seen occasionally amongst the indigenous population and also because of movement of population. It is, therefore, important that thoracic surgeons have knowledge of the disease, its characteristic features and its management.

2. Presentation and clinical features

In uncomplicated cases, that is those with intact (unruptured) cysts, patients may be asymptomatic. In such cases, the pulmonary hydatid cyst is discovered through chest radiography as an incidental finding. Only occasionally in uncomplicated cysts are there symptoms related to pressure by a large cyst surrounding the structure of the lung, pleura or mediastinal structures. In complicated cases, usually because of rupture of the cyst, symptoms are non-specific. Cough, chest pain, expectoration, haemoptysis and fever are the most common symptoms. Dyspnoea may be present in cases of large or multiple cysts.

2.1. Imaging Techniques

Typically, with an uncomplicated (unruptured) cyst, the chest X-ray shows a well-defined opacity, ho-

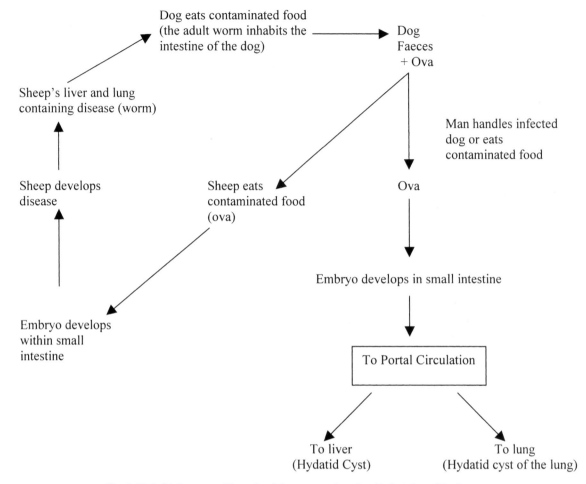

Fig. 1. Hydatid disease — life cycle of the worm and mode of infestation of the human.

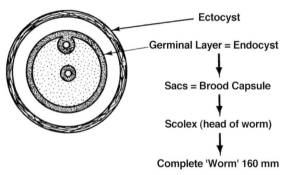

Fig. 2. Hydatid cyst.

mogenous in density and usually placed in the lower lobe of one lung. In complicated cases the radiological signs usually indicate air-fluid contrast either around the opacity or within it. The radiography may show a thin layer of air between the pericyst and ectocyst (meniscus signs) which indicate complication around the pericyst outside ectocyst (Fig. 2) and its communication with airways. When there is rupture of the cyst membranes into the bronchial tree, the cyst will appear as a cavity with a fluid level.

In some cases the chest radiograph shows a more diffuse type of lesion: neither a clearly definable cyst nor a peripheral pulmonary shadowing accompanied by pleural effusion. Plain chest radiograph together with history, symptoms and clinical examination can achieve diagnosis in over 90% of cases. When the cyst is in communication with the bronchial tree, its contents will be expectorated but contamination of the cavity can lead to infection or evolution to a microbial lung abscess.

CT scan, ultrasound and other imaging techniques add more information and are helpful in differential diagnosis. Such investigations should also be directed towards the liver. Rarely are ultrasonography and MRI used.

2.2. Laboratory tests

2.2.1. Sputum
Staining and microscopic examination of sputum may show parts of the parasite, which is diagnostic.

2.2.2. Casoni intradermal test
This is based on a similar principle to tests for tuberculosis. An intradermal injection of the antigen, i.e. sterilised hydatid fluid, into the anterior aspect of the forearm results within one hour in the production of a weal with erythema at the site of injection. Induration occurs 24–48 hours later. At the same time a control test is carried out of a similar volume of normal saline solution in the contralateral forearm. The site of the two injections should be compared to check the positivity of the test. It is, however, important to note that the test may remain negative in uncomplicated (unruptured) cyst despite existence of the disease.

There is some cross-reaction with some other parasites such as Taeniae and Schistosoma.

2.2.3. Complement fixation test (Weinberg reaction)
This test is based on detection-specific IgM which is present in 75% of cases, especially those with cyst membrane.

2.2.4. Blood test
There is no change in blood count in uncomplicated cases with intact cysts. However, when rupture occurs, white cell eosinophils of over 3% are believed to be almost always present.

3. Management

3.1. Prevention

In areas where there is a high prevalence of the disease, much can be done to reduce the incidence by education of the population (particularly dog owners), control of dogs, attention to hygiene and safety inspection within the meat industry.

3.2. Medical treatment

Mebenzadole and Albenzadole can achieve complete clinical response in a high percentage of small cysts, although there appears to be no clear selection criteria of patients who may achieve clear response. Also, the side effects of these drugs are considerable. The role of medication seems to be:
- in multiple cysts or those with rupture of the cyst at or before surgical treatment;
- in patients with incomplete eradication of the disease by surgery;
- in those with recurrent disease untreatable by further surgery.

3.3. Surgical treatment

The objectives of surgical treatment are:
- elimination of the parasite;
- eradication of lesions with preservation of maximum normal parenchyma;
- prevention of recurrence.

Regardless of the surgical method, it is important to employ measures which prevent rupture of the cyst and dissemination. This is achieved by:
- aspiration of the cyst at operation prior to its excision;
- injection of hypertonic saline solution into the cyst;
- lavage and suction of the residual cavity or residual area of adjacent pulmonary parenchyma using hypertonic saline solution.

It should be noted that the use of formaline or formaldehyde solution for prevention of contamination is not now practised because of its deleterious effect on tissue healing.

A variety of surgical methods may be used to excise the lesion. The goal is conservation of healthy parenchyma with removal of all disease.

3.3.1. Enucleation/cystectomy or pericystectomy
This is the simplest method and over 90% of cases can be treated in this way. Following thoracotomy the visceral pleura is incised and the pericyst opened. The shiny ecto- and endocyst is then enucleated; this is made easier by keeping the ventilation pressure low at the start. When the pericyst is opened higher, sustained pressure at the area of the cyst will assist the enucleation. Once the cyst is enucleated the remaining crater is cleaned, washed with saline and its wall approximated using absorbable sutures. Some surgeons prefer to excise the pericyst but this creates more air leak and blood ooze and its advantages have not been clearly demonstrated.

3.3.2. Wedge/segmental resection and lobectomy
The size of the cyst and the extent of parenchymal changes around the main lesion, together with the suspicion that the cyst may have ruptured or leaked through the pericyst, dictates the need for surgical excision of the cyst together with wedge, segment or lobe of the lung.

3.3.3. Bilateral lesion

When the topography of lesions permits access through a median sternotomy, this may be carried out. When access is difficult a staged operation at different times is preferable. The side containing larger cysts, or those at higher risk of rupture, should be dealt with first.

3.3.4. Medical therapy adjunct to surgery

The present trend is:

(a) for intact cysts: to use Mebendazole 7–10 days pre-operatively followed by a 30-day course.
(b) for cysts ruptured pre- or intra-operatively: to use Mebendazole 7–10 days before the operation followed by 3–6 months post-operatively.

3.3.5. Surgical results

The overall peri-operative mortality is less than 2% rising to about 5% when lung and liver are involved. Long-term surgical results are excellent. In Burgos et al.'s (1999) series of 240 patients treated surgically with 10–18 year follow-up, nearly 90% remained disease-free and over 92% had no recurrence of pulmonary hydatid.

3.3.6. Complications of surgery

Between 10% and 15% of patients develop post-operative complications, of which pneumothorax, empyema, wound sepsis, biliary fistula and bronchopleural fistula are important. Multiple cysts may develop at different sites. Extension of right lung cyst to liver necessitates simultaneous excision of cysts in both organs using thoracotomy or laparotomy. Alternatively thoracotomy and trans-diaphragmatic approach may be used.

Extension/rupture of the cyst to the pleural space creates hydro-pneumothorax of varying degree. Initial tube drainage is necessary followed by emergency thoracotomy in rare cases. This depends on the severity of bronchopleural fistula and the existence of active and living parasites.

References and further reading

Athanassiadi K, Kalavrouziotis G, Loutisidis A, Bellenis I, Exarchos N. Surgical treatment of echinococcosis by trans thoracic approach — A review of 85 cases. Eur J Cardiothorac Surg 1998; 14: 134–140.

Aubert M, Viard P. Étude statistique sur l'hydatidose. Pleuropulmonaire dans le basin Méditerranéen en 1982. À propos de 8,384 cas. Ann Chir 1983; 37: 74–77.

Burgos R, Varela A, Castedo E, Roda J et al. Pulmonary hydatidosis: surgical treatment and follow up of 240 cases. Eur J Cardiothorac Surg 1999; 16: 628–635.

Dogan R, Yuksel M, Cetin G, Suzer K, Alp M, Kaya S et al. Surgical treatment of hydatid cysts of the lung. Report on 1055 patients. Thorax 1989: 44: 192–199.

Gil-Grande LA, Boixeda D, Garcia-Hoz F, Barcena R et al. Treatment of liver hydatid disease with mebendazole: a prospective study of thirteen cases. Am J Gastroenterol 1983; 78: 584–588.

Khorasani AR, Saidi F, Roberts AJ. Surgical treatment of hydatid cyst. J Thorac Cardiovasc Surg 1987; 93: 636–637.

Morris DL, Dkes PW, Marriner S, Bogan J et al. Albendazole; objective evidence of response in human hydatid disease. JAMA 1985; 253: 2053–2057.

Zapatero J, Madrigal L, Lago J, Baschwitz B, Perez E, Candelas J. Surgical treatment of thoracic hydatidosis — A review of 100 cases. Eur J Cardiothorac Surg 1989; 3(5): 436–440.

K. Moghissi, J.A.C. Thorpe and F. Ciulli (Eds.)
Moghissi's Essentials of Thoracic and Cardiac Surgery

CHAPTER I.14

Emphysema and surgery of bullous emphysema

K. Moghissi

1. Introduction — Definition

The European Respiratory Society (ERS) defines emphysema in anatomical terms as "the permanent destructive enlargement of airspaces distal to the terminal bronchioles without obvious fibrosis". This is the generally agreed definition and accords with that of the World Health Organisation (WHO) and the American Thoracic Society. It should, nevertheless, be emphasised that such a structural and anatomo-pathologically based definition implies that the diagnosis of emphysema depends on tissue sampling and histological examination by the pathologist. In fact the clinical diagnosis of emphysema is difficult but its manifestations are close to those of chronic obstructive pulmonary disease (COPD), a clinical condition based on physiopathological changes seen in emphysema and chronic bronchitis. The ERS defines COPD in simple functional spirometric terms as "reduction in maximum expiratory flow and slow forced emptying of the lung which is slowly progressive and mostly irreversible to present medical treatment".

The structural changes found in COPD are those of emphysema and chronic bronchitis in variable mix.

2. Classification

2.1. Pathological classification

Pathologically emphysema has been classified into 3 subtypes.

- Panacinar emphysema (Syn Panlobular) consists of a large air space uniformly across the acinar unit. It is commonly associated with alfa antitrypsin deficiency.
- Centriacinar (Syn Proximal acinar, centrilobular) where abnormal air spaces are found together with apparently normal lung. The pathology primarily involves the respiratory bronchioles.
- Paraseptal (Syn distal acinar) is characterised by involvement of peripheral air spaces.

2.2. Clinical and surgical classification

A generally agreed classification useful to the clinician and relevant to the surgeon groups emphysema into the following categories (Dijkman, 1986).

2.2.1. Compensatory emphysema
This is not a true emphysema since there is no air space destruction; it is an over-inflation of the lung adjacent to areas of atelectasis when localised compensatory emphysema occurs in pulmonary infection and tumours or foreign body aspiration. In its more generalised form it is seen in residual lung after extensive pulmonary resection, such as pneumonectomy.

2.2.2. Diffuse obstructive emphysema
This type is a major cause of COPD and itself comprises two subtypes referred to as dry and wet emphysema. The main characteristics of these two subtypes are presented in Table 1.

Diffuse obstructive emphysema and its surgical treatment are described in chapter IV.2.

2.2.3. Bullous emphysema
This covers a range of conditions, at one end of which is a large bulla within an otherwise normal pulmonary parenchyma, and at the other end is bullous disease within a generalised obstructive emphysema.

Table 1

Subtypes of diffuse obstructive emphysema

Parameters	'Pink Puffer' syn. Type A (dry)	'Blue Bloater' syn. Type B (wet)
Symptoms:		
Dyspnoea	● At rest	● Less dyspnoea at rest
Cough	● Occasional	● Severe
Wheeze	● Usually absent	● Present
Sputum	● Usually scanty	● Copious
Cyanosis	● None	● Frequently present
Blood gases:		
P O$_2$	● May be slightly reduced	● Reduced <8K Pa
P CO$_2$	● Slightly reduced	● Elevated >6K Pa
Plain chest X-ray	● Diffuse over-inflation of lungs	● Moderate hyper inflation
	● Little/no fibrosis	● Fibrosis in lower lobes
	● Flat diaphragm	● No./little change of diaphragm
	● ↓ pulmonary vasculature	● ↑ central pulmonary vasculature
	● ↑ air space behind sternum	● ↓ or no air space behind sternum
Pathology	● Panacinar emphysema	● Centrilobular emphysema
Prognosis (longevity)	● Reasonable	● Poor

Key: ↓ = Reduced; ↑ = Increased.

3. Bullous emphysema and its surgical treatment

Bullous emphysema consists of single/multiple bullae associated with normal lung parenchyma. The condition may be discovered incidentally in a completely asymptomatic individual. The mode of presentation in symptomatic patients is dyspnea, or symptoms related to the complication of the bulla, e.g. pneumothorax or infection in the bulla.

Undisturbed, the bulla may assume a large size amounting to a huge air cyst with increasing breathlessness. Occasionally such cases present with an acute episode of disabling dyspnea mimicking tension pneumothorax and signalling a high pressure within the bulla displacing the mediastinum and greatly compressing the normal lung and blood vessels.

Diagnosis relies mainly on imaging.

Plain chest X-ray is characterised by:

- hyper-inflation showing on plain anterio-posterior view X-ray as low position of the diaphragm. At the mid-clavicular line the diaphragmatic shadow is usually level with the anterior end of the 7th rib. In emphysema the diaphragmatic shadow is at a lower level.
- flattening of diaphragmatic dome
- vascular changes characterised by:
  - reduction in number or size of pulmonary vessels;
  - distortion of vessels showing as excessive straightening of vascular marking;
  - localised or generalised trans-radiancy of lung.

In patients with a distinct large bulla the image is one of an air cyst, often defined by a thin but defined membrane border. A chest radiograph on inspiration and expiration can differentiate between generalised emphysema and a single compressive bulla. In the latter, expiration substantially reduces the volume of the hemithorax.

- Bronchography and angiography were used extensively in the pre-CT era to demonstrate the bullae and their effects on the normal parenchyma. They provide accurate information about compression of the bronchial tree and pulmonary vessels under the bulla. Angiographic evidence of crowding of the vessels still constitutes an important guide to patient selection, particularly when there is a question of determining multiplicity of bullae and their vascular effect, or in patients with bullae associated with generalised emphysema.
- A ventilation–perfusion isotope scan is carried out to evaluate the extent of the disease and the associated mismatch between air space and vasculature of the lung.
- Computed tomography has much advantage over simple radiography, particularly in differential diagnosis between bulla and pneumothorax and in identifying bullae not apparent on a plain X-ray.

3.1. Surgical treatment of bullous emphysema

3.1.1. Indications

Surgery is indicated in symptomatic patients and when a bulla occupies more than 30% of the hemithorax. Surgery is not indicated in asymptomatic patients and the best result is achieved in those with severe dyspnoea and in the presence of a giant bulla compressing normal parenchyma.

3.1.2. Methods

There are a number of methods to treat bullous emphysema.

- Surgical bullectomy. The principle of treatment is to excise the non-functioning, space-occupying bulla and to preserve functioning parenchyma. This will allow expansion of the lung under the bulla.
- The bulla if pedunculated may be clamped, ligated at its base (pedicle) and sutured. This will allow total excision without loss of any healthy lung tissue. This is particularly applicable to superficially placed bullae.
- A large bulla may be plicated or opened and its interior explored. If there are any visible small bronchial openings, they are clipped or sutured. Staples are then applied to the whole length of the base. Pleura, pericardial heterograft or Teflon pledglets may be incorporated into the staple to minimise air leaks.

Following bullectomy, parietal pleurodesis may be carried out. The operation may be done using standard or limited access thoracotomy or minimal access thoracoscopic surgery. In bilateral cases median sternotomy allows access to both sides. When one large or a number of smaller bullae occupy distinct anatomical pulmonary segments or lobes, it is best to perform standard resection, i.e. segmentectomy/lobectomy.

- Intracavitary (bulla) drainage. This is based on the method originally devised by Monaldi (1947). The principle is to inset a catheter into the bulla to reduce its tension and collapse its wall, allowing expansion of the lung under it. The method is specifically indicated in patients with severe symptoms but with poor general condition, which will not permit either bullectomy or standard resection. In this method the bulla is accessed via a small appropriately placed incision over the peripherally placed wall of the bulla. The wall of the bulla is reached, if necessary, by resection of a small portion of the overlying rib. A purse string-type stitch is inserted in the wall of the bulla. A catheter (preferably with a ballooned end) is then inserted into the bulla. Drainage of the bulla allows its deflation and expansion of the underlying lung; the pleural space is also drained. Chemical pleurodesis may be achieved using talcum powder (see section 4.4.2 in chapter I.22). The catheter and pleural drain are disposed of after cessation of the air leak.

References and further reading

American Thoracic Society. Standards for the diagnosis and care of patient with chronic obstructive pulmonary disease (COPD) and asthma. Ann Rev Resp Dis 1987; 139: 225–244.

Benfield JR, Cree EM, Pellett JR et al. Current approach to the surgical management of emphysema. Arch Surg 1966; 93: 59–70.

Ciba Guest symposium. Terminology definition and classification of chronic pulmonary emphysema and related conditions. Thorax 1959; 4: 286–299.

De Giacomo T, Venuta F, Rendina A, Della Rocca G, Ciccone AM, Ricci C, Coloni GF. Video assisted thoracoscopic treatment of giant bullae associated with emphysema. Eur J Cardiothorac Surg 1999; 15: 753–757.

Dijkman JH. Morphological aspects, classification and epidemiology of emphysema. Bull Eur Physiopathol Respir 1986; 22: 241–244.

Liu JP, Chang CH, Lin PJ, Chu JJ, Hsieh MJ. An alternative technique in the management of bullous emphysema. Thoracoscopic endoloop ligation of bullae. Chest 1997; 111: 489–493.

Liu HP, Chang CH, Lin PJ, Cheng KS, Wu YC, Liu YH. Emphysema surgery — loop ligation approach. Eur J Cardiothorac Surg 1999; 16: 40–43.

Menconi GF, Melfi FM, Mussi A, Palla A, Ambrogi MC, Angeletti CA. Treatment by VATS of giant bullous emphysema: results. Eur J Cardiothorac Surg 1998; 13: 66–70.

Moghissi K, Khoury S. Indications chirurgicales de l'emphysème bulleux. Rev Fr Mal Resp 1980; 8: 151–152.

Monaldi V. Endocavitary aspiration: its practical applications. Tubercle 1947; 28: 223–225.

Santambrogio L, Mossotti M, Baisi A, Bellaviti N, Pavoni G, Rosso L. Buttressing staple lines with bovine pericardium in lung resection for bullous emphysema. Scand Cardiovasc J 1998; 32: 297–299.

Siafakas NM, Verme P, Pride NB et al. On behalf of the Task Force, ERS consensus statement optimal assessment and management of chronic obstruction pulmonary disease (COPD). Eur Resp J 1995; 8: 1398–1432.

Wesley JR, Macleod WM, Mullard KS. Evaluation and surgery of bullous emphysema. J Thorac Cardiovasc 1972; 63: 945–955.

Witz JP, Roeslin N. La chirurgie de l'emphysème bulleux chez l'adulte: ses résultats éloignés. Rev Fr Mal Resp 1980; 8: 121–125.

K. Moghissi, J.A.C. Thorpe and F. Ciulli (Eds.)
Moghissi's Essentials of Thoracic and Cardiac Surgery

CHAPTER I.15

Pulmonary embolism (PE)

K. Moghissi

1. Introduction

By definition an embolus is an abnormal mass of unresolved material which is carried by the bloodstream from one part of the circulatory system to another.

In the case of pulmonary embolism, fragments of blood clot become detached from a venous propagated thrombus and are transported to the heart and hence to the pulmonary arterial system where they stop and cause obstruction and the arrest of circulation in that area.

The pathogenesis of PE is closely related to that of venous thrombosis, where in terms of aetiopathology, three groups of factors are operational (Virchow's triad):
- factors associated with blood flow;
- factors which affect the venous wall;
- factors related to blood clotting.

Once a thrombus is formed it can propagate when a portion becomes detached from the main mass and migrates as an embolus.

The incidence of pulmonary embolism in the general population and even following surgical operation is difficult to assess due to inaccuracy of diagnosis, inadequacy of records and lack of register of thrombo-embolic events for all operations. Those records and publications which are available relate to specific populations or a particular setting. This is illustrated by the literature review: Kumasaka et al. (1999) report the yearly incidence of thrombo-embolism as 0.28% in the Japanese population. In a retrospective analysis of data from patients admitted to University of Michigan Hospital, Proctor et al. (2001) found that about 2% developed thrombo-embolic events. Baeshko et al. (1999) recorded the incidence of postoperative PE in 14,833 patients

to be 1.2%. In this series 13% of all postoperative deaths were due to pulmonary embolism. Bergqvist et al. (1985) reported the incidence of death from PE amongst 5477 surgical patients in an autopsy material review to be 2.4%. A series reviewed by Gillies et al. (1996) found a 3% incidence of death from PE amongst surgical in-patients.

2. Presenting features and diagnosis

The clinical manifestation of PE can be one or a combination of the following: dyspnea, chest pain, haemoptysis, cyanosis, hypotension (state of shock), tachycardia and tachypnea. Some 10% of patients die at the onset of a massive PE. In these cases the diagnosis is a post-mortem event. In those who survive, the differential diagnosis is both problematic and often a matter of extreme urgency. A substantial number of those with massive PE who survive the initial event may be in such a critical cardio-respiratory state as to be unfit to undergo investigations other than simple tests which serve to exclude one of the many other cardio-respiratory catastrophes with similar presentations. Some of these patients only survive with the emergency establishment of cardio-pulmonary bypass. Presentation of PE may broadly be placed into 4 groups:
- Those patients who develop sudden chest pain, dyspnoea and shock may die within minutes of the crisis because of massive pulmonary embolism obstructing the pulmonary artery. The mechanism of the sudden death is possibly an acute haemodynamic disturbance.
- Patients with massive pulmonary embolism with severe symptoms and shock who are haemodynamically unstable but with energetic resuscitation can live for a short period of 1–2 hours. In

this group it is important to make the diagnosis and assess the severity and extent of the arterial obstruction in order to undertake the most suitable therapeutic measures. In these, symptoms alone make it difficult, if not impossible, to make the diagnosis of PE. Myocardial infarction will often have identical presentation and sometimes postoperative spontaneous pneumothorax can mimic pulmonary embolism. Electrocardiogram in established cases will show signs of right ventricular strain but the interpretation of ECG in the early phases of pulmonary embolism is difficult. Chest radiograph will generally show unilateral or bilateral hilar enlargement, reflecting dilatation of one or both of the pulmonary arteries with, at times, areas of pulmonary ischaemia.

- Patients with a sizeable, but not massive, pulmonary embolism will have pulmonary infarction with a definite clinical manifestation but with stable haemodynamic state. Pleuritic pain, dyspnoea of varying severity, cough, haemoptysis and pleural effusion are present singly or in concert. Radiological changes are pleural effusion, elevation of a hemidiaphragm and horizontal non-segmental linear opacities. In this group a comprehensive investigation to establish urgently the diagnosis of PE should be initiated.
- Some patients have repeated small emboli. Dyspnoea, intermittent chest pain on exertion and signs of cardiac failure are present and progress over months or years. In a few patients, episodes of embolisation may go unnoticed until the development of pulmonary hypertension and overt heart failure.

3. Diagnostic procedures

- Chest radiography: Initially chest radiography may only be useful to exclude other acute crises such as pneumothorax but it may not show any positive findings. Sometimes diminished pulmonary vascular marking in the area of embolus can be seen. After a few days abnormal findings at the area of the embolus, atelectasis, pleural effusion, consolidation, prominent pulmonary artery and shadowing can become apparent.
- Spiral CT: The primary evaluation of this technology for diagnosis of PE has shown encouraging results and its sensitivity in experienced hands appears to be superior to that of isotope ventilation perfusion (V/Q) scan.
- MRI: There is limited clinical experience in the

use of MRI whose place and indications in PE need yet to be established.
- ECG may show non-specific changes.
- Arterial blood gases: Decrease in arterial oxygen pressure (pO_2) and increase in carbon dioxide pressure (pCO_2) are the usual findings but these changes are not completely diagnostic.
- Radioisotope pulmonary scanning. Perfusion isotope scanning shows lack of arterial blood flow in the area of embolus. The method is particularly suitable in important pulmonary embolism when the chest X-ray may be quasi-normal. Ventilation (inhalation) isotope scanning is helpful in determining important ventilation/perfusion mismatch in the area of PE.
- Pulmonary arteriography is the most accurate method of indicating the existence of PE and its topography by filling defect at the site of embolus. However, there is a small percentage of false positives particularly in cases involving the segmental bronchus.
- Plasma D-dimer: This is a fibrin degradation product and its plasma levels rise in important venous thrombosis.

4. Management

4.1. Prophylaxis

This applies to cases in which risk factors can be identified and preventative measures can be undertaken. A prime example of this is postoperative thrombo-embolism in which two groups of factors, stasis and blood hyper-coagulability, are the known risk factors.

The measures advocated are:

4.1.1. Prophylaxis through anticoagulation
- Low-dose heparin. A number of studies have shown the efficacy of low-dose heparin injected subcutaneously to reduce the rate of postoperative deep vein thrombosis. This is administered at the dose of 5000 iu twice daily by subcutaneous injection. The prophylaxis should continue until mobilisation of the patient. However, the regimen should be flexible and be altered according to the patient's risk of deep vein thrombosis (DVT).
- Comparison between low molecular weight heparin (LMWH) given once a day (3500 iu bomparin) and unfractionated heparin (UFH) administered 5000 iu twice a day (Kakkar, 2000) indicated better protection with LMWH than with UFH.

- Dextran. A branched polysaccharide, Dextran is produced by bacteria and acts as an anticoagulant by interfering with platelet function and with the protein involved in clotting. Its prophylactic use has not received much attention because of the inevitable fluid overload which accompanies its administration.

4.1.2. Prophylaxis through reduction of stasis (mechanical means)
This includes:
- Elevation of lower limbs when lying in bed.
- Compression stocking. This is a simple, easily utilised method.
- Pneumatic compression. The method is probably as effective as the compression stocking but more difficult to use in practice.

4.2. Treatment

Initial treatment is one of resuscitation, the extent of which depends on the severity of the event and the resulting cardio-respiratory state of the patient. Symptom relief should be considered at this stage: analgesia for pain, high content inspired oxygen for hypoxia, maintenance of stable haemodynamic state and oxygenation, if necessary by mechanical devices, are on the list of priorities. Arterial and central venous pressure should be monitored. The extent of the initial investigation depends on cardio-respiratory and haemodynamic state and the choice of treatment is also governed by the prospect of survival beyond the initial collapse. The deciding factors are the clinical condition and haemodynamic stability of the patient.

4.2.1. Anticoagulants
Heparin remains the drug of choice in the initial stage of therapy. Its dose is governed by clotting time, which should reach and be maintained at 2–3 times the normal (i.e. normal clotting time × 2 to 3 = optimal therapeutic time). In practice an initial dose of 10,000 iu is given via a cental venous catheter followed by 1000 iu per hour. The activated partial thromboplastin time (APTT) is checked frequently in the first 24 h and should remain at 1.5–2 times the normal ratio. After 2–4 days warfarin is given in parallel with heparin which is continued for a further 3–4 days. The initial dose of warfarin is 10–20 mg. For 2–4 days both drugs are administered. During this time the heparin dose is controlled by APTT and that of warfarin by prothrombin. The

international normalized ratio (INR) should be kept in the therapeutic range of 2.0–3.0 times normal. The oral warfarin is then continued alone at a dose to achieve INR of 2–3 times normal.

Duration of oral therapy for anticoagulation depends on the existing risk factors and the incidence of previous thrombo-embolic events. According to the Research Committee of the British Thoracic Society (1992), this should vary from 3 months in those with no previous history/risk, to lifelong therapy for patients with multiple prior events.

4.2.2. Thrombolysis/thrombolytic agents
These agents are plasminogen converters to plasmin. Plasminogen is a naturally occurring protein which, when converted to plasmin, disposes of intravascular clots. At the present time there are three types of thrombolytic agents: streptokinase, urokinase and recombinant tissue plasminogen activator (rtPA).

For the past 30 years a number of studies have been carried out to assess both the place of thrombolytic agents in PE and also their merits compared with anticoagulants. The general consensus which has emerged following these studies is that thrombolytic agents are more effective than heparin in terms of rapidity of action to dispose of clots.
- There are more bleeding complications in patients treated by thrombolic agents than with anticoagulant regimens. This is particularly the case in postoperative cases.
- There is no convincing evidence to suggest the superiority of one thrombolytic agent over another.

4.2.3. Surgical management
The successful medical management of patients with PE has restricted indications of surgical embolectomy to:
- rare instances of patients with massive embolism and cardiac arrest who are successfully resuscitated after an acute episode using extra corporeal membrane oxygenator followed by embolectomy;
- patients with PE who are haemodynamically unstable or remain so despite medication;
- patients in whom thrombolysis is contraindicated.
  There are two techniques of pulmonary embolectomy:
(a) Percutaneous catheter technique. This consists of the passage of a balloon catheter from jugular or femoral vein, under radiological guidance, to reach the pulmonary artery and to extract the embolus. Alternatively an aspirating catheter is used to achieve suction of the clot. At the present

time experience in endo-vascular embolectomy is relatively small and its technology is still developing.

(b) Surgical embolectomy. Trendelenburg (1908) performed the first pulmonary embolectomy experimentally (in calf). Following this, and with observation of patients who had succumbed to PE, he proposed a method of embolectomy by rapid opening of the pulmonary artery via thoracotomy and extraction of the clot. Three patients treated in this manner died in less than 40 h. Kirschner (1924) performed the first successful pulmonary embolectomy with a long-term survival.

In 1960 Allison performed embolectomy on a young athlete with massive PE using total body hypothermia (20°C). The method employed was temporary interruption of circulation with caval occlusion. The patient made a good recovery. Since the advent of cardiopulmonary bypass using the extra-corporeal circulation technique in 1961 and 1962, pulmonary embolectomy has become technically feasible by all cardiothoracic surgeons familiar with the technique. Paradoxically, as the surgical embolectomy became technically available universally, the need for its use declined due to:

- the efficiency of medial treatment;
- a high mortality of pulmonary embolectomy, with the in-hospital mortality reaching near 50% (Stulz, 1994).

It must, however, be pointed out that published medical and surgical series are not comparable. All surgical series comprise a variable proportion of patients who were near, or at, cardiac arrest or whose operations were undertaken when other (medical) treatments had failed. Ideal patients for embolectomy are those with massive PE who are of a younger age group and are not in cardiac arrest. Many such patients are, in fact, given the benefit of medical treatment.

4.2.4. Associated surgical procedures

- Venous thrombectomy. This procedure was once strongly recommended and was undertaken in many early surgical embolectomies. The present consensus is that it is an unnecessary addition to embolectomy. Postoperative anti coagulation is used in some cases when there is arterial spasm in the limb in addition to venous thrombosis.
- Inferior vena caval interruption/percutaneous caval filtration. In early embolectomies there was a trend to ligate/plicate the inferior vena cava

(IVC) in order to prevent or reduce the incidence of recurrence of PE. With the development of the intra-luminal filter device there was a new enthusiasm to use caval filters. At present there is still controversy surrounding the use of caval filters but a subset of patients with PE seem to benefit from their deployment. These are:

- Patients with recurrent PE despite adequate anticoagulant and particularly those undergoing thrombolysis.
- Patients with free-floating thrombus.

There are a number of filters available for long- and short-term usage and the choice appears to be more of a matter of the experience of the operator than the device itself.

References and further reading

Baeshko AA, Shorokh GP, Molochko MI, Sheid AA, Klimovich VV. Post operative deep vein thrombosis of legs and pulmonary embolism (Article in Russian). Khirurgiia (Musk) 1999; 3: 52–58.

Bergqvist D, Lindblad B. A 30 year survey of pulmonary embolism verified at autopsy: an analysis of 1274 surgical patients. Br J Surg 1985; 72: 105–108.

British Thoracic Society Standards of Care Committee. Suspected acute pulmonary embolism: a practical approach. Thorax 1997; 52(Suppl 4): S1–S24.

Daily PO, Dembitsky WP, Iversen S et al. Risk factors for pulmonary thromboendarterectomy. J Thorac Cardiovasc Surg 1990; 99(4): 670–678.

Doerge H, Schoendube FA, Voss M, Seipelt R, Messmer BJ. Surgical therapy of fulminant pulmonary embolism: early and late results. Thorac Cardiovasc Surg 1999; 47(1): 9–13.

Gillies TE, Ruckley CV, Nixon SJ. Still missing the boat with fatal pulmonary embolism. Br J Surg 1996; 83: 1394–1395.

Hull RD, Raskob GE, Ginsberg JS, Panjo AA, Brill Edwards P, Coates G et al. A non-invasive strategy for the treatment of patients with suspected pulmonary embolism. Arch Intern Med 1994; 154: 289–297.

Kakkar V. The diagnosis of deep vein thrombosis using the 125I fibrinogen test. Arch Surg 1972; 104: 152–159.

Kakkar VV, Howes J, Sharma V, Kadziola Z. A comparative double-blind randomised trial of new second generation LMWH (bemiparin) and UFH in the prevention of post-operative venous thromboembolism. The Bemiparin Assessment Group. Thromb Haemost 2000; 83: 523–529.

Kirschner M. Ein durch die Trendelenburgsche Operation geheilter Fall von Embolie der Art. pulmonalis. Archiv für klinische Chirurgie, Berlin, 1924; 133: 312–359.

Kumasaka N, Sakuma M, Shirato K. Incidence of pulmonary thromboembolism in Japan. Jpn Circ J 1999; 63(10): 825–827.

Lilienfeld DE, Chan E, Ehland BA et al. Mortality from pulmonary embolism in the United States 1962–1984. Chest 1990; 98: 1067–1072.

Lilienfeld DE. Decreasing mortality from pulmonary embolism in the United States 1979–1996. Int J Epidemiol 2000; 29(3): 465–469.

Mayo JR, Remy–Jardin M, Muller NL, Remy J, Worsley DF, Hossein–Foucher C, et al. Pulmonary embolism: prospective comparison of spiral CT with ventilation–perfusion scintigraphy. Radiology 1997; 205: 447–452.

Meyer JA. Friedrich Trendelenburg and the surgical approach to massive pulmonary embolism. Arch Surg 1990; 125: 1202–1205.

Nyman U. Diagnostic strategies in acute pulmonary embolism. Haemostasis 1993; 23(Suppl): 220–226.

The PIOPED investigators. Tissue plasminogen activator for the treatment of acute pulmonary embolism. Chest 1990; 97: 528–533.

Prevention of fatal postoperative pulmonary embolism by low doses of heparin. An international multicentre trial. Lancet 1975; 2(7924): 45–51.

Proctor MC, Greenfield LJ. Thromboprophylaxis in an academic medical centre. Cardiovasc Surg 2001; 9(5): 426–430.

Remy–Jardin M, Remy J, Deschildre F, Artaud D, Beregi JP, Hossein–Foucher C, et al. Diagnosis of pulmonary embolism with spiral CT: comparison with pulmonary angiography and scintigraphy. Radiology 1996; 200: 699–796.

Research Committee of the British Thoracic Society. Optimum duration for anticoagulation for deep-vein thrombosis and pulmonary embolism. Lancet 1992; 340: 873–876.

Sharnoff JG. Results in the prophylaxis of postoperative thromboembolism. Surg Gynecol Obstet 1966; 123: 303–307.

Stein PD, Hull RD, Pineo G. Strategy that includes serial noninvasive leg tests for diagnosis of thromboembolic disease in patients with suspected acute pulmonary embolism based on data from PIOPED (Prospective Investigation of Pulmonary Embolism Diagnosis). Arch Intern Med 1995; 155: 2101–2104.

Stein PD, Goldhaber SZ, Henry JW, Millar AC. Arterial blood gas analysis in the assessment of suspected acute pulmonary embolism. Chest 1996; 109: 78–81.

Stulz P, Schlapfer R, Feer R et al. Decision making in the surgical treatment of massive pulmonary embolism. Eur J Cardiothorac Surg 1994; 8: 188–193.

Tai NR, Atwal AS, Hamilton G. Modern management of pulmonary emblism. Br J Surg 1999; 86; 853–868.

Trendelenburg F. Über die operative Behandlung der Embolie der Lungarterie. Arch Klin Chir 1908; 86: 686–700.

The UKEP Study Research Group. The UKEP study: Multicentre clinical trial on two local regimens of urokinase in massive pulmonary embolism. Eur Heart J 1987; 8: 2–10.

Ullmann M, Hemmer W, Hannekum A. The urgent pulmonary embolectomy; mechanical resuscitation in the operating theatre determines the outcome. Thorac Cardiovasc Surg 1999 Feb; 47(1): 5–8.

K. Moghissi, J.A.C. Thorpe and F. Ciulli (Eds.)
Moghissi's Essentials of Thoracic and Cardiac Surgery

CHAPTER I.16

Bronchopulmonary neoplasms

K. Moghissi

In this chapter we describe bronchopulmonary neoplasms under the following headings:

1. Primary lung cancer (bronchogenic carcinoma)
2. Bronchopulmonary tumours other than lung cancer
2.1 Rare primary malignant tumours
2.2 Secondary lung tumours
2.3 Benign bronchopulmonary neoplasms
2.4 Bronchial gland tumours (Adenomas)
3. Specific types of lung cancer
3.1 Small cell lung cancer (SCLC)
3.2 Superior sulcus tumour (Pancoast tumour)
3.3 Lung cancer presenting as a nodular lesion

1. Primary lung cancer

At the turn of the 20th century lung cancer was considered to be uncommon. By the millennium it was one of the commonest cancers worldwide, the most important malignant tumour of the male population in the western world and the world's most common malignancy in men and women combined (Parkin et al., 1993).

1.1. Incidence

There are variations in the incidence of lung cancer relating to age, sex, geography, environmental factors, occupational exposure to carcinogens and cigarette smoking. Worldwide there is a predominance in the male over the female population of lung cancer, at least partially explained by higher tobacco consumption in men, a trend which could easily reverse in view of the ever-increasing number of young women taking up the habit.

Geographically in the world, the highest rate is amongst black Americans followed by the Maoris of New Zealand, each with a rate in the range of 100–120 per 100,000 population. The lowest incidence is registered in India with ≤10 per 100,000 population. In Europe the countries with the highest and lowest rates are shown in Table 1.

In European countries there is a higher incidence of lung cancer in men than in women. The age prevalence is over 65 years and 45 years for males and females respectively. In the European Community the incidence of lung cancer for men is about 64 per 100,000 population and 8.2 per 100,000 population for women. Translated into numbers, this represents a total of about 135,000 men and 23,000 women yearly.

1.2. Aetiology and pathogenesis

For a number of years, epidemiological studies have drawn attention to an array of agents which appear to be involved in the development of lung cancer. Tobacco and cigarette smoking are the most tangibly important contributors to the disease. A variety of chemicals, biological, physical and radioactive ma-

Table 1

The highest and lowest incidence of lung cancer in European Countries

		For men Nr/100,000 (ASR)	For women Nr/100,000 (ASR)
Highest	1. Belgium	91.8	6.7
	2. Netherlands	89.2	7.3
	3. United Kingdom	82.1	18.6
Lowest	4. Spain	41.1	3.9
	5. Portugal	23.8	4.0

ASR: age standardised rate – Olsen (1995).

terials are also involved in the aetiology. In recent years, advances in molecular biology and genetics have presented the opportunity to study more closely the genetic factors in the pathogenesis of all cancer, including that of the lung (Mulshine et al., 1993; Carbone and Mina, 1992; Shields and Harris, 1993). It is understood that normal cell growth is controlled by a fine balance between the activities of two classes of genes: namely, proto-oncogenes which promote growth, and suppressor genes which inhibit growth. When mutationally altered, these two groups of genes are also responsible for uncontrolled cell proliferation. Oncogenes, the mutationally activated forms of proto-oncogenes, will stimulate growth and cell division through the inappropriate expression of proteins involved in signal transduction and positive regulation of the cell cycle. Mutational inactivation of tumour suppressor genes usually involves proteins involved in the negative regulation of the cell cycle and proliferation. The sequential accumulation of activating and inactivating mutations in these two main groups of genes eventually leads to uncontrolled growth. This classical and rather simplistic view of carcinogenesis would suggest that the pathogenesis of lung cancer, similar to that of many other malignant tumours, is a multi-stage process which begins with initiation and proceeds through promotion and conversion to progression, at which point the tumour disseminates and becomes widespread.

Initially, due to exposure to carcinogens, mutation of genetic material occurs. This is an irreversible molecular event, which paves the way to promotion in which the mutated cell clonally expands and acquires further mutations through the combined effects of carcinogen exposure and DNA replication of the resulting damaged genes. Progression and malignant conversion then follow, during which properties such as invasiveness and angiogenesis are acquired. The links between carcinogenic agents and the molecular events associated with lung cancer have been elucidated through the study of mutational hotspots in the lung tumours of smokers. The pattern of damage and mutation seen in such tumours closely matches that which can be experimentally induced with known tobacco smoke carcinogens such as benzyprene (Denissenko et al., 1996).

A number of oncogenes and tumour suppressor genes have been identified in human lung cancer development. The description and mechanism through which they play their role in lung cancer development is beyond the scope of this book. However, it suffices to mention that such oncogenes as K-*ras* (in adenocarcinoma), *erb*-B family (in non-small- cell lung cancer) and *myc* family (in small cell lung cancer) play various roles in lung carcinogenesis. Others including *p*53, *p*16, *FHIT* and *rb* (retinoblastoma) tumour suppressor genes are also implicated in tumorigenesis (Carbone and Mina, 1992; Harris 1993; Herndandez-Boussard et al., 1998).

1.3. Pathology

Lung cancer is considered to be a multi-step development. It arises from bronchial epithelial proliferation passing through the stage of hyperplasia and metaplasia to neoplasia. The changes from typical to atypical metaplasia leading to carcinoma in situ (epithelial neoplasia) appear to be the crucial step in carcinogenesis. A further step is the infiltration of the basement membrane and lymphatic involvement with local and metastatic spread.

1.3.1. Histology
The World Health Organisation's (WHO) histological classification (last reviewed in 1982), which is still in use, is based on light microscopy and distinguishes 4 major histological types: Squamous Cell, Small Cell, Adenocarcinoma and Large Cell. It also includes 4 other subsidiary types as shown on Table 2. (The 4 principal histological types are indicated in bold characters.)

Table 2

Histological classification of epithelial malignant tumours

1.	**Squamous Cell Carcinoma (Epidermoid Carcinoma):**
	(a) Variant: Spindle Cell (Squamous) Carcinoma
2.	**Small Cell Carcinoma:**
	(a) Oat Cell Carcinoma
	(b) Intermediate cell types
	(c) Combined Oat Cell Carcinoma
3.	**Adenocarcinoma:**
	(a) Acinar Adenocarcinoma
	(b) Papillary Adenocarcinoma
	(c) Bronchoalveolar Carcinoma
	(d) Solid Carcinoma with mucus formation
4.	**Large Cell Carcinoma:**
	(a) Giant Cell Carcinoma
	(b) Clear Cell Carcinoma
5.	Adenosquamous Carcinoma
6.	Carcinoid Tumours
7.	Bronchial Gland Carcinoma:
	(a) Adenoid Cystic Carcinoma
	(b) Muco-epidermoid Carcinoma
	(c) Other
8.	Others.

It is acknowledged that there is marked heterogenicity in each of the cell types as shown when morphometric, electron microscopic, immunohistochemical and molecular biological methods are used. A working classification for clinicians is to divide all epithelial malignant lung tumours into small cell (SCLC) and non small cell lung cancer (NSCLC). This division is based, amongst other considerations, on the fact that SCLC behaves more aggressively, responds more favourably to chemotherapy and is less amenable to resection at presentation. Some 80% of all cancers are NSCLC, with SCLC forming the remaining 20%.

The incidence of each cell type is greatly dependent on the sample of population and the source of the survey. As a general rule, the survey of surgical resection material will indicate a greatly higher ratio of NSCLC to SCLC than the review of bronchoscopic biopsy and autopsy samples. This is well documented by Muller (1995) who found that the proportion of squamous cell carcinomas and adenocarcinomas was 45% and 40% for surgical and 31% and 18% in autopsy material respectively; and 36% of the lung cancer in autopsy material was SCLC.

1.3.2. Staging and TNM classification
Staging is the evaluation of the extent of tumour in a patient. It is an essential measurement at presentation of a case and constitutes an important aspect of oncology with practical treatment implications. When staging is based on universally-agreed criteria, it provides a language of understanding amongst researchers and those involved in cancer therapy. It further allows correlation to be made between the extent of disease and the outcome of a given therapy serving as a useful prognostic guide.

Staging of lung cancer uses the tumour, node, and metastasis (TNM) system, which was first proposed by Denoix in 1941. Tumour (T) represents the primary tumour whose extent is conveyed by a numeric suffix. Node (N) denotes the regional lymph node involvement. Ipsilateral, contralateral and cervical extensions are taken into account and appropriately defined by a suffix of 1–3. By convention and universal understanding, thoracic lymph nodes, in relation to lung cancer, are mapped into a sequence of numbers representing 'stations' or regions within the lung and mediastinum. The mapping most comprehensively presented by Naruke et al. (1978) describes 14 stations (Fig. 1) on each hemithorax. Stations 1–10 are referred to as N2. These are the mediastinal nodes. Stations 11–14 are referred to as N1 which are peri-

bronchial. Metastasis (M) represents the metastatic spread. The basic principle of the TNM system remains unaltered to date, albeit with geographical and temporal variations. Updating occurs from time to time in the light of experience and result reporting. For instance, the American Joint Committee on Cancer (AJCC) and the Union Internationale Contre le Cancer (UICC) use the TNM classification but differ in some details. These differences neither interfere with understanding, nor contradict the primary goal of staging, which is the benchmark against which extent of disease is assessed.

Currently the most updated and universally accepted classification (see Tables 3, 4, 5 and 6) is one which is advanced by Mountain (1997) which in essence is similar to that of the most recent UICC classification (Sobin and Wittekind, 1997).

Note on stage grouping of small cell lung cancer. The clinical and histological characteristics of SCLC are very different from NSCLC. It is generally a rapidly growing tumour that metastasises easily, both to the lymph nodes and at distant sites. Although many investigators classify SCLC using the TNM system similar to that for NSCLC, a number of oncologists and clinicians employ a more practical classification for SCLC and group them into two categories: limited and/or extensive disease. By convention, limited disease is confined to one lung with no pleural or tracheal involvement even where there is peripheral mediastinal and supraclavicular lymph node spread. Extensive disease is defined as tumour which has spread beyond the primary tumour and regional lymph nodes to involve the pleura and distant organs.

Clinical and pathological stage grouping. Therapeutic decision making for lung cancer patients depends on information and overall results of clinical, radiological and endoscopic investigations with biopsy. These permit the establishment of histological type and TNM staging of the tumour which is referred to as cTNM. However, the true stage of a tumour can only be established at autopsy and/or at thoracotomy and after resectional surgery and following microscopic histological examination. This is referred to as pathological staging or pTNM (pT, pM). In practice, the more detailed and precise the pre-operative investigations, the narrower the difference between cTNM and pTNM will become. Note: the components of cTNM or pTNM are referred to as cT, cN and cM and pT, pN and pM respectively.

Lymph node station chart

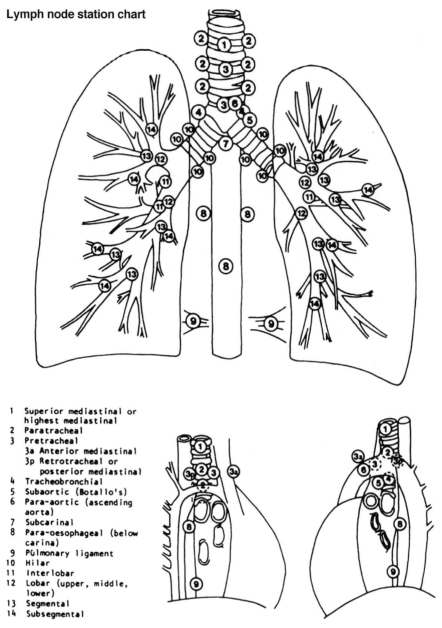

1   Superior mediastinal or
     highest mediastinal
2   Paratracheal
3   Pretracheal
     3a Anterior mediastinal
     3p Retrotracheal or
         posterior mediastinal
4   Tracheobronchial
5   Subaortic (Botallo's)
6   Para-aortic (ascending
     aorta)
7   Subcarinal
8   Para-oesophageal (below
     carina)
9   Pulmonary ligament
10 Hilar
11 Interlobar
12 Lobar (upper, middle,
     lower)
13 Segmental
14 Subsegmental

Fig. 1. Neruke et al. (1978) mapping of the lymph nodes.

1.4. Presentation and clinical features of lung cancer

Lung cancer may be completely asymptomatic and be discovered in the course of routine radiography (Fig. 2). The mode of presentation of symptomatic lung cancer patients may be:

- presentation with symptoms and signs of respiratory disease (see section 1.4.1 below)
- presentation with signs and symptoms of non-res-

piratory and metastatic disease (see section 1.4.2 below)
- presentation with non metastatic para-neoplastic symptoms (see section 1.4.3 below)

1.4.1. Lung cancer presenting with symptoms of respiratory disease (Figs. 3 and 4)

This is the commonest type of presentation. The patient, commonly a male of over 60 years of age, usually a heavy smoker, presents with:

Table 3

TNM Classification

T — Primary Tumour

TX   Primary tumour cannot be assessed, *or* tumour proven by the presence of malignant cells in sputum or bronchial washings but not visualized by imaging or bronchoscopy

T0   No evidence of primary tumour

Tis   Carcinoma in situ

T1   Tumour 3 cm or less in greatest dimension, surrounded by lung or visceral pleura, without bronchoscopic evidence of invasion more proximal than the lobar bronchus (i.e. not in the main bronchus)

T2   Tumour with any of the following features of size or extent:
- More than 3 cm in greatest dimension
- Involves main bronchus, 2 cm or more distal to the carina
- Invades visceral pleura
- Associated with atelectasis or obstructive pneumonitis that extends to the hilar region but does not involve the entire lung.

T3   Tumour of any size that directly invades any of the following: chest wall (including superior sulcus tumours), diaphragm, mediastinal pleura, parietal pericardium; or tumour in the main bronchus less than 2 cm distal to the carina but without involvement of the carina; or associated atelectasis or obstructive pneumonitis of the entire lung.

T4   Tumour of any size that invades any of the following: mediastinum, heart, great vessels, trachea, oesophagus, vertebral body, carina; separate tumour nodule(s) in the same lobe; tumour with malignant pleural effusion.

N — Regional Lymph Nodes

NX   Regional lymph nodes cannot be assessed

N0   No regional lymph node metastasis

N1   Metastasis in ipsilateral peribronchial and/or ipsilateral hilar lymph nodes and intrapulmonary nodes, including involvement by direct extension.

N2   Metastasis in ipsilateral mediastinal and/or subcarinal lymph node(s).

N3   Metastasis in contralateral mediastinal, contralateral hilar, ipsilateral or contralateral scalene, or supraclavicular lymph node(s).

M — Distant Metastasis

MX   Distant metastasis cannot be assessed

M0   No distant metastasis

M1   Distant metastasis, includes separate tumour nodule(s) in a different lobe (ipsilateral or contralateral)

---

1. The uncommon superficial spreading tumour of any size with its invasive component limited to the bronchial wall, which may extend proximal to the main bronchus, is also classified as T1.

2. Most pleural effusions with lung cancer are due to tumour. In a few patients, however, multiple cytopathological examinations of pleural fluid are negative for tumour and the fluid is non-bloody and is not an exudate. Where these elements and clinical judgement dictate that the effusion is not related to the tumour, the effusion should be excluded as a staging element and the patient should be classified as T1, T2 or T3.

Table 4

Stage Grouping

Stage	*T* factor	*N* factor	*M* factor
Occult carcinoma	TX	N0	M0
Stage 0	Tis	N0	M0
Stage I A	T1	N0	M0
Stage I B	T2	N0	M0
Stage II A	T1	N1	M0
Stage II B	T2	N1	M0
	T3	N0	M0
Stage III A	T1	N2	M0
	T2	N2	M0
	T3	N1, N2	M0
Stage III B	Any T	N3	M0
	T4	Any N	M0
Stage IV	Any T	Any N	M1

- **Cough**, which can be dry or productive. Smokers, who may suffer from bronchitis and morning cough, will often acknowledge that their cough has altered in character.
- **Wheeze**. In a patient who has not been previously subject to wheeze this symptom alone should raise suspicion particularly if the wheeze is both inspiratory and expiratory, is unilateral and does not disappear after coughing and clearing secretions. Wheeze is usually the manifestation of partial obstruction in the main or lobar bronchi.
- **Dyspnoea**. Most often dyspnoea relates to obstruction of a major bronchus and consequent pulmonary atelectasis. At other times dyspnoea may be related to replacement of healthy parenchyma by a mass of tumour. Occasionally pleural effusion accompanying pulmonary neoplasm will cause dyspnoea by reducing ventilatory capacity.

Table 5

Summary and quick reference: lung cancer staging

Factor	Clinical characteristics
TX	Positive cytology
T1	≤3 cm
T2	≥3 cm, main bronchus, ≤2 cm from carina, invades visceral pleura, partial atelectasis
T3	Chest wall, diaphragm, pericardium, mediastinal pleura, main bronchus ≤ 2 cm from carina, total atelectasis
T4	Mediastinum, heart, great vessels, carina, trachea, oesophagus, vertebra; separate nodules in same lobe
N1	Ipsilateral peribronchial, ipsilateral hilar
N2	Ipsilateral mediastinal, subcarinal
N3	Contralateral mediastinal or hilar, scalene or Supraclavicular
M1	Includes separate nodule in different lobe

Table 6

Summary and quick reference: Determination of stage from TNM factors

	$N0$	$N1$	$N2$	$N3$
$T1$	I A	II A	III A	III B
$T2$	I B	II B	III A	III B
$T3$	II B	III A	III A	III B
$T4$	III B	III B	III B	III B
Any M factor	IV	IV	IV	IV

- **Stridor**. Typically stridor results from obstruction of a main bronchus by tumour and its extension to the lower trachea.

- **Haemoptysis**. An important symptom. The amount may vary from staining of sputum to a large amount causing considerable cardiorespiratory embarrassment.

- **Pain**. Denotes the spread of tumour to the parietal pleura and chest wall. However, a paroxysmal attack of coughing in the elderly may cause rib fracture (cough fracture) with acute pain.

- **Respiratory tract and chest infection**. In many instances lung cancer presentation is in the form of bronchopulmonary infection. In some the episode of infection subsides after a course of antibiotics but some symptoms, such as cough, linger on. Chest radiograph then reveals the real

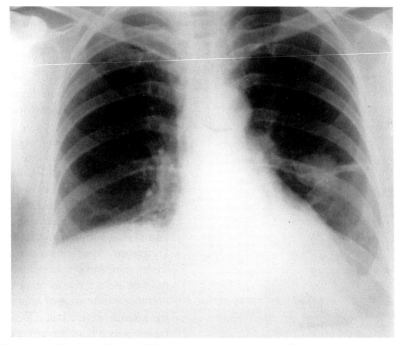

Fig. 2. Carcinoma of the lung (left lower lobe). An asymptomatic patient discovered at routine radiography.

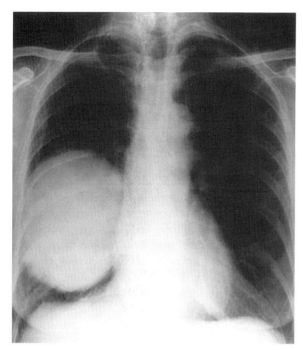

Fig. 3. Radiograph of a patient with bronchopulmonary cancer presenting with dyspnoea and chest pain. Note a large rounded opacity in the right lung.

cause which is usually a tumour with obstruction of the airway. Less commonly a peripheral tumour may involve the pleural surfaces with production of pleural effusion or even empyema as its consequence.

1.4.2. Presentation as non-respiratory disease and metastatic manifestation

In some cases of lung cancer, respiratory symptoms are absent or go unnoticed but symptoms referred to other systems are manifest. These are caused either by direct or metastatic involvement of intra- and/or extra-thoracic structures.

- **Superior vena caval syndrome.** This refers to signs and symptoms related to compression and obstruction of the superior vena cava by the tumour itself or through mediastinal lymph node involvement by the tumour which obstructs the venous return to the heart. (See SVC and superior mediastinal syndrome, section 4 in chapter II.3).

- **Brachial plexus neuralgia, Pancoast tumour and Horner's syndrome.** Pancoast tumour refers to a well-defined tumour at the apex of the chest usually from the apical/posterior segment of the upper lobe with infiltration of the chest wall, root of the neck and brachial plexus. This tumour was described in 1932 by Pancoast as superior sulcus tumour. The presentation relates to pain in the distribution of cervical (C_8) and first and second thoracic nerve roots (T_1 and T_2). There is also cutaneous temperature change and muscular atrophy of the shoulder and the arm innervated by nerves derived from the above spinal nerve roots.

- **Recurrent laryngeal nerve palsy.** In a few patients with lung cancer the first manifestation of the disease is hoarseness and/or bi-tonal voice

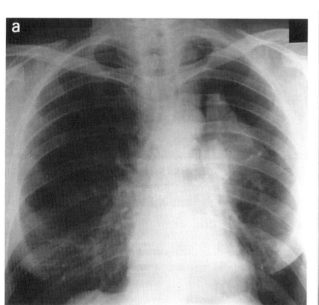
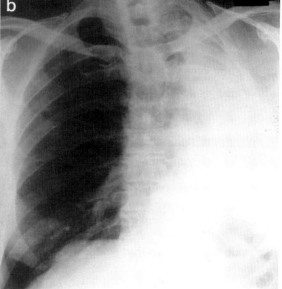

Fig. 4. (a) Radiograph of a patient with carcinoma of the bronchus presenting with haemoptysis and opacity in the left hilar region. (b) Chest radiograph of the same patient 14 years following pneumonectomy.

due to entrapment of the recurrent laryngeal nerve by the tumour, usually in the left upper lobe of the lung infiltrating the nerve directly or through involved metastatic mediastinal nodes as it loops around the aortic arch. Occasionally the recurrent laryngeal nerve on the right side is involved as it loops around the subclavian artery at the apex of the chest. Many patients with this mode of presentation are diagnosed following examination by an Otorhino-Laryngologist (ENT) to whom these patients are often first referred and are then X-rayed.

- **Phrenic nerve palsy**. This is usually discovered by chest radiography. The cause is usually involvement of the phrenic nerve, either by tumour and its infiltration (as the nerve runs over the pericardium at the root of the lung), or through the hilar lymph node affecting it over its course. It is worth emphasising that not all phrenic nerve palsies are neoplastic in origin; involvement of the nerve by calcified lymph nodes (e.g. tuberculosis) could have similar effects.
- **Chest wall involvement**. Direct involvement of the chest wall by cancer is common, particularly in peripheral lung tumours. Chest wall involvement may be limited to the parietal pleura and soft tissue or extend to bones with erosion of rib or, occasionally, sternum as a consequence. Pain is usually the primary manifestation and is accompanied by other symptoms and signs of respiratory disease.
- **Pleural effusion**. Pleural effusion in lung cancer patients may be the first manifestation of the disease. Direct tumour invasion of the visceral and/or parietal pleura may be the cause. Alternatively, the effusion may result from lymphatic obstruction. Sometimes the fluid is chylous, indicating obstruction of the intrathoracic duct.
- **Cardiac dysrhythmia**. The heart may be involved, usually through extension of the cancer to one of the pulmonary veins, the superior vena cava and/or right atrium. Various cardiac dysrythmia and/or atrial fibrillation are common manifestations of such involvement.
- **Pericardial involvement**. The pericardium is one of the commonest sites of direct metastatic involvement by primary lung cancer. Pericarditis, pericardial effusion and the resultant cardiac tamponade can occasionally be the initial clinical manifestation of lung cancer.
- **Dysphagia and oesophageal involvement**. Direct invasion of the oesophagus by lung cancer is uncommon and can produce dysphagia. Pos-

terior mediastinal malignant lymphadenitis and even massive involvement of these nodes usually causes displacement of the oesophagus without definite dysphagia. Rarely, left main bronchial cancer infiltrates the oesophagus directly and causes dysphagia which rapidly progresses to oesophago-airway fistula. Broncho-oesophago-scopic examination of such cases shows tumour both in the oesophagus and left main bronchus.

Extra-thoracic metastatic manifestation of lung cancer. Sooner or later in the course of its evolution, lung cancer metastasises to extra-thoracic organs, causing related symptoms and signs. Only occasionally does metastatic spread and its corresponding symptoms form primary manifestation and mode of presentation of the disease. However, lung cancer is the commonest source of metastatic disease in the western world.

That this mode of presentation is rare may be because in many organs, metastases remain silent for months before they become clinically relevant and symptomatic. The exception to this is metastatic disease of the central nervous system (CNS).

Central nervous system metastases (CNS). In some 10% of lung cancer patients there are CNS metastases and the same number develop secondaries in CNS during evolution of the disease. Small cell lung cancer is by far the most common histological type of metastasis in CNS. At autopsy some 40–50% of patients with lung cancer have CNS metastases (Wright and Delaney, 1989). However, a study involving 158 patients with NSCLC undergoing CT scan of the brain pre-operatively found 3% with positive scan (Kormas et al., 1992). Most symptoms of brain metastases are the consequence of an increase in intra-cranial pressure presenting as headache, nausea and vomiting.

Bone metastases. Some 25% of patients with lung cancer develop bone metastases with related pain. The spine, pelvis, femur and ribs are the most common sites. Such metastases are predominantly osteolytic causing pathological fracture, hypercalcaemia and neurological deficit. Occasionally bone metastases and their resulting symptoms and signs constitute the presenting mode of lung cancer.

Hepatic metastases. Liver metastases are usually discovered by CT and ultrasonography. Sometimes epigastric and right subcostal pain draw attention to the metastatic disease. Infrequently, painful hepatomegaly, the finding of a hard, tender mass on abdominal palpation or the presence of jaundice reveal the nature and extent of hepatic involvement.

Other visceral, skin and soft tissue metastases. Incidental metastatic disease is sometimes found during the investigation of lung cancer or other pathological condition. Skin and soft tissue metastases can occur in 1–2% of cases.

1.4.3. Presentation of lung cancer with non-metastatic para-neoplastic syndromes

Para-neoplastic syndromes (see Table 7) refer to a group of symptoms and signs which may appear in patients with lung cancer, but which neither relate directly to the respiratory system nor to local metastatic disease of the organs affected by the secondary tumours.

It is important to note that:

- Para-neoplastic syndromes are not specific to lung cancer though they are commonly associated with it.
- There is no relationship between the magnitude of tumour mass and the existence or severity of the para-neoplastic syndrome.
- Para-neoplastic syndromes can be associated with early stage cancer and, therefore, their diagnosis is of therapeutic relevance.
- Occasionally para-neoplastic syndromes are the presenting mode of lung cancer.
- Some 10% of patients with lung cancer can have manifestation of para-neoplastic syndrome.

1.5. Lung cancer treatment

It is generally accepted that for non-small cell types of lung cancer, the best and most appropriate method of treatment is surgical resection, when technically and oncologically feasible. In unresectable and inoperable cases other options have to be considered. There are now a number of therapeutic options, each for a specific set of indications. The most commonly used options for lung cancer therapy are:

- surgery (see section 1.5.1 below)
- radiotherapy (see section 1.5.2 below)
- chemotherapy (see section 1.5.3 below)
- laser therapy and other therapeutic methods (see section 1.5.4 below)

1.5.1. Surgical treatment of lung cancer

Historical background: Until the beginning of the 20th century, surgical access to the lung was not

Table 7

Para-neoplastic syndromes associated with lung cancer

1.	Endocrine: – Non-metastatic hypercalcaemia – Cushing syndrome – Syndrome of antidiuretic hormone – Carcinoid syndrome – Gynecomastia – Hyperthyroidism – Hypoglycaemia – Elevated levels of FSH and LH (follicle stimulating hormone and luteinising hormone)
2.	Neurological: – Encephalopathy – Subacute sensory neuropathy – Lambert-Eaton syndrome – Encephalomyelitis – Cancer-associated retinopathy
3.	Skeletal: – Clubbing – Hypertrophic osteoarthropathy
4.	Cutaneous: – Acquired hypertrichosis lanuginosa – Dermatomyositis – Acanthosis nigricans – Hyper-pigmentation – Erythema gyratum repens
5.	Haematological: – Anaemia – Thrombocytopaenic purpura – Leucocytosis
6.	Coagulopathy: – Disseminated intravenous coagulation – Thrombophlebitis
7.	Others: – Anorexia – Cachexia – Nephrotic syndrome – Vasculitis

a practical possibility because of the negative intrapleural pressure, which on opening of the chest, caused open pneumothorax. This phenomenon was aptly known at the time as "the pneumothorax problem". Some surgeons were able to carry out partial resection of the lung using a two-stage operation. In the first stage, pleural adhesions were created. This allowed a limited thoracotomy at the second stage over the area of pleural adhesion without total pneumothorax ensuing. The part of the lung to be resected was then exteriorised prior to excision.

The first pneumonectomy for cancer, reported by Graham and Singer (1933), was an important step in establishing surgical resection as the main method of treatment for primary lung cancer. For the next twenty years, pneumonectomy held its position as the operation of choice when surgical resection was contemplated. Since the 1950s lobectomy and lesser lung resection have been practiced. The introduction of sleeve resection, by Price-Thomas (1956), and its practice in lung cancer, heralded a new era of conservative pulmonary resection and parenchyma-saving operations.

The evolution of lung cancer surgery has depended on the parallel development of techniques for anaesthesia with the use of endotracheal intubation and positive pressure ventilation, which enabled surgeons to overcome the pneumothorax problem. Selective one lung ventilation, initially with the use of bronchial blockage followed by a variety of double lumen tubes, has facilitated surgical manoeuvres with a deflated lung.

General principles of pulmonary surgery for cancer. Resectional surgery for lung cancer tends to consider surgical anatomy of the lung as well as the oncological aspects of lung cancer. Close co-operation between the surgeon and the anaesthetist is crucial to match suitability of the patient to the proposed operation, its approach, extent of resection and any specific problems which could arise peri-operatively. *Oncological aspect.* Whilst, in all pulmonary resection, conservation of healthy parenchyma is the rule, in the case of cancer resection it should incorporate a safe margin of uninvolved lung tissue and bronchial stump. Only very small peripheral primary lung cancers may be resected with safety by segmental and wedge resections.

Bronchial stump: The margin of the bronchial stump should be macroscopically and microscopically free from tumour. Frozen section histology should be carried out at the time of resection in doubtful cases.

Dissemination and implantation of malignant cells must be an ever-present concern during pulmonary surgery for cancer. Care should be taken not to manipulate the tumour unnecessarily.

Peripheral lung tumour attached to the chest wall should be removed en bloc and not piecemeal unless there are insurmountable handicaps. Tumour involvement of major pulmonary vein branches should be handled with caution since detachment and tumour embolisation could result from pressure on the tumour in this situation. In some of these cases, where there is not a sufficient extra-pericardial length to enable a safe vascular ligation and division, sur-

gically or oncologically, the intra-pericardial route should be used for the purpose. This should be done before too much manipulation of the lung is undertaken.

Experience shows that nodal status is the most important determinant factor in the patient's long-term survival. Therefore, meticulous lymphadenectomy should be a mandatory part of cancer surgery as the presence of micro-metastases in lymph nodes is not unusual in bronchogenic carcinoma.

There is no place for incomplete resection for palliative purposes except on rare occasions and when there are compelling reasons at thoracotomy to adopt this option in lieu of no resection at all.

Indications for surgical treatment in lung cancer. For early stage lung cancer, surgical resection constitutes the most effective method of treatment and it is the therapy which achieves the highest rate of cure or long survival. However, this statement needs to be qualified and the qualification relates to the definition of early lung cancer. In the context of lung cancer therapy, early stage means:
- Stage 0   Tis N0 M0
- Stage I   A: T1 N0 M0
               B: T2 N0 M0
- Stage II   A: T1 N1 M0
               B: T2 N1 M0

It is to be noted that some physicians have defined early lung cancer as a locally infiltrating squamous cell carcinoma confined to the bronchial wall (Muller, 1988). Currently the depth of wall infiltration cannot be assessed pre-operatively, therefore this definition will have to be taken with understandable reservation.

It is important to specify that:
- Although stage classification refers to pathological (i.e. resection specimen) staging, obviously the submission to operation would have to be based on clinical staging.
- **Surgical treatment generally applies to non small cell lung cancer (NSCLC)** (see sections 1.3.2 and 3.1 in this chapter).

Stage 0 tumours: Tis N0 M0 and its treatment problem

In the absence of a screening programme, and at the present state of our practice, for most practitioners, stage 0 lung cancer is an incidental finding usually discovered by cytological examination of bronchial lavage sample at bronchoscopy or at routine sputum examination. Chest radiography is usually unhelpful and bronchoscopy using white light is unrevealing. It is suggested that by meticulous biopsy sampling there is the possibility of identifying lobar/segmental bronchial mucosal neoplasia responsible for shedding malignant cells. However, this is an elaborate undertaking and, until recently, has often had the disadvantage that the resection of such lesions presented the problem of potentially losing a functioning lobe or the whole lung if a bronchoplastic procedure were to be impractical. Developments in the field of fluorescence bronchoscopy and PDT can contribute to the diagnosis of stage 0 lung cancer and its treatment respectively. Fluorescence bronchoscopy potentially provides the visual localisation of malignant epithelial changes and directs the operator to biopsy any suspicious area (Lam et al., 1994). Endoscopic PDT (see section 6.2 in chapter IV.5) permits ablation of these superficial malignant lesions with high probability of cure (Cortese, 1986; Hayata et al., 1993). It is to be emphasised that, when technically possible, bronchoplastic procedures with/without PDT should be carried out. The cure rate of these occult carcinomas is high. However, it is generally observed that a high percentage of patients with treated occult carcinomas develop a new carcinoma in a different lobe/segment (Martini and Melamed, 1980). This underlines the point that resection of a large volume of the lung, in such patients with occult cancer, should be avoided. It also highlights the value of surveillance after treatment.

Stage I tumours: T1 N0 M0 and T2 N0 M0

These tumours are generally discovered as part of routine radiography or in the course of the investigation of other conditions. Sometimes haemoptysis may warrant a chest radiograph with demonstration of the tumour. In a high percentage of cases a less-than-pneumonectomy resection is technically and oncologically possible. Whether a stage I T1 N0 should still undergo a lobectomy, when a lesser resection with a wide healthy tissue margin is technically possible, is debatable. Nevertheless, two studies suggest an increased incidence of local recurrence in those who had less than lobectomy resection (Warren and Faber, 1994; Ginsberg and Rubinstein, 1995).

The 5-year survival rate after surgery in a mix (pT1/pT2 N0 M0) of stage I lung cancer is between 59–76%. When stratified between pT1 and pT2, the five year survival is between 76–83% for pT1 and 12–20% lower for pT2 (Lung cancer study group, 1987; Naruke et al., 1988; Schirren et al., 1995; Martini and Ginsberg, 1995).

Stage II tumours: T1–T2 N1 M0 and T3 N0 M0

Stage II tumours are resectable by lobectomy in the majority of cases and this type of resection remains the procedure of choice. Unlike stage I cancer, the T factor appears not to be a survival determinant factor but the involvement of lymph nodes at station N1 affects the survival of stage II cancer patients compared with N0 (stage I) patients. In a mix of T1–T2 and N1 patients, i.e. N1 in one or more stations, the 5-year survival of patients with stage II disease is about 40% (Lung cancer study group, 1987; Martini and Ginsberg, 1995). However, there is a difference in 5-year survival between single N1 and multiple N1 cases. In Martini et al.'s series (Martini et al., 1992) those with this difference was 14% (45% for single N1 versus 31% for multiple N1) There seems to be a worse prognosis for those with N1 in more than one station. There is no evidence that post-operative radiotherapy/chemotherapy can significantly affect survival in N1 disease. Also, such post-resection adjunct therapy could adversely affect the quality of survival (Martini et al., 1992). Stage II T3 N0 M0 survival is largely affected by the topography of the lesion, i.e., peripheral and chest wall or central.

Stage III tumours

Stage III lung cancer includes a range of advanced tumours, some of which are surgically and oncologically amenable to resection with survival benefit and even cure of the disease in a small number. Even in stage III A disease, the variation of T and N factors is such that prediction of life expectancy after surgical resection becomes clouded by the complexity of computation extrapolation. At one end of the gamut of III A is T3 N1 and at the other end is T1 N2. As a general rule, for a T3 tumour, the extent of N (N1–N2) is predictive of survival, and for tumours with N2 involvement, the extent of T (T1–T3) becomes an important prognostic value. In reality, stage III A tumours with mediastinal node (N2) have a worse prognosis than those with any T. In this scenario, it is difficult to present a survival rate after surgery. Nevertheless, an approximate 20% 5-year survival has been recorded by a number of authors (Maggi, 1988; Goldstraw et al., 1994) for patients whose N2 is discovered at operation (pN2) where pre-operative investigation, including mediastinoscopy, failed to show nodal (mediastinal) involvement. At present the results of surgery in pre-operatively diagnosed N2 disease cannot be stated with any degree of accuracy. For one thing, many surgeons and oncologists, including the author, consider these cancers to be inoperable in the presence of mediastinoscopy-proven N2 disease. Therefore, carefully planned induction chemotherapy or chemo/radiotherapy should be employed. It seems also a rational prerequisite that only those who have responded to such induction therapy should be offered surgical resection. Review of literature on the subject of stage III N2 disease reveals that 3- or 5-year survival figures from different centres are neither consistent (because of a number of variables) nor reproducible by other centres (De Leyn et al., 1999). Management of stage III NSCLC with N2 is, therefore, still the subject of controversy. There is, however, better agreement for stage III A T3 N1 tumours.

Currently there is no evidence to suggest that stage III B tumours (N3) would benefit from surgical resection with or without chemo/radiotherapy.

Selection of patients for pulmonary resection in lung cancer. The selection of patients for pulmonary resection is of paramount importance in order to minimise the number of unnecessary thoracotomies, reduce operative and peri-operative morbidity and mortality and improve survival and quality of life. The selection process considers 3 basic issues:

1. The general condition of the patient and fitness for the proposed operation. Determination of risk factors can be predictive of early operative results, which relate to morbidity and mortality.
2. Oncological aspect considers the extent of disease and its metastatic spread. This involves clinical staging using TNM classification and determines the oncological operability status. Post-resectional pathological staging is more accurately predictive of the long-term results of resection and in certain circumstances may indicate the need for post-operative therapy.
3. Extent of resection. This has an important effect on quality of survival and requires inclusion in the selection process of the patient.

Fitness for surgery and risk factors
- **Age**: Extension of life expectancy in recent years has resulted in a parallel increase in the number of elderly lung cancer sufferers. A number of studies have now shown that an individual of age >70 will have greater incidence of concomitant cardiovascular and other diseases with a higher operative and post-operative risk of complication. However, age per se does not constitute

a major risk factor, although generally, elderly patients require greater pre-operative work-up and more intensive post-operative care. Selection for surgery is made on the basis of the individual patient's suitability and not age alone (Gebitekin et al., 1993; Thomas et al., 1994).
- **Cardiovascular system risk factors**: Patients with previous myocardial infarction and/or co-existing coronary arterial disease present with higher surgical resection risk. Thorough cardiological assessment, including coronary angiography, should be carried out in cases with ischemic changes on ECG or with severe angina. Patients with coronary arterial disease and operable lung cancer should be judged independently for each procedure and be offered surgery if they qualify for each operation. The decision as to which of the operations should be carried out first is a matter of choice and subject to discussion by the team of oncologist, cardiologist and surgeon (Thomas et al., 1994). The presence of lung cancer does not exclude the operation of coronary revascularisation nor is the existence of coronary arterial stenotic lesion a contraindication to lung resection. In some cases the two operations may be carried out in one procedure (Rao et al., 1996; Danton et al., 1998).
- **Respiratory system risk factors**: Pulmonary function greatly influences both early and later results of surgical resection for lung cancer. Therefore, pre-operative measurement is important for two reasons. In the immediate post-operative phase, an increased functional demand is made on the residual parenchyma. Since quality of life after recovery from operation is largely dependent on remaining pulmonary function, the more extensive the pulmonary resection, the more elaborate the pulmonary function testing needs to be.

Time and financial constraints demand rationalisation of the extent of functional investigation of patients prior to resectional surgery and many surgical centres have adopted minimal functional standards for a given extent of resection. Such thresholds are based on experience and literature review.

The British Thoracic Society standard-of-care document (BTS recommendations to respiratory physicians, 1998) recommends the following pulmonary function investigations:
- All patients should have spirometry. No further respiratory function tests are required for lobectomy if the post-bronchodilator FEV_1 is >1.5

litres and for pneumonectomy if the post-bronchodilator FEV$_1$ is >2.0 litres.
- For pneumonectomy patients with spirometry below the above figures, a quantitative isotope perfusion scan, full pulmonary function testing including transfer factor and also measurement of oxygen saturation on air at rest should be undertaken.

There is evidence that patients with a calculated post-operative value of FEV$_1$ less than 40% (of the predicted value) and transfer factors of less than 40% are at risk of higher post-operative complication and higher mortality.

Cardiovascular assessment

Apart from history taking and clinical investigation, the minimum cardiovascular assessment requirement for patients undergoing resectional surgery are:
- pre-operative ECG;
- echocardiogram for those with cardiac murmur;
- patients with myocardial infarction need a 6–8 week infarct-free interval before lung resection is undertaken.

1.5.2. The role of radiotherapy in lung cancer treatment

The role of radiotherapy in the treatment of lung cancer is considered under:
(a) External Beam Radiotherapy (EBR) (see below)
(b) Brachytherapy and intra-operative radiotherapy (see below)

External Beam Radiotherapy (EBR). EBR is used in the following circumstances:
- with curative intent
- in palliation
- prophylactic/pre-operative
- post-operatively
- in conjunction with chemotherapy in small cell lung cancer (SCLC)

EBR with curative intent

This is reserved for a limited number of stage I and II patients with NSCLC who either refuse surgical operation or cannot be offered surgery. More often patients with stage III A or III B are candidates. There is no "standard" radiotherapy regimen for NSCLC and most suggested schedules are derived from experience and/or based on empirical criteria. A study by the Radiation Therapy Oncology Group (RTOG) demonstrated the effect of total dose on response when a total dose of 40 Gy, 50 Gy or 60 Gy was given as 2 Gy per fraction. There was better local control associated with a higher dose (Perez et al., 1982, 1986) although this caused the expected higher toxicity. The 5-year survival result of EBR with curative intent is reported to be 6% for stage III B ascending to 32% for stage I: (Zhang et al., 1989; Kaskowitz et al., 1993). It must however be realised that in stage I and II tumours, there is inevitably an element of bias in selection since generally, only patients unsuitable for surgical resection are offered EBR. Also, depending on the mix of cases and regimen used, different results can be expected.

Palliative EBR

The role of EBR in unresectable tumours is to control symptoms. EBR can relieve haemoptysis and pain due to skeletal involvement and can also alleviate dyspnoea when this is due to major bronchial obstruction and atelectasis. For palliation, a lower dosage is used than in EBR with curative intent. Many of the regimens use 30 Gy spread over 2 weeks (Scarantino, 1985; Salazar et al., 1993) but there is no consensus on the optimal regimen, i.e. dose/fraction, number of fractions and interval between fractions.

The Medical Research Council (MRC) in the UK has conducted a number of trials addressing the issue of impact of these variables on palliation of symptoms. One study showed no difference between 30 Gy in 10 fractions over 2 weeks as opposed to 17 Gy in 2 fractions of 8.5Gy in one week (Bleehen, 1991).

Post-operative radiotherapy

The role of EBR in patients who have complete surgical resection of their tumour is yet to be defined despite a number of trials devoted to the issue. Overall, there appears to be no survival advantage to be gained from EBR post-operatively. An MRC multicentre trial did not show any advantage in post-operation radiotherapy to T1–2 N1 cases (Stephens et al., 1996). However, in subgroups of patients, there is a decrease in local and regional recurrence of tumour. There may also be some survival benefit to resected patients with N2 disease. At the present state of our understanding, and based on available data, there is no evidence to advise routine post-operative radiotherapy for patients who have had complete resection, nor is there a place for EBR in stage I tumours. It does, however, have a place for T3 chest wall tumours and in N2 disease.

Pre-operative EBR

The pre-operative role of EBR relates to the down-staging of tumours to achieve a higher rate of resectability and survival benefit but the measurement of beneficial effects is difficult. General observation and experience backed by some evidence indicates the resectability rate may be increased in some stage III tumours although whether pre-operative EBR can offer survival benefit is questionable. In the case of superior sulcus tumour, pre-operative radiotherapy is practiced by a number of groups (Shaw et al., 1961; Dartevelle and Macchiarini, 1995).

Endobronchial Radiotherapy. Advances in technology and radiation protection in recent years have been responsible for renewed interest in endoluminal brachytherapy. Brachy technique is classified under low dose rate (LDR) delivering 0.4–2 Gy/h and high dose rate (HDR) >12 Gy/h. The radiation dose is delivered via a catheter which is placed through the flexible bronchoscope (see interventional bronchoscopy, chapter IV.3). This method is used for endoluminal projecting tumours causing obstruction and atelectasis. Treatment can be given to patients having had previous EBR for palliation of haemoptysis or dyspnoea and also for small endobronchial tumours when neither surgery or EBR is indicated.

Side-effects and toxicity of Radiotherapy

"To have another operation I will, but to have radiotherapy again I will not" said a patient who after recurrence of his resected tumour had a full course of EBR. This reaction illustrates that, at its worst, radiotherapy is perceived by some patients as being every bit as invasive as thoracotomy.

Symptoms during the course of EBR are:
Early complications:

- fatigue, exaggeration of existing cough and sputum
- dysphagia due to oesophagitis is often present and can be associated with weight loss. Antacid and antispasmodic will alleviate early oesophageal complications.

These symptoms are temporary and tend to subside after a few weeks.

- skin manifestations; i.e. hyperaemia and erythema still occur even with modern equipment

Delayed/late complications:

- Radiation pneumonitis. This collateral damage occurs usually 1–3 months post-treatment and can lead to pulmonary fibrosis. Total dose, fractional regimen and particularly irradiation volume influence the severity of this complication. Steroids with/without antibiotic help to reduce the extent of damage.
- Continued oesophagitis can lead to stricture occurring several months after termination of treatment. There may also be motor disturbance of the oesophagus. At an early stage, anti-spasmodic will help. Later oesophagoscopy and dilatation may become necessary.
- Cardiovascular. Radiation can induce pericarditis, myocardial functional impairment and ischemic changes due to coronary stenotic lesions. This risk is elevated by high-dose (>40 Gy) EBR.
- Myelopathy: Early in the course of high-dosage thoracic radiotherapy, spinal cord damage can occur with paraesthesia. Later on myelitis and necrosis of the cord may ensue, leading to the worst case scenario of paresis and paraplegia.

Note on Fractionation in Radiotherapy

- Classical fractionation:
  single treatment/day 1.8–2 Gy
- Split course:
  daily fraction for 1–2 weeks,
  rest period for 2–4 weeks,
  then daily fraction dose
- Hypofractionation:
  less than 4 fractions/week of 3–5 Gy
- Hyperfractionation:
  higher number of fractions but smaller dose/fraction: e.g. 2–3 fractions/day (1–1.3 Gy) × 5 days for 60 Gy over 5 weeks or more for 6.5 Gy (mean)
- Continuous hyperfractionated accelerated radiation therapy (CHART):
  1.5 Gy, 3 times/day with minimal interfraction interval of 6 hours = total of 40–54 Gy

1.5.3. Chemotherapy in lung cancer

The role of chemotherapy in lung cancer is discussed under 2 headings:

(a) in non-small cell lung cancer (see section 1.5.3.1 below)
(b) in small cell lung cancer (see section 1.5.3.2 below)

Chemotherapy in non-small cell lung cancer. The rationale of the use of chemotherapy in NSCLC is that, at presentation, over 60% of patients will have unresectable and disseminated tumours and some of the remaining have sub-clinical metastases. Theoretically an appropriate chemotherapeutic agent could improve symptoms and/or offer survival benefit.

However, before embarking on such a therapy, its aims for each particular case should be identified and the benefits and drawbacks considered. In practice, chemotherapy for NSCLC is used either for symptom relief with/without survival benefit in patients with extensive and unresectable tumour or as an adjunct to surgery in potentially resectable cases.

In the past 40 years there has been a considerable advance in the synthesis and manufacture of powerful chemotherapy agents. There have also been several trials involving different schedules and drug combination regimens.

There appears to be no agreed standard schedule of chemotherapy for advanced and inoperable NSCLC. Most regimens include Cisplatin and many have also vinca alkaloids and Ifosfamide (e.g. VIP, Vindesine Ifosfamide Platinum regimen).

Neither does there seem to be evidence based on randomised trials to indicate that either a single agent or combination chemotherapy can achieve palliation of symptoms and/or survival benefit to advanced cases of NSCLC when compared with non-specific supportive care (Woods et al., 1990; Kaasa et al., 1991). One of the greatest problems of chemotherapy for NSCLC is toxicity, although there are other complications, all of which are more pronounced when the treatment is not organised or monitored properly (Thatcher et al., 1995).

Chemotherapy in small cell lung cancer (SCLC). From 20 to 25% of the lung cancer population have SCLC but only a very small proportion, probably no more than 5%, may be suitable for surgical resection. Chemotherapy has, therefore, been the mainstay of treatment for this type of tumour.

Chemotherapeutic agents for SCLC are similar to those for NSCLC.

Although there is no particular standard scheme or recommended regimen, combination therapy is more effective than single agent administration. The two regimens most frequently used are:
- CAV (cyclophosphamide, adriomycin and vincristin)
- EP (etoposide and cisplatin)

There is definite overall survival benefit in patients who receive chemotherapy versus those who do not. This benefit is more pronounced in patients with limited rather than extensive disease. The overall survival for 2 and 5 years in a large series from the UK (Souhami and Law, 1990) has been reported to be 5.9% and 3% respectively. This is in line with other reported large series.

Complications of chemotherapy. All chemotherapeutic agents have side effects and can present with associated early or late complications. These are more pronounced in some patients than others. Nausea, vomiting and loss of appetite are common occurrences and are associated more with cisplatin than other agents.

Steroid, dexamethasone and serotonin antagonists are of substantial help.

Myelo suppression is a more serious complication with potential for infection and bleeding.

Peripheral neuropathy, nephrotoxicity, mucosal ulceration and a number of other complications can result from the cytotoxicity of a variety of chemotherapeutic agents. These complications usually occur early in the course of treatment. There are other complications which occur after completion of chemotherapy. These consist of cardiomyopathy, pulmonary fibrosis and central nervous system toxicity. An important complication is a tendency for the development of a second malignancy, including in the lung itself. Late cardiorespiratory complications can be of significance in patients who receive induction chemotherapy followed by surgery. In these an increasing and unexpected degree of post-operative respiratory restriction might follow, months after resection, which may be out of proportion to the extent of resection.

References and further reading

Bleehen N. Inoperable non small cell lung cancer (NSCLC). A Medical Research Council randomised trial of palliative radiotherapy with two fractions and ten fractions. Br J Cancer 1991; 63: 265–270.

British Thoracic Society recommendations to respiratory physicians for organising the care of patients with lung cancer. Thorax 1998; 53 (Supp I): 51–58.

Carbone PP, Mina JD. The molecular genetics of lung cancer. In: Advances in Internal Medicine. Mosby Year Book Inc 1992; 37: 153–171.

Cortese DA. Bronchoscopic photodynamic therapy of early lung cancer. Chest 1986; 90: 629–631.

Danton MHD, Anikin VA, McManus KG et al. Simultaneous cardiac surgery with pulmonary resection: presentation of a series and review of literature. Eur J Cardiothorac Surg 1998; 13: 667–672.

Dartevelle P, Macchiarini P. Cervical approach to apical lesion. In: Pearson GF et al. (eds.), Thoracic Surgery. Churchill Livingstone 1995; 99: 887–897.

Denissenko MF, Pao A, Tang M, Pfeifer GP. Preferential formation of benzo[a]pyrene adducts at lung cancer mutational hotspots in *p*53. Science 1996; 274: 430–432.

Denoix PF. Enquête permanente dans les centres anticancéreux. Bull Inst Nat Hyg 1941; 1: 70–75.

Gebitekin C, Gupta NK, Martin PG et al. Long term results in the elderly following pulmonary resection for non small cell lung carcinoma. Eur J Cardiothorac Surg 1993; 7: 653–656.

Ginsberg RJ, Rubinstein LV. Randomised trial of lobectomy versus limited operation for T1 N0 non small cell lung cancer. Cancer Study Group. Ann Thorac Surg 1995; 60: 622–623.

Goldstraw P, Mann G, Kaplan D, Michael P. Surgical management of non small cell lung cancer with ipsilateral mediastinal node metastases (N2 disease). J Thorac Cardiovasc Surg 1994; 107: 19–28.

Graham EA, Singer JT. Successful removal of the entire lung for carcinoma of the bronchus. JAMA 1933; 101: 1371.

Harris C. *p*53: at the crossroads of molecular carcinogenesis and risk assessment. Science 1993; 262: 1980–1981.

Hayata Y, Kato H, Konoka C. et al. Photodynamic therapy in early stage lung cancer. Lung Cancer 1993; 9: 287–294.

Herndandez-Boussard TM and Hainaut P. A specific spectrum of *p*53 mutations in lung cancer from smokers: review of mutations compiled in the IARC *p*53 database. Environ Health Perspectives 1998; 106: 385–391.

Kaasa S, Lund E, Thorud E et al. Symptomatic treatment versus combination chemotherapy for patients with extensive non small cell lung cancer. Cancer 1991; 67: 2443–2447.

Kaskowitz L, Graham MV, Emami B et al. Radiation therapy done for stage I non small cell lung cancer. Int J Radiat Oncol Biol Phys 1993; 27: 517–523.

Kormas P, Bradshaw JR, Jaysingham K. Pre-operative computed tomography of the brain in non-small cell lung carcinoma. Thorax 1992; 47: 106–108.

Lam S, MacAulay C, Le Riche JC et al. Early localisation of bronchoscopic carcinoma. Diagn Ther Endosc 1994; 1: 75–78.

De Leyn P, Vansteenkiste J, Deneffe G et al. Results of induction chemotherapy followed by surgery in patients with stage III A N2 NSCLC: Importance of pre treatment mediastinoscopy. Eur J Cardiothorac Surg 1999; 15(5): 608–614.

Lung Cancer Study Group. Post operative T1 N0 non small cell lung cancer squamous versus squamous recurrences. J Thorac Cardiovasc Surg 1987; 94: 349.

Maggi G. Results of radical treatment of stage III A non small cell carcinoma of lung. Eur J Cardiothorac Surg 1988; 2: 329–335.

Martini N, Melamed MR. Occult carcinomas of the lung. Ann Thorac Surg 1980; 30: 215.

Martini N, Burt ME, Bains MS et al. Survival after resection in stage II non small cell lung cancer. Ann Thorac Surg 1992; 24: 460.

Martini N, Ginsberg RJ. Lung cancer surgical management. In: Pearson FG, Deslauriers J, Ginsberg RJ et al. (eds.). Thoracic Surgery. Churchill Livingstone Inc 1995; 690–741.

Mountain CF. The new international staging for lung cancer. Surg Clin North Am 1987; 67: 925.

Mountain CF. Revision in the international system for staging of lung cancer. Chest 1997; 111: 1710–1717.

Muller KM. Early cancer of the lung. Recent Results Cancer Res 1988; 106: 119–130.

Muller KM. Lung cancer: Morphology. In: Carcinoma of the lung. SG Spiro (ed.). Eur Respiratory Monograph Vol 1. 1995; Eur Resp Soc J: 50–71.

Mulshine JL, Treston AM, Brown PE (eds.). Initiators and Promoters of lung cancer. Chest 1993; 103 (suppl): 45–115.

Naruke T, Goya T, Tsuchiya R, Suemasu K. Prognosis and survival in resected lung carcinoma based on the new international staging system. J Thorac Cardiovasc Surg 1988; 96: 440–447.

Naruke T, Suemasu K, Ishikawa S. Lymph node mapping and curability at various levels of metastasis in resected lung cancer. J Thorac Cardiovasc Surg 1978; 832–839.

Olsen JH. Epidemiology of lung cancer in carcinoma of the lung (European Respiratory Monograph). SG Spiro (ed.), Eur Respir J 1995; 1–18.

Osterlin K. Chemotherapy in small cell lung cancer in Carcinoma of the lung. Spiro SG (ed.), European Respiratory Monograph 1995; Vol 1: 306–331.

Pancoast HK. Superior pulmonary sulcus tumour: Tumour characterised by pain, Horner's syndrome, destruction of bone and atrophy of hand muscles. JAMA 1932; 99: 1391–1396.

Parkin DM, Pisani P, Ferlay J. Estimate of the worldwide incidence of eighteen major cancers in 1985. Int J Cancer 1993; 54: 594–606.

Perez CA, Stanley K, Grundy G et al. Impact of irradiation technique and tumour extent in tumour control and survival of patients with unresectable non oat cell carcinoma of the lung. Report by the Radiation Therapy Oncology Group. Cancer 1982; 50: 1091–1099.

Perez CA, Bauer M, Edelstein S et al. Impact of tumour control on survival in carcinoma of the lung treated with irradiation. Int J Radiat Oncol Biol Phys 1986; 12: 539–547.

Price-Thomas C. Conservative resection of the bronchial tree. J R Coll Surg Edinb 1956; 1: 169.

Rao V, Todd TRY, Weisel RD et al. Results of combined pulmonary resection and cardiac operation. Ann Thorac Surg 1996; 62: 342–347.

Salazar OM, McDonald S, Van Houtte P et al. Lung cancer. In: Rubin P, McDonald S, Qazi R (eds.). Clinical Oncology for medical students and physicians. Philadelphia: WB Saunders Co. 1993; 645–665.

Scarantino CW (ed.). Lung cancer diagnostic procedure and therapeutic management with special reference to radiotherapy. Berlin: Springer–Verlag 1985.

Schirren J, Krysa S, Trainer S et al. Surgical treatment of lung cancer. In: European Respiratory Monograph Vol I. Spiro SG (ed.) 1995; 1: 212–240.

Shaw RR, Paulson DL, Kee JL Jr. Treatment of the superior sulcus tumour by irradiation followed by resection. Ann Surg 1961; 154: 29.

Shields PG, Harris CC. Principle of carcinogenesis chemical. In: Devita VT, Helman S, Rosenberg SA (eds.). Cancer: Principle and practice of oncology. Philadelphia: JB Lippincott Co 1993; 200–212.

Sobin LH and Wittekind C (eds.). UICC TNM classification of malignant tumours, 5th ed. New York: Wilsey-Liss (A John Wiley and Sons Inc publication), 1997.

Thomas P, Piraux M, Jacques LF et al. Clinical patterns and trends of outcome of elderly patients with bronchogenic carcinoma. Eur J Cardio Thorac Surg. 1998; 13: 266–274.

Souhami RL, Law K. Longevity in small cell lung cancer a report to The Lung Cancer Committee of the United Kingdom co-ordinating committee for cancer research. Br J Cancer 1990; 61: 584–589.

Stephens RJ, Girling D, Bleehen N, Moghissi K et al. The role of post operative radiotherapy in non small cell lung cancer: a multi-centre randomised trial in patients with pathologically staged T1–T2 N1–2 M0 disease. Medical Research Council lung cancer working party. Br J Cancer 1996; 74: 632–639.

Thatcher N, Ranson M, Anderson H. Chemotherapy in non small cell lung cancer. In: Carcinoma of the lung. Spiro SG (ed.), European Respiratory Monograph. 1995; Vol 1: 269–305.

Thomas P, Giudicelli R, Guillen JC et al. Is lung cancer surgery justified in patients with coronary artery disease? Eur J Cardiothorac Surg 1994; 8: 287–292.

Warren WH, Faber LP. Segmentectomy versus lobectomy in patients with stage I pulmonary carcinoma. Five years survival patterns of intrathoracic recurrence. J Thorac Cardiovasc Surg. 1994; 1087–1093.

WHO International histological classification of tumours No 1 Histological typing of lung tumour. 2nd ed. Am J Clin Pathol. 1982; 77: 123–136.

Woods RL, Williams CJ, Levi J et al. A randomised trial of Cisplatin and Vindesine versus supportive care only in advanced non small cell lung cancer. Br J Cancer. 1990; 61: 608–611.

Wright DC, Delaney TF. Treatment of metastatic cancer to the brain. In: De Vita VT Jr, Hellman S, Rosemberg SA (eds.) Cancer principle and practice of oncology. Philadelphia: PA Lippincott. 1989; 2245–2261.

Zhang HX, Yin WB, Zhang LY et al. Curative radiotherapy of early operable non small cell lung cancer. Radiotherapy Oncol 1989; 14: 89–94.

2. Bronchopulmonary tumours other than lung cancer

Under this heading are described a group of heterogeneous bronchopulmonary neoplastic lesions, some of which are definitely malignant, others benign and a third subgroup are benign with malignant potential. A classification acceptable and useful to pathologists, oncologists and surgeons is unrealistic and not relevant to the scope of this book. For descriptive purposes we use the following grouping and elaborate on those tumours which have surgical relevance:
2.1 Rare primary malignant tumours.
2.2 Secondary malignant lung tumours.
2.3 Benign bronchopulmonary tumours.
2.4 Bronchial gland tumours.

2.1. Rare primary malignant tumours

2.1.1. Pulmonary blastomas

This rare tumour develops from embryonic tissue and was first described by Barrett and Barnard in 1945. In many cases the tumour contains a mixture of epithelial and mesenchymal elements. They are slow-growing but have some potential for metastasis formation. When symptomatic, presentation is akin to carcinoma. Otherwise, in about 40% of cases the tumour is found in routine chest radiography in the peripheral pulmonary parenchyma beyond the broncho-

scopic field of vision. The nature of the tumour is revealed at thoracotomy. CT-guided needle biopsy is advisable when the patient is unfit for thoracotomy.

The result of surgical resection is good and is attended by long survival (about 40–50% 5-year survival).

2.1.2. Carcino-sarcoma

This rare tumour contains both carcinoma and sarcoma components. Frequently it presents as a tumour within the main bronchus with resultant cough and haemoptysis. In other cases the tumour is diagnosed following chest radiography. Carcino-sarcoma is a malignant tumour capable of development of metastases. Surgical resection is the treatment of choice with expected 5-year survival of about 30%.

2.1.3. Primary Hodgkins

Primary Hodgkins of the lung may be present as multiple nodular disease in one or both lungs; rarely, tumour can be endobronchial. Apart from a very rare subset which can be diagnosed bronchoscopically, the overall majority require lung biopsy for their identification. Resection with/without adjunct chemotherapy has been used in those with limited local disease.

2.1.4. Non-Hodgkins lymphomas

This is an extremely rare condition often presenting as an asymptomatic nodular pulmonary lesion. The cell type is usually B type. The diagnosis is made by tissue biopsy and the treatment of choice is surgery adjunct to chemotherapy.

2.1.5. Plasma cell tumour

These are groups of malignant neoplasms derived from the proliferation of plasma cells secreting immunoglobulin, the most common member of which is multiple myeloma. Solitary plasma cell tumour (plasmacytoma) is extremely rare and may be endo-tracheo-bronchial or within the pulmonary parenchyma presenting as a pulmonary nodular lesion. Resectional surgery is the treatment of choice. About 50% of cases eventually develop multiple myeloma (Woodruff et al., 1979). Adjuvant radiotherapy seems to confer a further benefit.

2.1.6. Primary sarcoma of the lung:

These are amongst the rarest of lung tumours and are subdivided into:
(1) Soft tissue sarcoma
(2) Chondrosarcoma

(3) Osteosarcoma

They are all malignant but with differing degrees of malignancy.

Soft tissue sarcomas have a number of subtypes according to their constituent cells, of which Leiomyosarcoma is the commonest and malignant haemangiopericytoma the least frequent in the subtypes. The majority of patients are symptomatic at presentation with respiratory disease symptoms. Asymptomatic patients are detected radiologically with a solitary mass on the chest radiograph. Surgical resection, when complete, is attended by 44–69% 5-year survival (Jansen et al., 1994; Bacha et al., 1999). There is no evidence that chemo/radiotherapy could have an impact on results.

Chondrosarcoma and osteosarcomas are extremely uncommon pulmonary neoplasms. They present as a solitary mass on chest radiograph. Treatment, when possible, is surgical resection.

2.1.7. Malignant melanoma

Malignant melanoma of the lung is a very rare tumour. Both the origin of the tumour and whether the tumour is a primary malignant lung tumour are disputed.

2.1.8. Germ cell tumours

Both malignant and benign varieties (Teratomas) are extremely rare. The malignant variety may be an extension of the mediastinal Teratomas. The treatment of choice is chemotherapy.

2.1.9. Chorinocarcinoma

This tumour is extremely rare and presents as a large pulmonary mass. A characteristic of this tumour is its vascularity, which is prone to cause haemoptysis.

Summary of rare (uncommon) primary malignant tumours of the lung

For the practising thoracic surgeon, most of these tumours present as a solitary pulmonary mass and may even remain undiagnosed until thoracotomy or video-assisted thoracoscopic surgery. Large tumours require standard resection. Local excision may suffice for small nodular tumours. Frozen section should be carried out in pre-operatively undiagnosed cases. Those tumours which are symptomatic present with symptoms common to many neoplastic lesions including lung cancer. Some tumours may be visible at bronchoscopy and diagnosed by bronchial biopsy. Rarely such tumours as germ cell tumours and lymphomas may not require surgical treatment but will necessitate surgical biopsy to ascertain the diagnosis.

2.2. Secondary malignant lung tumours (pulmonary metastases)

In the past 15 years, attention has been focused on the importance of an aggressive surgical approach to pulmonary metastases and experience has shown that in some patients long-term survival can be achieved. It is, however, important to lay down selection criteria in order to offer metastatectomy to those who could predictably benefit from surgical metastatectomy.

Cancer from many organs can metastasise in the lung. The most important of these are:
- breast cancer
- colon cancer
- renal carcinoma
- osteogenic and soft tissue sarcoma
- non-seminomatous germ cell tumours

Two aspects of pulmonary metastases and their surgical treatment require consideration:
(a) Oncological aspects (see section 2.2.1 below)
(b) Thoracic surgical aspects (see section 2.2.2 below)

2.2.1. Oncological aspects

From the oncological viewpoint the following are of therapeutic and practical relevance:
- Evidence of total clearance of the tumour at the primary site and lack of local recurrence.
- Knowledge of the size, number and topography of pulmonary metastatic lesions.
- Absence of metastatic deposits in any other organs or parts of the body.
- Information on histology, evolution of the tumour, natural history and date of the primary treatment (medical or surgical), as well as the staging at the time of the treatment.

It is important to establish tumour-free intervals, i.e. time lapse between the eradication/excision of the primary tumour and the occurrence of pulmonary metastases. It is also helpful to take into account the speed of tumour doubling.

2.2.2. Thoracic surgical aspect

It is necessary to know the precise size, number, topography and extent of pulmonary metastases. Knowledge of pleural and lymphatic involvement is relevant. The presence of pleural effusion per se may not be a contraindication if the parietal pleura is not infiltrated or involved.

Total excision of all pulmonary lesions is the minimum requirement. It follows that pre-operative and predicted post-operative pulmonary function must be taken into account.

Surgical approach should be planned with the knowledge that:

- There is often discrepancy between the number of metastases as perceived by the most accurate CT image and findings at thoracotomy when, at times, pulmonary palpation reveals a greater number of metastases.
- VATS may not be a safe technique for pulmonary metastatectomy particularly when there are multiple deep-seated tumours.
- Extent of lung resection in pulmonary metastatectomy can vary according to a number of factors. The experience suggests that in many cases the metastases can be locally excised. At other times, wedge and segmental resection may suffice. Conservation with excision of all the metastases should be the aim. The use of NdYAG laser for metastatectomy combines local excision with a safety margin as well as control of air leak and haemostasis (Moghissi, 1990).
- In bilateral pulmonary metastatectomy, sternotomy (mediastinotomy) and/or bilateral staged thoracotomy using muscle-sparing thoracotomy will have a special place, particularly if laser is used to locally excise the tumour.
- Chemotherapy influences the progress of some tumours and the pattern of metastasis. It also has a role in conjunction with pulmonary metastatectomy. The influence of chemotherapy on osteogenic secondaries has been documented and shows that, when used post-operatively after the primary operation, it can reduce the incidence and number of secondaries in the lung.

2.3. Benign bronchopulmonary tumours

These are rare tumours, presenting often as pulmonary nodules with heterogenous tissue of origin. Most are benign, some can develop locally and few have malignant potential. A rational classification appears to be one suggested by Liebow (1952) which, with minor variations, is used by most authors. This classification groups the benign bronchopulmonary tumours according to their tissue of origin (Table 8).

2.3.1. Benign bronchopulmonary tumours of unknown origin

- Hamartoma of the lung

Albrecht (1904) introduced the term Hamartoma to describe a disorganised arrangement of tissue which normally presents in an organ. In the case of the lung, the lesion appears as a tumour consisting of tissues that normally make up the bronchus but which are arranged abnormally.

According to the above description, a hamartoma is a malformation but it is in fact a true neoplasm. The tumour is benign but it does grow slowly in size and very rarely becomes malignant (Poulsen et al., 1979).

Pulmonary hamartomas are composed predominantly of fibrous tissue, cartilage and epithelial cells. They are sometimes named by the adjective of their most dominant component. Since cartilage is the dominant tissue in many of the pulmonary hamartomas they are often referred to as cartilaginous hamartomas. In an overall majority of cases the tumour is in the substance of the lung where it appears as a rounded or lobulated pulmonary nodule, in which case the patient is asymptomatic. The lesion in an accidental X-ray finding appears as a pulmonary

Table 8

Benign bronchopulmonary tumours

Unknown origin (2.3.1)	Epithelial (2.3.2)	Mesodermal (2.3.3)		Miscellaneous (inflammatory) (2.3.4)	Neurogenic (2.3.5)
		Vascular	Bronchial		
Hamartoma	Papilloma	Angiomas: – Haemangioma – Lymphangioma – Haemangioendothelioma	Fibroma	Xanthoma	Neurofibroma
Clear cell tumour Teratoma (developmental)	Polyps	Lymphangiomyomatosis Haemangiopericytoma Arteriovenous fistula (malformation) Sclerosing haemangioma	Chondroma Lipoma Leiomyoma Granular cell (myoblastoma) tumour	Amyloid tumour Pseudolymphoma	Neuroma Neurilemoma

nodule. The definitive diagnosis of such a lesion is often made at exploratory thoracotomy/excision enucleation. The tumour is endobronchial in less than 20% of cases, causing pulmonary collapse due to bronchial obstruction.

Local excision or enucleation is the standard treatment. A small incision is made in the pulmonary parenchyma overlying the tumour which is easily enucleated. A few absorbable stitches and/or fine clips check the bleeding and air leak if present.

A frozen section should be carried out to exclude malignancy of the excised lesion. The endobronchial variety may be dealt with by bronchoscopic resection.

- Clear cell tumours

This is an extremely rare tumour and usually presents as a solitary nodule in the periphery of the lung. Originally described by Liebow and Castleman (1971), the tumour is benign but with the rare potential of malignant evolution. As the name implies the tumour is formed of clear cells akin to renal carcinoma and containing abundant glycogen. Local excision is usually curative. Immunohistochemical analysis should distinguish primary clear cell tumours from secondary renal cell carcinoma; however, the cells of origin of these tumours are uncertain.

- Pulmonary teratoma

This tumour is composed of undifferentiated tissue which is usually discovered on X-ray as a cavitation with possible calcification.

2.3.2. Epithelial tumours

(a) **Papillomas:**

Benign bronchial papillomas are rare and seen most commonly in children either as single or multiple tumours. The aetiology of papillomas is obscure but there is some evidence to suggest viral infection as a cause. Endoscopic resection is not usually advised on account of the high rate of recurrence and the possibility of malignant changes. Bronchoscopic laser resection (NdYAG laser) has been reported with good early to intermediate results (3–5 years). In some cases the sheer number of papillomas over the whole length of trachea make their surgical resection impossible.

(b) **Polyps:**

These tumours are endobronchial and probably inflammatory in origin. Bronchoscopic resection using NdYAG laser is the treatment of choice and is attended by cure.

2.3.3. Mesodermal tumours

These are classified under:

(a) vascular tumour (see below)
(b) bronchial tumour (see below)

Vascular (mesodermal) tumours.

- Angiomas

Under this heading 3 types of tumour are described: haemangioma, lymphangioma and haemangioendothelioma.

- Haemangiomas: These vascular tumours are found either in the upper airways or the lung.

Subglottic and upper tracheal haemangiomas characteristically occur in infants and tend to obstruct the airway. Tracheostomy is necessary in some cases to relieve the obstruction. Tracheo-bronchial haemangiomas are diagnosed bronchoscopically and are treated by radiotherapy for the upper trachea and by laser therapy for bronchial tumours.

Pulmonary haemangiomas are, in the majority of cases, a manifestation of hereditary Telangiectasia syndrome (Rendu–Osler–Weber disease).

- Lymphangiomas: The mode of presentation of these tumours is similar to tracheo-bronchial haemangioma and they can be managed in a similar fashion.

- Haemangioendothelioma is a solid tumour in infancy but the bronchial haemangioendothelioma may present as a pedunculated tumour.

- Lymphangiomyomatosis

This tumour presents as a multi-nodular pulmonary lesion which can involve a lobe or entire lung bilaterally. Clinical presentation of lymphangiomyomatosis may be pneumothorax and/or chylo-pneumothorax. Resectional surgery, when possible, is the treatment of choice.

- Arteriovenous fistula

This lesion is a malformation in which the branches of the pulmonary artery within the lung connect with those of the pulmonary veins without intervening capillaries. On chest radiograph the lesion presents as an opacity within the pulmonary parenchyma. CT scan of the thorax will define the outline of the feeding vessels. It is associated with hereditary Telangiectasia (Rendu–Osler–Weber syndrome) and effectively constitutes a right to left shunt with cyanosis, polycythaemia and pulmonary hypertension. Treatment is resection of the lesion with minimum of parenchyma.

- Haemangiopericytoma

This arises from capillary pericytes. It is often an asymptomatic lesion found on chest radiography, at times reaching over 10 cm in size. Both benign and malignant varieties are reported. Resection is the treatment of choice. The tumour is vascular and intra-operative bleeding can be a problem.

- Sclerosing haemangioma

This tumour has a number of histological sub-types and is generally benign, presenting as a nodular lesion in the periphery of the lung. The question of malignancy should be considered in the multi-nodular variety. Resectional surgery is intended as curative.

Bronchial (mesodermal) tumours.

{ Fibroma,
Lipoma,
Leiomyoma,
Chondroma

These tumours are described under a single heading because of their common features.

All four present as either:
(a) a peripheral pulmonary nodule which remains asymptomatic and is detected radiologically; or
(b) an endobronchial tumour which can be mildly symptomatic with a clear chest radiograph when small or with signs of atelectasis when they exert luminal obstruction.

Leiomyomas have more of a tendency to present as a pulmonary nodule or a mass than the fibromas or lipomas.

When peripheral, conservative resectional surgery should be undertaken and is attended by cure. Video-assisted thoracoscopy is one way to achieve this.

Endobronchial tumours may be treated bronchoscopically by excision or laser evaporation.

Leiomyoma can occasionally progress and behave in a malignant fashion even when histological features suggest otherwise.

- Granular cell tumour (syn. Myoblastoma)

Formerly known as myoblastoma. From the surgical point of view there are at least two varieties of this condition:
(a) Intra-pulmonary which presents as a solitary nodule;
(b) endo-tracheo-bronchial which involves principally the lower airway. The cell origin is probably granular degeneration of perineural fibroblasts in the endo-luminal variety; the patient is usually symptomatic with episodes of cough, wheeze and/or haemoptysis. Local excision or bronchoplastic operation with preservation of parenchyma is the choice treatment when possible. Recurrence is rare.

2.3.4. Miscellaneous (mesodermal) tumours

Whether members of this group should be considered as tumour in the sense of neoplasm is debatable. They do present as tumour in the clinical and imaging sense of the word and are often referred to as pseudo-tumour. They are:

- Xanthoma: a tumour-like post-inflammatory lesion composed of foam, spindle cells and lymphocytes. It presents as a pulmonary nodule and is locally excised to exclude a malignant tumour.
- Amyloid tumour: a tumour-like lesion appearing as a pulmonary nodule or, rarely, in the bronchi. Pulmonary nodules are usually excised.
- Pseudolymphoma: This tumour presents as a nodular lesion in the lung. A variety of this same tumour is giant lymph node hyperplasia (Castleman's disease) presenting as a circumscribed mediastinal node hyperplasia. Histologically, the tumour is composed of lymphoid cells with germinal centre. This lesion appears to have some potential for malignancy and should be excised.

2.3.5. Neurogenic tumours

These include neurofibroma, neuroma and neurilemoma. They are rare and generally occur in the main tracheo-bronchial tree. They can be resected bronchoscopically but preferably should be resected surgically because of the possibility of recurrence following bronchoscopic resection.

2.4. Bronchial gland tumours (adenomas)

A small number of tumours, accounting for some 5% of bronchopulmonary neoplasms, were previously grouped together and referred to collectively as adenomas. However, the term adenoma is inappropriate since it implies a benign tumour, whereas the behaviour of most members of this group is malignant. Also, many tumours in this group arise from bronchial glands; therefore, it seems logical to describe such tumours as bronchial gland tumours (adenomas) in order to appreciate the old term in its newest concept. The members of this group are:

2.4.1 Carcinoid tumours
2.4.2 Adenoid cystic carcinoma (syn. cylindroma)
2.4.3 Mucoepidermoid carcinoma

2.4.4   Mixed tumours of the bronchial tree

2.4.5   Bronchial mucous gland adenoma

2.4.1. Carcinoid tumours

These are by far the most common of the bronchial gland neoplasms but they form 2–4% of all pulmonary neoplasms and they belong to the neuroendocrine group of tumours similar to that of small cell lung cancer. Both clinically and pathologically, they are divided into two subgroups: atypical and typical, both of which arise from Kulchitsky cells of the bronchial mucosa.

The relationship between typical and atypical carcinoids and small cell lung cancer is well documented. Paladugu et al. (1985) suggest classifying Kulchitsky tumours into three categories in descending order of malignancy: typical carcinoid, atypical carcinoid and small cell lung cancer. They are all neuroendocrine neoplasms, which belong to the amine precursor uptake decarboxylase (APUD) group of tumours.

The typical variety forms 90% of all carcinoids. It is slow growing with less potential of metastasis (probably 5–10%). The less common atypical variety is a true malignant tumour; these metastasise in 60–70% of cases.

- Mode of presentation

In the majority of cases the tumour arises from the main or lobar bronchi with early appearance of symptoms. Clinical manifestation is akin to that of bronchogenic carcinoma: cough, wheeze (unilateral), dyspnoea, haemoptysis and chest pain may be present. Carcinoid syndrome described by Thorson et al. (1954) may be present in only about 5% of cases. This consists of: attacks of flushing, tachycardia, faintness, bronchospasm; heart valvular disease, abdominal pain and diarrhoea. The first bronchial carcinoid associated with the syndrome was described in 1956 (Kincaid-Smith and Brosst, 1956). Carcinoid syndrome has been attributed to 5-hydroxytryptamine, its precursor 5-hydroxytryptophan, and its breakdown product 5-hydroxyindoleacetic acid (which can be identified in urine), kallikrein, bradykinin and other catecholamines released by the tumour.

The diagnosis is based on chest radiograph and CT scan, often showing atelectasis, consolidation and infection when the tumour is central. Some 10–15% of carcinoids present as a peripheral pulmonary mass and remain asymptomatic. These will only be detected radiologically. In the majority (85–90%) of cases when the tumour arises from a major lobar or main bronchus, the diagnosis can be made bronchoscopically. It is important to note that tumour projecting into the lumen is usually covered by normal mucosa and that a deep biopsy is required to reveal the pathology on histological examination. It is also worth mentioning that carcinoid tumours can be very vascular and may bleed seriously when a biopsy sample is taken. This is particularly relevant for those bronchoscopists who do not use the rigid instrument (with its provision of good suction facilities). Mediastinoscopy is performed when there is evidence of mediastinal lymphadenopathy.

- Treatment

Complete resection is the only effective mode of therapy for carcinoids. The treatment options are:

Endoscopic interventions: Endoscopic interventions (diathermy/laser) are not adequate for excision of carcinoids as these tumours are largely extraluminal and extent of infiltration cannot be entirely assessed bronchoscopically. However, such interventional bronchoscopic procedures are useful in patients who are not fit for pulmonary resection even though there is a risk of recurrence.

Bronchotomy: Bronchotomy and resection of tumour is ideal when it can be practiced. It is best to carry out thoracotomy and excise the involved airway or appropriate segments when parenchyma is involved. The author believes that this is only possible in small tumours involving the main bronchi. It is important to check the excision margin by frozen section. Such a frozen section sample needs to incorporate some lung tissue as well as bronchial tissue, when the tumour arises from a segmental bronchus.

Formal resection: The rule should be to conserve pulmonary parenchyma by sleeve resection (bronchoplastic procedure) whenever possible and check completeness of resection by frozen section (Jensik et al., 1974; Aberg et al., 1981; Ribet et al., 1993). It should be noted that all bronchoplastic procedures (sleeve resection included) are subject to development of bronchial stenosis. In practice, the majority of cases require lobectomy, but pneumonectomy may (rarely) be needed to achieve a complete resection. This should be carried out when lesser excision is not feasible. Segmental, wedge and local excision can be undertaken in peripheral lesions only presenting as pulmonary nodules.

Small peripheral tumours may be excised locally, particularly by YAG laser in order to bring an added margin of safety to neighbouring parenchyma (Moghissi et al., 1989, 1990). Long-term results depend on a number of factors, such as the size and type of tumour (typical–very atypical) and regional lymph node involvement (which should be treated in the same way as in carcinoma). The 5–10-year survival for typical carcinoid can be as high as 87–100%, but for atypical tumour it is 50–65%.

Radiotherapy appears to have little effect on this tumour and the effect of chemotherapy in advanced cases with metastases remains unimpressive.

Carcinoid syndrome associated with bronchial carcinoid totally subsides when successful resection is performed. Drug treatment is guided towards inhibiting the synthesis of hormones (e.g. L-methyldopa) or preventing the release of seratonin (e.g. methysergide) or of anti-kallikrein (e.g. corticosteroids).

2.4.2. Adenoid cystic carcinomas

These tumours have been variously described as bronchial cylindromatous adenomas, bronchial mucous gland adenomas and mixed bronchial tumours. The name cylindroma was coined by Billroth (1859) to describe tumours of the eye arising from the lachrymal gland and since has been likened to tumours in other parts of the body with similar microscopic appearance. In the case of the airway the name cylindroma was used because growth of the tumour occurs in long cylinders of cells. Characteristically the tumour arises in the trachea and main stem bronchi from mucous-secreting cells of the tracheo-bronchial glands. Adeno-cystic tumours are slow growing but have definite malignant properties in that they expand locally, involve the lymphatics and produce distant metastases into the lungs, liver, kidneys, brain and skin. Symptoms are those related to airway obstruction such as wheeze, stridor, cough and haemoptysis. Bronchoscopic examination reveals the tumour as a circumscribed mass with a pedicle and covered with pinkish epithelium. Biopsy provides the histological diagnosis. CT scan and MRI determine the extent and depth of the tumour.

The treatment of choice is resection which, if complete, can achieve cure.

Radiotherapy alone is not an effective method for complete cure but, as an adjunct to surgery, it is useful either pre-operatively, to reduce the extent of the tumour and the size of lymph nodes locally, or post-operatively in those where resection may be incomplete.

No effective chemotherapeutic agent has been reported to be useful in controlling the disease.

Special cases of adenoid cystic tumours of the trachea

With these tumours, symptoms arise late and many cases are beyond surgical scope at presentation. Resection and end-to-end anastomosis, when possible, is the treatment of choice. A large (6 cm) portion of trachea may be circumferentially excised with reconstruction involving an end-to-end anastomosis (Grillo and Mathisen, 1990; Sharpe and Moghissi, 1996). We have converted the total circumferential defect to a partial defect which is then bridged using a composite patch of Marlex mesh (Moghissi, 1975). In some cases the tumour involves the lower trachea, carina and both main bronchi (bifurcation). In such cases, resection of bifurcation and reconstruction can be carried out with very good long-term survival (see chapter II.1 on tracheal surgery).

Main stem or lobar bronchial disease may be dealt with by sleeve resection, lobectomy and appropriate broncho-plastic procedures. Recurrent and/or unresectable tracheo-bronchial adenoid cystic carcinoma causing major obstruction may be treated using NdYAG laser, photodynamic therapy or a combination of both (Sharpe et al., 1996; Moghissi et al., 1997, 1999).

2.4.3. Mucoepidermoid carcinoma

This tumour arises in the trachea or main bronchi (main stem/lobar). In the majority the symptoms are cough, wheeze and haemoptysis. Chest radiograph may show a nodular lesion. At one time this tumour was regarded as benign but experience shows that the tumour may become malignant (Yousem and Hochholzer, 1987). Greater cellularity and frequent mitotic figures are characteristic of its higher malignant potential. Surgical excision with bronchoplasty is the treatment of choice and has a good prognosis in those with low-grade malignant potential. High-grade tumours should be considered and treated as carcinomas.

2.4.4. Mixed tumours of the tracheo-bronchial tree (mixed benign tumours)

These tumours resemble mixed tumours of the salivary glands. Histologically the tumour is composed of epithelial and connective tissue components. They present as polypoid pedunculated or sessile growths with a tendency of local and deep invasion. Local excision and conservative parenchyma saving should be the treatment aim. However, bronchoscopic excision is not advisable since the tumour can reoccur.

2.4.5. Bronchial mucous gland adenoma

This is a true benign tumour composed of mucous-secreting cells forming a microcyst. The tumour usually grows into the lumen of the airway and can present as a nodular lesion on X-ray. Alternatively, the radiograph may be entirely normal. When the tumour causes luminal obstruction, which it occasionally does, there is resultant atelectasis. The tumour is usually accessible to bronchoscopic detection. The aim of treatment is parenchyma-saving conservative surgery through bronchotomy, broncho-plastic procedures or even bronchoscopic excision using laser. Laser therapy is only permissible if there is a definite histological diagnosis and when the tumour can be totally ablated by the bronchoscopic intervention.

References and further reading

Aberg T, Blondas T, Nou E et al. The choice of operation for bronchial carcinoids. Ann Thorac Surg. 1981; 32: 19.

Albrecht E. Über hamartoma. Verch Dtsch Path Ges 1904; 7: 153.

Bacha EA, Wright CD, Grillo HC et al. Surgical treatment of pulmonary sarcoma. Eur J Cardiothorac Surg. 1999; 15: 456–460.

Barrett NR, Barnard WG. Some unusual thoracic tumours. Br J Surg 1945; 33: 447.

Billroth T. Beobachtungen über Geschwulste der Speicheldrüsen. Virchow Arch A Pathol Anat Histopathol 1859; 17: 197.

El Jamal M, Nicholson AG, Goldstraw P. The feasibility of conservative resection for carcinoid tumours: is pneumonectomy ever necessary for uncomplicated cases? Eur J Cardiothorac Surg 2000; 18: 301–306.

Fink G, Krelbaum T, Yellin A, Bendayan D, Saute M, Glazer M, Kramer MR. Pulmonary carcinoid: presentation, diagnosis and outcome in 142 cases in Israel and review of 640 cases from the literature. Chest 2001; 119: 1647–1651.

Gould VE, Warren WH. Epithelial tumours of the lung. Chest Surg Clin N Am 2000; 10: 709–728.

Grillo HC, Mathisen DJ. Primary tracheal tumours: treatment and results. Ann Thorac Surg 1990; 49: 864–868.

Jansen JP, Mulder JJS, Wagenaar SS et al. Primary sarcoma of the lung: a clinical study with long-term followup. Ann Thorac Surg 1994; 58: 1151–1155.

Jensik RJ, Faber LP, Brown CM et al. Bronchoplastic and conservative resectional procedures for bronchial adenoma. J Thorac Cardiovasc Surg 1974; 68: 556–565.

Kincaid-Smith P, Brosst JJ. A case of bronchial adenoma with liver metastases. Thorax 1956; 11: 36.

Liebow AA. Tumours of the lower respiratory tract. Atlas of tumour pathology, Section V, Fascille 17. Armed Forces Institute of Pathology. Washington, DC, 1952.

Liebow AA, Castleman B. Benign clear cell (sugar) tumours of the lung. Yale J Biol Med 1971; 43: 213–222.

Martini N, Vogt-Moykopf I (Eds.). Thoracic surgery: frontiers and uncommon neoplasms. Vol 5: International Trends in Thoracic Surgery. St Louis: CV Mosby, 1989.

Maziak DE, Todd TR, Keshavjee SH, Winton TL, Van Nostrand P, Pearson FG. Adenoid cystic carcinoma of the airway: thirty-two year experience. J Thorac Cardiovasc Surg 1996; 112: 1522–1531.

Moghissi K. Tracheal reconstruction with a prosthesis of Marlex mesh and pericardium. J Thorac Cardiovasc Surg 1975; 69: 499–506.

Moghissi K. Local excision of pulmonary nodular (coin) lesion with non-contact Yttrium Aluminium Garnet laser. J Thorac Cardiovasc Surg 1989; 97: 147–151.

Moghissi K. Experience with limited lung resection with the use of laser. Lung 1990; Supp: 1103–1109.

Moghissi K, Dixon K, Hudson E, Stringer MR, Brown S. Endoscopic laser therapy in malignant tracheobronchial obstruction using sequential NdYAG laser and Photodynamic Therapy. Thorax 1997; 52: 281–283.

Moghissi K, Dixon K, Stringer MR et al. The place of bronchoscopic Photodynamic Therapy (PDT) in advanced unresectable lung cancer: experience of 100 cases. Eur J Cardiothorac Surg 1999; 15: 1–6.

Muller KM. Lung cancer morphology in carcinoma of the lung. European Repiratory Monograph. SG Spiro (ed.), Eur Resp J 1995; 50–71.

Paladugu RR, Benfield JR, Pack HY et al. Bronchopulmonary Kulchitzky cell carcinoma. A new classification scheme by typical and atypical carcinoid. Cancer 1985; 55: 1303.

Porte HL, Metoif DG, Leroy X et al. Surgical treatment of primary sarcoma of the lung. Eur J Cardiothorac Surg 2000; 18: 136–142.

Poulsen JT, Jacobson M, Francis D. Probable malignant transformation of a pulmonary hamartoma. Thorax 1979; 34: 557.

Prommegger R, Salzer GM. Long term results of surgery for adenoid cystic carcinoma of the trachea and bronchi. Eur J Surg Oncol 1998; 24: 440–444.

Ribet M, Gosselin B, Gambiez L, Frere L. Bronchial carcinoids. Eur J Cardiothorac Surg 1993; 7: 347–350.

Sharpe DAC, Dixon K, Moghissi K. Endoscopic laser treatment for tracheal obstruction. Eur J Cardiothorac Surg 1996; 10: 722–726.

Sharpe DAC, Moghissi K. Tracheal resection and reconstruction. A review of 82 patients. Eur J Cardiothorac Surg 1996; 10: 1040–1046.

Thorson A, Biorck G, Bjorkman G et al. Carcinoid of the small intestine with metastases to the liver, valvular disease of the right side of the heart (pulmonary stenosis and tricuspid regurgitation without septal defect), peripheral vasomotor symptoms, broncho constriction and unusual type of cyanosis: a clinical and pathological syndrome. Am Heart J 1954; 47: 795.

Woodruff PK, Whittle JM, Malpas JS. Solitary plasmacytoma I extramedullary soft tissue plasmacytoma. Cancer 1979; 43: 2340.

Yousem SA, Hochholzer L. Mucoid epidermoid tumour of the lung. Cancer 1987; 60: 1346.

3. Specific types of lung cancer

3.1. Small cell lung cancer (SCLC)

Small cell lung cancer forms some 20–25% of all lung cancer. This proportion is, however, subject to variation and the population which is sampled. The two extremes of the range are surgical versus post-mortem (<1%–>30% respectively) series.

The main characteristics of SCLC are:

- Extremely high grade of malignancy.
- Diagnosis made most often through metastases or from the bronchoscopic recovery of malignant cells by brush rather than biopsy.
- Under light microscopy the tumour is highly cellular and almost devoid of stroma. The cells resemble lymphocytes, the cytoplasm is scanty and the nucleus has a coarse and abundant chromatine.
- 3 varieties of small cell lung cancers are recognised according to their histological features:
  – Oat cell = about 85%
  – Intermediate small cell type
  – Combined squamous–small cell? = about 15%
- Hormone-like substances are found in the small cell carcinoma originating from cells similar to those of neuroendocrine systems. These are related to endocrine cells of Kulchitsky type in the bronchi.

Management: SCLC behaves as a systemic disease. This fact became apparent early in the development of surgical treatment for lung cancer.

Until the late 1960s, all patients with resectable lung cancer, irrespective of the histological subtypes, including those with small cell lung cancer, were submitted to surgical resection. However, the result of 10 years' followup in a study by the Medical Research Council (Fox and Scadding, 1973) which compared surgery alone versus radiotherapy in limited disease showed the disadvantage of surgery compared with radiotherapy. In fact no patients in the surgical arm of randomisation survived 5 years.

At present chemotherapy remains the mainstay of therapy for SCLC. Multi-drug chemotherapy is used as multiple cycles. External beam radiotherapy of the chest and cranium is added to chemotherapy by some centres, usually after 3–4 chemotherapy courses.

- Currently two subsets of patients (making up less than 5% of total SCLC) may receive surgical treatment:
  (a) Those presenting as nodular lesion in the periphery of the lung diagnosed at operation or after resection. These will have a high rate of 5-year survival. In the most recent series (Rea et al., 1998), chemotherapy is added post-operatively as an adjunct to surgical resection.
  (b) Those with limited thoracic disease who receive induction chemotherapy who are then submitted to surgery.

This subgroup is comprised of:

- Patients in whom surgery is used as a salvage operation. These are patients who have had chemotherapy but still have residual tumour at the primary site, or those with recurrence of tumour at the primary site after a good response (Sheperd et al., 1991).
- Patients in whom induction chemotherapy is used as a "down staging" programme. In this group a 38–40% (estimated) 5-year survival has been reported (Salzer et al., 1990).

3.2. Superior sulcus tumour (Pancoast tumour)

This refers to a type of lung cancer which arises from the apex of the upper lobe with a tendency of growing through the thoracic inlet towards the root of the neck. The tumour is slow-growing but expands locally to invade the brachial plexus sympathetic chain and the stellate ganglion. The upper ribs and thoracic vertebral column become involved sooner or later.

The tumour, with its distinct clinical features, was first described by Pancoast in 1932. The presentation is one of pain, Horner syndrome (unilateral enophthalmos, ptosis, miosis, dryness of face and the upper extremities, and atrophy of hand muscles). The presence of Horner syndrome denotes involvement of the sympathetic chain whereas other neuromuscular signs indicate brachial plexus invasion. Most of these tumours are squamous cell type and their histological diagnosis can be quite difficult. CT-guided needle biopsy, thoracoscopy and/or surgical biopsy may have to be employed to obtain histological identification. The work-up should incorporate neurological examination and electromyography as well as angiography (venous and arterial) of root of the neck vessels.

3.2.1. Treatment

Surgical treatment with intended cure/long survival involves adjuvant radiotherapy. There appears to be no prevailing opinion as to whether radiotherapy should be pre-or post-operative. The recommended dose is 30–45 Gy. This may be administered 4–6 weeks before or after surgery. The operation needs to be en bloc and extensive to allow complete excision of all tumour and the involved structures. In practice this means all or some of the following: excision of first rib (or any other involved ribs), part of the body of the upper thoracic vertebrae, intervening soft tissues of chest wall, involved nerve roots, portion of the lower trunk of brachial plexus, appropri-

diac ischaemic and/or valvular disease which requires surgical treatment, poses questions regarding which operation should be carried out first and whether there is a place for both operations to be carried out concomitantly.

1.2.3. Respiratory system assessment

Clinical and functional tests should be carried out to determine the suitability of the patient for the proposed surgery.

Previous history of airway and pulmonary parenchymal diseases will be reflected on pulmonary function test results. Spirometry, diffusion capacity (carbon monoxide) and arterial blood gas analysis are a necessity for all major thoracic surgical cases even though there are difficulties to correlate the measured parameters with the level of risk involved. Bernard et al. (2000) prospectively studied 500 patients undergoing lung resection and stratified them into 4 groups according to the severity of post-operative complications. They identified those having extensive lung resection or bronchoplastic procedures with FEV_1 less than 80% of the predicted value to be at the highest peri-operative risk of complication. Nevertheless no hard and fast rule can be proposed since ventilatory performance represents only one of the trio components (i.e. ventilation, perfusion and diffusion) in global respiratory function. But FEV_1 is an important indicator: a level of 0.8-1 L in an adult is considered to be the limit of operability for major thoracic surgery.

Ferguson (1995) suggested the predicted post-operative diffusing capacity to be the strongest single predictor of complication and mortality after lung resection. For practical purposes, spirometry, diffusion capacity and arterial blood gas analysis should be considered when assessing suitability for major thoracic surgery.

1.2.4. Other systems assessment

Clinical evaluation should cover general examination of other systems. Good clinical history-taking will be a guide to initiate further investigation to elucidate coexistence of pathologies other than those of cardiovascular and respiratory systems. In some instances, nutritional assessment is of importance in order to correct deficiencies prior to admission for operation.

2. Admission and preparation for surgery

In elective surgery the diagnostic investigations and pre-operative assessment will have been completed and admission takes place a day prior to operation for pre-operative examination and preparation.

2.1. Pre-operative examination

Upon admission patients need a thorough clinical examination of their cardiovascular, respiratory and other systems to check for changes since the pre-operative assessment and to record base-line observations.

- Routine blood tests should be carried out to check the patients' blood count and biochemical profile. All patients should have their blood group identified as part of their assessment. Blood should be cross-matched and kept on standby in case of need.
- Pre-operative antero-posterior and, in some cases, lateral view chest X-ray should be taken. This is important in order to identify changes since the previous assessment and to have a base-line pre-operative image for comparison with post-operative films.
- A pre-operative ECG recording should be carried out.

2.2. Psychological aspects and information

Medical staff of the thoracic surgical unit should undertake the task of psychological preparation according to the customs, habits and mental attitude of their patients. Many thoracic surgical operations are carried out for cancer and most patients are understandably frightened and depressed when faced with the possibility of having thoracic surgery for cancer. The surgeon must find time to establish a relationship of trust and understanding with the patient. The truth must be conveyed to the patient in the kindest possible way by the surgeon, or a senior member of his team who knows the case and has been involved in discussion regarding management. This person should provide clear, sympathetic and precise information about the treatment options and the intended operation. The risks and benefits of treatment should also be discussed with the aim of helping the patient to come to terms with his/her condition and develop hope for the future. The patient should be informed about the state in which he/she will be returning to the intensive therapy unit or the ward after the operation. By doing so he/she will not be too alarmed by intravenous fluid infusion, blood transfusion, intercostal drains and blood-stained material drained.

2.3. General hygiene

Whilst nurses are expected to attend to the general hygiene of patients under their care, certain specific areas need to be addressed by the medical staff. Mouth and dental hygiene have a special place in thoracic surgery as dental bacteria along the air passages may be one of the major sources of post-operative infection.

2.4. Nutrition

Unlike patients with obstructive, oesophageal lesions, patients undergoing general thoracic and pulmonary surgery are not, as a rule, in need of special nutritional preparation, i.e. they do not need artificial feeding or supplementary nutrition. Nevertheless, it must be realised that there is a link between the nutritional state and immunological competence of the body and resistance to infection. Patients with potential or actual sepsis should receive a high protein and calorie content diet.

2.5. Physiotherapy

All patients undergoing thoracic surgery should be introduced to chest physiotherapy before the operation. The objectives are:
- Harmonious deep breathing which increases the effective tidal volume.
- Effective coughing to allow deep-seated secretions to be expectorated.

Physiotherapy is even more important in those with chronic obstructive pulmonary disease (COPD) and bronchiectasis with mucopurulent sputa. These patients need a period of rehabilitation and chest physiotherapy pre-operatively either by the primary care team near their home or as an out-patient at the thoracic unit. Peri-operative physiotherapy then starts on admission.

2.6. Antibiotic prophylaxis

Prophylactic antibiotics are of value in pulmonary surgery, especially for patients undergoing major pulmonary resection. In the event of infection being present pre-operatively, the infecting organism should be identified and appropriate antibiotics administered therapeutically. Despite the advice of many that a single intravenous administration will suffice to prevent infective complications in most cases, experience, backed by trials, shows that such a regimen can only reduce the rate of post-operative wound sepsis. In fact, most trials indicate that the rate of pleuro-pulmonary infection, which in thoracic and pulmonary surgery is of major concern, is not affected by a single dose. The author believes a course extended to 3 days (i.e. the day of operation and two further days post-operatively) is the optimal regimen which will also reduce the rate of pleuro-pulmonary infection. In cases of impending infection, collection and examination of sputum (or secretion) will guide further antibiotic therapy.

2.7. Venous thrombosis prophylaxis

Patients with a previous history of thrombophlebitis (phlebo-thrombosis) should be given low-dose heparin prophylaxis and antiembolic stockings. For other patients this prophylactic measure should be considered according to the age and mobility of the patient, related clinical history and type of surgical procedure.

2.8. Skin preparation

Preparation of the skin has a special importance in thoracotomies for the following reasons:
- Thoracotomy skin incision is extensive. Both the skin and the wound are exposed over a relatively long period during the operation.
- Many patients undergoing pulmonary surgery suffer from neoplastic disease which influences the immunological competence of the host.

Different techniques exist and each surgeon has his/her own routine of skin preparation. The author has employed the following methods for a number of years with satisfaction:
- The skin over the anterior aspect of the chest from the clavicles down to the umbilicus and over the corresponding posterior area is shaved. (The author is aware of the controversy about shaving but lack of a controlled trial (at the time of writing) in this aspect compels rejection of the argument against it).
- The patient bathes prior to operation.
- The chest and abdomen are washed with soap and water an hour or so before the operation.
- The skin over the chest and upper abdomen is painted with a solution of 1–2% iodine,[1] in 70% alcohol.

---

[1] In cases of known allergy to iodine, an alternative disinfectant such as cholorhexidine in alcohol solution may be used.

- The iodine paint is wiped off with 70% alcohol solution.
- A sterile towel is wrapped over the painted area.
- The patient is sent to the operating theatre with the sterile towel still on his chest; this is removed in the anaesthetic room. In the operating theatre a further disinfectant solution is used to carry out the cleaning of the skin prior to placing towels in position.

2.9. Information and consent for operation

This is an important aspect of the pre-operative undertaking. A doctor who understands the patient, knows the case and is articulate should inform the patient about the operation, its risks and the peri-operative potential complications.

In the experience of the author, an overall majority of medical negligence claims emanate from misinformation, misunderstanding and lack of proper explanation by the medical staff.

References and further reading

Bernard A, Ferrand L, Hagry O et al. Identification of prognostic factors determining risk groups for lung resection. Ann Thorac Surg 2000; 70: 1161–1167.

Bernard A, Pillet M, Goudet P, Viard H. Antibiotic prophylaxis in pulmonary surgery. A prospective randomised double-blind trial of flash cefuroxime versus forty eight hour cefuroxime. J Thorac Cardiovasc Surg 1994; 107(3): 896–900.

Ferguson MK, Reeder B, Mich R. Optimising selection of patients for major lung resection. J Thorac Cardiovasc Surg 1995; 109: 275–283.

Forster R, Toth S, Redman K et al. A prospective risk analysis of contemporary thoracic surgery. Eur J Cardiothorac Surg 1996; 10: 641–648.

Gibetekin C, Martin PG, Satur CM et al. Results of pneumonectomy for cancer in patients with limited ventilatory function. Eur J Cardiothorac Surg 1995; 9: 347–351.

Gonzalez RP, Holevar MR. Role of prophylactic antibiotics for tube thoracostomy in chest trauma. Am Surg 1998; 64(7): 620–621.

Kohman LJ, Meyer JA, Ikins PM et al. Random versus predictable risks of mortality after thoracotomy for lung cancer. J Thorac Cardiovasc Surg 1986; 91: 551–554.

Kreter B, Woods M. Antibiotic prophylaxis for cardiothoracic operations. Meta-analysis of thirty years of clinical trials. J Thorac Cardiovasc Surg 1992; 104: 590–599.

Miller JR. Thallium imaging in pre-operative evaluation of the pulmonary resection candidate. Ann Thorac Surg 1992; 54: 249–252.

Nooyen SM, Overbeek BP, Brutel de la Riviere A, Storm AJ. Langemeyer JJ. Prospective randomised comparison of single-dose versus multiple-dose cefuroxime for prophylaxis in coronary artery bypass grafting. Eur J Clin Microbiol Infect Dis 1994; 13(12): 1033–1037.

Varela G, Novoa N, Jiminez MF. Influence of age and predicted forced expiratory volume in 1 second on prognosis following complete resection of non small cell lung cancer. Eur J Cardiothorac Surg 2000; 18: 2–6.

Veterans Affairs Total Parenteral Nutrition Cooperative Study Group. Perioperative total parenteral nutrition in surgical patients. N Eng J Med 1991; 325: 525–532.

Wertzel H, Swoboda L, Joos-Wurtemberger A, Frank U, Hasse J. Perioperative antibiotic prophylaxis in general thoracic surgery. Thorac Cardiovasc Surg 1992. 40: 326–329.

Woods M, Tillman D. Antibiotic prophylaxis in cardiothoracic surgery. Hosp Pharm 1992; 27(404): 406–407.

K. Moghissi, J.A.C. Thorpe and F. Ciulli (Eds.)
Moghissi's Essentials of Thoracic and Cardiac Surgery
© 2003 Elsevier Science B.V. All rights reserved

CHAPTER I.18

Pulmonary resection — general principles

K. Moghissi

1. Introduction

Accesses to the chest have been described previously (chapter I.4). In whatever way the thoracic cavity is approached the aim is to first visually explore and then expose the target organ prior to carrying out surgical procedure.

A rib spreader is inserted and the intercostal space is widened to the required width. The chest and lung are then thoroughly examined. In the presence of pleural effusion the volume is noted and a sample taken for microbiological studies before aspiration (suction) and disposal. The lung parenchyma is next examined from the apex down to the base. This is followed by examination of the root and fissures. Particular attention is paid to the anterior aspect of the hilum and freedom of the major vessels from invasion by the pathological process as well as lymphadenopathies.

Except for biopsy or wedge excision, all pulmonary resections are based first on the dissection of the corresponding bronchovascular structures. In practice, this means that the pulmonary vascular branches are divided between ligatures individually and the bronchi are closed separately. In pneumonectomy the main pulmonary artery, the two main pulmonary veins (superior and inferior), and the main bronchus at, or just below, the division of the trachea have to be dealt with.

In lobectomy the branches of the pulmonary artery and vein to the lobe concerned are to be divided between ligatures. With minor anatomical variations on each side the number of pulmonary arterial branches to a lobe equal the number of its constituent segments. In lobar resection the artery to the lobe can be dealt with before it gives off segmental branches. In segmental resection these have to

be dealt with individually because they are given off separately from the trunk of the main lobar artery. The vein to a lobe is a single one which then divides. Therefore, the lobar vein can be divided between ligatures, as a single structure, before its division. Likewise, the bronchial branch to a lobe is given off as a single trunk which then divides and, therefore, the lobar bronchus can be dealt with separately.

The segments are the smallest pulmonary anatomical unit which can be excised. They receive a single arterial branch, one or two veins and a single bronchial branch. In segmentectomies these are dealt with individually.

2. Dissection and ligation of vessels

With minor variation, the anatomical arrangement of the pulmonary arterial and venous systems are similar for the right and left lung.

There is a superior and an inferior pulmonary vein on each side.

On the right side, the superior vein is concerned with the upper and the middle lobe. On the left it gives off branches to the upper lobe proper and the lingula. The inferior pulmonary vein on either side is concerned with the lower lobe. The veins are anterior structures of the hilum and are surrounded by a pericardial cuff. The inferior vein can be easily identified in the antero-inferior aspect of the lung within the inferior pulmonary ligament on each side. The superior pulmonary vein is adjacent and inferior to the pulmonary artery.

Like veins, the main pulmonary artery is an anterior structure on both sides.

After giving off segmental branches to the anterior and apical segments of the upper lobe, the main artery passes posteriorly and turns into the oblique

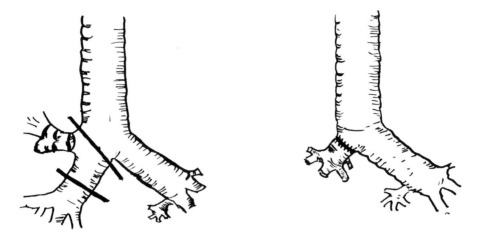

Fig. 1. Right upper lobectomy sleeve resection.

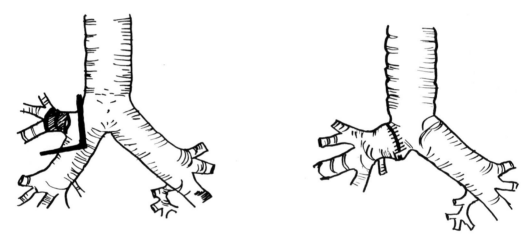

Fig. 2. Right upper lobectomy with wedge resection of the main bronchus.

fissure to run along its axis. Therefore, the segmental arterial branches, except for the upper lobe, are given off from the pulmonary arterial trunk in the oblique fissure. As a general rule, the arterial trunk in the fissure is overlaid by the pleura and lymph nodes. The latter are a good landmark. The branches of the pulmonary artery are ligated and divided. The veins are dealt with in a similar fashion. It is a wise precaution to suture the main pulmonary artery and the main trunks of the pulmonary veins in addition or as an alternative to ligating them.

In certain circumstances intrapericardial division of pulmonary vessels is mandatory as there may not be an uninvolved length outside of the pericardium to allow extrapericardial division as described above. It is imperative to suture vessels when they are to be divided intrapericardially. Simply tying them off is a recipe for disaster which happens only once

to a patient and should never happen to a surgeon. In recent years stapling devices have been used by many to deal with pulmonary vessels safely and efficiently.

3. Bronchial closure

It is best to clamp the bronchus distal to the line of incision. The alternative of dividing the bronchus between two clamps will produce crushing of the tissues at the site of the closure. The two edges of the bronchial cut are stitched together and the bronchial opening is closed. Staplers are used by many surgeons which have been shown to be safe and easy to apply. To categorically state which is the best method of bronchial closure and what suture material is the most appropriate is neither scientific nor particularly useful. Each surgeon has been trained

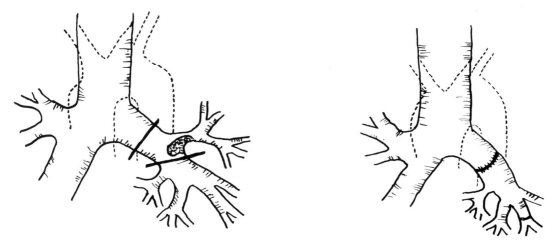

Fig. 3. Left upper lobectomy sleeve resection.

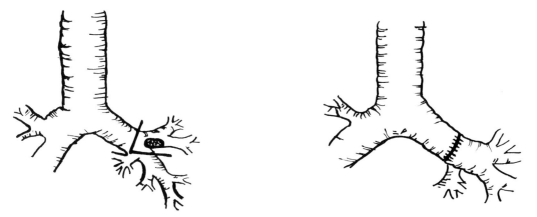

Fig. 4. Left upper lobectomy with wedge resection of the main bronchus.

to use a particular method and will continue to practice it unless it proves unsatisfactory. A trainee surgeon should be familiar with hand sewing as well as stapling, bearing in mind, however, that staplers may not always be available. The author's method is to hand sew and approximate without crushing the two edges of bronchial section and employ interrupted non-absorbable sutures. Many surgeons have a method of covering the bronchial stump with living tissues in cases of pneumonectomy, with the aim of reducing the risk of broncho-pleural fistula formation. Pedicle intercostal graft, pleura, pericardium and pedicle omental graft have been extensively used for this purpose. The author has used the pedicle graft of the pericardium for many years and has, as a result, had no cases of bronchopleural fistula following pneumonectomies in a 10-year period (over 140 consecutive cases).

3.1. Additional tips on pulmonary resection

- It is easier to divide pulmonary and pleural adhesions when the lung is ventilated rather than using the alternative of collapsing the lung. Therefore, at the start of the operation with the lung expanded, adhesions are divided and exploration (both visual and by palpation) is done. The lung is then collapsed for further exploration.
- It is easier to separate and dissect the lobes of the lung by incising the adhesion and the pleura in the fissures when the lung is expanded and ventilated.
- The way to mobilise a very adherent lung which is attached to the chest wall is to strip the parietal pleura with the lung (i.e. extrapleural mobilisation) from the chest wall and then enter the pleural space proper in a convenient place where the lung is free, usually on the mediastinal aspect of the lungs.

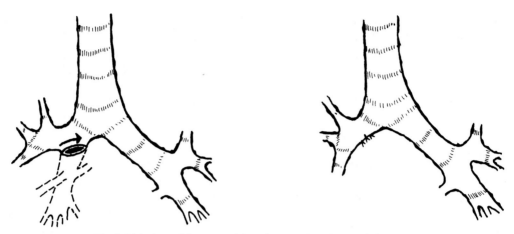

Fig. 5. Right lower lobectomy with wedge resection of the main bronchus.

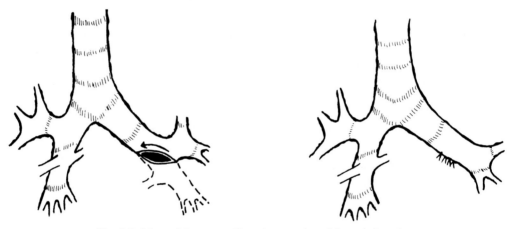

Fig. 6. Left lower lobectomy with wedge resection of the main bronchus.

- Following the bronchial closure it is a wise precaution to test the closure against a ventilation pressure of 30–40 cm water. This pressure is generated by the anaesthetic machine through the endotracheal tube, whilst 500 ml of warm (body temperature) saline is poured into the pleural space to submerge the stump and thus demonstrate any air leak.
- It is important to handle the lung with extreme gentleness since trauma or rough manipulation will result in air leak and/or pulmonary contusion, either/both of which will prolong recovery.
- Electro-diathermy and coagulation should not be used near the bronchial stump; bleeding vessels should be ligated or sutured.

4. Bronchoplastic procedures

These operations are designed to offer an economic resection of the lung by preserving the healthy pulmonary parenchyma whilst allowing the surgical excision of a diseased bronchus. In physiological terms the tissues which are responsible for effective ventilation (i.e. parenchyma) are conserved, whereas a part of the dead space is excised. In practice this is achieved by excision of a bronchus without resection of its distal lung tissue or by bronchial excision in excess of the corresponding pulmonary parenchyma.

The common bronchoplastic procedures are as follows:

4.1. Bronchial excision without pulmonary resection

4.1.1. Excision of the carina and main bronchi (syn. Bifurcation excision)

This operation is carried out in cases of localised tumour of the carina and main bronchi, which are benign or slow growing malignant but as yet non-invasive. Adenoid cystic carcinoma is an indication, par excellence, for this operation. In expert hands it is attended by good results in patients who are in a desperate respiratory situation. The operative access is via right posterolateral thoracotomy.

The excision of the lower trachea, carina and the bifurcation is carried out, followed by reconstruction of the airway. This consists of joining the residual right and left bronchi to one another and to the trachea. (See chapter II.1 on tracheal surgery.)

4.1.2. Excision of the right or left main bronchus without pulmonary excision

A lesion, generally a benign tumour, can be excised from the right or left main bronchus, together with the circumferential excision of a portion of the bronchial wall, followed by reconstruction.

4.2. Upper lobectomy with sleeve bronchial resection (Figs. 1 and 3)

The principle of sleeve resection is to excise the upper lobe of the lung together with the sleeve of the main bronchus and then to reconstruct the bronchial tree by joining the trunk of the lower lobe bronchus to the trachea. On the right side this is easily achieved because the upper lobe bronchus branch is given off very near the horizontal plane of the carina. Therefore, after ligation and division of the Azygos vein, the carina, the intermediate and right upper lobe bronchi are individually encircled, and whilst the lung is collapsed (contralateral ventilation), division and anastomosis are carried out.

4.3. Other broncho-plastic procedures

There are numerous possibilities of broncho-plastic procedures in which a portion of the main bronchus, with a lobe of the lung, is excised and the reconstruction is carried out by swinging the remaining lobar bronchus to join with the trachea or available healthy bronchi. In some the whole circumference of the bronchus is excised and re-implantation of the residual bronchi is undertaken. In others partial circumferential excision takes place followed by reconstruction as required (Figs. 2 and 4, 5 and 6).

In all plastic procedures, it is wise to provide a protective cover to the anastomosis by pericardium or pleura. In some cases intercostal pedicled graft can be provided for covering.

CHAPTER I.19

Post-operative management of patients undergoing pulmonary and general thoracic surgery

K. Moghissi

1. Introduction

The aims of post-operative care are:
- Restitution of the vital activities of the body temporarily disturbed by anaesthesia and surgical trauma.
- Restoration of the lung function which, in turn, is dependent on full expansion of the residual lung tissue.
- Assisting the body's local and general efforts to repair the surgical wounds.
- Prevention of complications.
- Preparation of the patient physically and psychologically for return to his/her own environment and occupation.

Patients are usually transferred from the operating theatre to the recovery room, which is an integral part of the theatre suite, where they remain until they are fully conscious and until spontaneous breathing and a satisfactory cardiovascular state has been established.

2. Transfer to the ward

Before return to the ward (or ITU) a bed is prepared to receive the patient. Provision of oxygen, adjustable suction machine with connecting catheter, and tubes (for clearing the airways) near the bed are essential. Pressure-adjustable pleural suction equipment and appropriate tubing should also be readily available as suction may have to be applied to the drainage system. Transfer of the patient from trolley to bed must be effected with minimum discomfort. During this procedure care must be taken to see that attachments such as intravenous drips and pleural drains are not displaced or disconnected. The tube leading from the pleural drain to the underwater containers (see pleural drain, chapter I.21) must be clamped during lifting, otherwise fluid and air enters the chest due to negative intrapleural pressure. Alternatively, the drainage container should be kept below the level of the patient's chest. Once the patient is in bed, the drainage containers are placed below the patient's chest without any clamp applied to the drainage tube.

It must be emphasised that when there is a considerable air leak, drainage tubes should not be clamped for a long period of time. During transfer of the patient, the drainage containers should be supported by a holder near the foot of the bed or carried un-clamped and held at a level lower than that of the bed. Failure to do so will result in:
(a) pneumothorax, or even a tension pneumothorax, and
(b) mediastinal and surgical subcutaneous emphysema.

The following should be noted:
- A written report detailing the type of operation, number and position of pleural drains and other attachments to the patient must be given to the nurse receiving the patient in the ward.
- Written instructions regarding blood and fluid transfusion and supply and rate of oxygen should also be given to the nurse.
- Post-operative drugs, analgesics and other medication should be written up.
- Instructions regarding the pleural drains are most important. The requirement of suction pump and pressure required should be indicated.

3. Base-line observations and monitoring

3.1. Initial observations

Nursing staff record observations of the patient's vital functions and monitor the basic physiological parameters on return from operating theatre to the ward. These will usually include:
- State of consciousness: auditory and visual response.
- Temperature.
- Respiration: rate and ease of breathing or ventilatory state when on mechanical ventilation. Saturation on pulse oxymetry.
- Circulatory system: Heart rate, arterial and central venous pressure and electrocardiogram.
- Pleural drains: The volume of blood in the container and air leak.
- ECG, temperature, arterial blood gas and oxygen saturation are monitored as required according to the initial stability of the patient's condition.

It is mandatory to stress the importance of recording base-line observations particularly regarding the rate of bleeding and air leaks from pleural drains.

3.2. Monitoring

3.2.1. Cardiovascular state
Cardiovascular state is monitored by recording pulse rate and its volume, arterial and central venous blood pressure (CVP), and the general state of venous filling, skin colour and its temperature. These parameters should be recorded and charted at regular, frequent intervals depending on patient requirement. The duration and frequency will depend on patient progress and stability of their condition. In a stable condition the pulse remains regular and steady (or slightly raised) and arterial and central venous pressure remain within normal limits. The patient's extremities will become warm soon after return to the ward. It is important to be particularly aware of early circulatory complications. A fall in central venous pressure with an increase in pulse rate is an earlier sign of bleeding than a fall in arterial blood pressure which manifests itself later. It follows that placement of a CVP line is an important precautionary measure enabling nursing staff to monitor the patient.

3.2.2. Respiration
The rate, depth and mode of breathing of the patient are recorded and particular attention is paid to:

- Upper respiratory obstruction and respiratory embarrassment by secretions.
- Position of the patient: the patient is propped up in bed as soon as possible to improve diaphragmatic movement
- Pulse oximetry is continued until a stable condition is maintained for 1-2 hours and arterial blood gas analysis is repeated if clinically deemed necessary.

It is worthwhile to emphasise that:
- Respiratory system monitoring and care of the pleural drains go hand-in-hand.
- Management of pleural drains has been fully covered (chapter I.21). Therefore, the drains must always be examined and their functional state re-evaluated when there is deterioration of respiratory function.

3.2.3. Nervous system
General neurological survey includes:
- Assessment and monitoring of level of consciousness
- Auditory and visual response to command
- Pupillary reaction to light
- Sensory and motor function
- EEG recording and other more sophisticated tests which should be undertaken when there are indications to do so.

3.2.4. Functional state of other organs
It is important to pay attention to the following:
- Urinary output and signs of bladder distension which can produce restlessness and irritation.
- Nausea, vomiting and abdominal distension.

4. Post-operative management

4.1. Monitoring of vital functions

The above-mentioned monitoring of vital functions is carried out at regular intervals. The frequency of monitoring in the first 3–4 post-operative days depends on the progress and stability of the patient's condition.

4.2. Chest X-rays

An early post-operative portable chest radiograph is taken and examined with particular attention to:
- Full expansion of the residual ipsilateral or contralateral lung and state of the pneumonectomy space, as applicable.
- Position of the chest drains.

- Existence of haemopneumothorax.
- A chest radiograph is usually taken every day when the drainage tubes are in situ, which normally means for 2–3 days following pulmonary resection and 1–2 days for other thoracic surgical operations. Occasionally, drains will have to remain for a longer period, in which case routine daily chest radiography has to be modified. When the drains are removed, lung expansion is checked a few hours later by a further radiograph, and following this, a chest radiograph is taken when the patient is discharged from the hospital.

4.3. Pain management

Thoracotomy wound is painful and relief of pain constitutes an important part of post-operative management following chest surgery. The patient has to breathe deeply to maintain continued pulmonary expansion and by doing so will experience more pain; therefore, the natural reaction to such pain is to breathe shallowly which in turn reduces the tidal volume. This results in even more rapid breathing and increased pain because of the frequency of respiratory movements. Analgesics should be given to alleviate this pain. However, too much analgesic can upset respiration by adversely affecting the respiratory centre as well as suppressing the cough reflex. It is worthwhile to note that a patient who becomes restless, excited and even aggressive may be suffering from anoxia and that further doses of sedatives and analgesics will only make the situation worse. Pain relief after thoracotomy has been the subject of many research-based publications culminating in abandoning the use of repeated intermuscular injections as the administration route. It has also renewed the interest in pre-emptive and intra-operative procedures, which aim to reduce administration of analgesics post-operatively. The basic principle is that opioids are administered post-operative by the following methods which may be used alone or in conjunction with non-steroidal anti-inflammatory preparation.

4.3.1 Intravenous bolus dose of analgesic repeated at intervals

4.3.2 Intravenous infusion at a controlled rate by nursing staff

4.3.3 Patient-controlled analgesia (PCA): This is a convenient system requiring minimal nursing staff intervention. In effect patients administer

their own drugs. The dose (both loading and maintenance) is established by the anaesthetist following which the programmed system is self-regulating.

4.3.4 Epidural catheter administration: The catheter is inserted (thoracic or lumbar, epidural 'space') using lipid insoluble opioid. It is important that the catheter is placed expertly. The method requires frequent nursing supervision and on the whole is used most effectively in the high dependency ward.

4.3.5 Regional analgesia: There are several methods of pain relief which rely on nerve blocks by analgesic administration in or around the intercostal nerve and para-vertebral space.
  - The block may, with advantage, be initiated intra-operatively with a catheter placed extra-pleurally at and around the site of thoracotomy. Both intercostal and sympathetic nerve block can follow infusion of analgesic.
  - Intra pleural analgesia: This method uses a catheter placed at operation between parietal and visceral pleura around the thoracotomy incision into which is infused Bupivacaine 0.25–0.5% with Epinephrine.
  - Cryoanalgesia: This method is used at operation by applying cryoanalgesic probes under direct vision to intercostal nerves
  The thoracic surgical team should adopt a method or combination of methods which can be practiced within the unit taking into account type of surgery and structure of peri-operative care of the unit. Options of pain control after the operation should be discussed with the patient, whose input should assist in the choice of an acceptable method.

4.4. Blood, fluid and nutrition

- Blood: Many patients undergoing lung and thoracic surgery require blood transfusions during the operation but they may continue to lose blood in the first 24–48 hours post-operatively which should be replaced if necessary.
- Fluid and nutrition: Most patients undergoing non-oesophageal thoracic surgery can take oral fluid a few hours after operation. Normal food intake can begin on the first post-operative day; initially a light diet, and then a normal high-calorie, high-protein diet is given. In the early post-operative pe-

riod a chart should record fluid intake and output. It is important not to over-transfuse and overload the patient with fluid. In the absence of gastrointestinal complications, intravenous infusion should be discontinued on the first or second post-operative day.

4.5. Physiotherapy

Breathing exercise, coughing and expectoration should start a few hours after the operation when the patient is fully conscious and able to cooperate. In the early stages, deep breathing and gentle coughing are all that is required in pulmonary surgery. Continuous expansion of the residual lung and clearance of airways should be monitored clinically and radiologically.

Unless there are specific contraindications, the patient can sit in a chair by the side of the bed on the first post-operative day. The presence of pleural drains and intravenous drip should not constitute a problem or contraindication for the patient's mobility. When drips and other attachments have been removed, the patient can be fully mobilised, initially walking with supervision and help. A single drain attached to an underwater sealed system can be carried by the patient. Alternatively the tube may be connected to a flutter valve (see intercostal tube drainage, section 4.4.1(b) in chapter I.22).

4.6. Medication

- Analgesics: These have already been referred to. It is clear that opioid need not be continued for more than a few days. In practice, when drainage tubes have been removed, milder oral analgesics should be given.
- Cardiac drugs: Post-operative dysrhythmic events are not uncommon amongst elderly patients undergoing pneumonectomy. The events should be investigated by ECG recording and appropriately dealt with by suitable medication. There is no evidence that prophylactic digitalisation will prevent the onset of post-operative atrial fibrillation. However, observation and experience suggests that some patients, such as those requiring pericardial resection and/or intra-pericardial excision of pulmonary veins, may benefit from digitalisation initiated at operation.
- Antibiotics: These should be provided prophylactically or, in some cases, therapeutically as

indicated. For therapeutic purposes the organism will have to be identified.

4.7. Laboratory tests

Full blood count, serum electrolytes and urea and biochemical profile analysis should be carried out early after operation and repeated at intervals. Urine tests for proteins and sugar should also be carried out post-operatively. Sputum samples should be sent to the laboratory at intervals for microbiological study and for testing sensitivity to antibiotics. If there are purulent expectorations or abnormal discharges, additional tests should be undertaken as necessary.

4.8. Further post-operative care

Once monitoring devices, drainage tubes and attachments are disposed of many patients will remain in the hospital for a day or two (or longer according to circumstances) for rehabilitation prior to discharge. Early discharge (2–3 days after surgery) or attempting to carry out a major thoracic operation as a day case can only be practical when the primary care system has been effectively structured and when the thoracic surgical centre can have an open access policy for patients. In the 3–4 week post-operative period, the following issues need to be addressed and parameters measured:

- Body temperature recording twice a day for 7–10 days.
- The wound requires inspection and complications need to be evaluated and treated accordingly.
- Chest X-ray is required to check continuing lung expansion and normal progress of pneumonectomy space (see Fig. 3 in chapter I.21).
- Physiotherapy: Besides chest physiotherapy, general movement and increased level of activity should be encouraged. Attention should be paid to shoulder movement especially on the thoracotomy side. A 'frozen' shoulder with pain and limitation of movement can complicate postero-lateral thoracotomy; this may be the result of pain and patient reluctance to carry out shoulder movement exercise.
- Medication:
  - Analgesics and sedatives: Even at the time of discharge, the majority of patients require mild analgesics.
  - Sedatives and hypnotics may be essential to some patients. Occasionally after thoracotomy a patient becomes so exhausted as to require se-

dation in order to relax and sleep. This dramatically improves their mental and physical state.

- A number of patients with cancer of the lung develop post-operative depression, occasionally with a definite psychosis, which requires appropriate therapy.
- It is not unusual for a patient to require therapeutic digitalis preparations. Fluid retention associated with impending or overt heart failure requires diuretic therapy with potassium salt supplement.
- Bronchodilators: Many pulmonary and thoracic surgical patients suffer from COPD and need various bronchodilators. Some are specifically prone to bronchospasm and experience asthmatic attacks which need special handling and administration of bronchodilators and steroids.
- Mucolytic drugs: In many patients bronchial secretions are thick and 'sticky' following operation. This is particularly the case in smokers and bronchitic patients. Mucolytic agents may be used with benefit in such cases to reduce the viscosity of the sputum and help expectoration.

Arrangement for follow-up prior to patient discharge: Clear notification should be given to the primary care/community care organisations regarding the patient's care in the community. Also, follow-up for the patient should be clarified at the thoracic surgical unit by the surgical team.

References and further reading

Benumof JL. Anaesthesia for thoracic surgery. Philadelphia: WB Saunders, 1987.

Bimston DN, McGee JP, Liptay MJ, Fry WA. Continuous paravertebral extrapleural infusion for post-thoracotomy pain management. Surgery 1999; 4: 650–656.

Cook TM, Riley RH. Analgesia following thoracotomy: a survey of Australian practice. Anaesth Intensive Care 1997; 5: 520–524.

Doyle E, Bowler GM. Pre-emptive effect of multimodal analgesia in thoracic surgery. Br J Anaesth 1998; 80: 147–151.

Gruber EM, Tschernoko EM, Kritzinger M et al. The effects of thoracic epidural analgesia with bupivacaine 0.25% on ventilatory mechanics in patients with severe chronic obstructive pulmonary disease. Anesth Analg 2001; 4: 1015–1019.

Insel PA. Analgesic antipyretic and anti-inflammatory agents. In: Hardman JG, Limbird LE, Molinoff PB, Ruddon RH, Gilman AG (eds.), Goodman and Gilman's The pharmacological basis of therapeutics (9th ed.). New York: McGraw-Hill 1996; p. 637.

Khan IH, McManus KG, McCraith A et al. Muscle-sparing thoracotomy: a biomechanical analysis confirms preservation of muscle strength but no improvement in wound discomfort. Eur J Cardiothorac Surg 2000; 18: 656–661.

Kruger M, McRae K. Pain management in cardiothoracic practice. Surg Clin North Am 1999; 79: 387–400.

Mahon SV, Berry PD, Jackson M, Russel GN, Pennefather SH. Thoracic epidural infusions for post-thoracotomy pain: a comparison of fentanyl–bupivacaine mixtures versus fentanyl alone. Anaesthesia 1999; 54: 641–646.

Moorjani N, Zhao F, Tian Y et al. Effects of cryoanalgesia on post-thoracotomy pain and on the structure of the intercostal nerves: a human prospective randomised trial and a histological study. Eur J Cardiothorac Surg 2001; 20: 502–507.

Pelton JJ, Fish DJ, Keller SM. Epidural narcotic analgesia after thoracotomy. South Med J 1993; 86: 1106–1109.

Perttunen K, Nilsson E, Heinonen J et al. Extradural, paravertebral and intercostal nerve blocks for post-thoracotomy pain. Br J Anaesth 1995; 75: 541–547.

Sabanathan S, Richardson J, Mearns AJ. Efficacy of continuous intercostal bupivacaine for pain relief after thoracotomy. Br J Anaesth 1993; 71: 463–464.

Sandler AN. Post-thoracotomy analgesia and perioperative outcome. Minerva Anestesiol 1999; 5: 267–274.

Sullivan E, Grannis FW Jr, Ferrell B, Dunst M. Continuous extrapleural intercostal nerve block with continuous infusion of lidocaine after thoracotomy: a descriptive pilot study. Chest 1995; 108: 1718–1723.

Tovar EA. One-day admission for major lung resections in septuagenarians and octogenarians: a comparative study with younger cohort. Eur J Cardiothorac Surg 2001; 20: 449–454.

Zieren HU, Muller JM, Hamberger U et al. Quality of life after surgical therapy of bronchogenic carcinoma. Eur J Cardiothorac Surg 1996; 10: 233–237.

there is no other condition which can present with such a dramatic clinical picture of sudden collapse and exsanguination. Action has to be immediate and directed to arresting the bleeding. Fortunately, this event is not a common occurrence but, unfortunately, if it does occur there is little time before the patient dies from exsanguination.

2.4. Management of post-operative haemorrhage

In the case of reactionary haemorrhage, a central venous pressure line is usually in situ and the pressure is monitored and recorded every 10–15 minutes with review of vital signs. A repeat chest radiograph is taken to monitor intra-thoracic collection of blood clot. In a typical case of intra-thoracic haemorrhage, this shows pulmonary collapse with an ill-defined opacity or haziness in that hemithorax. Continuous ECG recording (visual display) is set up and record is made for review every 30 minutes. Blood gas analysis is carried out as appropriate and oxygen saturation monitored with continuous oximetry. Drainage containers are changed as required and the volume of drained blood is recorded every 15 minutes. Blood transfusion is continued and the volume adjusted to cover the loss through the drains and according to the central venous pressure.

Other therapeutic measures are as follows:
• The patient is reassured and suitably sedated.
• Oxygen is administered to raise the oxygen level of inhaled gas.
• Intravenous fluid/blood is carefully adjusted. Care should be taken not to overload.
• A urinary catheter is inserted and intake/output is monitored.

If the condition of the patient improves and the volume of bleeding reduces, the conservative policy may be continued for 2–3 hours when the whole situation should be reviewed. When improvement does not occur, plans should be made to return the patient to the operating theatre for exploration and arrest of haemorrhage. In early post-thoracotomy cases with intercostal tube in situ, this usually requires thoracotomy opening.

In cases of late discovery of intra-thoracic bleeding and secondary haemorrhage, imaging techniques (X-ray and ultrasonography) are used to localise the site of bleeding. Tube thoracostomy is tried initially with/without thoracoscopic exploration. When an intercostal tube is inserted and the initial blood clot is drained, the rate of bleeding should be checked. This, together with progress of the clinical condition

of the patient, is the deciding factor as to whether the conservative or a more radical line (i.e. thoracotomy or VATS) is to be pursued.

In cases of massive haemorrhage, the drainage tube is clamped immediately and the thoracotomy wound should be opened. The patient will only be saved by the speedy arrest of haemorrhage.

3. Haemoptysis

Frank haemoptysis should be distinguished from blood-stained sputum (phlegm with streaks of blood) and also from fluid which could be haemorrhagic.
• Blood-stained sputum a day or two after operation is not unusual and can be due to residue from bronchial bleeding at the stump. Its continuation should be monitored and, if necessary, checked bronchoscopically. Blood-staining of sputum due to thrombo-embolism is usually associated with pain and breathlessness.
• Post-resection expectoration of haemorrhagic fluid is usually associated with early development of broncho-pleural fistula. This should be investigated urgently in partial pulmonary resection (lobectomy) and as a matter of emergency in pneumonectomy.
• Late post-operative haemoptysis is often associated with infection and occurs in patients with infective complications in the post-operative period. The bleeding is either from a bronchial artery or, more seriously, due to broncho-vascular fistula. Chest radiography, CT scan and bronchoscopy are important methods of investigation. Management should consider first aid and emergency measures which are guided towards clearing the airway, oxygenation and replacement of lost blood volume (see haemoptysis, chapter IV.4).

4. Cardiovascular complications

4.1. Cardiac complications

Serious cardiac complications such as myocardial infarction occur occasionally, usually early after major thoracotomies. Abnormalities of rhythm, particularly atrial fibrillation, commonly complicate pulmonary surgery in the older age group of patients and in cases where the pericardium is incised or excised (intra-pericardial ligation and division of vessels). In a typical case, atrial fibrillation develops some 48–72 hours after the operation and the patient becomes hypotensive, dyspnoeic and may present with low cardiac output syndrome. Digitalisation deals with the problem and experience shows that prophylactic digitalisation in predisposed patients substantially reduces the incidence of this complication. Other types of dysrhythmic complications need accurate diagnosis and appropriate treatment.

4.2. Vascular complications

- Thrombophlebitis of superficial veins of the hands and arms following intravenous administration of drugs, infusion of solutions and extravasation of irritant substances, though painful and unpleasant, presents no danger of embolisation. Deep vein thrombosis is an important cause of morbidity because of migration of thrombus and pulmonary embolus and infarction. Routine prophylactic use of low-dose heparin has diminished, although not completely removed, this post-operative complication.
- Arterial embolisms following pulmonary surgery originate from two sources:
  - Migration of tumour/clot arising from pulmonary veins during operation.
  - Blood clot and particles such as calcium which could be present in the heart prior to the operation originating from the left heart at operation or due to haemodynamic changes (e.g. atrial fibrillation) after the operation.

5. Respiratory complications

5.1. Respiratory insufficiency

- Immediately after the operation, respiratory complications are related to general anaesthesia and obstruction of the airways by excess bronchial secretions, vomitus or blood with subsequent atelectasis.
- Early after the operation patients with limited respiratory reserve, the emphysematous and those with chronic obstructive pulmonary disease (COPD) may present with respiratory insufficiency which, in practical terms, means hypoxia and carbon dioxide retention.

Clinical manifestation of anoxia after pulmonary surgery can be focused on:
- The central nervous system with excitement and aggression and then confusion and drowsiness.
- The respiratory system with breathing being rapid and shallow and then becoming periodic and finally stopping totally.

- The cardiovascular system where there is initially an increase in the heart rate with slight rise in blood pressure followed by bradycardia and final cardiac arrest.

Carbon dioxide retention after pulmonary surgery has important damaging effects on:
- The central nervous system with anxiety, disorientation, coma and then carbon dioxide narcosis.
- Respiratory system: Breathing is initially deep and then becomes rapid and shallow.
- Circulatory system: Initially there is tachycardia followed by slow heart rate culminating in cardiac arrest. These cardiac changes are associated with hypertension, bounding (full) pulse, warm and sweating skin.

5.1.1. Aetiology of post-operative respiratory insufficiency

The main causes of respiratory insufficiency after pulmonary surgery may be classified under three headings:
- Inadequacy of ventilation: These include airway obstruction of any kind (e.g. retention of secretions), neuromuscular such as paralysis of the diaphragm and pneumothorax.
- Inadequacy of pulmonary parenchyma:
  - Through lack of sufficient parenchyma because of volume excision in excess of that which the patient's pulmonary function permits.
  - Pre-existing parenchymal diseases such as pulmonary fibrosis, emphysema and post-operative pneumonitis.
  - Post-operative pulmonary atelectasis or too great a volume of air leak amounting to loss of a high proportion of the tidal volume.
- Inadequacy of perfusion, including heart failure and pulmonary arterial thrombosis or embolism.

5.1.2. Management

Clinical, radiological and laboratory tests are carried out to:
- Confirm the diagnosis
- Evaluate the severity of respiratory insufficiency
- Establish the aetiology
- Obtain the baseline objective data which can be useful to assess the result and progress of the treatment.

Treatment should be based on aetiological diagnosis. However:
- First aid measures must be undertaken in severe cases whilst assessing the situation; this consists of:

– Clearance of the airways
– Rechecking the pleural drains to ensure their function
– Provision of oxygen in the inspired air (40–50%)
– Proceeding with tracheostomy or assisted ventilation, if necessary.

5.2. Sputum retention

In the early post-operative days, retention of sputum in some patients can cause considerable problems as secretions are tenacious and difficult to expectorate. Thoracotomy pain, repeated administration of analgesics and general fatigue bring about in some patients, particularly heavy smokers, a state of mental and physical exhaustion leaving the patient unable to expectorate. This can lead to pulmonary infection and/or respiratory insufficiency.

Sputum retention must be treated actively and energetically by physiotherapy before respiratory failure develops. Humidifiers and nebulisers are used as appropriate with administration of mucolytic agents to reduce the viscosity and stickiness of secretions. Expectorants are helpful, particularly those containing mucolytic agents and bronchodilators. Antibiotics are prescribed when infection is present.

If these measures are not successful, repeated bronchoscopic aspiration and tracheostomy (mini/standard) may be required. The latter should be considered when bronchoscopy becomes a frequent necessity when there are clear indications of impending respiratory failure and before the need for the procedure becomes imminent.

5.3. Bronchospasm

Immediately after operation, i.e. during recovery from anaesthesia, severe bronchospasm may occur, requiring the administration of bronchodilators and/or hydrocortisone. Later bronchospasm may be associated with an increase in secretions and partial obliteration of small bronchi; bronchitics are particularly prone to this complication. It is relevant to point out that a small bronchopleural fistula can simulate bronchospasm.

Bronchodilators will alleviate a mild bronchospasm though steroids may have to be used in some patients.

6. Infective pneumonitis and lung abscess

Infective complications of pulmonary surgery are often the consequence of retention of bronchial secretion and, to a large extent, are preventable. Daily auscultation is important and examination of the chest radiograph alone is not sufficient. Positive findings on X-ray film means that consolidation has already developed. When the diagnosis of infection is made, the treatment is undertaken by:
- Administration of appropriate antibiotics based on sputum micro-organism sensitivity
- Regular chest physiotherapy
- High calorie and protein nutrition
- In the case of lung abscess or the expansion of infection to the pleural space, appropriate surgical measures are undertaken.

7. Atelectasis of the residual lobe or segment after partial pulmonary resection

When the residual lung does not expand or it collapses after its earlier expansion, respiratory difficulties and pleural space infection will occur. The most important causes of pulmonary collapse after lung surgery are:

7.1. Bronchial obstruction due to retention of secretions

When a large area such as a lobe of the lung collapses, the diagnosis can be made clinically and confirmed radiologically. There is usually respiratory difficulty, pulse rate is rapid and there may be fever. Examination reveals lack of chest movement on the affected side and the absence of breath sounds in the area concerned. Abnormal added sounds such as rhonchi or wheeze may also be heard on auscultation. Chest radiograph confirms a typical picture of the lack of 'aerated' parenchyma and the retraction of the mediastinum towards the collapsed lung.

If atelectasis is not extensive, re-expansion is achieved by rigorous physiotherapy, humidification of air, administration of expectorants and mucolytic agents. Bronchoscopic suction is required if the lung fails to re-expand. This is usually carried out under local (topical) anaesthesia, preferably with the use of the rigid bronchoscope with the patient in his/her own bed (see Fig. 2 in chapter I.2, and section 2.1.2 in chapter IV.3). In this way the patient and his/her drains (if in situ) are not disturbed. Despite extensive use of the flexible fibreoptic instrument and the ease and frequency of its practice by physicians (bronchoscopists), this author believes bronchoscopy in this situation should be carried out employing the rigid instrument and by a member of the surgical team. This is because:

– During the procedure the patient can be ventilated through the open-ended instrument.
– The bronchoscopy may reveal abnormalities diagnosable by surgeons since they would appreciate more readily the anatomy of bronchial stump.

7.2. Collapse due to pneumothorax

Early in the post-operative phase, air leaks from the intersection of the pulmonary segments and lobes are evacuated by drains which are left in the pleural space until all leaks stop and full expansion of the lung is obtained. The malfunction of drains due to a faulty system, poor connections, blockage of the drains or the patient lying on the connecting tubes are the most frequent cause of early post-operative pneumothorax. A residual cushion of air in the pleural space at the apex, or sometimes at the base, in the absence of visible air leaks from drains signifies malfunction or malposition of the drainage tube. It can also be the cause of continuous air leak. Effort should be made to expand the lung by effective drainage and active physiotherapy. A functionally useless drainage tube should be removed and replaced by a functioning one.

Later post-operative pneumothorax may be due to a smaller air leak or bronchopleural fistula. The possibility of spontaneous pneumothorax should also be borne in mind.

8. Pleural space complication

8.1. Pneumothorax

This has been referred to above (section 7.2 of this chapter).

8.2. Pleural effusion

Sero-sanguinous fluid may collect in the pleural space after pulmonary surgery. In the case of pneumonectomy, this is part of the natural pneumonectomy space behaviour (see pleural space after lung resection, section 4.1 in chapter I.21). In the case of partial pulmonary resection, effusion can cause collapse of the lung and will embarrass ventilation of the residual lung. In this case the causes may be:

- Malfunction and malposition of tube when the drains are in situ
- Continuous leak of lymphatic fluid and blood ooze and fluid collection when the drains have been removed. Except for pneumonectomy cases, the fluid should be evacuated from the chest either by pleural aspiration or tube drainage. The choice of method depends on the volume and consistency of the fluid. Once fluid is removed, an X-ray is taken to assess lung expansion.

In pneumonectomy cases, if there is a suspicion of infection, a sample of fluid should be aspirated and despatched to the laboratory for microbiological study and sensitivity to antibiotic. A further X-ray taken a few days later will monitor the presence or absence of recurrence. The cause of fluid should be investigated, particularly in a case of recurrence.

8.3. Post-resection pleural space infection

Pleural space infection is a serious post-operative complication, which, when not fatal, can affect quality of life and prolong postoperative recovery. Alternatively, it may lead to lifelong disabling chronic sepsis. To a great extent the outcome of pleural space infection depends on the presence or absence of broncho-pleural fistula (BPF) and the effectiveness of therapy which is undertaken. A number of other factors affect the success or failure of treatment. These are:

– The type of micro-organisms involved and their sensitivity to antibiotic.
– General and nutritional state and immunological competence of the patient.
– The extent of resection.
  General principles of management
This consists of control of local and general infection and expansion of the residual lung in lobectomy cases and measures to prevent recurrence.

The control of local infection can only be achieved by evacuation of the purulent material and sterilization of the space. In patients with fistulae, the control of the infection is linked with closure of fistulae. Expansion of the residual lung in partial pulmonary resection depends not only on the quality of parenchyma but on clear airways.

In all pleural space infection in cancer patients it is important to exclude the presence of tumour in the bronchial stump, residual lung and/or pleural space.

Pleural space infection is discussed under:
8.3.1 Space infection in partial pulmonary resection
8.3.2 Space infection in pneumonectomy

8.3.1. Space infection in partial pulmonary resection

- Empyema without fistula is generally the consequence of persistent residual pleural space after resection followed by infection. Initially the lung fails to expand fully to occupy the hemithorax and a pneumothorax is visible on the chest X-ray. Sometimes the lung expands fully but then subsequently collapses and fails to re-expand, leaving space which persists only to become infected. Presentation is one of fever with signs of infection, and chest X-ray shows the presence of effusion in the pleural space with/without pneumothorax.

- In empyema with broncho-pleural fistula, the onset is usually gradual. In some cases incessant air leak and persisting air space herald the development of space infection. Fever, leucocytosis and expectoration of purulent blood-stained sputum with air leak beyond 7 days should draw attention to BPF. In this regard it is important to check the integrity of tube drainage and examine the sputa. It is also necessary to carry out bronchoscopy and to visually examine the bronchial stump. In fistula cases bronchoscopy shows the opening at the site of the bronchial stump through which the contents of the pleural space bubble out.

  It should be re-emphasised that such post-operative bronchoscopies should be carried out by a thoracic surgeon experienced in bronchoscopy who is aware of the surgical anatomy of the stump.

- Management

  In post-lobectomy empyemas without BPF, evacuation of purulent fluid and sterilization of the space usually allows expansion of the lung and control of infection, provided that chronicity has not taken place. When the visceral pleura is covered over by fibrin and fibrous 'skin', the lung is not able to expand despite effective evacuation of purulent effusion even when the space is sterilised. In practical terms the management protocol for early post-operative empyemas are:

  – Assessment bronchoscopy, to exclude BPF.
  – Tube thoracostomy drainage. This, in many cases, is the first step. Such a drain should be appropriately placed in the most dependent part of the collection, free from fibrous septa and loculation, and connected to underwater sealed drainage system (UWSDS). Ultrasonographic and thoracoscopic method may be used to achieve accurate placement of the tube. Thoracoscopy has the advantage of visual exploration and debridement prior to drainage.
  – Supportive treatment. This consists of antibiotic administration, chest physiotherapy and maintenance of nutritional state. In the absence of BPF and lack of fibrous tissue deposition over the pleura, the lung will expand with eradication of infection.

When the lung fails to expand, steps should be taken to achieve expansion by pleural decortication, thoracoscopically (VATS), via limited access or standard thoracotomy approaches.

In post-lobectomy BPF, the management consists of:

– Provision of adequate drainage via intercostal tube drain.
– Administration of appropriate antibiotic based on sensitivity of the organisms.
– Physiotherapy and bronchial toilet if necessary by repeated bronchoscopy aspiration.
– Effort to expand the lung and eliminate redundant space.
– Closure of fistula by bronchoscopic measures (application of sodium hydroxide 20% or biological glue to the stump) when the fistula opening is 1–2 mm^2.
– Thoracoscopy, thoracotomy, decortication and closure of fistula when the fistula is larger than 1–2 mm^2.

8.3.2. Space infection in pneumonectomy cases

Pneumonectomy space infections have the following characteristics:

- They are uncommon without broncho-pleural fistulae.
- They can become a chronic ongoing sepsis.
- They may occur months or even years after the initial operation.

Broncho-pleural fistula (BPF) has an incidence of 5–10% depending on the disease and general condition of the patient. They are more frequently encountered than in lobectomies or segmental resections, one reason being the empty pleural space which surrounds the bronchial stump in pneumonectomy. Factors influencing BPF in pneumonectomies are multiple:

- Host factor: Patients with poor cardiorespiratory performance, those in malnutritional state and the immuno-compromised are more susceptible.
- Type of disease: Resections in some conditions such as tuberculosis, bronchiectasis and fungal infection are more prone to this complication.
- Technical (iatrogenic) factors:
  – Devascularization of the stump at operation
  – Careless dissection or crush clamping of main

bronchus proximal to the line of division
– Disease involvement of the bronchial margin (e.g. incomplete resection in cancer patients)
– Faulty closure of the bronchial stump
– Pleural space infection and peri-bronchial stump abscess

In cases where BPF develops immediately after operation, there is a sudden deterioration in the patient's respiration with dyspnoea, tachypnoea and expectoration of watery, blood-stained sputa. Chest radiograph will show a reduction of the level of fluid in the pneumonectomy space (see Fig. 4 in chapter I.21) and patchy infiltration in the residual lung.

- Presentation in cases occurring a few weeks after surgery is one of chest infection with purulent and old, blood-stained expectoration.
- In patients who develop BPF months or years after pneumonectomy, repeated chest infection with intermittent discharge from the site of the scar, or a 'sinus' at the 'dependent' part of the scar and intermittent leaking may be indicative.

Management:

Early post-operative cases can be diagnosed readily and require prevention of spillage from the pneumonectomy space into the airway of the residual lung, which is achieved by tube thoracostomy inserted into the space and appropriate measures necessary to check infection and stabilise the general and cardio-respiratory state of the patient.

In all post-pneumonectomy cases, a complete work-up is necessary to evaluate the size of the fistula, the content of the pneumonectomy space and the type of pathogens involved. The principles of further management are:

- Bronchoscopy, which is essential not only for evaluation of the fistula but also for checking of pathology (e.g. recurrence of tumour).
- Complete evacuation of purulent effusion from the chest.
- Sterilisation of the space by pleural lavage with an antiseptic solution or antibiotic (see empyema, chapter I.25). Lavage is discontinued when space infection is cleared after a period of 2–3 months. It should be noted that the systemic administration of antibiotic in chronic empyema after pneumonectomy has no relevance except for control of infection in the contralateral lung or for other coincidental infection (e.g. urinary).

Once the pneumonectomy space is totally evacuated and sterilised, a decision should be made to treat the fistulous opening and prevent recurrence.

Treatment is achieved by closure of the fistula by either bronchoscopic method or via surgical intervention:

- Bronchoscopic method consists of the use of preparations such as NaOH (sodium hydroxide) 20% or Fibrin sealant which is applied to the fistulous opening through the bronchoscope. In either method, prior drainage and sterilisation of the space is necessary. Also, the method can only succeed when the fistula is small.
- Operative method is based on exposure of the bronchial stump surgically via thoracotomy and repair of the fistula.

A broncho-pleural fistula occurring early in the post-operative recovery phase of pneumonectomy with a clean space is best treated by operation. This consists of re-opening the thoracotomy wound, cleaning the pleural space of debris and carrying out a thorough toilet of the space with an antiseptic/antibiotic solution (e.g. Neomycin). The bronchial stump is then refreshed and carefully re-sutured. BPF occurring later can also be treated by surgical repair with the proviso referred to previously. However, access to the bronchial stump through the original thoracotomy wound may not be possible, particularly in a left-sided BPF. Trans-sternal, trans-pericardial approach provides satisfactory access to the stump on both sides, allowing cleaning, debridement and excision of the fistulous stump in either of the operative methods. Application of intercostal, diaphragmatic and/or pedical pericardial graft provides an added security to the suture line. The pleural space is drained.

Prevention of recurrence:

This is largely dependent on obliteration of the redundant pleural space. It is relevant to emphasise that in cases of empyema and BPF after a lobectomy, the redundant space is usually filled by the expanding lung following drainage of effusion and closure of the fistula. In pneumonectomy cases, the space will remain vacant and, despite its drainage and sterilisation, there is a risk of recurrence. It follows that various methods have been proposed to obliterate or reduce the extent of the space.

- Thoracoplasty: Once a common practice, it has only a limited application, possibly in conjunction with other methods and in conditions such as tuberculous BP.
- The greater omentum transplantation has both the advantage of its large mass and copious vascular supply.

- Transposition of large thoracic wall muscles into the space.

Summary of BPF:
- Every effort should be made to prevent/reduce the risk of space infection and development of BPF.
- Appropriate investigations should be set up to diagnose as early as possible these complications.
- Drainage of space and its sterilisation should be undertaken.
- Bronchoscopic/operative methods are used to close the fistula.
- In operative cases of closure of the fistula, the suture line and the stump should be protected by homologous tissue coverage.
- In lobectomy patients, the residual lung should be fully re-expanded, thus obliterating the pocket of air and reducing the risk of recurrence.
- In pneumonectomy cases, the space should be obliterated after drainage and sterilisation of the space together with fistula closure. In many cases, closure of the fistula and obliteration of space can be achieved at one operation (e.g. closure and omental transplant).

9. Other complications of pulmonary surgery

9.1. Alimentary tract complications

Nausea and vomiting may occur early after the operation. These usually subside by the end of the first 24 hours. When persistent, the cause must be investigated.

The common cause is distension and dilatation of the stomach which can be of an acute onset. Decompression by aspirating through a nasogastric tube, together with intravenous infusion for a day or two, usually deals with the problem. A thorough and frequent examination of the abdomen should be made in order to diagnose a coincidental intra-abdominal catastrophe such as perforation of a duodenal ulcer or appendicitis.

A great number of patients in hospital develop minor bowel irregularities. In some this becomes very distressing; in others, especially the elderly, the bowel action may stop and faecal impaction occurs.

9.2. Genitourinary complications

Urinary retention is not unusual in the early post-operative phase. Contributing factors are:

- In male patients, some degree of prostatic enlargement
- Post-operative pain inhibiting the start of micturition
- Analgesics given repeatedly
- The inability to start micturition when in bed.

If normal micturition has not occurred 12–18 hours after operation, despite encouragement, a urinary catheter is passed and the urine is drained. Later in the post-operative phase, retention of urine or overflow incontinence should be more carefully investigated.

Urinary infection, dysuria, haematuria and the frequency of micturition may occur after pulmonary surgery and the cause should be investigated.

Renal failure: This complication occasionally occurs after extensive pulmonary and chest wall surgery, such as thoracoplasty, particularly when an extensive operation has been complicated by haemorrhage, hypotension and/or shock. The manifestations are anuria or oliguria, rise in the blood urea and metabolic acidosis. Renal failure occurs early in the post-operative phase and the diagnosis should be made taking into account the history of the operative events.

Menstrual disturbances: Early in the post-operative phase, many young women start a rather heavy menstrual period, irrespective of the expected date. This is not really a complication but is worthy of mention as it can cause anxiety which only requires reassurance.

9.3. Neurocerebral complications

Neurological complications are rare after a pulmonary operation and only a few can be directly attributed to surgery.
- Hemiplegia and hemiparesis can occur as a result of the migration and cerebral vascular embolisation of the tumour or clot particles from the pulmonary vein as a result of operative manipulations. This complication is usually noticed soon after operation or early in the post-operative phase. Occasionally, neurological complications occur later on due to cerebral embolus, haemorrhage or metastatic deposition of a tumour in the brain. Early secondaries in the vertebral column cause bone destruction/vertebral collapse and neurological disturbances with severe pain and paralysis.
- Mental confusion and temporary personality changes are occasionally encountered following

extensive pulmonary surgery in older patients, particularly those who may have suffered some degree of post-operative hypoxia.

9.4. Thoracotomy wound complications

The approach for standard pulmonary resection is postero-lateral thoracotomy. Thoracotomy wound complications prolong hospitalisation and have a demoralising effect on the patient when they have already had a long stay in hospital. Certain features of the thoracotomy wound need consideration:
- The wound is usually extensive, and when repaired, it should be airtight.
- Repair of the wound involves several layers of muscular suturing. All these muscles are constantly active and under strain by breathing and other movements.
- On the anterior of the chest, intercostal spaces are wider and the ribs and their cartilages are covered by a thinner layer of soft tissues. In addition, the anterior part of the wound is the lowest and most dependent part when the patient is sitting up or standing. Therefore, there is a greater tendency for fluid or pus in the wound to gravitate and escape from this area.

Early wound complications may develop soon after operation. They are:
9.4.1 Wound disruption
9.4.2 Wound haematoma
9.4.3 Wound bleeding
9.4.4 Collection of purulent fluid
9.4.5 Sepsis and wound discharge
9.4.6 Other complications of the wound

9.4.1. Wound disruption
Wound disruption may affect all muscular layers, including intercostals, in which case there is a total disruption (burst chest). Similarly, individual muscular layers of the thoracotomy wound may break down. Dehiscence of the intercostal layer is diagnosed by the presence of surgical emphysema and applying the palms of the hands over the thoracotomy area firmly and by a palpable impulse on palpation of the chest when the patient coughs. This is due to the sudden exit of air and fluid from the pleural space under the skin. Total disruption of the intercostal layer of the wound can also be diagnosed radiologically. A normal post-thoracotomy chest radiograph shows the intercostal space, e.g. the 5th interspaces, to be narrower than the spaces above and below or the numerically identical space on the opposite

side. When there is a disruption of the intercostal layer, the reverse is the case, i.e. the thoracotomy interspace becomes wider.

Any wound disruption which involves the intercostal space should be taken seriously and treated urgently by re-opening, exploration and re-closure of the thoracotomy wound. An early disruption of muscular layers should, in principle, be dealt with by early exploration and operative repair since the muscle edges will retract, and approximation and suturing becomes more difficult later on.

Late disruption of the thoracotomy wound is usually associated with, and results from, infection and does not usually involve the intercostals and deeper layers of muscle. Most commonly, the superficial muscles and skin layers are involved. When such disruption is clean and limited in extent, a few through-and-through (deep tension) sutures are all that is required. A more extensive and deeper wound disruption requires cleaning, debridement and formal closure. If the muscle layers cannot be individually identified, one layer of interrupted through-and-through skin sutures will suffice. In this case the stitches are left 10–14 days before being removed. During this time the patient can be at home and recalled for inspection and removal of stitches provided that his/her general condition is satisfactory.

9.4.2. Wound haematoma
This may or may not be associated with wound disruption. In addition to the bulging in the wound, which is palpable, the patient experiences a painful tension in the wound. Aspiration with a wide bore needle and a syringe is only successful when there is liquefaction and in the absence of blood clots. Most often it is necessary to open an area of the wound from the skin down to the haematoma to evacuate the blood clot. A drain may be inserted down to the area to allow evacuation and healing from the depth.

9.4.3. Wound bleeding
In some patients there is oozing from the surface of the wound. A pressure dressing usually deals with the ooze; otherwise a deep skin suture tied over a piece of gauze will successfully control this.

9.4.4. Collection of purulent fluid
Collection of purulent fluid in the layers of the thoracotomy wound may be of two origins. When deep in the wound, fluid or pus can be an extension of pleural effusion. In effect this is an 'empyema necessitatis' which has not as yet reached the skin. As the fluid

(or pus) originated from the pleural cavity, the pleura needs draining to evacuate the collection. In some cases the wound has to be drained separately as well. Both drains have to be connected to the underwater sealed drainage system unless there is evidence that the collection is in a confined space which is not connecting to the general pleural cavity.

Another source of fluid (or pus) collection in the wound is from an infected haematoma. Signs and symptoms of an inflammatory swelling are present, the severity of which depends on the volume of fluid and the extent of sepsis.

9.4.5. Sepsis and wound discharge

Wound sepsis is defined as the presence of pus with or without micro-organisms. Deep wound sepsis has already been referred to above (section 9.4.4 in this chapter). When the collection is subcutaneous, it usually discharges to the surface through the gap in the line of incision.

For sepsis in the deep layer of the wound, aspiration and/or drainage allowing evacuation should be undertaken. If there is, in addition, wound disruption and sloughing, the wound should be re-opened and cleaned with an antiseptic solution such as aqueous solution of 1/5000 chlorhexidine or cetrimide in the first instance. Closure is then carried out later when the sepsis has subsided. When there is superficial sepsis, the lowest, most dependent part of the infected area is opened up to allow for discharge. When there is evidence of a 'tunnel' under the skin, the infection may be high in the uppermost part of the wound tracking down, in which case it may be necessary to:

(a) Leave an elongated drain under the skin in the 'tunnel' with its gradual shortening and then removal when healing is completed; or

(b) Re-open the skin, clear the area of necrotic material and re-close with or without a drain.

The basic principles of treatment of a discharging thoracotomy wound are to:

- Leave a wide channel for the exit of purulent material
- Pay attention to the peculiarities of the thoracotomy wound already referred to previously, and the fact that a discharge appearing on the surface may not only originate from a deep 'well' and a purulent reservoir which could go as deep as the pleural space, but also may communicate with side tracks which will be tunnelling widely under the chest wall's muscular layers.

If there is a discharging sinus the track has to be outlined radiologically by sinography. The source should be identified, together with the track, which should be opened, and then excised. The wound is then cleaned before its closure directly or by second intervention.

9.4.6. Other complications of the wound

Apart from the pain during the process of wound healing, which can last for a few weeks, many patients feel abnormal sensations which are more of a discomfort than pain. The knowledge of these is important to all those (resident staff, general practitioners) who come into contact with these patients. Per se these sensations are mostly unimportant but reassurance gives the convalescing patient peace of mind.

- Hypo-aesthesia and anaesthesia are generally felt at the anterior end of the wound and the upper quadrant of the abdomen.
- Pins-and-needles sensation is also felt at or around the anterior end of the scar.
- Sensation of swelling around the thoracotomy wound is a common complaint of the patient 4–6 weeks after the operation. The sensation is located at the anterior end of the wound, the costal margin, the hypochondrial and part of the epigastric region. Usually, examination of the area involved shows no real abnormality.
- All of these sensations usually disappear after 2–3 months and the patient needs reassurance only.

Pain:

Even when, as usually is the case, the thoracotomy wound heals satisfactorily, there is pain and discomfort in and around the wound for the first 10–12 post-operative days. At first there are several factors responsible for pain of which the important ones are:

- Stretching of the intercostal space by the retractor
- Pleuritis which accompanies thoracotomy wound healing
- The soft tissue wound pain
- The intercostal nerve pain

A patient's response to a thoracotomy wound and scar pain is variable; some hardly require any analgesics after 48 hours, while others go on complaining of pain for months or even years after the operation. Generally, by the time the wound is healed and the patient is being discharged from hospital, no great pain is experienced and only mild analgesics are required in small dose for 1–2 weeks. When the pain is persistent and severe it can constitute a real problem. Of all the wound complications this may be the most difficult to deal with. Scar pain is brought to attention by the patient after the wound is completely healed, usually without any complication. The site of the pain mostly, but not always, corresponds to the areas supplied by one or more intercostal nerves. Thorough examination of the scar and the chest should be carried out for possible abnormalities affecting the chest wall, such as an early recurrence of neoplastic involvement when the original thoracotomy had been for carcinoma.

Pleural effusion sometimes is accompanied by pain and its aspiration relieves the patient. In many instances, however, no cause can be found for wound or chest pain. In some patients anxiety and psychological strain are undoubtedly contributory factors adding a strong emotional component. Thoracotomy scar pain is treated by:

- Analgesics together with mild sedation.
- In a few cases the psychological pain can be abolished by placebos.
- Intercostal nerve infiltration by local anaesthetic and hydrocortisone in some patients with typical intercostal neuritis is effective in abolishing the pain temporarily and, occasionally permanently.
- In those patients who have received temporary relief, if there is evidence that the pain, in spite of analgesics, is interfering with the patient's quality of life, and particularly when there is evidence of involvement of the nerve by neoplasia, chemical or surgical neurectomy is indicated.

In recent years specialist pain clinics have taken charge of this aspect of wound complications. However, close co-operation between the surgical team and pain specialist is required for the benefit of the patient.

References and further reading

Abruzzini P. Trattamento chirurgico delle fistole del broncho principale consecutive a pneumonectomia per tubercolosi. Chir Toraci 1961; 14: 165–171.

Duan M, Chen G, Wang T, Zhang Y et al. One stage pedicled omentum majus transplantation into thoracic cavity for treatment of chronic persistent empyema with or without bronchopleural fistula. Eur J Cardiothorac Surg 1999; 16: 636–638.

El-Gamel A, Tsang GMK, Watson DCT. The threshold for air leak stapled versus sutured human bronchi: an experimental study. Eur J Cardiothorac Surg 1999; 15: 7–10.

Hollaus PH, Huber M, Lax F, Wurnig PN. Closure of bronchopleural fistula after pneumonectomy with a pedicled intercostal muscle flap. Eur J Cardiothorac Surg 1999; 16: 181–186.

Hollaus PH, Lax F, Wurning PN, Janakieve D et al. Videothoracoscopic debridement of the post pneumonectomy space in empyema. Eur J Cardiothorac Surg 1999; 16: 283–286.

Hollaus PH, Huber M, Lax F, Wurnig PN, Bohm G, Pridun NS. Closure of bronchopleural fistula after pneumonectomy with intercostal muscle flap. Eur J Cardiothorac Surg 1999; 16: 181–186.

Hollaus PH, Lax F, El-Nashef BB. Natural history of bronchopleural fistula after pneumonectomy: a review of 96 cases. Ann Thorac Surg 1997; 63: 1391.

Kalweit G, Feindt P, Huwer H et al. The pectoralis muscle flaps in the treatment of bronchial stump fistula following pneumonectomy. Eur J Cardiothorac Surg 1994; 388–362.

Klepetko W, Taghavi S, Perezcenyi A et al. Impact of different coverage techniques on incidence of post pneumonectomy stump fistula. Eur J Cardiothorac Surg 1999; 15: 758–763.

O'Neill PJ, Flanagan HL, Mauney MC, Spotnitz WD, Daniel TM. Intrathoracic fibrin sealant application using computed tonfluoroscopy. Ann Thorac Surg 2000; 70: 301–302.

Pairolero PC, Amold PG, Pichler JM. Intrathoracic transposition of extrathoracic skeletal muscle. J Thorac Cardiovasc Surg 1983; 86: 809–817.

Porhanov V, Poliakov I, Kononenko V et al. Surgical treatment of 'short stump' bronchial fistula. Eur J Cardiothorac Surg 2000; 17: 2–7.

Regnard JF, Alifano M, Puyo P, Fares E, Magdeleinat P, Levasseur P. Open window thoracostomy followed by intrathoracic flap transposition in the treatment of empyema complicating pulmonary resection. J Thorac Cardiovasc Surg 2000; 120: 270–275.

Rendina EA, Venuta F, Ciriaco P, Ricci C. Bronchovascular sleeve resection: technique, peri-operative management, prevention and treatment of complications. J Thorac Cardiovasc Surg 1993; 106: 73–79.

Smolle-Jüttner F, Beuster W, Pinter H, Pierre G et al. Open window thoracostomy in pleural empyema. Eur J Cardiothorac Surg 1999; 38: 355–358.

Spiliopoulos A, de Perrot M, Licker M, Murith N, Robert J. Successful closure of postpneumonectomy bronchopleural fistula with latissimus dorsi island flap and closed-chest irrigation. Scand Cardiovasc J 2000; 34: 92–94.

Stamatis G, Martini F, Freitag L, Wencker M, Greschuchna D. Transsternal transpericardial operations in the treatment of bronchopleural fistulas after pneumonectomy. Eur J Cardiothorac Surg 1996; 10: 83–86.

Topcuoglu MS, Kayhan C, Ulus T. Transsternal transpericardial approach for the repair of bronchopleural fistula with empyema. Ann Thorac Surg 2000; 69: 394–397.

CHAPTER I.21

Pleural space and its drainage

D.A.C. Sharpe

1. Introduction

The lungs and the chest wall are elastic structures which are normally separated by a thin film of fluid. The lungs have a natural tendency to recoil and collapse. Their physiological position is maintained by surface tension between the chest wall and the lung. As a result there is a sub-atmospheric pressure within the pleural space varying between -5 mmHg and -10 mmHg with normal respiration.

This can be measured using a transducer and electronic pressure recorder or by connecting the needle inserted into the pleural space to a simple manometer such as the Maxwell box (Fig. 1).

When the pleural cavity is in communication with air at normal atmospheric pressure, from either an air leak within the chest or a penetrating wound, the lung will collapse. This phenomenon proved to be a barrier to open intra-thoracic surgery until the advent of endotracheal intubation and positive

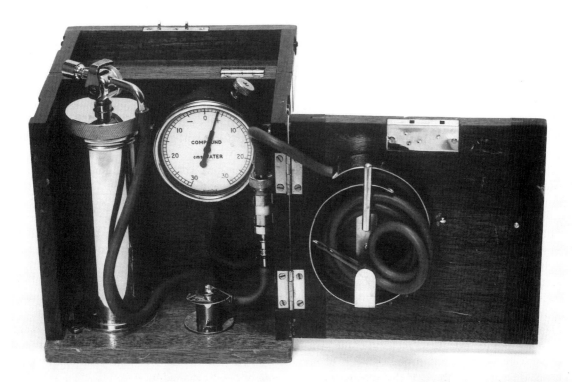

Fig. 1. The Maxwell Box.

pressure ventilation. Maintenance of subatmospheric intra-thoracic pressure and expansion of the lung is essential for normal function of the lung.

2. Pleural drainage

To drain the pleural space the system must allow fluid or air out of the pleural space but not their return to the space. This is usually achieved with an underwater sealed drainage system in which the water acts as a one-way valve. During inspiration the water does not allow air or fluid to pass up the tube into the subatmospheric pressure pleural space. During expiration, as the pressure in the pleural space rises above atmospheric pressure, or during coughing, air or fluid is freely expelled through the water. Valve systems such as the Heimlich system are occasionally employed for the same purpose.

2.1. Method for drainage of the pleural space

2.1.1. Equipment
- Local anaesthetic and needles long enough to achieve anaesthesia all the way to the pleural cavity (the needle from the centre of a venous access catheter is often longer than standard needles of the same gauge).
- A sharp blade to cut the skin and blunt forceps, such as 'Roberts', to penetrate the pleural space.
- Dressings, towels and antiseptics to allow the procedure to be carried out in a sterile field.
- A chest drain (which are sized according to the French Gauge).
- An underwater sealed drainage system. These are commercially available and contain all of the appropriate connections to the chest drain.

2.1.2. Technique of pleural drain insertion
(a) Determine the site and side for insertion of the drain using a recent chest X-ray. This is usually just anterior to the mid-axillary line at the level of the nipple (5th intercostal space).
(b) Surgically prepare and drape the chest at the site of chest drain insertion.
(c) Anaesthetise the skin and subcutaneous tissues down to the ribs, the periosteum of the rib and the intercostal muscles. Remember to allow sufficient time for the local anaesthetic to act.
(d) Make a 2 to 3 cm transverse incision in the skin at the point of drain insertion. Using a blunt clamp, dissect down through the subcutaneous tissues, just over the top of the rib.

(e) Puncture the pleura with the clamp and put a gloved finger into the incision to avoid injury to other organs and to clear clots and adhesions. (Fig. 2).
(f) Clamp the proximal end of the chest drain then advance it into the pleural space using the tract created by the finger. If this is difficult to negotiate, clamp the end of the drain in the forceps and use this to aid entry to the pleural space. A sharp instrument should not be introduced into the pleural space.
(g) Unclamp the drain and look for fogging of the plastic and listen for breath sounds.
(h) Connect the drain to the underwater sealed bottle.
(i) Suture the tube in place and dress the wound
(j) Take a chest X-ray to confirm that the drain is in good position and has performed its function.

2.2. Management of chest drains

Suction should be applied to the drain if either the fluid within the pleural space is not spontaneously evacuated or if the lung fails to expand to fill the pleural space. When the lung is fully expanded, suction can be discontinued from the drain and the patient mobilised. There is no need to routinely apply suction to a drain. The drainage bottle should be kept below the height of the chest otherwise fluid will siphon from the drain back into the chest.

The amount and nature of any fluid draining from the chest should be noted. This may be necessary hourly following thoracic surgery. Similarly, the amount of air leakage and the time of the last air bubble to pass the drain should also be noted. These two measures will guide the timing of removal of the drain.

Intrinsically, drains are painful; the pleura is an acutely sensitive structure with a rich nerve supply. The intercostal nerves cannot effectively be protected from either the insertion of the drain or the resultant pressure it causes. Analgesia with all thoracic surgery is a key issue; failure to cough and the resulting atelectasis and collapse can be disastrous in this group of patients who almost invariably have a degree of respiratory impairment. The importance of adequate analgesia should not be underestimated. This can be achieved by a variety of local methods such as local intercostal block, paravertebral catheter inserted at the time of surgery or epidural. They can be supplemented by systemic analgesics and patient controlled analgesia systems (PCAS). The use

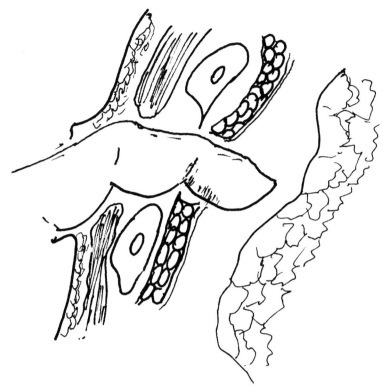

Fig. 2. Technique of chest drain insertion. Note a finger in the pleural space.

of anti-inflammatory drugs in patients undergoing pleurodesis is controversial since they block the very thing pleurodesis is attempting to achieve.

2.3. Removal of chest drains

"When should I remove a chest drain?" When it has completed its function. In the case of drains inserted to drain fluid, this should have reduced to less than 50 ml per day. In air leakage, they should be removed 24 hours after the last bubble has passed. Chest drain removal is painful for the patient. Adequate loading with systemic analgesia or the application of short-acting agents such as Entenox is obligatory. The technique used is to ask the patient to take a deep breath in and hold while the chest drain is rapidly removed from the chest. The previously inserted purse string is then used to close the defect in the chest wall. The site is checked by asking the patient to cough; any air leakage will be heard as a whistling sound. If this is identified, the wound should be sealed initially with an occlusive dressing and then secured with further sutures.

3. Common problems

3.1. The lung fails to expand

- Check that the drain is in the chest past the break in the radio-opaque line that marks the last drainage hole.
- Check that the drainage equipment is correctly connected and is not kinked. Suction equipment, if attached, must be checked to be working (if connected and switched off, it will block the exit of air from the system effectively clamping the drain, blocking off any possible exit of accumulated air from the system).
- Can the lung expand? Is it bound down by a pathological process i.e. empyema or malignancy?
- Is the airway to the lung blocked, i.e. by malignancy or foreign body?
- Is the air leakage so massive that routine suction cannot keep pace? If this is the case, consider the use of a high volume suction device such as a Thompson pump.

3.2. Persistent air leakage

- Is there a drainage hole outside the chest cavity and in the subcutaneous tissues?
- Is air leaking in around the chest drain?
- Are all of the connections to the underwater seal tight?
- Is there a defect in a structure which is unlikely to heal spontaneously, i.e. bronchus, oesophagus?
- Was the initial diagnosis correct? Has the drain been inserted into a giant bulla?

3.3. Massive (apparent) haemorrhage

Hopefully, not a frequently encountered problem but one witnessed by all thoracic surgeons.
- The commonest cause is the drainage of a large bloody effusion. In these cases, despite the loss of what appears to be litres of blood, the patient appears to be well. Classically, such an effusion will not clot and simple observation is usually all that is required.
- The second commonest cause is a transected intercostal vessel. These will tend to stop spontaneously with conservative management. Occasionally an exploratory thoracotomy and a simple oversew is required.

- Penetration of the heart is much rarer, although one should bear in mind that intrathoracic disease processes causing pulmonary collapse can markedly alter the geometry of the intrathoracic anatomy. Ventricular fibrillation rapidly follows insertion of a drain. Clamp the drain and resuscitate the patient. Penetration of a great vein or artery should be similarly treated. In all cases it is advisable to seek the urgent help of the cardiothoracic surgical team who may need to perform an emergency thoracotomy.

3.4. When should I clamp a drain?

Only when catastrophic amounts of blood are pouring down it from penetration of a major vascular structure, There are no other indications to undertake this dangerous practice outside a regional cardiothoracic surgical unit.

4. Drains in special circumstances

4.1. Pulmonary resection (i.e. lobectomy)

Usually two drains are placed within the cavity following lung resection (Fig. 3). These are anterior, which passes to the apex of the chest and drains air,

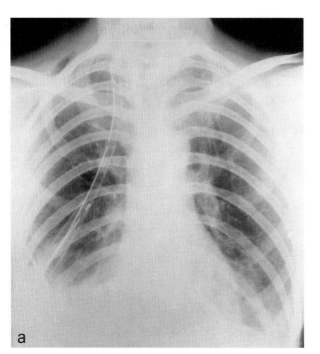 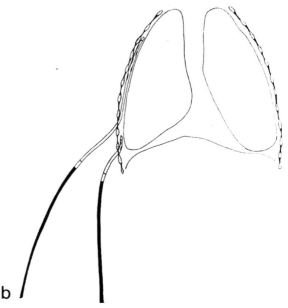

Fig. 3. Pleural drains in situ after lobectomy, (a) chest X-ray, (b) diagram. Notice the position of the drainage tube and in (a) the expansion of the residual lung.

and posterior, at the base of the lung to drain blood. They are usually placed on low-pressure suction following extubation of the patient on the operating table. They are removed when they have completed their function. Usually the basal drain is removed on the first post-operative day and the apical drain taken off suction. The apical drain is removed 24 hours after the last air bubble is passed.

4.2. Pneumonectomy

Drainage of the pleural space following pneumonectomy is radically different from all other circumstances. The aim is to maintain the mediastinum in the central position to prevent torsion of the heart about the great vessels. In some instances, the cavity is not drained at all; more usually a single drain is passed and clamped. Unclamping of this drain allows equalisation of pressures within the chest. Numerous

regimes have been described; the most common is to unclamp the drain for one minute each hour. The drain is usually removed 24 hours after completion of surgery.

4.3. Pleuropulmonary sepsis

There is no 'policeman' within the chest to fulfil the role of the omentum. Within the thoracic cavity the body deals with sepsis and inflammation by walling off the cavity with fibrous tissue. The resulting stiff walled structures are difficult to treat, requiring either total excision with operations such as decortication of the lung or prolonged drainage. In these circumstances the drain, which should reach the apex of the cavity, is removed in a staged process over a number of weeks a few centimetres at a time. Sinograms are often used to track the size of the cavity.

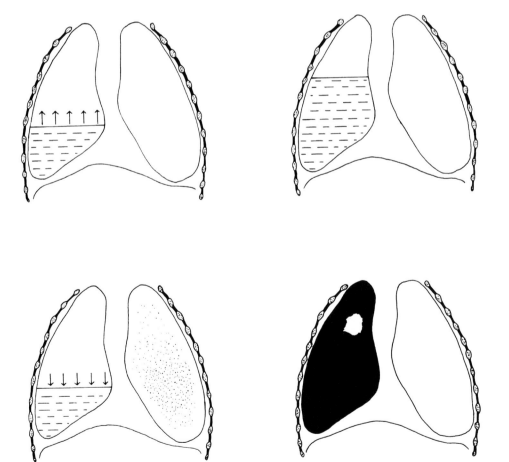

Fig. 4. Schematic of the pleural space after pneumonectomy, (a) the fluid in the pneumonectomy gradually ascends, (b) after a month or so the fluid has risen to a higher level, (c) in cases of broncho-pleural fistula, the level of fluid descends once again, (d) normally after many years the pleural space is practically obliterated.

4.3.1. Ultrasound guidance

Fluid collections within the chest can be identified through the chest wall by ultrasound or by the use of computerised axial tomography. This enables the radiologist to mark optimal sites for drain insertion. The radiologist will often use a pigtail catheter for drainage of the pleural cavity. These should be managed as any other drain and removed when they have completed their task.

Editor's Note:

- Post-pneumonectomy space (Fig. 4).
  Soon after operation (48 hours after drainage tube removal) the space contains a small amount of fluid but mostly air. During the next few days and weeks, the air is absorbed and fluid increases. The pneumonectomy space then shrinks in all its diameters by flattening of the chest wall, ascending of the diaphragm and mediastinal shift towards the operation side. There also follows hyperexpansion of the residual lung.
  After many years the space is no larger than the size of a closed fist. This reduction in volume is achieved by:
  – Elevation of the diaphragm
  – Atrophy of the intercostal muscle and approximation of the ribs
  – Movement of the mediastinum towards the pneumonectomy space
  – Descent of the apex of the thorax.

In addition, deposition of fibrin and fibrous tissue formation forms a thick layer inside the bony chest. Increase in the size of the space on chest X-ray after the initial reduction must be taken as a sign of bronchopleural fistula.

- Post-pneumonectomy syndrome
  In some post-pneumonectomy cases displacement of the mediastinum is accompanied by symptoms of airway obstruction. The term 'post-pneumonectomy syndrome' refers to the condition in which patients present with dyspnoea, cough and stridor and radiological evidence of displacement of the mediastinum with tracheo-bronchial distortion and partial lung herniation. Bronchoscopic examination is important to show the distortion and the possible extrinsic obstructive aetiology (or tracheo-bronchial malacia).
  The condition predominantly develops after right pneumonectomy with a variable interval. It is important to note that the radiological appearance of severe mediastino-tracheal deviation can exist in asymptomatic patients, particularly those who undergo operations for non-malignant conditions who have a long survival.
  Repositioning of the mediastinum using tissue expanders in the pleural space appears to offer good results in some cases. A tracheo-bronchial stent may have to be used, particularly in the presence of malacia, to ensure patency of the airway lumen and firmness.

KM

CHAPTER I.22

Pneumothorax

K. Moghissi

1. Introduction

Pneumothorax is the collection of air in the pleural space with resulting collapse of the lung.

2. Classifications

Pneumothoraces can be classified in a number of ways:

2.1. According to mechanism of their occurrence

- Spontaneous
- Traumatic
- Accidental/iatrogenic
- Induced/therapeutic

2.2. Depending on free movement of air into and from the pleura

- Closed pneumothorax: air enters the space but has no possibility of exit.
- Open pneumothorax: air can get into and out of the pleura. Entry and exit of air may be through the tracheo-bronchial tree or via an opening in the chest wall (e.g. penetrating wound).
- Valvular pneumothorax: air can enter the pleura during inspiration but cannot escape through the same opening during expiration.
- Tension pneumothorax: in a valvular pneumothorax a great volume of air can enter the pleural space and will create a considerably high pressure in the space, which displaces the mediastinum and will interfere with cardiovascular functions, particularly the venous return.

In effect, tension pneumothorax creates an emergency situation which is particularly dangerous in infants and children causing hypoxia and low car-diac output which culminates in cardiorespiratory arrest.

3. Terminology

A number of lesions are commonly associated with or play a role in the aetiology of pneumothoraces.
- Blebs are a small, 2 to 2.5 cm, collection of air under the visceral pleura, macroscopically looking like a soap bubble. They are due to rupture of subpleural alveoli, mostly at the apex of the lung and are often surrounded by adhesions attaching the lung to the parietal pleura. The parenchyma away from the bleb may be totally normal.
- Bullae are larger collections of air which are usually associated with emphysema although they may be found in the otherwise normal lung. Bullae result from rupture of the alveoli, some of which become large and space occupying.

Rupture of blebs and bullae are important causes of pneumothorax.

4. Spontaneous pneumothorax

4.1. Aetiology

A sudden and unexpected escape of air from the lung into the pleural space may have the following underlying causes:

4.1.1. Congenital abnormality
This occurs in children and young adults. Rupture of sub-pleural blebs, congenital air cyst or distended alveoli are the usual causes.

4.1.2. Acquired lung diseases
- Emphysematous bullae: The commonest cause of pneumothorax in adults is rupture of emphyse-

matous bullae. Bullae vary in size from small to large. In the latter case, there may be gradual increase in volume to form a large air cyst occupying over 50 to 60% of the entire hemithorax and compressing underlying lung tissues. Whereas the rupture of blebs cause pneumothorax with minor/moderate escape of air, rupture of a large air cyst may cause a continuous air leak amounting to a broncho-pleural fistula.

• Other air cysts and cavities
  Apart from emphysematous bullae leakage of air from a variety of other air cysts can be the cause of spontaneous pneumothorax. These include:
  – Air cyst which follows staphylococcal abscess
  – Air cysts formed as a consequence of tuberculous cavity
  – Neoplastic cystic lesions/air cysts associated with neoplasms
  – Pneumothorax associated with acquired immune deficiency syndrome (AIDS) secondary to pneumocystis carini pneumonia.

In some conditions such as bronchial asthma, pneumothorax can occur because of high pressure in terminal bronchi and alveoli, particularly when there is a bronchiolar obstruction due to thick mucous plugs.

4.2. Clinical features

Spontaneous pneumothorax is usually an acute event and presents with:
• Pleuritic pain.
• Dyspnoea.
• Cough which is usually unproductive.
• Raised venous pressure when a right-sided pneumothorax is under tension.

In small pneumothoraces, symptoms gradually disappear within two to three hours; in larger ones the symptoms remain. When there is a tension pneumothorax, cyanosis appears and the neck veins become distended. This situation is a prelude to fall in cardiac output and imminent cardiorespiratory failure. Mediastinal shift is evident by the displacement of the trachea from its midline position towards the healthy side (Fig. 1).

On examination of the chest, physical signs are related to the magnitude of the pneumothorax. Breath sounds are reduced or absent and there is a varying degree of hyper-resonance on percussion. A chest radiograph confirms the diagnosis of pneumothorax by the presence of air in the pleural space with absence of lung markings and collapse of the lung. At times there is an associated pleural effusion. Mediastinal

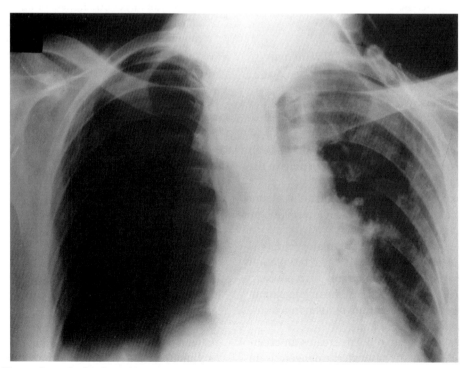

Fig. 1. Chest radiograph of patient with complete pneumothorax of the right side with shift of the mediastinum to the left.

shift is usually present in large pneumothoraces. CT scan demonstrates pneumothorax and it also shows the texture of pulmonary parenchyma away from pneumothorax.

The progress of the patient after spontaneous pneumothorax depends on several factors:
- Size of the pneumothorax and the degree of lung collapse.
- Pre-existing pathology in the lung.
- Age of the patient and respiratory function.
- Duration of the pneumothorax.
- Infective complication in the pleural space.

The following points should be borne in mind:
- A lung which has been greatly collapsed for a number of days or weeks may be difficult to expand and could well require decortication (see section 5.5 in chapter I.25).
- A collapsed lung is prone to infection.
- An empty pleural space (with collapsed lung) to which air has access is like a pool of stagnant water which is already contaminated and therefore ready to become infected.

4.3. Complications of pneumothorax

Spontaneous pneumothorax may be complicated by the following:
- Tension pneumothorax.
- Haemothorax (spontaneous haemo-pneumothorax).
- Infection, resulting in pyopneumothorax.
- Pneumo-mediastinum and surgical subcutaneous emphysema.
- Persistent air leak and bronchopleural fistula.

4.4. Treatment of spontaneous pneumothorax

The principal aims of the treatment of pneumothorax are as follows:
4.4.1 Evacuation of air from the pleural space and re-expansion of the lung
4.4.2 Maintenance of re-expansion and prevention of recurrence

4.4.1. Evacuation of air from the pleural space can be achieved by

(a) Chest aspiration (thoracentesis).
(b) Intercostal tube drainage (tube thoracostomy).
(c) Thoracoscopic treatment.
(d) Thoracotomy.

Thoracoscopic and thoracotomy methods are applicable when, in addition to evacuation of air, exploration of space and additional diagnostic and/or therapeutic measures are intended.

(a) Thoracocentesis. Needle aspiration to evacuate air form the pleural space is not a satisfactory method and, at most, can be applied to a small percentage of shallow pneumothoraces. It has to be repeated frequently and is labour intensive for medical and nursing staff. It may be argued that if the pneumothorax is so small as to require a single aspiration, it does not require any intervention at all.

(b) Intercostal tube drainage. This method is satisfactory for the great majority of spontaneous pneumothoraces. When properly applied, an intercostal drain allows evacuation of air at the desired rate. This is the method of choice in the majority of first time pneumothoraces. Compared with chest aspiration, tube drainage is not only a more satisfactory method of evacuating air but is also a more certain way of ensuring the expansion of the lung and monitoring the progress.

To be successful it is necessary to take account of the following:

The intercostal tube should be placed in the most appropriate place. This is usually in the apex of the chest where air rises to collect (unless it is loculated and walled off by adhesions). Although insertion of an intercostal tube through the 2nd intercostal space anteriorly and directed to the apex will assure satisfactory drainage, experience shows that tube thoracostomy is managed more easily when it is placed through the axillary line which also avoids the breast and subsequent scarring which is particularly important in the female patient.

When the tube is in place and is connected to the underwater drainage system the patient is asked to cough. Evacuation of air as a bubble indicates satisfactory drainage. As the air exits and the lung expands, patients often experience sharp chest pain requiring analgesics. The pleural drain system is left without suction for a few minutes and evacuation of air occurs when the patient coughs. After a short period the pleural drain is connected to low grade suction. The patient's chest is X-rayed to check the position of the drain and the state of the lung expansion. It is important that the drainage system is managed correctly and efficiently, as success of the treatment depends on this.

The use of drains fitted with a flutter valve such as the Heimlich device (1968) is a convenient way to provide mobility to patients. This, however, has many disadvantages particularly when patient progress is not monitored appropriately. One problem associated with the use of the valve is that the rate of air leak cannot be assessed. Also, this type of thoracostomy tube drainage cannot be left unsupervised. This fact may not be generally appreciated. Additionally, flutter valves are also subject to blockage or malfunction in the presence of pleural fluid or blood. The author believes that all thoracostomy tube drainage should at first be connected to a standard underwater sealed system. After a day or two, if the lung is expanded and air leak minimal (i.e. present only on suction or coughing), the drain may be connected to a flutter valve. If it is planned for patients to be discharged from hospital, arrangement should be made for supervision at home with visits to the surgical/medical centre for X-ray and re-evaluation every two or three days with the provision of an open access service. It should be noted that a patient with a standard sealed drainage system can also be mobile by simply carrying the under water sealed (UWS) drainage system.

Further management of the patient with an intercostal drain is as follows.

If the lung expands and there is no air leak on suction, then the tube is left *in situ* but the drainage container is detached from the suction apparatus. The patient is allowed to carry his underwater sealed system or the tube may be connected to a flutter valve system. When there is no air leak or swing in the underwater rod of the drainage system the drain is withdrawn. A chest radiograph should be taken after a few hours and the maintenance of the expansion assured. The patient is examined again clinically and radiologically the following day and, providing the lung has remained expanded, the treatment of the pneumothorax is concluded.

If the lung does not expand following the intercostal tube drainage one or all of the following may be the cause:

- There may be bronchial secretions or a mucous plug that obstructs the airways and prevents inflation of the lung. Active physiotherapy and/or bronchoscopic aspiration will usually succeed in expanding the lung.
- Sometimes there is fibrinous (or fibrous) deposition over the surface of the lung (visceral pleura). This is like a crust preventing expansion of the underlying lung. This complication usually occurs in a longstanding pneumothorax which is either not diagnosed early or not properly managed. In some of these cases the lung may be covered by a thick fibrous skin

and can only expand after it is decorticated (see decortication, section 5.5 in chapter I.25).

- In some pneumothoraces the air leak may be so extensive that residual air remains in the pleura in spite of extraction via the pleural drain, i.e. the rate of air leak is in excess of the rate of evacuation of air. This indicates that the intercostal tube drainage method is not a suitable method of treatment for the case and thoracoscopy and/or standard thoracotomy is required to explore the chest and deal with the air leak.

(c) Thoracoscopic treatment. In a case of pneumothorax, thoracoscopy may be employed to:

- identify the cause of pneumothorax/explore pleural space.
- divide adhesions which prevent lung expansion and to seal leaks from the lung.
- excise bullae
- carry out pleurodesis.

Indications for thoracoscopic treatment include:

- Recurrent pneumothoraces.
- Patients requiring pleurodesis or other intervention, in addition to chest drainage, such as excision of bullae or control of air leak.
- When tube thoracostomy is judged unsuitable or has failed to expand the lung.
- Persistent air leak.

The major contra-indications of thoracoscopic treatment are:

- Dense and widespread adhesions making thoracoscopic procedure technically difficult or not possible
- Multiple bullous disease with considerable air leak (broncho pleural fistula).
- Chronic infected pneumothorax

(d) Thoracotomy. This is generally used when, in addition to drainage, there is a need for assuring the maintenance of expansion of the lung which cannot be achieved by pleural drainage alone.

The indications for thoracotomy and drainage in spontaneous pneumothorax are similar to thoracoscopy and video-assisted thoracoscopic operation. However, there are contra-indications to thoracoscopic treatment (see above) and many experienced surgeons feel more comfortable carrying out minithoracotomy using a minimal access, muscle-sparing method.

In practice, for a simple first time pneumothorax, tube thoracostomy should be used. A complicated pneumothorax should be treated using thoracoscopic or thoracotomy method.

4.4.2. Maintenance of lung re-expansion and prevention of recurrence: Pleurodesis

Pleurodesis is a procedure whereby the two layers of the pleural membrane are made to adhere to one another with resultant obliteration of the pleural space (pleural symphysis), The basic principle of pleurodesis is to create an inflammatory reaction followed by adhesions which in turn bring about pleural symphysis. Various methods may be used to achieve pleurodesis. These are:

- Introduction by injection of an irritant substance into the pleural space. A number of chemicals such as camphor oil and silver nitrate were originally advocated. Presently tetracycline is commonly used.
- Thoracoscopic methods.
  Thoracoscopy and poudrage to treat pneumothorax has been in use for over 40 years. The procedure consists of exploratory thoracoscopy as a first step, followed by thoracoscopic division of adhesions and excision of bullae. Insufflation of talcum power/or iodised talcum power over the surface of the visceral pleura is carried out using an insufflator or similar device. Talcum powder alone or in association with iodine will achieve pleurodesis by initiating an inflammatory reaction.
- Other thoracoscopic methods.
  Thoracoscopy may be employed to carry out partial parietal pleurectomy using standard endoscopic instrumentation or laser photoradiation to carry out partial pleurectomy (see section 6 in chapter IV.5, laser in cardiothoracic surgery and video assisted thoracoscopic surgery).
  Alternatively, abrasion of parietal pleura may suffice to achieve partial pleurodesis.
- Thoracotomy pleurodesis. With the development of thoracoscopic surgery the indications for thoracotomy in spontaneous pneumothorax are becoming restricted to:
  - Cases in which the hemi-thorax needs to be explored prior, and in addition, to pleurodesis, and there are compelling reasons for this not to be done by thoracoscopic methods.
  - Cases requiring intervention other than pleurodesis. Such procedures may not always be easily carried out by thoracoscopic operations. Amongst these are large air leak and bronchopleural fistula.

- When thoracoscopy is technically not feasible.
  The thoracotomy approach and the choice of access are determined by the type of procedure which is envisaged to be undertaken in the chest. In practice, it is prudent to use thoracotomy in bullous disease complicated by broncho-pleural fistula.

Such thoracotomies will be limited access and use muscle-sparing techniques. At thoracotomy, adhesions which create loculation are divided. The required procedure is then carried out with partial pleurectomy or pleural abrasion to achieve pleurodesis. Pleural drains are suitably placed prior to closure. Pleurectomy consists of peeling off the parietal pleura from the inner chest. It is easier to carry out pleurectomy at the apex and lateral aspect of the chest wall. Pleurectomy of the mediastinal pleura is more difficult to perform.

Note on pleurodesis:

Historical note:
In the book Chest Diseases by Perry and Holmes–Sellors (1963) the principle and method of pleurodesis are described as follows:
"Simple closed pleurodesis — The principle of closed pleurodesis is to set up an artificial pleurisy by means of irritants introduced through the thoracoscopy cannula. A variety of irritants has been used including 0–5% camphor in arachis oil, iodized talc, blood, hypertonic glucose and silver nitrate."

- Chemical pleurodesis is a painful procedure and the patient can continue to have pain for several days requiring strong analgesics in the first two to three days. There is often a low-grade fever 24 to 48 hours after chemical pleurodesis. This is not usually an infective fever. However, it is a wise precaution to administer a single bolus of intravenous antibiotic at the time of operation (e.g. Cefuroxime 1.5 g). It is important to emphasize that after pleurodesis there often develops a small amount of pleural effusion. This will not usually require aspiration or drainage. Following pleurodesis, the drainage tube is removed when the air leak has ceased, the lung is expanded and there is no evidence of air space which indicates residual pneumothorax.

4.4.3. Summary of treatment of spontaneous pneumothorax

- In acute and for a first time pneumothorax, intercostal tube drainage will usually suffice.
- Thoracoscopy or video-assisted thoracoscopic surgery (VATS) is used:

- When exploration of the pleural space is required.
- In patients requiring bullectomy or other intervention.
- In those requiring pleurodesis.
- In chronic and repeated recurrent pneumothoraces.

Thoracotomy is considered:

- When the lung fails to expand despite proper and adequate drainage.
- In patients with persistent air leak.
- When it is considered that VATS is unsuitable for the case.

The choice between thoracoscopy and thoracotomy depends on the circumstances of the case and the experience of the surgeon as well as the general condition of the patient. A simple thoracoscopic exploration and poudrage can be carried out under sedation and local anaesthesia. To achieve pleurodesis it is neither desirable nor necessary to carry out total parietal pleurectomy. Partial pleurectomy or pleural abrasion/scarification suffices in the majority of cases.

References and further reading

Cardillo G, Facciolo F, Corzani F, et al. Recurrences following treatment of primary spontaneous pneumothorax: the role of redo-video thoracoscopy. Eur J Cardiothorac Surg 2001; 19: 396–399.

Feito BA, Rath AM, Longchampt E, Azorin J. Experimental study on the in vivo behaviour of a new collagen glue in lung surgery. Eur J Cardiothorac Surg 2000; 17: 8–13.

Macchiarini P, Wain J, Almy S, Dartvelle P. Experimental and clinical evaluation of a new synthetic, absorbable sealant to reduce alveolar air leaks in thoracic operations. J Thorac Cardiovasc Surg 1999; 117: 751–758.

Massard G, Thomas P, Wihlm OM. Minimally invasive management for the first and recurrent pneumothorax. Ann Thorac Surg 1998; 66: 592–599.

Matthew T, Spotnitz W, Kron IL, Tribble CG, Nolan SP. Four year experience with fibrin sealant in thoracic and cardiovascular surgery. Ann Thorac Surg 1990; 50: 40–44.

Perry KMA, Holmes–Sellors T. Chest Disease. London: Butterworth, 1963.

Robson K, Emmerson PA. Pneumothorax. In: Perry KMA and Sellors TH (eds.), Chest Disease (Vol. 1). London: Butterworth, 1963; p. 318.

Shackcloth M, Poullis M, Page R. Autologous blood pleurodesis for treating persistent air leak after lung resection. Ann Thorac Surg 2001; 71: 1402–1403.

Sharpe DAC, Dixon K, Moghissi K. Spontaneous haemopneumothorax: a surgical emergency. Eur Resp J 1995; 8: 1611–1612.

Sharpe DAC, Dixon K, Moghissi K. Thoracoscopic use of laser in intractable pneumothorax. Eur J Cardiothorac Sug 1994; 8: 34–36.

Vanderschueren RGJRA. Le talcage pleural dans le pneumothorax spontané. Poumon Coeur 1981; 37: 273–276.

Viallat JR, Rey F, Astoul P, Boutin C. Thoracoscopic talc poudrage pleurodesis for malignant effusion: a review of 360 cases. Chest 1996; 110: 1387–1393.

Wain JC, Kaiser LR, Johnstone DW, Yang SC, Wright CD, Friedberg, Feins RH, Heitmiller RF, Mathisen DJ, Selwyn MR. Trial of a novel synthetic sealant in preventing air leaks after resection. Ann Thorac Surg 2001; 71: 1623-1628; discussion 1628–1629.

K. Moghissi, J.A.C. Thorpe and F. Ciulli (Eds.)
Moghissi's Essentials of Thoracic and Cardiac Surgery
© 2003 Elsevier Science B.V. All rights reserved

CHAPTER I.23

Pleural effusion

K. Moghissi

1. Introduction

The pleural space contains a small volume of serous fluid. Normally this amounts to about 20 ml and acts as a lubricant between the visceral and parietal pleura. In a healthy person there is a constant flow of fluid into the pleural space followed by its reabsorption; this is in the order of 5 to 10 litres/day and there is usually a balance between the entry of fluid into the space and absorption from it. Much of the absorbed fluid enters the lymphatic channels. Any imbalance in the movement of fluid, resulting from deficiency of absorption and/or excess fluid production, will create an accumulation of fluid and the development of pleural effusion.

It is traditional to differentiate between transudate and exudate. The transudate is supposed to be protein free or, at most, to contain small amounts of protein compared with exudate. However, transudate does in fact contain some proteins of smaller molecules, namely albumin and some of the globulins. Exudate contains larger protein molecules and fibrinogen but since fibrinogen deposits as fibrin, the aspirated fluid many not necessarily contain high fibrinogen levels. An effusion is considered an exudate if the fluid to serum ratio of protein is greater than 0.5 and the lactic acid dehydrogenase ratio is greater than 0.6.

2. Clinical manifestation

Whether the pleural effusion is due to primary pleural disease or secondary to another condition, it is the volume of the effusion which determines the existence and/or severity of the symptom. However, clinical manifestations of primary pleural effusion are related to the fluid itself and its volume, whereas in secondary effusion, the manifestations of the primary condition may predominate.

- Of the symptoms, dyspnoea is present in nearly all cases and its severity is proportionate to the volume of fluid. Other symptoms, such as pain and cough, often accompany dyspnoea, the former particularly in rapidly developing effusion and in diseases affecting the parietal pleura.
- Physical signs of fluid are dullness on percussion and absent or reduced breath sounds. (The percussion is so distinct that the adjective 'stony' dullness on percussion has become synonymous with a great collection of fluid in the chest). When the mediastinum is displaced the trachea moves with it and its displacement can be gauged above the suprasternal notch on palpation. Occasionally, an effusion in the right chest may produce raised jugular venous pressure without evidence of heart failure.

Less than 200 to 300 ml of fluid in the interlobar area or anteriorly may not be clinically manifest.

3. Investigation

3.1. Clinical examination

General clinical examination, including present and past medical history, is particularly important in elucidating the cause of pleural effusion. It is not unusual for a patient with a carcinoma of the breast treated several years previously to develop malignant pleural effusion and it is also commonly acknowledged that pleural effusion can be a manifestation of many non-neoplastic systemic diseases and in cases of heart failure.

3.2. Laboratory tests

General laboratory tests, such as blood count and biochemical profile, are not specific to elucidate the aetiology but are helpful in diagnosis and management of patients with pleural effusion.

3.3. Specific investigations

3.3.1. Imaging

- Plain chest radiograph: Postero-anterior and lateral view chest X-ray gives an indication of the volume and location of the fluid within the chest.
- Computerised tomography: This helps to eliminate super-imposition of structures and can more precisely show the image of the underlying lung.
- Ultrasonography: Differentiates between pulmonary consolidation and pleural effusion, demonstrates septa and loculation and therefore provides guidance to the best drainage point.
- Nuclear medicine: ventilation scanning may be helpful in some cases such as broncho-pleural fistula following pneumonectomy
- Magnetic resonance imaging: has limited application in pleural effusion. It is however helpful to demonstrate associated mediastinal disease.

3.3.2. Examination of the fluid

Thoracocentesis allows recovery and examination of the effusion. Most neoplastic fluids are in excess of 1 litre. In benign cases the volume rarely reaches this amount. The fluid may be straw coloured, blood-stained, haemorrhagic and purulent. Besides traumatic injury and some rare cases of spontaneous haemothorax, blood stained effusion is usually associated with malignancy but this is by no means the rule. Straw coloured, odourless fluid is a characteristic of a transudate, whereas exudates are generally cloudy because of the presence of cells and high protein concentrations. A chronic empyema is thick and creamy in consistency and has a variably offensive odour depending on the type of organism.

- Biochemical analysis of fluid provides some guidance to its aetiology.
  The concentration of glucose in the fluid can be of particular diagnostic significance. Glucose <60 mg/l is found in tuberculous pleuritis, neoplasia, rheumatoid disease and pneumonic effusion. Amylase level is elevated in pancreatitis and in malignant effusion. A rise in triglyceride level is characteristically found in chylous effusion (level >110 mg/dl).
- Cytology of the fluid: Most transudates contain a few white cells; all exudates have above 1000 white cells/ml. The type of cells found in the effusion has some relevance to its aetiology. Neutrophils are the predominant cells in pleurisy associated with pneumonia and in pulmonary infarction. Lymphocytes predominate in tuberculosis, lymphomas and some malignancies. Haemorrhagic effusions contain red cells. A count above 100,000/ml is caused by frank bleeding in the pleura, and is usually associated with traumatic injury. Malignant cells are often found in malignant effusion but their absence in aspirated fluid does not exclude malignancy.
- Microbiological study of the fluid is important for the diagnosis of empyema and infective pleural disease. It is relevant to note that it is difficult to recover tuberculosis bacilli (mycobacterium tuberculosis) in a fresh preparation of tuberculous effusion; bacilli can be cultured in only 30% of tuberculous pleural effusions.

3.3.3. Bronchoscopy

All cases of pleural effusion should have bronchoscopy to eliminate endobronchial lesions.

3.3.4. Pleural biopsy

Provision of pleural tissue sample is often necessary to establish the aetiology of the pleural effusion/pathology. This may be obtained by needle/punch biopsy instruments (Abrams, 1958; Moghissi, 1961) or using thoracoscopy technique.

- When the closed or blind method is used, a higher pleural yield is obtained with an instrument which provides a larger biopsy. A number of needle and punch biopsy instruments have been devised and used since 1950s. In thoracoscopic technique, the biopsy material is obtained under vision. Even before the re-emergence of thoracoscopy and the evolution of video-assisted thoracoscopic surgery (VATS), physicians and surgeons for many years employed thoracoscopy for exploration of the pleural cavity and tissue sampling.
- Thoracoscopic biopsy is reserved for those cases in which the pleural effusion remains undiagnosed after other diagnostic methods have been exhausted. It is relevant to emphasise that in some cases at least, thoracoscopy should be used sooner rather than later in order to resolve the diagnostic dilemma.
- Open pleural biopsy employs a mini-thoracotomy to obtain tissue samples. An incision is made over the area previously mapped out by appropriate imaging in order to achieve optimal results. However, indications for thoracotomy are restricted to

cases in which there are pleural adhesions (pleural symphysis) and in the absence of fluid.

Both thoracoscopy and mini-thoracotomy biopsies are best undertaken under general anaesthesia although they can be carried out under local anaesthetic and sedation.

It is important to emphasise that biopsy material should be examined both histologically and microbiologically (culture).

4. Management of pleural effusion

Every effort should be made to diagnose the aetiology and nature of the effusion in order to plan and undertake appropriate treatment. From the therapeutic viewpoint pleural effusion may be classified into two major categories: (1) benign and (2) malignant, each with subsets as follows.

4.1. Benign effusion

Management options in benign effusions are:
- Medical treatment with/without pleural aspiration.
- Pleural drainage.
- Exploration and evacuation of the pleural cavity of fluid and debris followed by pleurectomy and decortication.

A benign effusion may respond to medical therapy alone. This is particularly the case in those with transudate fluid. An exudative benign effusion, in which the pleura is involved in the disease process, may also respond to medical treatment, e.g. tuberculous pleural effusion, particularly when the lung itself is not grossly diseased. In some cases a large volume effusion will require pleural aspiration/drainage in addition to medication. Occasionally a benign pleural effusion will need surgical intervention using either VATS or standard thoracotomy. In these cases, the development of fibrinous and fibrous septa causes loculation of the fluid. There is also collapse of the lung and formation of a thick crust of fibrin and fibrous tissue over the visceral pleura. In such cases medication alone even with evacuation of the fluid will not achieve expansion of the lung. Therefore, surgical exploration and decortication becomes necessary.

It should be emphasized that when exploration is carried out, frozen section biopsies of the pleura and the underlying lung should be taken to exclude neoplasia.

4.2. Malignant effusion

Distinction should be made between:
4.2.1 Cases which can be surgically treated with curative intent.
4.2.2 Cases requiring palliation.

4.2.1. Treatment of malignant effusions with curative intent
The most common cause of malignant effusion in male patients is lung cancer. In female patients, lung cancer is also an important cause but breast tumour heads the list. In a small percentage of patients with lung cancer, the effusion is not caused by pleural involvement and pleuro-pulmonary resection can be attended by long survival. This also is the case in early stage pleural mesothelioma.

4.2.2. Palliative treatment of malignant effusion
From a practical point of view, the palliation of malignant pleural effusions should be considered under two headings:
(a) Those in which the lung is potentially expandable after drainage.
(b) Cases in which the underlying lung and visceral pleura is covered with thick layers of fibrin and fibrous crusts or tumour tissue which prevents lung expansion. These are referred to as trapped lung.

(a) Palliation for those with potentially expandable lung: The aims are:
– Expansion of the lung
– Prevention of recurrence of effusion.

These aims may be achieved by drainage of the fluid followed by pleurodesis either by surgery or medical method. In some cases, expansion of the lung can only be achieved by the additional procedure of decortication which needs surgical intervention.
- Surgical method: The re-emergence of thoracoscopy as video-assisted thoracoscopic surgery (VATS) has meant that many cases which, in the past, required standard or 'limited' thoracotomy may be able to undergo VATS exploration, aspiration of the fluid and pleurectomy to achieve pleurodesis. When the visceral pleura is covered by fribrin and fibrous tissue the imprisoned lung requires decortication which provides opportunity for full expansion.
The indications for surgical decortication/pleurectomy in malignant effusion are:

– Large volume effusion in which the aetiopathology is in doubt despite having employed all less invasive methods of investigation.
– Patients with loculated effusion.
– Patients whose visceral pleura is overlaid by thick fibrin/fibrous skin.

In practice, the protocol for surgical pleurectomy and decortication is as follows:

– The chest should be evacuated of effusion and debris and a frozen section histology sample despatched to the laboratory as appropriate and when required.
– Decortication is carried out, which may be difficult if the visceral pleura contains tumour involving the lung. Attention is paid to air leakage which can easily impede the successful result.
– Parietal pleurectomy is then carried out. This brings about pleural symphesis (pleurodesis).
– Chest is closed with one/two pleural drains in the chest

• Complications of surgical drainage and pleurodesis are:
  – Non-expansion of the lung due to inadequate decortication and/or trapped lung.
  – Continuous and prolonged (more than one week) air leak amounting to broncho-pleural fistula
  – Implantation of tumour to the chest wall tracking through drainage tubes/incision.

• Medical (non-surgical) method of drainage and pleurodesis

The rationale for pleurodesis rests on the principle of eliminating the pleural space by creating pleural symphysis; that is complete adherence of visceral to parietal pleura, ideally, after evacuation of fluid and when the lung is fully expanded or is potentially expandable. Such pleural symphysis (pleurodesis) may be achieved by instillation of a sclerosing agent which provokes an inflammatory reaction, adhesion and fibrosis between parietal and visceral pleura. Many chemicals, when instilled into the pleural cavity, will achieve pleurodesis with variable success rate. Every method of pleurodesis has a side effect. In most cases this consists of pain which requires alleviation by injectable analgesic for 1 to 2 days and fever which usually subsides after 3 or 4 days without antibiotics.

Many agents have been used to achieve pleurodesis in malignant effusions.

– Chemotherapeutic (anti-cancer) agents: Instillation of a variety of chemotherapeutic (cytotoxic) agents into the pleural space has been used since the mid 1950s to control effusion. The optimal regimen and dose of drugs seems to be subject to trial and error.

– Tetracycline: This method was first introduced by Rubinson and Bolooki in 1972. Success of tetracycline in achieving pleurodesis in malignant effusion is variably reported to be between 30% and 94% (mean 70%). Our technique is as follows:

Drain the effusion slowly over a period of 12 to 24 hours by tube thoracostomy and then remove the drain. Postero-anterior and a lateral view X-rays are taken to check lung expansion.

1 to 1.5 gram Tetracycline (15 to 20 mg/kg b/w) in 50 ml of water for injection is prepared, to which is added 20 ml of 1% lignocaine for injection.

The solution is injected into the pleural space towards the apex of the chest. Appropriate analgesic is administered by intramuscular injection for one or two days.

Patient is discharged after 3 to 4 days following chest radiograph demonstrating continuous expansion of lung.

Patient is followed up in the outpatient clinic 3 to 4 weeks later.

– Pleurodesis using corynebacterium parvum (CP): Malignant pleural effusions have been controlled by interpleural instillation of CP. The claim that such intrapleural injection will affect the malignant disease by the immunostimulation effect of CP is rather speculative. The success rate in controlling recurrent effusion is about 60 to 70%. A randomised trial of CP and tetracycline has shown no difference between the two in so far as control of effusion is concerned.

– Talcage Pleurodesis: This method uses talc alone or mixed with iodine to achieve pleural symphysis. The success rate is about 90% and more successful in comparison with tetracycline (Fentiman et al., 1986). Our personal preference for all types of malignant effusion, except in trapped lung, is to use talcage with iodine.

The preparation of iodized talc is made of 50 mg of iodine in 2.5 ml of ether solution mixed with 9.9 gram of sterile talc. The ether evaporates during mixing and the iodized talc remains in powder form. Our method of talcage is one of the following:

Method A: Thoracoscopic technique: with the patient under general anaesthetic and using double lumen tube ventilation. Thoracoscopy is performed and the fluid is aspirated from the pleura. Fibrous/fibrinous septa, if present, are divided. The surface of the lung is sprayed with talc using a powder blower (insufflator) or similar device to spray the powder over the lung. An intercostal tube is then placed into the pleural space to drain air after which the lung is expanded using positive pressure ventilation. Twenty-four hours later the tube is removed, if chest X-ray is satisfactory.

The development of VATS techniques means that many cases previously diagnosed and treated surgically using thoracotomy are explored and treated by the thoracoscopic method. The pleural space is explored and, if required, a biopsy is taken for frozen section and confirmation of the diagnosis. The fluid is then evacuated and pleurectomy or poudrage is carried out to achieve pleurodesis.

Method B: An intercostal tube is inserted into the chest to drain the fluid over a 24-hour period. This is followed by instillation of a suspension made of iodized talc (similar to method A) in 50 ml of water for injection. The suspension is injected into the intercostal tube followed by 50 ml of sterile water. The tube is then clamped for 24 hours. During this time the patient is placed in different positions to allow powder suspension to deposit over the pleural surface. The clamp is then removed and the intercostal tube retained for a further 24 hours before removal.

(b) Malignant effusion with trapped lung: One of the therapeutic problems of chronic malignant effusion is identification of the state of the collapsed lung under the effusion. For the purpose of treatment policy it is important to know firstly whether the lung has the potential of expansion with or without decortication once the fluid is evacuated. This evaluation is not easy with the use of imaging techniques alone. In our experience, in the majority of malignant effusions, decortication is possible if involvement of visceral pleura by the tumour is not widespread.

We advocate thoracoscopic (VATS) exploration in order to evacuate fluid and make a decision on therapeutic options which are:

(a) Thoracoscopic evacuation of fluid, decortication and pleurodesis. In some cases debulking of the tumour (e.g. in mesothelioma) may be performed.
(b) Conversion to thoracotomy and surgical pleurodesis or pleuro-pulmonary resection.
(c) Limited pleurectomy/poudrage.

In a case of trapped lung, the objectives of the treatment should be clearly identified. If no pul-

monary functional recovery can be expected, then the arguments in favour of therapeutic intervention need to be based on quality-of-life parameters. Therapeutic options are:

• Parietal pleurectomy with no active intervention on the lung (but short term 24 to 72 hours drainage). The rationale of this method is that many such patients have permanently lost the function of that lung and there will be no possibility of lung expansion under the "crust" of the tumour. It is surprising that, in some cases, the fluid collection remains stable and the patient continues with a reasonable quality of life.

• Establishment of pleuro-peritoneal shunt:
The apparatus comprises two silicone tubes interposed by a pump chamber. One of the tubes or catheters is inserted into the chest, the other into the abdomen. The whole equipment is placed subcutaneously with the pump lying on the costal margin near the sternum. The method is attended by a number of complications and its efficacy in true trapped lung cases is questionable. Some reports indicate the method to be useful with high success rates, however, neither theoretically nor from experience can I share the enthusiasm of some surgeons for this method. The reason being that when a lung is so trapped as to have no possibility of re-expansion, the evacuation of fluid and its delivery into the peritoneum will have no contribution to make to pulmonary function and has the disadvantage of introducing malignant cells into the peritoneal cavity.

References and further reading

Abrams LD. A pleural biopsy punch. Lancet 1958; 1: 30–31.

Adler RH, Sayek J. Treatment of malignant pleural effusion: A method using tube thoracostomy and talc. Ann Thorac Surg 1976; 22: 8–12.

Boutin C, Rey F, Gouvernet J. Malignant mesothelioma: Prognostic factors in a series of 125 patients studied from 1973–1987. Bulletin de l'Academie National de Medicine 1992; 176(1): 105–114 (Discussion 115–117).

Canto A, Ferrer G, Romagosa MD, et al. Lung cancer and pleural effusion: Clinical significance and study of pleural metastatic location. Chest 1985; 87: 649.

Cope C, Bernhardt H. Hook needle biopsy of pleural, pericardium, peritoneum and synovium. Am J Med 1963; 35: 189–195.

Decker DA, Payne WS, Bernatz PE, Pairolero P. Significance of a cytologically negative pleural effusion in bronchogenic carcinoma. Chest 1978; 74: 640.

De Francis N, Klosk E, Albano E. Needle biopsy of the parietal pleura: A preliminary report. N Engl J Med 1955; 252: 948–949.

Fentiman IS, Rubens RD, Hayward JL. A comparison of intracavitary talc and tetracyclin for the control of pleural effusion secondary to breast cancer. Aur J Cancer Clinic Oncol 1986; 22: 1079–1081.

Garcia JP, Richard WG, Sugarbaker DJ. Surgical treatment of malignant mesothelioma. In: Kaiser A, Kron B, Spray C (Eds.), Mastery of cardiothoracic surgery. Philadelphia: Lippincot Raven, 1998.

Genc O, Petrou M, Ladas G, Goldstraw P. The long term morbidity of pleuroperitonal shunts in the management of recurrent malignant effusions. Eur J Cardiothorac Surg 2000; 18: 143–146.

Grossebones MW, Arif AA, Goddard M, Ritchie AJ. Mesothelioma — VATS biopsy and lung mobilization improves diagnosis and palliation. Eur J Cardiothorac Surg 1999; 16: 619–623.

Hussain SA. Pleuroperitoneal shunt in recurrent pleural effusions. Ann Thorac Surg 1986; 41(6): 309–311.

Little AG, Kadowki MH, Ferguson MK, Staszek VM, Skinner DB. Pleuroperitoneal shunting alternative therapy for pleural effusions. Ann Surg 1988; 208: 443–450.

Little AG, Ferguson MK, Harvey M, et al. Pleuroperitoneal shunting for malignant pleural effusion. Cancer 1986; 58: 2740–2743.

McLeod DT, Claverley PMA, Millar JW, Horne NW. Further experience of coryne bacterium pavum in malignant pleural effusion. Thorax 1985; 40: 515–518.

Mestitz P, Purves MJ, Pollard AC. Pleural biopsy in the diagnosis of pleural effusion: A report of 200 cases. Lancet 1958; 2: 1349.

Moghissi K. A new type of pleural biopsy instrument. Br Med J 1961; 1: 1534.

Moghissi K. The malignant pleural effusion: tissue diagnosis and treatment in International Trends. In: J Deslauriers, LK Lacquet (Eds.), General Thoracic Surgery (Vol. 6), Management of Pleural Diseases J. St. Louis: The CV Mosby Company, 1990; pp. 397–408.

Ostrowski MJ. An assessment of the long-term results of controlling the reaccumulation of malignant effusion using intracavitary bleomycin. Cancer 1986; 57: 721–727.

Rubinson RM, Bolooki H. Intrapleural teracycline for malignant pleural effusion: A preliminary report. South Med J 1972; 65: 647–649.

K. Moghissi, J.A.C. Thorpe and F. Ciulli (Eds.)
Moghissi's Essentials of Thoracic and Cardiac Surgery
© 2003 Elsevier Science B.V. All rights reserved

CHAPTER I.24

Chylothorax

K. Moghissi

1. Introduction

Chylothorax is the accumulation of an excess of lymphatic fluid and/or the presence of chyle in the pleural space. It is commonly the result of a leak from the thoracic duct or one of its major tributaries and branches. Chyle is a mixture of intestinal lymph with chylomicron (true chyle) and lymph originating from the lymphatics of the lungs, abdominal wall and viscera and the lower limbs. It is an odourless alkaline, milky white liquid with the following composition:

- Water
- Electrolytes similar in concentration to plasma
- Lipids as much as 210 mmol/l
- Protein: 50% of that of plasma concentration
- Lymphocytes (mostly T-cell) numbering 4000–6000/ml

Normally some 100 to 150 ml/h of chyle passes through the thoracic duct which is the principal channel for its transport (Fig. 1). This can increase 4- to 5-fold after meals.

2. Anatomy

The thoracic duct originates from the cisterna chyli. It passes through the posterior mediastinum and ends at the left jugular-subclavian vein junction. Cisterna chyli is 5 to 7 cm long and 2 to 3 cm wide. It is situated adjacent to the 1st and second lumber and 12th thoracic vertebrae just to the left of the right crus of the diaphragm and behind and right of the aorta. The thoracic duct is usually a single channel which ascends into the chest through the aortic hiatus of the diaphragm between the 12th and 10th thoracic vertebrae and to the right of the aorta. In the thorax, the duct remains adjacent to the vertebral column on the right anterior aspect of vertebral bodies behind the oesophagus between the aorta and the azygos vein. At the level of the 5th thoracic vertebra the duct passes to the left behind the aortic arch and ascends to the neck behind the left carotid sheath and the jugular vein. In the upper chest and neck the duct lies to the left of the oesophagus. It is important to note that:

- There are a number of variations to the above anatomical arrangement.
- There are communicating channels between the thoracic duct and intercostal and azygos system of veins.
- There can be 2 or 3 lymphatic ducts instead of a single one (in 40–50% of individuals).
- The thoracic duct is an extra-pleural structure.

3. Aetiology of Chylothorax

The common causes of chylothorax are:

3.1. Neoplastic infiltration

Neoplastic infiltration of the duct causing obstruction or its compression, usually by malignant and occasionally by benign tumours. Lymphomas, lympho-sarcomas and lung cancer are the usual culprits.

3.2. Laceration of the duct

Laceration of the duct by blunt and penetrating injuries of the neck and chest. The mechanism in blunt trauma is through hyperextension of the vertebral column causing rupture of the duct.

3.3. Accidental surgical injuries

The anatomy and relationship of the duct to other structures in its passage from the abdomen to its air leak, otherwise the patient will certainly develop surgical emphysema and/or pneumothorax.

5.5.1. Post-operative management

Decortication, especially if done in chronic empyema, may cause considerable intra- and perioperative blood loss from the pleural surfaces. Care has to be taken to prevent bloody pleural secretions from coagulating in the drainages.

Provided their general situation permits it, patients must have active physiotherapy and early mobilisation. Young children particularly must be watched for a chest deformity which can follow a chronic empyema with a longstanding lung collapse and which is perpetuated by postoperative pain causing the children not to ventilate the operated side properly.

If there are thick secretions in the tracheo–bronchial tree in patients who are unable to expectorate, bronchoscopic aspiration and lavage should be thorough. If the intervention is carried out under a short general anaesthesia, the therapeutic effect can be improved by intubation and inflation of the lung under positive pressure.

- Antibiotics should continue for seven to ten days.
- In tuberculous empyema, anti-tuberculous drugs are continued for six months to a year.
- Drainage tubes are removed when the lung is expanded, if there is no air leak and if the discharge is less than 100 ml/24 hours without bacteriological evidence of empyema.

Severe sepsis accompanying empyema has long been considered as a contraindication for decortication. Thoracotomy and subsequent eradication of the septic focus, however, must be regarded as a life-saving procedure as soon as other measures have failed. In most cases also these severely septic patients will recover quickly as soon as the cause of their infectious process has been abolished. Surgery in these cases may be difficult due to the impossibility of even short-time single lung ventilation and to an encreased tendency for bleeding (e.g. in patients requiring hemofiltration) (Renner et al., 1998; Pothula and Krellenstein, 1994).

5.6. Open window thoracostomy

In complicated Stage III empyema, an empyema necessitatis may make primary closure of the chest after decortication impossible. Another indication for open window thoracostomy are patients in whom open chest drainage after rib resection has proved ineffective, but who would not tolerate decortication. Rarely, a severely necrotizing process at the pleura or the total absence of a dissection plane make efficient decortication impossible. Also in these cases open window thoracostomy can achieve a cure.

There are two different options of thoracic fenestration:

- Delayed closure of a standard thoracotomy,
- Open window for long-term drainage.

5.6.1. Delayed closure of a standard thoracotomy following decortication

Operation: If the soft tissues of the chest wall are involved into the infectious process showing gross cellulitis and necrotic areas, a primary closure of a thoracotomy following decortication is inadvisable. In these cases, the thoracotomy is left open while a light packing of the wound with saline soaked dressing is done. Positive pressure ventilation has to be kept up until the chest wall has been closed as otherwise the lung would collapse.

The dressings are changed every day, if necessary, necrectomy is performed. Once clean granulative tissue has formed, two drainages are inserted and the thoracotomy is closed. Usually this can be done within a few days after decortication.

5.6.2. Open window for long-term drainage

The intervention is carried out under general anaesthesia in a lateral decubitus position. A 15 to 20 cm longitudinal incision is made over the point of maximum extent of the empyema sac. Keeping in mind the possible necessity of later myoplastic closure the latissimus dorsi muscle should be severed as far distally as possible or dissected at its distal insertions.

Usually, a rib resection is required to enter the chest. After opening and sucking out the empyema cavity its lateral extent is evaluated by finger palpation. Extrapleural mobilization of the lateral wall of the empyema sac is then carried out and two to four ribs are resected to an extent of about 10 to 15 cm, carefully stitching the intercostal vessels. The lowermost point of the empyema cavity must drain freely. The cavity is mechanically cleared of debris and fibrin and the borders of the skin are loosely sutured to the osseous 'frame' of the window or to the margin of the empyema sac. The window is loosely packed with dressings soaked in saline.

During the first postoperative days, dressings are changed daily, which can be conveniently done on the ward. Once the window is well established, the patient is discharged for outpatient care and changes of dressings every two or three days. If there is no bronchopleural fistula, the patient may even do much of the treatment by himself, carefully cleaning the thoracostomy by applying water under the shower. Gradually, these windows will shrink, leaving a more or less pronounced crater in the chest wall.

If necessary, myoplastic closure can be done as soon as there is no more evidence of empyema (Renner et al., 1998; Smolle–Jüttner et al., 1992).

References and further reading

Chin NK, Lim TK. Controlled trial of intrapleural streptokinase in the treatment of pleural empyema and complicated parapneumonic effusions. Chest 1997; 111: 275–279.

Ferguson AD, Prescott RJ, Selkon JB, Watson D, Swinburn CR. The clinical course and management of thoracic empyema. QJM 1996; 89: 285–289.

Galea JL, De-Souza A, Beggs D, Spy, T. The surgical management of empyema thoracis. J R Coll Surg Edinb 1997; 42: 15–18.

Laisaar T, Puttsepp E, Laisaar V. Early administration of intrapleural streptokinase in the treatment of multiloculated pleural effusions and pleural empyemas. Thorac Cardiovasc Surg 1996; 44: 252-256.

Landreneau LR, Keenan RJ, Hazelrigg SR, Mack MJ, Naunheim KS. Thoracoscopy for empyema and hemothorax. Chest 1996; 109: 18–24.

LeMense C, Strange C, Sahn SA. Empyema thoracis. Therapeutic management and outcome. Chest 1995; 107: 1532–1537.

Martella AT, Santos GH. Decortication for chronic postpneumonic empyema. J Am Coll Surg 1995; 180: 573–576.

Pothula V, Krellenstein DJ. Early aggressive surgical management of parapneumonic empyemas. Chest 1994; 105: 832–836.

Renner H, Gabor S, Pinter H, Maier A, Friehs G, Smolle–Jüttner FM. Is aggressive surgery in empyema justified? Eur J Cardiothorac Surg 1998; 14: 117–122.

Silen ML, Naunheim KS. Thoracoscopic approach to the management of empyema thoracis. Indications and results. Chest Surg Clin N Am 1996; 6: 491–499.

Smolle–Jüttner F, Beuster W, Pinter H, Pierer G, Pongratz M, Friehs G. Open-window thoracostomy in pleural empyema. Eur J Cardiothorac Surg 1992; 6: 635–638.

Thurer RJ. Decortication in thoracic empyema. Indications and surgical technique. Chest Surg Clin N Am 1996; 6: 461–490.

Wait MA, Sharma S, Hohn J, Dal–Nogare A. A randomized trial of empyema therapy. Chest 1997; 111: 1548–1551.

Weissberg D, Refaely Y. Pleural empyema: 24–year experience. Ann Thorac Surg 1996; 62: 1026–1029.

CHAPTER I.26

Pleural neoplasms

K. Moghissi

1. Introduction

Primary neoplasms of the pleura originate from mesothelial and/or submesothelial connective tissues of the pleura. They are uncommon compared with other chest tumours. Secondary neoplasms are metastatic deposits from primary tumours of the lung, breast, ovary and many other sites. Until recently, and prior to advances in immuno-histochemistry methods, there was confusion and debate about histogenesis of primary pleural tumours. This confusion is apparent in publications by the variation in terminology used by different authors for a given tumour, which in turn reflects the pleomorphism and heterogeneity of histological features of these tumours. In this chapter we describe pleural neoplasm under:

- Benign
- Malignant

2. Benign pleural tumours

2.1. Lipomas, angiomas, endotheliomas and cysts

These are rare but are seen from time to time. They are generally asymptomatic and are discovered by incidental imaging abnormalities.

Lipomas are the commonest of this group and are usually found against the chest wall. A lipoma placed anteriorly in the costo-diaphragmatic angle may be mistaken for Morgagni hernias. Video-assisted thoracoscopy can diagnose and also provide a minimal access approach to excision of some.

2.2. Benign localised fibrous tumour of the pleura

This tumour has been variously described as fibrous pleural mesothelioma, benign mesothelioma, pleu-

ral fibroma and localised (solitary) mesothelioma. The tumour represents just over 15% of all benign intrathoracic tumours (Schworm et al., 1991). It is usually a solitary mass of variable size, from 2 cm to over 35 cm in its greatest diameter and can often arise from visceral or less often from parietal pleura. At presentation, 40 to 50% of patients are asymptomatic with mean age of about 50 years. When symptomatic, dyspnoea, pain, cough and rarely haemoptysis may be present individually or in concert. Clubbing of fingernails, and hypertrophic osteo-arthropathy are also commonly observed. Recurrent episodes of hypoglycaemia are found in as high as 14% of patients (Rena et al., 2001). This is due to an increase in IGF-II insulin-like output, which enhances glucose utilization and reduces IGF-I which regulates response to hypoglycaemia. Chest radiograph often shows a single well defined mass and CT of thorax indicates the usually homogeneous and very occasionally heterogenous nature of the tumour. Magnetic resonance imaging demonstrates the fibrous character of the mass. Bronchoscopy may show only extrinsic pressure of a larger tumour on the adjacent bronchial tree. Diagnosis is sometimes established by CT-guided needle biopsy but usually at operation. Thoracoscopy is an important diagnostic tool. Surgical excision is the only treatment and in many cases the tumour is removed at exploration. If the tumour is attached or arises from the visceral pleura, it is excised with a wedge resection of the adjacent lung. Those which arise from the parietal pleura are excised without chest wall excision.

Surgical excision is usually attended by cure with no risk of recurrence. Even in tumours whose histology shows high indices of suspicion for malignancy (England et al., 1989) recurrence is extremely unusual. When pre-operative biopsy is not obtained, the histology is established post-surgically. The diagnosis is confirmed by immuno histochemistry. Localised fibrous tumours are negative for keratin, S-100 and positive for vimentin. CD34 antibody staining is a more sensitive test for diagnosis of the tumour. It is important to note that the trio signs of clubbing of fingernails, osteo-arthropathy and recurrent episodes of hypoglycaemia will disappear after a successful operation. In one patient in Rena et al.'s (2001) series, clubbing returned 10 years after surgical excision. The chest X-ray then showed recurrence of the tumour which was re-excised successfully with repeat loss of clubbing.

2.2.1. Note on pleural plaques

Pleural plaques are thickened, raised circumscribed patches of pleura, 1 to 2 cm in length. Predominantly they are seen over the diaphragmatic surface of the pleura as shiny looking elevations with, at times, calcification. Many plaques are found at autopsy or during the course of intrathoracic operation. Histologically, they consist of dense collagen fibres with no inflammatory cells or vascularisation. Calcification can occur throughout the plaque. There is no evidence of relationship between plaques and mesothelioma. However, early stage mesothelioma and plaques can look alike when calcified plaques are demonstrable on X-ray plate. Note that calcification of patches of tuberculous pleuritis, empyema and old blood clot can also appear on chest radiograph but these usually are unilateral whereas the plaques are generally bilateral.

2.3. Malignant fibrous pleural tumour

England et al. (1989) in a review study suggested existence of solitary malignant fibrous pleural tumour and proposed the following criteria of malignancy:
– Abundant cellularity and pleomorphism,
– Nuclear atypia,
– More than four mitoses per ten high power field,
– Large necrotic or haemorrhagic area,
– Associated pleural effusion.

It is important to note that many solitary fibrous tumours, which by the above criteria are classed as malignant, do not behave aggressively and the patients are cured following surgical excision. In some cases with follow up of 20 years or more (on retrospective review using the above criteria) patients remained well with no tumour recurrence, thus providing evidence that cyto-histological criteria in this tumour is not a predictor of malignant behaviour.

3. Malignant mesothelium (diffuse malignant mesothelioma)

Malignant mesothelioma (MM) is by far the commonest of the pleural tumours and arises from mesothelial cells of visceral or parietal pleura.

Some authors describe a diffuse and a localised form of MM, however, the present day general view, to which I subscribe, regards the localised type of malignant mesothelioma as an aggressive (malignant) form of fibrous pleural tumour (described in section 2.3 above). Under the heading malignant mesothelioma we describe the diffuse form of this malignant tumour whose association with asbestos is well established and documented.

3.1. Asbestos

Asbestos means "unquenchable" or "inextinguishable", i.e. indestructible. It was used in Finland over 4000 years ago to make pottery. It is a mixture of silicate of iron, magnesium nickel, calcium and aluminium occurring naturally in the form of fibres. There are four main types of asbestos fibres:
– Chrysotile (serpentine asbestos) used in heat resistant textiles,
– Amosite (brown in colour) with long fibres of as much as 25 to 30 cm used in heat insulation,
– Crocidolite (blue asbestos) used in pipe packing,
– Anthophyllite (white asbestos) used for coating welding rods.

3.2. Pathology

Diffuse malignant mesothelioma (MM) consists of an extensive sheet of tumour which arises from visceral or parietal pleura, peritoneum and occasionally other serous membranes. Pleural MM runs an insidious course and is discovered when the disease is in its advanced stage in which case the inner chest wall and the lung are covered by a thick leather-like avascular looking material with interspersed nodules of softer tumour. In this situation the lung is contracted under the crust of the tumour showing no respiratory movement even on high pressure ventilation, A variable volume of blood stained effusion usually separates the visceral from parietal pleural sheets of tumour. In yet more advanced cases, there is also expansion of the tumour to the pericardium, diaphragm and chest wall with rib erosion followed by the muscles of the chest wall. The relationship between malignant mesothelioma and asbestos has been known for many years based both experimentally and on epidemiological grounds. One of the characteristics of the disease is the latent period between exposure/inhalation of asbestos particles and development of the disease, which can run to 30 or 40 or more years. Histologically, the tumour is composed of three types of cells in different proportions. Based on the predominance of the cell types three varieties of malignant mesotheliomas are recognised:

- Spindle cell sarcomatoid
- Tubular papillary epithelial
- Mixed spindle and epithelial

About one half of cases are of epithelial cell type and the other half are divided between sarcomatoid and mixed types.

Differential diagnosis between malignant mesothelioma and other tumours, notably adenocarcinoma, on standard histological staining techniques and using simple light microscopy is difficult. Histochemistry and electron microscopic methods are used for diagnosis. Immunohistochemistry stains contain antibodies. Mesothelioma stains positive for vimentin (antigen) and cytokeratin (antigen). They stain negative for carcino-embryonic antigen (CEA). Sarcomas do not stain positive for cytokeratin. Electron microscopy demonstrates the ultra structure and is an important diagnostic tool.

3.3. Stage classification

There have been several classifications, none totally satisfactory. The UICC classification (Sobin and Wittekind, 1997) using the TNM system (Table 1) appears most consistent and is used here.

3.3.1. Pleural mesothelioma staging
Rules for classification. The classification applies only to malignant mesothelioma of the pleura. There should be histological confirmation of the disease. The following are procedures for assessing T, N and M categories:

T categories	Physical examination, imaging, endoscopy, and/or surgical exploration
N categories	Physical examination, imaging, endoscopy, and/or surgical exploration
M categories	Physical examination, imaging, and/or surgical exploration

Regional lymph nodes. The regional lymph nodes are the intrathoracic, scalene and supraclavicular nodes.

Table 1

TNM Classification (Sobin and Wittekind, 1997)

T – Primary Tumour

TX	Primary tumour cannot be assessed
T0	No evidence of primary tumour
T1	Tumour limited to ipsilateral parietal and/or visceral pleura
T2	Tumour invades any of the following: ipsilateral lung, endothoracic fascia, diaphragm, pericardium
T3	Tumour invades any of the following: ipsilateral chest wall muscle, ribs, mediastinal organs or tissues
T4	Tumour directly extends to any of the following: contralateral pleura, contralateral lung, peritoneum, intra-abdominal organs, cervical tissues

N – Regional Lymph Nodes

NX	Regional lymph nodes cannot be assessed
N0	No regional lymph node metastasis
N1	Metastasis in ipsilateral peribronchial and/or ipsilateral hilar lymph nodes, including involvement by direct extension
N2	Metastasis in ipsilateral mediastinal and/or subcarinal lymph node(s)
N3	Metastasis in contralateral mediastinal, contralateral hilar, ipsilateral or contralateral scalene or supraclavicular lymph node(s)

M – Distant Metastasis

MX	Distant metastasis cannot be assessed
M0	No distant metastasis
M1	Distant metastasis

pTNM pathological classification. The pT, pN and pM categories correspond to the T, N and M categories.

Stage grouping

Stage I	T1	N0	M0
	T2	N0	M0
Stage II	T1	N1	M0
	T2	N1	M0
Stage III	T1	N2	M0
	T2	N2	M0
	T3	N0, N1, N2	M0
Stage IV	Any T	N3	M0
	T4	Any N	M0
	Any T	Any N	M1

Summary: Pleural mesothelioma

T1	Ipsilateral pleura
T2	Ipsilateral lung, endothoracic fascia, diaphragm, pericardium
T3	Ipsilateral chest wall muscle, ribs, mediastinal organs or tissues

T4   Direct extension to contralateral pleura, lung, peritoneum, intra-abdominal organs, cervical tissue

N1   Ipsilateral peribronchial, ipsilateral hilar

N2   Ipsilateral mediastinal, subcarinal

N3   Contralateral mediastinal or hilar, scalene or supraclavicular

3.4. Clinical features

The clinical presentation is insidious, the patient being asymptomatic at the early stage of the disease. Symptoms appear only when there is relatively large effusion or the tumour has progressed to such an extent as to interfere with respiratory mechanism. Dyspnoea and pain are the primary and predominant manifestations of the disease resulting from chest wall involvement and pleural effusion. Haemoptysis is uncommon, hoarseness, dysphagia and Horner's Syndrome appear in some cases indicating spread of the tumour to extra pleural structures. Physical signs relate to the presence of effusion and loss of lung expansion on ventilation. Diagnosis is suspected by radiological appearances of fluid and/or thickening of the inner chest wall. In some cases CT scan and MRI can detail more precise changes. Confirmation of the diagnosis is made by biopsy and tissue diagnosis.

Blind or radiologically guided needle and/or punch biopsies can provide tissue sample but not always sufficient for definite diagnosis. Thoracoscopic exploration of the pleural space provides visual evidence of the tumour and suitable samples for histology. Open biopsy may have to be performed using mini-access limited thoracotomy in some cases when thoracoscopy is not feasible or is unhelpful.

3.5. Treatment

None of the standard cancer treatment methods alone or in combination have thus far succeeded to change the course of this disease significantly or its fatal outcome. However, surgery and radiotherapy in particular and chemotherapy in some cases have an important place in palliation of symptoms.

3.5.1. Surgical operation

Parietal pleurectomy alone, pleurectomy decortication and extensive radical pleuro-pneumonectomy cover the range of operations advocated for MM.

- Pleurectomy alone aims at providing palliation particularly related to arrest of recurring malignant pleural effusion by the creation of pleurodesis combined with pleural debulking. This procedure can easily be carried out via VATS or limited muscle-sparing thoracotomy.

- Combined pleurotomy and decortication aims at debulking the tumour and releasing the imprisoned lung from its thick sheet of tumour, thus allowing its expansion. In ideal situations the parietal pleura is excised to a great extent and the lung expanded fully with creation of pleurodesis. Decortication in mesothelioma is only partially possible and only when the tumour can be peeled off which is not always the case without producing extensive air leak. It is, therefore, important not to be 'carried away' and cause air leaks to such an extent that the lung will have no chance of re-expansion.

- Pleuro-pneumonectomy. This is an extensive operation, which aims to provide an *en bloc* resection of the tumour covered lung, parietal pleura, and ipsilateral diaphragm and hemipericardium. The approach is essentially through postero-lateral thoracotomy, when necessary, with extension towards the umbilicus (thoraco-abdominal) and/or appropriate separate contra incision. Bleeding can be a problem. Therefore, diathermy and/or various thermal lasers have been used to limit blood loss. The author prefers the use of Neodymium YAG laser in its contact and non-contact mode which combines 'cutting, evaporation coagulation and charring' (Moghissi et al., 1994).
  Careful dissection is important to avoid injury to blood vessels and mediastinal structures.

The pericardium and diaphragm need reconstructing after excision using Gortex, Dacron or other suitable material. The operation is attended by high mortality and morbidity (12–30%).

3.5.2. Radiotherapy

Local pain can be controlled by radiotherapy. However, extensive and widespread chest wall involvement needs a high radiation dose, which can be prohibitive because of toxicity. This is particularly relevant to heart, oesophagus and spinal cord. Radiotherapy after surgical treatment can also be useful in chest wall involvement or recurrence.

3.5.3. Chemotherapy

An array of agents have been used and are being tried alone or in combination in an effort to find a regimen which may improve quality of life and offer survival benefit. Cisplatin, Doxorubicin and Mitomycin are used by various worked trials in different combinations.

One of the difficulties of appraisal of results is that the natural history of the disease is, in many cases, one of slow growing tumour some patients surviving five years with no treatment other than supportive therapy. It follows that only a trial covering a large number of patients for five to ten years and by committed centres is likely to achieve useful answers.

3.5.4. Supportive drugs and palliation of effusion

This consists of palliation of symptoms and prevention of recurrence of effusion using simple methods (see malignant pleural effusion, section 4.2 in chapter I.23). Some studies carried out in the 1980s suggest that some patients can survive five years without specific oncological therapy with a good to reasonable quality of life.

3.5.5. Combination (trimodality) treatment

A regimen consisting of combined radical surgery (pleuro-pneumonectomy), radiotherapy and chemotherapy in various mixes has been followed by some centres (Achatz et al., 1989; Sugarbaker et al., 1991; Grondin and Sugarbaker, 1999; Maggi et al., 2001). Evaluation of effectiveness and comparison of this treatment protocol with a simpler method of pleurectomy decortication is difficult because of the lack of evidence-based study. One of the difficulties relates to unpredictability of the natural progression of the disease even without specific treatment. It is, however, possible to suggest that stage I of the disease and epithelial cell type will be a better candidate for a curable intent treatment. Trimodality treatment seems to offer a long survival in stage I disease and in some patients in stage II.

3.5.6. Other treatment

Treatments which have been advanced in the hope of finding an alternative to the 'standard treatment' methods are:

- Immunotherapy. Intrapleural interferon has received attention either alone or with chemotherapy. Preliminary results show some success.
- Photodynamic therapy with surgery has been tried showing encouraging results in terms of delayed recurrence.

3.5.7. Conclusion

At the time of writing, except for early stage disease, treatment should concentrate on patient quality of life and avoidance of methods which have a high mortality and morbidity. A debulking procedure consisting of pleurectomy decortication and pleurodesis is the choice method for the majority at presentation and achieves reasonable palliation. This may be carried out by VATS method. In selected patients with stage I tumour trimodality treatment can be recommended.

References and further reading

Achatz R, Beba W, Ritschler R, et al. The diagnosis, therapy and prognosis of diffuse malignant mesothelioma. Eur J Cardiothoracic Surg 1989; 3: 445–448.

Brisellis M, Mark EJ, Dickersin GR. Solitary fibrous tumours of the pleura. 8 new cases and review of 360 cases in the literature. Cancer 1981; 47: 2678–2689.

Edwards JG, Abrams KR, Levermen JN, et al. Prognostic factors for malignant mesothelioma in 142 patients: validation of CALGB and EORTC prognostic scoring system. Thorax 2000; 55: 731–735.

England DM, Hochholzer L, McCaughey WTE. Localised benign and malignant fibrous tumours of the pleura. Am J Surg Pathol 1989; 13: 640–658.

Flint AQ, Weiss SW. CD34 and Keratin expression distinguishes solitary fibrous tumour (fibrometothelioma) of pleural from desmoplastic mesothelioma. Human Pathol 1995; 26: 428–431.

Grondin SC, Sugarbaker DJ. Pleuropneumonectomy in the treatment of malignant pleural mesothelioma. Chest 1999; 116: 4505–4545.

Ho L, Sugarbaker DJ, Skarin AT. Malignant Pleural Mesothelioma. Cancer Treat Res 2001; 105: 327–373.

Kuku O, Parker DL. Diagnosis and management of asbestosis. Minn Med 2000; 83(11): 47–49.

Law MR, Gregor A, Hodson ME, et al. Malignant mesothelioma of the pleura: A study of 52 treated and 63 untreated patients. Thorax 1984; 39: 255–254.

Maggi G, Casadio C, Cianci R, et al. Trimodality management of malignant pleural mesothelioma. Eur J Cardiothorac Surg 2001; 19: 346–350.

Moghissi K. Lasers in broncho-pulmonary cancer. Radiol Oncol 1994; 28: 359–364.

Peto J, Decarli A, La Vecchia C, et al. The European Mesothelioma epidemic. Br J Cancer 1999; 79: 666–672.

Procopio A, Strizzi L, Guiffrida A, et al. Human malignant mesothelioma of the pleura: new perspective in diagnosis and therapy. Monaldi Arc Chest Dis. 1998; 53: 241–243.

Rena O, Dilosso PL, Papalia E, et al. Solitary fibrous tumour of the pleura: surgical treatment. Eur J Cardiothorac Surg 2001; 1a: 185–189.

Schworm MD, Saeger HD, Hiirle M, et al. Benign and pleural tumour. Chirurg 1991; 62: 213–216.

Sobin LH and Wittekind CH. International Union Against Cancer TNM Classification of malignant tumours (5th ed). Wiley–Liss Publications, 1997.

Sugarbaker DJ, Heher EC, Lee TH, et al. Extrapleural pneumonectomy, chemotherapy and radiotherapy in the treatment of diffuse malignant pleural mesothelioma. J Thorac Cardiovasc Surg 1991; 102: 10–14.

Takahashi K, Yosuida J, Nishimuro M. Extrapleural pneumonectomy for diffuse malignant pleural mesothelioma: a treatment
option in selected cases? JPN J Thorac Cardiovasc Surg
2001; 49: 89–93.

Utley JR, Parker JC, Hahn RS, et al. Recurrent benign fibrous
mesothelioma of the pleura. J Thorac Cardiovasc Surg 1973;
65: 830–834.

Trachea, Mediastinum, Chest Wall and Diaphragm

CHAPTER II.1

The trachea

K. Moghissi

1. Surgical anatomy

The trachea commences in the neck below the cricoid cartilage at the level of the 6th cervical vertebra and extends into the thorax where it divides into the left and right bronchi, at the manubri-sternal junction, level with the body of the 4th thoracic vertebra. The adult trachea measures 12 to 13 cm, its diameter varies between 1.5 to 2.5 cm and its patency is assured by 18 to 22 incomplete rings of cartilage (approximately two rings per centimetre). The cartilages are C shaped; the gap in the rings lies posteriorly and is closed by a sheet of smooth muscle, which is in contact with the oesophagus. This allows expansion of the latter during the ingestion of food. The division of the trachea into two bronchi is indicated internally by a midline ridge, the carina, which is situated between the opening of the two bronchi. In the supine position, with the head extended, about half of the trachea is in the neck and the other half in the thorax. However, when the head is flexed, a greater length of the trachea becomes intramediastinal.

The cervical trachea is superficial and subcutaneous but as it descends to the chest it becomes more deeply situated and in contact with the manubrium 3.5 to 4 cm from the surface.

Anatomical relations of the trachea in the neck are, from above downwards: the thyroid isthmus which lies over the 2nd, 3rd and 4th cartilaginous rings, the innominate artery which crosses the trachea below the thyroid isthmus from left to right and the innominate vein passing over the trachea, itself covered by the thymus gland. Posteriorly, the trachea is in close contact with the oesophagus with the recurrent laryngeal nerves, one on each side, in the groove between the trachea and oesophagus. Lat-

erally, first the lateral lobes of the thyroid then the carotid sheath lie on each side of the trachea.

In the chest, the common carotid artery, the mediastinal pleura and the left lung lie on the left side of the trachea, whilst on the right of the trachea lie the mediastinal pleura and the right lung. The arch of the aorta on the left and the azygos vein on the right, pass over the left and the right main bronchi, respectively, and flank the lower trachea on each side.

Much of the blood supply of the trachea is in common with the oesophagus and is derived from branches of superior and inferior thyroid arteries, bronchial arteries and contributions from the costocervical trunk and subclavian arteries. These branches contribute to form a longitudinal arterial network running on either side of the lateral aspect of the trachea. Venous return is through the inferior thyroid plexus and branches accompanying the arteries to reach the innominate veins.

Lymphatics of the cervical trachea drain into the postero-inferior group of deep cervical glands. The lymph from the thoracic trachea drains into the mediastinal glands in the posterior part of the superior mediastinum. It is to be noted that there are paratracheal lymph nodes scattered along the anterior aspects of the trachea; these are particularly abundant near its bifurcation. These glands communicate with one another and with the deep cervical glands.

On endoscopic examination, the interior of the trachea shows corrugations caused by the cartilaginous rings. The division of the trachea, the carina, is seen as a sharp ridge between the openings of the two bronchi.

2. Investigatory methods in tracheal diseases

The clinical manifestations of tracheal lesions are those of upper airway obstruction, namely dyspnoea, wheeze and stridor of varying severity. Haemoptysis occurs in neoplastic cases, or as a result of ulceration and granulation tissue formation in benign lesions. History taking and clinical examination should draw attention to tracheal obstruction and its possible aetiology. A chest radiograph often shows no abnormalities but in severe obstructions it may demonstrate pulmonary non-specific inflammatory signs. Negative chest X-ray findings should be borne in mind by all who rely on X-ray reports for the management of their patients. *In the presence of symptoms, patients must be investigated further,* even when the chest radiograph is apparently normal.

Other radiological techniques such as air contrast radiography, tomography, CT scan, magnetic resonance imaging and barium swallow studies are useful in furnishing the anatomical definition and extent of lesions.

2.1. Tracheobronchoscopy

This is the essential investigation. It provides visual definition of the lesion and its level and is the means of obtaining tissue diagnosis. Caution must be exercised in performing bronchoscopy and particularly in biopsying some highly vascular lesions as this can result in bleeding and/or serious respiratory obstruction.

In stenotic tracheal lesions, tracheobronchoscopy using a rigid bronchoscope is the most important examination. The rigid instrument will permit inspection and assessment of the size and other characteristics of the lesion as well as allowing an initial dilatation, improving the airway, if necessary. In the opinion of the author, tracheoscopic examination for those cases requiring resection and reconstruction should be carried out by the surgeon who proposes to undertake the operation.

At tracheobronchoscopy the following should be evaluated and recorded:
- Endoscopic length of the trachea from the cords to the carina,
- Extent of the endotracheal lesion,
- Distance between the carina and lower limit of the lesion,
- Distance between the upper limit of the lesion and the cords.

If there is tracheal stenosis, dilatation is carried

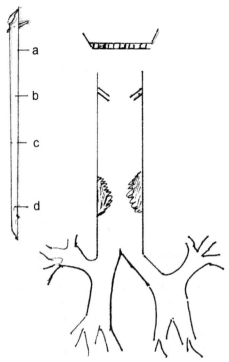

Fig. 1. Left: tracheal measurement for surgical/endoscopic procedures. Right: marking on the bronchoscope (see text). All measurements are in cm. (a) to (b) = carina to lower limit of tracheal lesion, (b) to (c) = the extent of the lesion, (c) to (d) = the upper limit of the lesion to the cords. (d) to end of the bronchoscope + cords to upper alveolus.

out sufficiently to allow passage of the bronchoscope through it in order to examine the trachea fully. A simple method to carry out this evaluation is to introduce the rigid bronchoscope into the trachea down to the carina and mark that point on the bronchoscope with a marker pen level with the upper alveolus (a). The instrument is then withdrawn gradually and markings are made on the bronchoscope as follows:
- At the lower limit of the lesion (b),
- At the upper limit of the lesion (c),
- At the level of the vocal cords (d).

Using this method (Fig. 1) the distance is measured in centimetres on the bronchoscope:

(a) to (d) = Total length of the trachea,
(a) to (b) = Carina to the lower limit of the lesion,
(b) to (c) = Length of the lesion,
(c) to (d) = Upper limit of the lesion to the cords.

In cases of tracheomalacia, tracheoscopy is best carried out under topical anaesthesia or general anaesthesia with the patient breathing in order to appreciate the collapse of the trachea. This occurs in the expiratory phase of respiration and is of diagnostic characteristic.

3. Congenital lesions of the trachea

Serious congenital anomalies are incompatible with survival and generally escape the clinician's attention because of their early fatal outcome. These include tracheal atresia and agenesis which are often associated with other anomalies. A less serious group is comprised of stenotic lesions ranging from web-like strictures to long segment congenital chondromalacias with or without a compressive vascular ring. These are not uncommon. In their severe form these lesions present as a serious neonatal respiratory distress syndrome which are investigated and diagnosed. In their milder form they manifest as cases of neonatal stridor which often recover spontaneously by the age of 2 or 3 years. Such babies may have stridor, paradoxical wheeze and feeding difficulties. Radiological investigations are usually of assistance in the elimination of mediastinal and pulmonary lesions as the cause of the respiratory distress. Diagnostic tracheobronchoscopy has to be performed by an experienced operator, who can recognise neonatal tracheal anomalies when seen through the neonatal (infant and infant small) bronchoscope.

Obstruction by webs and limited stenotic lesions may be relieved endoscopically.

External compressions by vascular rings or tumour can be effectively dealt with by surgery.

In many tracheal lesions of the neonate, tracheostomy may be the only possible life saving measure when the anatomical position of the lesion permits such an undertaking. Direct surgery on the neonatal trachea is difficult and hazardous even in experienced hands. These cases should be referred to centres with experience in handling paediatric airway problems (Grillo et al., 2002).

4. Traumatic injuries of the trachea

Penetrating injuries by a sharp instrument are occasionally encountered in civilian life, sometimes occurring accidentally. The tracheal wound such as that caused by a sharp knife, may be repaired by primary suturing. Such a wound is generally found in the cervical portion of the trachea. At times the trachea may have been severed completely in which case the lower segment may retract and disappear down into the mediastinum. Iaterogenic instrumental perforations of the trachea are now very rare but

accidental tear of the lower trachea at the level of the carina during placement of a double lumen endotracheal tube is occasionally seen. This type of tear is noticed at the start of thoracic operation. Diagnosis can be made bronchoscopically and repair can be undertaken by direct suturing, if necessary reinforced by a Teflon/Dacron pericardial patch. Mediastinal tracheal penetrating lacerations are extremely uncommon, except in cases of war injury.

Blunt traumatic injuries are not uncommonly encountered following road traffic accidents. These usually involve tearing of the lower trachea, above or together with the laceration of one of the main bronchi. Sometimes the injury may remain undiagnosed until later development of stenotic lesion.

Clinical presentation of tracheal injuries may vary according to the presence of associated injuries:

- Shock is sometimes present together with dyspnoea and haemoptysis.
- Surgical subcutaneous and mediastinal emphysema is almost always demonstrable.
- Persistent pneumothorax with a large air leak indicates main bronchial involvement.

Chest radiography indicates mediastinal emphysema and haematoma with possible pneumothorax. CT scan and, in difficult cases, MRI help to establish the diagnosis and indicate the level of the injury.

Tracheobronchoscopy should always be performed for the precise diagnosis of the injury and its anatomical extent and location.

Emergency repair of a tracheobronchial rupture should be carried out after rapid preliminary preparation and the insertion of an intercostal tube for drainage of pneumothorax. Cervical tracheal injuries can be dealt with through a neck incision. A right posterolateral thoracotomy through the 4th intercostal space provides a satisfactory approach for all lower tracheal and main bronchial lacerations. When the injury involves the lower trachea and the left main bronchus, a right thoracotomy is still the best approach. Only when the distal left main bronchus at the level of the upper lobe is ruptured is a left thoracotomy required.

5. Post-intubation tracheal injuries

These are lesions which occur as a complication of endotracheal intubation notably following tracheostomy and assisted ventilation. The incidence of post-intubation injuries varies in different centres with differing techniques and methods of respiratory support. The type and anatomical location of tracheal lesions are important considerations with respect to their management.

According to their anatomical position, post-intubation tracheal lesions may be classified as follows:

5.1. Subglottic lesions

These lesions are at or just below the cricoid cartilages and are produced by:
(a) Endotracheal tubes causing ulceration and scarring,
(b) High tracheostomy and injury to the first tracheal cartilage,
(c) Pressure and ulceration from an ill-fitting tracheostomy tube,
(d) In some instances, subglottic lesions (infracricoid) are caused by the shelf-like backward displacement of the anterior wall of the trachea above the tracheostomy opening.

5.2. Stomal lesions

These appear at or about the tracheostomy opening. Factors involved in this type of lesion are:
- Too large an opening,
- Infection,
- Heavy connecting tubes exerting pressure against the tracheal wall, leading to necrosis and scarring.

5.3. Infrastomal lesions

These occur some 2 to 4 cm below the site of the tracheostomy. The majority are stenotic in type. Occasionally, the rings of cartilage are replaced by fibrous tissue which does not protrude into the lumen, but creates softening and loss of rigidity (tracheomalacia).

The pressure of the sealing cuff has much to do with the causation of injuries at this site.

5.4. Lower tracheal lesions

These lesions are placed 3 to 4 cm above the carina and are generally caused by trauma inflicted by the end of the tracheostomy tube.

5.5. General discussion on aetiology of post-intubation tracheal injuries

Factors that cause post-intubation tracheal injuries in different locations are largely the same but with a different degree of emphasis for each one of the sites. These include:

- Infection, particularly those caused by Gram-negative organisms,
- Pressure necrosis with ulceration,
- Faulty techniques of intubation,
- Heavy connectors and tubing which cause movement of the tracheostomy tube with consequent ulceration, granulation tissue formation and scarring,
- Poor management of tracheostomy, including infection and trauma inflicted by suction catheters.

5.6. Pathology and clinical manifestation

The evolution of post-intubation tracheal injuries begins with traumatic inflammation and infection and progresses through ulceration and granulation tissue formation to the formation of stenotic scarring. At times, this evolution is further complicated by erosion of the posterior tracheal wall with tracheo-oesophageal fistula as its consequence. At other times, it is anterior wall erosion which creates trachea to innominate artery fistula. Post-intubation injuries usually present themselves as obstructions of the trachea.

Patients with minor injuries not leading to tracheal ulceration and severe obstruction may remain asymptomatic. This is particularly the case when the patient is young and has good pulmonary function. When present, symptoms are related to upper airway obstruction. Dyspnoea, wheeze and stridor are the usual manifestations.

In the early stage of stenosis or in ulceration and granulation, cough, bloodstained sputum and difficulty in expectorating are common symptoms. Chest radiography may be unhelpful. Tracheal tomography, CT scans and MRI may provide diagnosis of the severity and location of the stenosis. Tracheoscopy (bronchoscopy) is the most important diagnostic tool.

5.7. Treatment

Once the diagnosis is made, a decision must be taken on the most appropriate treatment for a particular patient. This decision should take into account:
- Degree of disability and severity of symptoms,
- Age and general condition of the patient,
- Type of lesion, its extent and its anatomical location.

Therapeutic modalities are:

5.7.1. Resection and reconstruction

In a fit patient with limited stenosis and/or tracheo-malacia this constitutes the treatment of choice and, in expert hands, it will have little or no mortality. Re-stenosis is a possibility (between 2 to 4% of cases).

5.7.2. Bronchoscopic dilatation and excision

Bronchoschopic dilation and excision is coupled with medication to assist prevention of re-infection and granulation tissue formation (e.g. antibiotics, corticosteroids). This method is not successful in tight and established stenosis accompanied by a degree of malacia

5.7.3. Endoscopic laser treatment using non-contact mode Nd YAG laser

This method is likely to succeed providing that:

(a) Tracheal cartilages have not been destroyed to any great extent,

(b) There is no tracheo-malacia above/below the stenotic lesion.

5.7.4. Tracheal stent

In some cases with debilitated patients and those not responding to other conservative treatment methods (e.g. laser), placement of a stent may have to be considered (see tracheo-bronchial stent, chapter II.2).

5.7.5. Permanent tracheostomy

This method may have to be adopted in some cases with subglottic stenosis or in extensive tracheomalacia. In the latter case, the tracheostomy tube functions both as a stent, preventing the collapse of the wall during expiration, and also as a bypass of the larynx if necessary. Ideal for this purpose is the Montgomery-T tube (see chapter II.2).

6. Tracheomalacia

The term denotes softening of the trachea. The condition presents a condition which is associated with some changes in tracheal cartilage, and elongation of the posterior membranous wall. The ensuing functional abnormality is an exaggerated reduction of tracheal calibre during expiration and coughing. In some instances, there is a definite herniation of the posterior wall into the tracheal lumen with, at times, quasi-total obstruction of the tracheal lumen. The condition was originally described by Herzog (1954) and Nissen (1954) in patients with chronic bronchitis due to an alteration of elastic fibres.

6.1. Aetiology

- Congenital: Congenital tracheomalacia is associated with segmental cartilaginous deficit, congenital vascular rings and anomolous vascular ring.
- Post-intubation: This occurs usually with stenotic lesions and sometimes without actual stenosis.
- Post-operative: After successful tracheal reconstruction this may be post infective.
- Extrinsic compression: Cases of thyroid goitre, particularly those with mediastinal extension, may compress the lower trachea above the bifurcation and produce malacia. These have been well-documented. However, other anterior mediastinal tumours can also produce a similar effect.
- Emphysema and chronic obstructive pulmonary disease (COPD): The original description of tracheo-bronchial malacia was based on observation in such cases and the aetiology appears to relate to deficiency of the cartilage.

6.2. Presentation/Diagnosis

The characteristic presentation is an extreme expiratory wheeze and stridor with, at times, a barking cough. The differential diagnosis from asthma should be made particularly in emphysematous and chronic bronchitics.

- Clinical examination may not be specific except when the malacia is in the cervical trachea which then can be observed and palpated.
- Spirometric tracing is characteristic in showing a break in the expiratory phase of spirometry. This is presented as a plateau which corresponds to functional obstruction due to collapse of the airway.
- Radiology: Chest radiography, tracheal tomography and CT may be totally normal except for some cases associated with a mediastinal pathology and "sabre trachea." Dynamic imaging using video tracheography is useful to indicate both the existence of narrowing and its level.
- Tracheo-bronchoscopy: This is the most useful investigation, particularly when combined with videoscopic recording. Rigid and/or flexible fibreoptic bronchoscopy should be performed using topical anaesthesia or under general anaesthesia with the patient breathing normally without muscle relaxant. Typical malacia will be seen as the collapse of the tracheal wall in the expiratory phase of breathing. Videoscopic recording of the tracheobronchoscopy, when possible, has the

advantage of allowing further study and examination.

6.3. Management

6.3.1. Resection
Post-intubation tracheomalacia affecting a short segment may be resected, particularly when associated with stenosis. Characteristic of this combination is that, when the easily dilated segment is satisfactorily entered by the rigid bronchoscope, the area collapses almost immediately after withdrawal of the instrument proximally.

6.3.2. External splinting
The principle is based on that which was originally described by Herzog (1954) and Nissen (1954). That is stiffening of the posterior membranous part of the trachea. The operation is suitable for malacia associated with emphysema and chronic bronchitis. In the original operation autologous pieces of bone (rib) or cartilaginous "rings" were used. Others have since used Marlex mesh and silicone stents secured to the trachea by stitches (Rainer et al., 1968).

6.3.3. Internal splinting (stenting)
A short segmental malacia may be dilated with the use of Montgomery T stents. This is particularly suitable in younger patients with post-intubation malacia without severe obstruction. The stent may be removed after 12 to 18 months. This method of temporary stenting is also satisfactory in cases resulting from external compression (e.g. goitre with sabre sheath deformity).

6.4. Summary and conclusion on tracheal malacia

- Symptoms of expiratory obstruction should be distinguished from stricture, stenotic lesions and asthma.
- Diagnosis of airway malacia relies on spirometry, dynamic tracheography and endoscopy.
- Aetiological factors should be taken into account when treatment options are considered.
- Conservative therapy, particularly in young patients, should take priority. Temporary stenting using Montgomery T tube should be considered, as many cases, apart from those associated with emphysema and chronic airway disease with extensive malacia, will benefit from such conservative therapy and major surgical operation can be avoided.

7. Neoplasms of the trachea

7.1. Primary tumours

Primary tracheal neoplasms are rare. This is testified by the fact that Grillo and Mathisen (1990) reported 198 cases of tracheal tumours treated during a 27 year period at Massachusetts General Hospital (Boston, USA), and Perelman and Korolova (1987) from the Soviet Union reported on 90 patients of which, unusually, 45 were benign. Sharpe and Moghissi (1996) presented only16 surgically resected cases seen during a 20 year period from a cardio thoracic centre in the UK concerned with 1 to 1.5 million population. These were amongst 82 tracheal lesions (19.5% of all lesions).

More recently Schneider et al. (2001) presented their experience of 16 patients seen during a 26 year period.

The majority of tracheal tumours are malignant; only some 10% are benign.

- Papillomas are the commonest of the benign tumours. They are most frequently encountered in the neonate and children and are generally multiple, usually spread along the length of the trachea. The larynx and bronchial tree can also become involved. The aetiology of the lesion is unknown but viral infection has been implicated as the causative agent. Papillomatous lesions of childhood usually regress at puberty. Their management in neonates and children is difficult. Tracheostomy is usually required, particularly when the larynx is involved. Interventional bronchoscopy, such as repeated laser fulguration is useful to relieve respiratory distress and remove the larger lesions with malignant potential.
- Carcinoid is a relatively common tumour included amongst the benign tumours. Although in the past all carcinoids were considered as being benign lesions, they are in fact, generally of low malignant property and some are definitely invasive and are behaviourally malignant.
- Squamous cell carcinomas and adenoid cystic carcinomas are two of the commonest malignant tracheal tumours. The latter has been known as "cylindroma" and usually progresses slowly. It infiltrates the submucosa more extensively than the surface epithelium and also metastasises, notably in bones and lungs. Resection is attended by over 70% five years survival (Prommegger and Salzer, 1998).
- Rarer types of tracheal tumours are: mucoepider-

mal carcinomas, haemangioma, chondroma and chondrosarcomas.

The commonest feature of all tracheal neoplasms is the tendency to develop airway obstruction. The mode of presentation in all consists of cough, wheeze, dyspnoea and stridor. Haemoptysis appears as a consequence of tumour necrosis and early in haemangioma as a primary clinical presentation. Plain chest radiograph may be unremarkable except for those lower tracheal tumours which impinge on the right upper lobe bronchial opening producing pulmonary segmental or lobar collapse and pneumonitis. In severe tracheal stenosis, lateral X-ray, air tomography or CT scan reveals the lesion. MRI is helpful to indicate changes in the soft tissue brought about by tumour invasion. Tracheobronchoscopy establishes the diagnosis and provides samples for histology.

7.2. Secondary tumours

The commonest secondary tumour affecting the lower trachea is bronchial carcinoma extending usually from the right main bronchus to the carina and the lateral wall of the trachea. Cancer of the larynx commonly involves the upper trachea, particularly those cancers which recur after resection or radiotherapy. Carcinoma of the oesophagus and thyroid can extend into the trachea causing obstruction. Malignant oesophago-tracheal fistula is a common occurrence in advanced cancer of the cervical oesophagus.

The clinical presentation of secondary tumours is one of upper airway obstruction together with other symptoms related to the primary tumour.

7.3. Management of Patients with Tracheal Tumours

7.3.1. Surgical treatment

Following investigation, assessment is made of the operability of the lesion which in turn is dependent on extent of the tumour. The operative approach is dependent on the site of the lesion. This can be cervical, mediastinal, cervicomediastinal or thoracic. It is therefore important to define the anatomical site of the lesion endoscopically.

Benign tumours are usually amenable to resection and reconstruction with end-to-end anastamosis. Some tumours are pedunculated, others are sessile. In either form, a limited resection can usually be undertaken. Carcinoid tumour, though usually described amongst benign tumours, should be considered as potentially malignant and treated as such by resection.

Malignant tumours should be offered surgical resection as a primary choice. An end-to-end anastomosis is possible without undue difficulty after excision of 4 to 5 cm of the trachea. In some patients, it is necessary in the course of preparation, to carry out a preliminary tracheostomy to provide acceptable ventilation whilst the work-up process is in progress. The author prefers laser fulgaration, which can be carried out instead of tracheostomy as a first step towards complete resection and reconstruction. In using YAG laser in these pre-operative cases, care should be taken to limit radiation to the exophytic tumour without effect to the surrounding tissue. This is to avoid vascular damage to the healthy portion of the trachea.

Surgery for secondary malignant tracheal tumours is particularly relevant in cases of extension of lung cancer to the lower trachea and in patients with differentiated papillary or follicular thyroid cancer. Lung cancer spreading from the right upper lobe in particular can involve the lower trachea. To surgically excise these tumours one option is complete pneumonectomy with carinal and lower tracheal circumferential excision followed by reconstruction. A simpler procedure is lobectomy and partial circumferential excision of the lower trachea followed by reconstruction and, if necessary, with patch grafting. The author's method in selected cases is to place a patch of Marlex mesh covered with a pedicle graft of pericardiam over the tracheo-bronchial defect (Figs. 2a and b). This does not involve too many anastomoses and the long-term results are satisfactory. (Sharpe and Moghissi, 1996). In the case of tracheal involvement by thyroid tumour, circumferential resection and end-to-end anastamosis is usually achievable.

- Mortality of resection and reconstruction in a large series of primary tracheal tumours is reported in the published literature to be between 5% and 17%. The range is accounted for by the extent of resection, location of tumour and general condition, including respiratory function, of the patients.
- Benign tumours are usually limited in extent requiring a less extensive resection than malignant lesions and are, therefore, expected to have a lesser mortality.
- Tracheal surgery for malignant and benign cases is also attended by non-fatal complications which are:

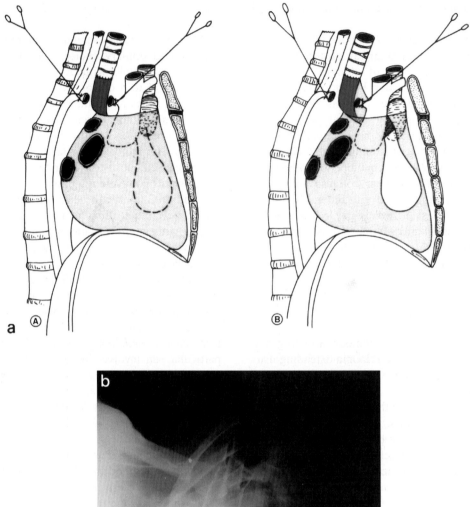

Fig. 2. (a) (A) A lateral view of the right hemithorax shows the tracheal defect covered over with Marlex mesh. The heavy interrupted line indicates the outline of the pedicle graft of pericardium to be prepared. The azygos vein is ligated and divided. (B) The pericardial patch attached to its pedicule is passed beneath the superior vena cava. It is sutured to the trachea over the Marlex mesh. (b) Chest radiograph of a patient 10 years after right pneumonectomy with carinal and lower right lateral wall of trachea and patch graft (Marlex/pericardial).

- Wound (anastomotic) dehiscence,
- Local wound infection,
- Pulmonary infection,
- Granulation tissue formation causing tracheal stenosis.

Long term results of surgery. Benign tumours are usually cured by a successful operation. Adenoid cystic carcinomas have an excellent prognosis with a five year survival rate of 70% or more. The survival rate is considerably lower in squamous cell carcinomas. In Perelman and Korolova's (1987) series, the five year survival after resection for squamous cell carcinoma was 15%. In the Massachusetts General Hospital series (Grillo and Mathison, 1990) 34% of patients survived between three to 15 years. The stage of disease influences survival.

7.3.2. Non-Surgical Treatment of Tracheal Tumours
Patients with benign tumours not suitable for surgical resection can be offered endoscopic treatment. Prior to the availability of lasers, these tumours were resected endoscopically using a rigid bronchoscope and bronchial biopsy forceps. In some cases, electrocautery was used. Since the widespread use of laser, these tumours can be adequately treated with its use. For malignant, unresectable/inoperable tracheal tumours, or those with recurrence after resection, the aim should be good-quality palliation with as long a survival as possible. Desobliteration of the airway is undertaken to relieve dyspnoea. There should also be therapeutic measures in place to prevent and treat infection by antibiotics and airway clearance.

Radiotherapy. Both squamous cell carcinoma and adenoid cystic carcinoma are radiosensitive although there are cases which present with early recurrence following radical radiotherapy. The author's personal experience indicates that response to radiotherapy in adenoid cystic carcinoma is short-lived.

Endoscopic lasers (see also Lasers in Cardiothoracic Surgery, chapter IV.5). NdYAG laser is the most appropriate type of laser for treatment of bulky endotracheal obstructive lesions with acute asphyxiating signs. Its effect is rapid and improvement of respiration immediate.

Benign tumours can be successfully treated using the non-contact mode of NdYAG laser with a good prospect of cure and long survival (Sharpe and Moghissi, 1996). Treatment can be repeated in both malignant and benign cases.

The author's experience suggests that photodynamic therapy (PDT) is a more appropriate type of laser therapy for malignant endoluminal tumours in achieving desobliteration as well as long lasting results. However, in bulky tumours, I prefer to de-bulk the obstructive tumour using NdYAG laser and follow this six to eight weeks later with PDT

Implantation of stent. The most appropriate indication of stenting is in extrinsic stenotic lesions caused by compression of the trachea. The choice of stent depends on the extent and location of the obstruction (see chapter IV.3, interventional bronchoscopy).

8. Tracheal operations

8.1. Introduction

Tracheal operations cover a range of procedures from simple emergency tracheostomy to complicated resection of tracheal bifurcation for cancer followed by reconstruction. In all tracheal surgery, the primary goal is the provision of a reliable airway. Reliability does not stop with the provision of respiratory airway but also many subsidiary but important functions such as expectoration of normal and abnormal secretions from the lung, active participation in coughing and phonation.

For all operations on the trachea, consideration should be given to a number of issues such as:
- Aim of the procedure,
- Level and localisation of the pathology,
- Access,
- Repair after the surgical procedure.

It is not within the scope of this chapter to describe all tracheal operations but to provide the principle of more common procedures on the trachea.

8.2. Tracheostomy

Tracheostomy is one of the oldest surgical operations which has been in use throughout the ages for different objectives. Early tracheostomies were carried out for the relief of upper airway obstructions. Since the development of respiratory support techniques the majority of tracheostomies are performed for the purpose of assisted (artificial) ventilation.

8.2.1. Indications
Tracheostomy is used for the following:
I   Bypassing obstructed upper airways
II Ventilatory assistance which may be required for:

- Patients with respiratory failure
- Neurological conditions affecting the respiratory muscles
- Severe cases of thoracic wall injuries with paradoxical breathing and an unstable chest
- Respiratory complications of cardiac operations and pulmonary resection
- Patients with severe pulmonary infection

III   For aspiration of bronchial secretions:
- In pulmonary suppurations
- Following lung resection when the patient is unable to clear the airways with physiotherapy alone and when repeated and frequent bronchoscopy may have to be carried out.

Timing of the tracheostomy is dependent on several factors such as the clinical condition of the patient and whether an endotracheal tube is already in place. It has been said that the time for tracheostomy is when the clinician debates whether or not to perform tracheostomy.

8.2.2. Preparation

It is important to prepare the patient and the family, explaining the reason for tracheostomy, the nature of the procedure, its risk and possible complications.

The operation is facilitated when in addition to the tracheostomy set the following instruments are added:
- One self-retaining (Neislander type) retractor,
- Tracheostomy (dilating) forceps,
- One blunt (skin/cricoid) hook,
- Suction machine, tubing and a sterile suction catheter must not be forgotten.

8.2.3. Tracheostomy tubes

A variety of plastic tubes are available with or without inflatable cuffs. In addition, silver tracheostomy tubes are an option. A selection of sterile plastic tubes with inflatable cuffs should be ready at the start of the operation. At operation, a cuffed tube should be inserted; this is mandatory when assisted ventilation is to be undertaken. This tube may later be changed to a non-cuffed tube or a silver type tube as required. The size of the tracheostomy tube employed depends on the size of the patient's trachea. The size of endotracheal tube used by the anaesthetist at the start of the operation may be taken as a guide in selecting the size of tracheostomy tube (Table 1).

8.2.4. The operation

Tracheostomy is generally carried out in an operating theatre under general anaesthesia administered

Table 1

Sizes of tracheostomy tubes

Endotracheal tube size	Tracheostomy tube size	External diameter (mm)
7	30	10
7.5	30–32	10–11
8	31–33	11–11.5
9	36–38	12–13

through the endotracheal tube. In certain circumstances the operation may have to be carried out under local anaesthesia in an intensive care unit with the patient placed on his bed.

- The patient is positioned supine on the operating table with the neck hyper extended by placing a sandbag, inflatable bag or pillow under the shoulders. Surgical drapes are placed to cover the whole of the patient with the exception of the neck from the lower border of the mandible down to the upper border of the sternum vertically and the lateral borders of the neck transversally.
- Skin incision is made either as:
  (a) Vertical incision 4 to 6 cm from the lower border of the thyroid cartilage downwards towards the suprasternal notch.
  (b) Transverse collar incision 4 to 5 cm long, a finger breadth (1.5 to 2 cm) below the cricoid cartilage (Fig. 3a).

The platysma is incised and the pre-tracheal strap muscle fibres are split in the midline and retracted laterally using the self-retaining retractor to expose the thyroid isthmus which is then divided. The pre-tracheal fascia is divided to expose the tracheal cartilages and the site of the tracheostomy (usually between the 2nd and 3rd cartilage) is selected (Fig. 3b). Before incising the trachea, the following pieces of apparatus are brought near the operative field:
- Tracheostomy tube with its introducer in situ,
- Syringe for inflation of the cuff of the tube,
- Suction catheter connected to suction tubing and machine for tracheal suction when the opening is made,
- Container for collection of secretions,
- Length of tubing and connectors for the attachment of the tracheostomy tube to the anaesthetic machine.

The endotracheal tube is withdrawn by the anaesthetist to above the site of the proposed tracheal incision. The trachea is then incised (Fig. 3c) between the 2nd and 3rd tracheal ring and a small portion of the cartilage (about 5 mm) is excised to allow easy

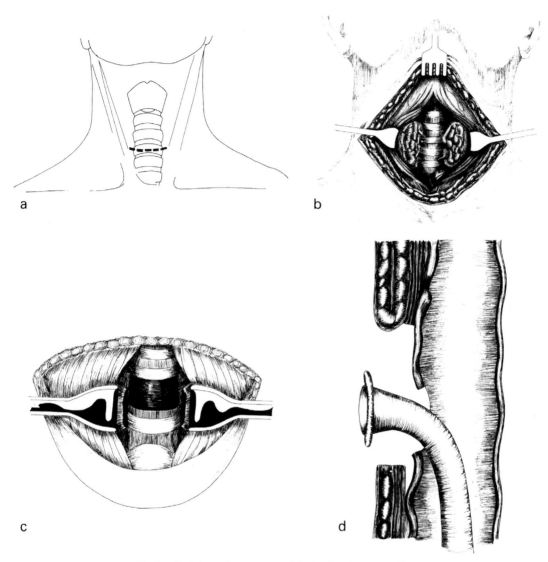

Fig. 3. a to d shows the sequence of the tracheostomy operation.

insertion of the tracheostomy tube. The opening is enlarged and the tracheal dilator is introduced into the trachea. It is important not to excise too much of the cartilage in adults, and not to excise any in children. The trachea is cleaned of secretions by suction and a sample is collected for microbiological studies.

A tracheostomy tube is introduced (Fig. 3d) and the cuff is inflated to fit the lumen without any air leak. The tracheostomy tube is next connected to the anaesthetic apparatus and the original endotracheal tube is completely withdrawn. One skin stitch may have to be applied to approximate the excess incision. A dry gauze is applied just over the incision and the tracheostomy tube is secured by lateral tapes.

8.2.5. Management of Tracheostomy

Management of tracheostomy involves:
- Care of the equipment,
- Humidification,
- Tracheobronchial aspiration of secretions,
- Microbiological monitoring and prevention of infection,
- Nutrition,
- Extubation.

Care of the equipment. This includes the tracheostomy tube and its accessory attachments which connect the patient's respiratory tract to the ventilator. It also includes the management of the tracheostomy tube and inflatable cuff.

The main points are:

- The provision of support for the connectors and additional tubing in order to prevent trauma and necrosis of the tissues, particularly at the site of the stoma.
- The sealing cuff should allow a combination of a high volume of inflation with a low pressure. The inflation should be just sufficient to occlude the lumen of the trachea in order to stop a leak between it and the tracheal wall (i.e. minimum occluding volume).

Humidification. Inspired air must be humidified with water vapour at body temperature. Dryness of inspired air causes drying of secretions and reduces the natural mucosal decontamination and disinfection. The patient who is on assisted ventilation receives humidified inspired air via an inline humidifier incorporated into the ventilator system. For others, a humidifier or nebuliser should be provided.

Tracheobronchial aspiration. This must be carried out with aseptic precautions. The suction must be brief (5 to 10 seconds). The frequency of aspiration must be judged according to the volume of secretions and with the consideration that:

(i)   Each suction manoeuvre is a traumatic event.
(ii) With the patient receiving assisted ventilation the assistance cannot be interrupted too frequently or for too long.
(iii) For the suction to be effective, good physiotherapy and humidification is necessary. The injection of 2 to 5 ml of sterile normal saline through the tracheostomy tube into the trachea before aspiration helps the procedure.

The technique of tracheal aspiration and the equipment used are both important:

- Suction catheters should not be so soft as to bend and curl easily in the trachea since these would be ineffective and thereby give the impression of lack of secretions.
- The catheter should not be connected directly to the suction machine. This provides uncontrolled negative suction pressure. The addition of a Y or T connector or the provision of a catheter with a finger hole allows the control which is necessary.
- Aspiration is applied during the withdrawal of the catheter.
- The catheter is changed after each aspiration.

Microbiological monitoring and prevention of infection. A sample of secretion should be dispatched to the microbiological laboratory for identification of organisms, culture and sensitivity to antibiotic, daily in the early post-operative period and later every 2 or 3 days. It is not advisable to use prophylactic antibiotics since the development of resistant organisms is likely to occur. In addition, fungal infection may also supervene. However, in the presence of infection an appropriate antibiotic regimen should be undertaken.

Nutrition. In many patients with tracheostomy and assisted ventilation it is not possible to proceed with normal alimentary tract nutrition. It must not, however, be forgotten that a patient who is on ventilatory assistance requires adequate nutrition. Parenteral and/or enteral methods of feeding may be used according to metabolic demands and the expected duration of artificial feeding.

Extubation. The extubation of the tracheostomy is considered when the patient is strong enough to breathe spontaneously, respiratory function is satisfactory and sputum can be expectorated normally. The following points are relevant with respect to extubation.

In most adults and in many children the tracheostomy tube is removed without complication. The tracheostomy wound is cleaned, swabbed and a dry dressing applied. The stoma usually heals within a week. It is the practice of the author to bronchoscope every patient who has had tracheostomy when the tube has been removed and the stoma healed. Some advise bronchoscopy before the tube is finally removed only if the tracheostomy has been in place for more than 2 to 3 weeks. In young children and sometimes in adults, the tracheostomy tube cannot be removed at once and it is necessary to proceed with extubation in stages, gradually using smaller tubes.

8.2.6. Complications of tracheostomy

Some complications arise essentially from faulty operative techniques, others from faulty post-operative management, whilst a third group develop as a result of a combination of factors (Table 2).

Operative complications. Apart from haemorrhage and accidental injury to neighbouring structures during the operation, malpositioning of the incision and the tracheostomy opening are responsible for some complications which appear at a later stage.

A tracheostomy incision and opening, when placed too high, is hazardous and risks injury to the 1st tra-

Table 2

Tracheostomy complications

Type of complication	Time of appearance	Common cause	What to do
(1) Haemorrhage	At operation Early post-op Late (infection)	Technical error (accident) Reactive ? innominate artery	Check and arrest Check: take urgent expert advice
(2) Tube displaced	Early post-op	Faulty technique Inadequate post-op management	Recognise and replace
(3) Tube blockage	Early + Later	Dryness Inadequate suction Copious secretion	Recognise and change tube
(4) Aspiration of food	Early	Incoordination of swallowing Neurological	Delay feeding Inflate sealing cuff
(5) Infection	Early + Later	Faulty nursing technique Cross infection	Check sterilisation technique Upper respiratory Toilet
(6) Pulmonary collapse	Early + Later	Cross-infection Dryness Mucous plug	Recognise Bronchoscopy and aspiration
(7) Tracheal injuries	Early + Late	Faulty technique Sealing cuff pressure Necrosis Infection	Recognise and treat, see section 1 in this chapter

cheal ring and the cricoid cartilage, with subsequent chondritis and subglottic stenosis. An incision which is too low will cause difficulties in the changing of the tube and will also promote its displacement during flexion of the neck. In addition, such an incision can cause compression of the innominate artery between the intubated trachea and the sternal manubrium with a risk of fistula forming between the trachea and the innominate artery.

Post-operative complications.
- *Accidental extubation*
  In individuals with a short and thick neck this complication can arise, particularly when the patient is restless and not carefully observed. If the patient is receiving artificial ventilation this complication can be fatal.
- *Post-operative haemorrhage*
  Haemorrhage may occur from inside or outside the lumen. Bleeding from mucosal vessels generally stops an hour or two after the operation. During this time, particular care is needed to ascertain that the airways are clear. Pre-tracheal bleeding must be investigated and checked.
- *Tube obstruction*
  In patients with copious thick secretions, the tra-

cheostomy tube may become obstructed early after operation. This may go unnoticed by an inexperienced nurse even during endotracheal suction or in a patient connected to a pressure controlled ventilator.

Aspiration of food particles in patients with a non-inflatable cuff tube can occur in the early post-operative period. In some patients oral feeding has to be tried cautiously after 4 or 5 days. If there is evidence of spillage the inflatable cuff tube may have to be used with the balloon inflated during meals. Alternatively, enteral feeding via a fine tube may be used.
- *Pulmonary infection*
  Upper respiratory and pulmonary infection is one of the commonest, and potentially fatal, complications. Gram-negative organisms, notably Pseuduomonas aeruginosa are particularly troublesome and difficult to eradicate.
- *Pulmonary collapse and atelectasis*
  A number of patients with tracheostomy have copious secretions. In some, dry secretions form a plug of cerumen, an encrusted material which obstructs segmental, lobar or even a main bronchial lumen, resulting in atelectasis and pulmonary collapse. Humidification, with effective physiother-

apy and tracheal suction, usually prevents this
complication. Bronchoscopic suction is nevertheless required in some cases and may be carried
out through the tracheostomy stoma.

• *Tracheal injuries*
Tracheo-oesophageal fistula, tracheomalacia and
tracheal stenosis are rare complications. Pressure
necrosis caused primarily by the sealing cuff has

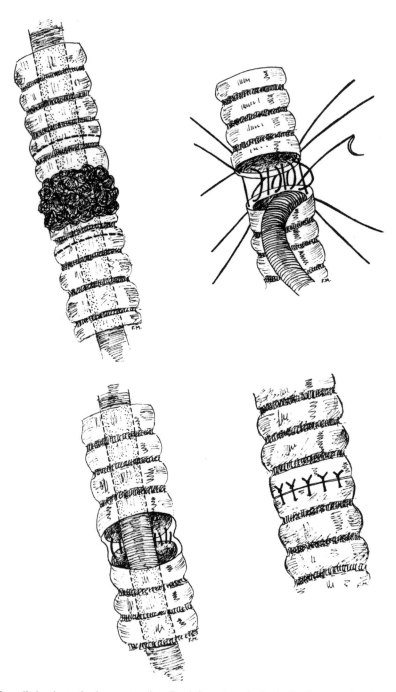

Fig. 4. Management of ventilation in tracheal reconstruction. Top left: endotracheal tube in place, passing through the lesion. Top right:
Tracheal lesion is excised. Ventilation is continued through endotracheal tube (B) introduced in the lower tracheal segment. Posterior
wall is reconstructed. Bottom left: The tube (B) is removed from the lower trachea after completion of posterior wall reconstruction and
the original tube (A) is passed down the trachea. Bottom right: anterior wall reconstruction is completed (see text).

been responsible for many reported cases. Granuloma and firm fibrous stricture can form at the site of the tracheostomy because of faulty technique. These manifest themselves when the tracheostomy tube is removed.

8.3. Percutaneous mini-tracheostomy

8.3.1. Introduction

This refers to a tracheostomy which is established through a short 1–1.5 cm skin incision. In practice, a short vertical skin incision is made down from the lower border of the cricoid. The trachea is entered by a wide-bore catheter covered needle. A guide wire is then passed into the tracheal lumen over which sequentially larger diameter dilators are introduced over the wire until the required size opening is obtained. The tracheostomy tube is next advanced into the trachea over the dilator.

Percutaneous tracheostomy was introduced in the 1960s. In the 1980s its use gained popularity and its indications widened to include those of standard tracheostomy.

The advantages of percutaneous tracheostomy are: its simplicity and the rapidity and ease of its placement. Besides rare fatality, the complications of percutaneous tracheostomy include haemorrhage, false route and pneumothorax.

9. Tracheal reconstruction

9.1. Approaches

Almost all operations on the trachea can be carried out using one of two approaches:

- Cervical and/or cervicomediastinal approach. This consists of an anterior collar incision with a downwards vertical extension over the sternum which can be divided. This allows mobilisation of the whole of the trachea and both bronchi, together with excision of a large part of the cervical trachea followed by its reconstruction.
- Right posterolateral thoracotomy approach through the 4th intercostal space. This approach allows good mobilisation of a great portion of the trachea and both main bronchi, together with excision of the lower trachea and the two main bronchi followed by reconstruction.

9.2. Anaesthesia and ventilation during the operation

One of the basic technical problems in tracheal surgery is the maintenance of adequate oxygenation of the patient during the operation without hindrance to the surgeon by the presence of the endotracheal tube. Cardiopulmonary bypass technique can be used, but heparinisation is a disadvantage and pulmonary complications a hazard. Problems of ventilation during resection and reconstruction of the trachea can be overcome by the use of a double endotracheal ventilation circuit as follows (Fig. 4):

- Circuit A: Consists of the standard (single lumen) endotracheal intubation at the start of the anaesthesia. The tip of the tube is placed above the lesion when it cannot pass through the stenotic segment. Alternatively, an existing tracheostomy tube may be used for the purpose of ventilation at the start of the operation. This endotracheal tube is connected to the anaesthetic machine in the usual way.
- Circuit B: An endotracheal tube is connected to separate sterile airway tubing ready at hand on the instrument trolley to be used later on during the operation.

At the start of the operation, circuit A is used, as in standard anaesthetic technique. When the trachea is incised by the surgeon and the lesion is being excised, the endotracheal tube (A) is withdrawn to well above the line of incision, but below the cords, and its use for ventilation, for the time being, is discontinued. Next, the endotracheal tube of circuit B is introduced by the surgeon (through the surgical field) into the lower tracheal segment (below the lesion which is excised) down to the left main bronchus. The patient's ventilation is maintained through this tube. The posterior layer of the tracheal anastomosis is carried out and completed first without hindrance from either of the endotracheal tubes. Following this the endotracheal tube of circuit B is withdrawn completely and the endotracheal tube of circuit A is pushed down the airway and placed into the trachea across the posterior suture line. The ventilation is now maintained through this (the original tube A). The anterior layer of the anastomosis is next completed. Note that the switch between circuit A and B, and vice versa, should be carried out swiftly and after pre-oxygenation of the patient.

The same principle is applied for tracheal bifurcation resection — lower trachea, carina and main bronchi (Fig. 5).

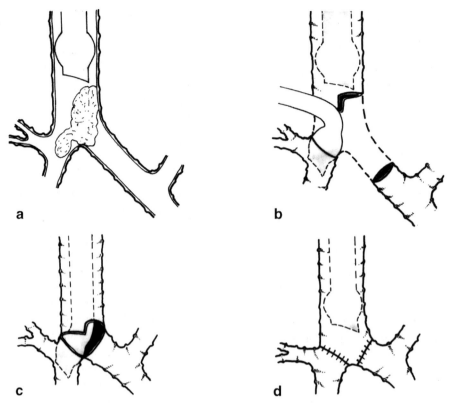

Fig. 5. Diagram illustrating the management of ventilation for bifurcation resection. Step a: an endotracheal tube is inserted into the trachea by the anesthetist above the lesion or through the obstruction after dilation. Step b: the anterior wall of the trachea is incised and the endotracheal tube (A) is withdrawn to above the lesion. A second endotracheal/endobronchial tube (B) is introduced through the incised anterior wall of the trachea to the right main bronchus below the lesion. Step c: the lesion is excised and the posterior wall of the trachea reconstructed. The second endotracheal tube (B) is removed and tube (A) is forwarded through the trachea to the right main bronchus. Step d: the anterior wall is repaired and the endobronchial tube (A) is placed in the trachea (see text).

9.3. Important technical points

During mobilisation of the trachea, attention should be paid to:
(a) Recurrent laryngeal nerves which should not be damaged,
(b) Vascularization of the trachea.

Anastomosis is carried out using non-absorbable suture material such as prolene 3/0. Flexion of the neck gives additional length and allows anastomosis to be carried out without tension. After the operation, drainage of the mediastinum should be carried out and the drains connected to an underwater sealed system of drainage.

In circumferential excision of tracheal lesions resulting in a limited (4 or 5 cm) defect, a direct end-to-end anastomosis can be carried out with good results. For more extensive defects, tracheal prostheses may be employed. Whilst tracheal prostheses, such as Marlex mesh/pericardium for patch graft-

ing have proved satisfactory, the use of prosthesis for extensive circumferential defects have been, by and large, disappointing and are not attended by sustained good results. Recently alternative tracheal prosthesis have been tried with some success particularly in children (Elliot et al., 1996).

References and further reading

Altman KW, Wetmore RF, Marsh RR. Congenital airway abnormalities requiring tracheostomy: A profile of 56 patients and their diagnosis over a 9 year period. Int J Paediat Atorhino Laryngol 1997; 41(2): 199–206.

Bodenham AR, Diament R, Cohen A, Webster N. Percutaneous dilatational tracheostomy on the intensive care unit. Anaesthesia 1991; 46: 570–572.

Borro JM, Chirivella M, Vila C, et al. Success for revascularisation of large isolated tracheal segments. Eur J Cardiothorac Surg 1992; 6: 621–623.

Cheng E, Fee WE. Dilatation versus standard tracheostomy: A meta-analysis. Ann Otol Rhinol Laryngol 2000; 109: 803–807.

Cooper JD., Grillo HC. The pathological study. Ann Surg 1969; 334–348.

Dumon JF. A dedicated tracheo-bronchial stent. Chest 1990; 97: 328–332.

Dyet JF, Moghissi K. Role of venography in assessing patients with superior vena caval obstruction caused by carcinoma for bypass operations. Thorax 1980; 35: 628–630.

Elliot MH, HaWMP, Jacobs JP, et al. Successful tracheal homograft. Eur J Cardiothorac Surg 1996; 10: 702–712.

Fanton A, Ripamonti D. A non-derivative, non-surgical tracheostomy: The translaryngeal method. Intensive Care Med 1997; 23: 386–392.

Fisher L, Duane D, Lafreniere L, et al. Percutaneous dilational tracheostomy: a safer technique of airway management using a microlaryngeal tube. Anaesthesia 2002; 57: 253–255.

Furman RH, Backer CL, Dunham ME, et al. The use of balloon expandable metallic stent in the treatment of paediatric tracheomalacia and bronchomalacia. Arch Otolaryngo P Head & Neck Surg 1999; 125: 203–207.

Garrillo HC. Tracheal tumours: surgical management. Ann Thorac Surg 1978; 26: 112–125.

Graham JS, Mulloy RH, Sutherland FR, Rose S. Percutaneous versus open tracheostomy: A retrospective cohort outcome study. J Trauma 1996; 41: 245–250.

Grillo EH, Spain DA, Bumpous JM, et al. Percutaneous dilatational tracheostomy for airway control. Am J Surg 1997; 174: 469–473.

Grillo HC, Mathisen DJ. Primary tracheal tumours: Treatment and results. Ann Thorac Surg 1990; 49: 67–77.

Grillo HC. Tracheal tumours: Surgical management. Ann Thorac Surg 1978; 26: 112–125.

Grillo HC, Wright CD, Vlahakes GJ, et al. Management of congenital tracheal stenosis by means of slide tracheoplasty or resection and reconstruction, with long-term follow-up of growth after slide tracheoplasty. J Thorac Cardiovasc Surg 2002; 123: 145–52.

Harvey-Smith W, Busch W, Northrop C. Traumatic bronchial rupture. Am J Roentgenol 1980; 134: 1189–1193.

Herzog H. Erschlaffung und expiratorische Invagination der Membranosen teile der intrathorakalen Luftrhore und der Hauptbronchienals ursache der asphyktischen Anfalle beim Asthma bronchiale und bei der chronischen asthmoiden Bronchitis des Lungemphyseme. Schweiz Med Wochenschr 1954; 84: 217–219.

Horvath P, Hecin B, Hruda J, et al. Intermediate-to-late results of surgical relief of vascular tracheobronchial compression. Euro J Cardiothorac Surg 1992; 6: 366–371.

Houston HE, Payne WS, Harrison EG Jr., Olsen AM. Primary cancers of the trachea. Arch Surg 1969; 99: 132–40.

Jackson C. Tracheostomy. Laryngoscopy 1909; 90: 430–436.

Jacobs JP, Quintessenza JA, Andrews T, Burke RP, et al. Tracheal allograft reconstruction: The total North American and Worldwide paediatric experience. Ann Thorac Surg 1999; 68: 1043–1052.

Jeretzki A, Bethea M, Wolff M, et al. A rational approach to total thymectomy in the treatment of myasthenia gravis. Ann Thorac Surg 1977; 24: 120–130.

Johnston HR, Loeber N, Hillyer P, et al. External stent for repair of secondary tracheomalacia. Ann Thorac Surg 1980; 30: 291–296.

LoCicero J III, Costello P, Campos CT, et al. Spiral CT with multiplanar and three-dimensional reconstructions accurately predicts tracheobronchial pathology. Ann Thorac Surg 1996; 62: 811–817.

Makarewicz R, Mross M. Radiation therapy alone in the treatment of tumours of the trachea. Lung Cancer 1998; 20: 169–174.

Mathisen DJ. Primary tracheal tumour management. Surg Oncol Clin N Am 1999; 8: 307.

Matthews HR, Hopkinson RB. Treatment of sputum retention by mini tracheostomy. Br J Surg 1984; 71: 147–150.

Maziak DE, Todd RTJ, Keshavjee SH, et al. Adenoid cystic carcinoma of the airway: 32 years experience. J Thorac Cardiovasc Surg 1996; 112: 1522–1532.

Moghissi K, Dixon K, Hudson E, et al. Endoscopic laser therapy in malignant tracheo-bronchial obstruction using sequential NdYAG laser and Photodynamic Therapy. Thorax 1997; 52: 281–283.

Moghissi K. Tracheal reconstruction with a prosthesis of Marlex mesh and pericardium. J Thorac Cardiovasc Surg 1975; 69: 499–506.

Montgomery WW. Suprahyoid release for tracheal stenosis. Arch Otolaryngol. 1974; 99: 255–260.

Neville WE. Prosthetic replacement of the trache. In: Grillo HC and Eschapass H (Eds.), International Trends in General Thoracic Surgery (Vol. 2). Philadelphia: WB Saunders 1987; p. 138.

Nissen R. Tracheoplastic zur Beseitigung der Erschlaffung des Membranosen teils der intrathorakalen Lufthore. Schweiz Med Wochenschr 1954; 84: 219–221.

Nomori H, Kaseda S, Kobayashi K, et al. Adenoid cystic carcinoma of the trachea and main stem bronchus: A clinical histopathological study. J Thorac Cardiovasc Surg 1986; 96: 271–277.

Perelman MI, Korolova NS. Primary tumours of the trachea. In: Grillo HC and Eschapass EH (eds.), International Trends in General Thoracic Surgery (Vol. 2). Philadelphia: WB Saunders 1987; pp. 91–110.

Perelman MI, Burukov JV, Gudovski LV, et al. Surgery of trachea and bronchus. Ann Surg 2001; 1: 30–35.

Peterffy A, Konstantinov IE. Resection of distal tracheal and carinal tumours with the aid of cardiopulmonary bypass. Scand Cardiovasc J 1998; 32: 109–112.

Prommegger R, Salzer GM. Long-term results of surgery for adenoid cystic carcinoma of the trachea and bronchi. Eur J Surg Oncol 1998; 24: 440–4.

Rainier HG, Newby JP, Kelble DL. Long term results of tracheal support surgery for emphysema. Chest 1968; 53: 765.

Refaely Y, Weissberg D. Surgical management of tracheal tumours. Ann Thorac Surg 1997; 64: 1429–1432.

Regnard JF, Fourquier P, Levasseu RP, et al. Results and prognostic factors in resection of primary tracheal tumours: A retrospective multi-centre study. J Thorac Cardiovasc Surg 1996; 111: 808–814.

Salassa JR, Pearson BW, Payne WS. Gross and microscopic blood supply of the trachea. Ann Thorac Surg 1977; 24: 100–107.

Sasaki S, Hara F, Oowa T, et al. Esophegeal tracheoplasty for congenital tracheal stenosis. J Pediatr Surg 1992; 27: 645–649.

Schneider P, Schirren J, Muley T, et al. Primary tracheal tumours: experience with 14 resected patients. Eur J Cardiothorac Surg 2001; 20: 12–8.

Sharpe DAC, Moghissi K. Tracheal resection and reconstruction: A review of 82 patients. Eur J Cardiothorac Surg 1996; 10: 1040–1046.

Sharpe DAC, Dixon K, Moghissi K. Endoscopic laser treatment for tracheal obstruction. Eur J Cardiothorac Surg 1996; 10: 722–726.

Tomaselli F, Maier A, Sankin O, et al. Successful endoscopical sealing of malignant esophageotracheal fistulae by using a covered self-expandable stenting system. Eur J Cardiothorac Surg 2001; 20: 734–738.

Velmahos GC, Gomez H, Boicey CM, et al. Bedside percutaneous tracheostomy: Prospective evaluation of a modification of the current technique in 100 patients. World J Surg 2000; 24: 1109–1115.

Wang MB, Berke GS, Ward PM, et al. Experience with percutaneous tracheostomy. Laryngoscopy 1992; 102: 157.

Weber AL, Grillo H. Tracheal lesions — Assessment by conventional films, computed tomography and magnetic resonance imaging. Isr J Med Sci 1992; 28: 233–240.

Westphal KI, Byhahn C, Rinne T, Wilke HJ. Tracheostomy in cardiosurgical patients. Surgical tracheostomy versus Ciaglia and Fantoni methods. Ann Thorac Surg 1999; 68: 486–492.

CHAPTER II.2

Tracheobronchial stenting

K. Moghissi

1. Introduction

The purpose of tracheobronchial stenting is to restore the patency of the airway which is compromised by disease. The main indication for placement of a stent is in malignant tracheobronchial stenotic lesions. However, stents are also used in some specific cases of benign stenosis. A variety of stents are now available for tracheal, tracheobronchial and bronchial strictures. Both the selection of patient and the choice of stent require careful consideration and planning.

As a general rule selection is made on the basis that:
- The lesion is not suitable for resection and airway reconstruction,
- The patient's general condition does not permit resection/reconstruction operation to be undertaken.

2. Type of stents

The many varieties of stent are categorised into three main types (Fig. 1):
- Tracheal stents,
- Tracheo-bronchial/bifurcation stents and tubes,
- Bronchial stents.

2.1. Tracheal stents

These are comprised of:

2.1.1. T-tubes
These are exemplified by the well-known Montgomery T tube (stent) (Fig. 1), which is made of silicone and is essentially a tracheostomy tube whose vertical component extends both below and above the horizontal portion. They are used to treat tracheal stenosis at all levels. A surgical tracheostomy is a prerequisite for the Montgomery tube.

Advantages of the T tubes are:
- Stability of their position once placed. Dislocation is extremely rare and their migration is near impossible.
- They can function as a tracheostomy when the horizontal portion is open or can be used for tracheo-bronchial suction through the opening. They also permit speech when the horizontal limb is plugged.
- They provide support for the collapsing trachea (tracheomalacia).

2.1.2. Straight tracheal tubes
These tubes need to have a mechanism to hold them in position within the trachea. They are inserted endoscopically and do not require a tracheostomy.
- The Dumon tube (Novatech, Abayone, France) is made of silicone with a series of studs on the outside. Displacement of the Dumon tube is rare and is usually associated with precise indications and selection since it is held in position by contact pressure and, in some cases, the existence of malacia prevents proper fitting.
- Orlowski stent (Rusch–Kernen, Germany) consists of steel wire rings embedded in silicone. The rings are intended to provide stiffness and also hold the stent in position. Its indications are for malignant stricture or firm benign stenotic lesions.

2.2. Tracheo-bronchial/bifurcation stents

These are T–Y or Y shaped tubes. When in the trachea, the Y portion sits astride the carina. The indications for placement of these stents are lower

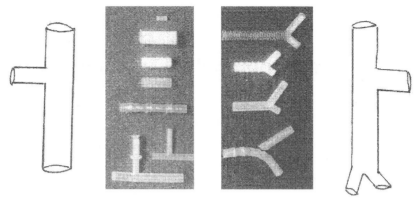

Fig. 1. Tracheo-bronchial stents (left to right): Montgomery T tube, selection of tracheo-bronchial stents, selection of bifurcated stents, Montgomery bifurcated stents.

tracheal stenosis extending to one or both bronchia. There are two varieties of these tubes, namely T–Y and Y-shaped. The T–Y tube has a horizontal limb which is fashioned into a tracheostomy stoma. The Y tube has no horizontal limb and relies on good fitting over the bifurcation of the trachea for its positional stability. When fitted properly T–Y tubes are easier to manage because the horizontal limb acts as a tracheostomy and provides better stability for the tube remaining in position.

• Westaby T–Y tubes (Hood Company, Pembroke, MA, USA): This tube is made of firm plastic/silicone and is useful for elongated stenotic lesions involving the trachea and main bronchi. It is cur-

Table 1

The characteristics of the currently available stents

Name	Reference	Important characteristics	Advantages/disadvantages
Dumon	Dumon, 1990 Dumon et al., 1996	• Coated silicone tube with studs • Various lengths and diameter • Radio-opaque variety available • Rigid bronchoscopy required	• Suitable for malignant + benign cases • Not suitable for malacia • Migration possible
Montgomery	Montgomery, 1965	• Soft silicone rubber • T-tube is very stable, can be left for months • Tracheostomy as well as stent	• Suitable for malignant + benign cases • Suitable for malacia • Can be replaced with ease • Mucous secretion retention is rare
Westeby T–Y tube	Westeby et al., 1982	• Relatively rigid plastic/silicone • Suitable for elongated stenosis • Rigid bronchoscopy required	• Used in malignant cases • Retention of secretion + (requires frequent cleaning)
Gianturco	Simond et al., 1989 George et al., 1990	• Originally made of Z wire • Can be placed by flexible fibreoptic bronchoscope	• Granulation tissue • Perforation • Fatigue fracture possible • High rate of failure
Wallstent	Monier et al., 1996	• Woven metal surrounded by layer of polyurethane • Requires rigid bronchoscopy	• The cover prevents growth of granulation tissue • Suitable for malignant + benign stenosis
Ultraflex strecker	Strecker et al., 1990 Becker, 1990	• Originally made from Tantalum, now made from Nitinol (wire filament) • Available covered with polyurethane or uncovered • Can be placed by flexible fibreoptic bronchoscope	• Suitable for malignant + benign cases • Permits axial and radial movements of wire filaments • Adapts well to distorted lumen

rently available in three diameters. Insertion needs experience and the use of a rigid bronchoscope.
- Hood bifurcated stent: is a soft silicone tube and insertion requires rigid bronchoscopy skill. Its use has not been popular in Europe.
- Dynamic (Rusch) stent: is a bifurcated stent made of silicone. It has a flexible posterior membrane which protrudes inwards during coughing increasing the efficiency of expectoration. This stent is useful for a range of conditions from tracheo-oesophageal fistula to long stenosis involving the trachea and main stem bronchi.

2.3. Bronchial stents

There is now a plethora of endobronchial stents made of silicone rubber, stainless steel mesh and metal embedded in silicon (Table 1). Many are made in different diameters to fit in different bronchial "sizes". Some are expandable after they are inserted.
- Bronchial stent with flange (Hood Pembroke Laboratories): are straight tubes with a shorter flange at both ends helping to stabilise the position once they are fitted. They are not in common use (at least in Europe).
- Straight studded tube (Dumon) stent: is made of coated silicone with little studs on the outside. This stent is by far the most utilised stent in Europe and is available in various lengths and diameters. The range is such that in most cases they can be fitted into the trachea and bronchi. A bifurcated Dumon Stent has also been produced.
- Gianturco stent: is a stainless steel wire, shaped like a cylinder. The stent is held in a cartridge which discharges it to the target position.
- Wall stent (Schneider–Pfizer, Switzerland): is a woven filament of stainless steel alloy.
  In stents made of stainless steel mesh or filaments, the wire elements are held in a porous material and expand after insertion to a predetermined diameter. The disadvantage of the porous stent in cancer cases is that the tumour can grow through the wire mesh and obstruct the lumen of the stent. However, there are modified metallic stents in which the wire filaments are covered with a plastic material to prevent tumour in-growth.
- Ultraflex Strecker stent: is a nitinol stent in a knitted design which allows axial and radial movement of the wire filaments. This stent has been used for malignant and benign strictures and sealing oesophago-airway fistula.
- Modified Gianturco stent: is now available in

which the wire is covered thus preventing growth through the pores.

3. Placement of tracheo-bronchial stent

3.1. General principles

- The patient will have had full investigation, including imaging, and diagnosis.
- Pulmonary function assessment; at least Peak Expiratory Flow and FEV_1 is required. This allows evaluation of the effectiveness of the function of the stent.
- The rigid bronchoscope is best used in all cases, and is mandatory in most. The flexible instrument can be used for placement of some stents (Gianturco).
- General anaesthetic, administered by an anaesthetist experienced in bronchoscopy, is usually required.
- Assessment of the stenotic lesion and its dilatation is a necessary pre-requisite in all patients with stenosis. Bulky tumours may be given pre-stent NdYAG (Neodymium Yitrium Aluminium Garnet) laser treatment to facilitate stent placement.
- Position of the stent should be checked bronchoscopically after its placement.
- Most stents need cleaning and clearing from secretions, blood and debris every 3 or 4 months.
- Patients need to be monitored and have, at least, one repeat peak flow and FEV_1 measurement after placement of the stent, and at follow-up.

3.2. Preliminary assessment

Besides investigation related to the aetiology of the tracheo-bronchial lesion and imaging, specific endoscopic assessment of the airway is a mandatory requirement. It is important to record the location and extent of the lesion within the trachea and to evaluate the diameter of the inner trachea and to assess the length, consistency and diameter of the stricture. This assessment is best achieved by rigid bronchoscopy carried out under general anaesthetic. If necessary the stricture should be dilated thus allowing a more complete assessment of the required parameters.

It is necessary to accurately measure:
(a) The endoscopic length of trachea between the vocal cords and the carina,
(b) Distance between the cords and the upper border of the lesion,
(c) The extent of the stenotic lesion,

metal stent for recurrent tracheal obstruction. Lancet 1990: 335: 582–584.

Heitz M, Bolliger CT. Tracheo bronchial insertion of the dynamic (Rusch) stent. J Bronchol 1997; 4: 250–254.

Monnier P, Murdy A, Stanzel F, et al. Wallstent for the palliative treatment of inoperable tracheo-bronchial cancer: A prospective multi centre study. Chest 1996; 110: 1161–1168.

Montgomery WW. T Tube tracheal stent. Arch Otolaryngol 1965; 82: 320–321.

Nashef SA, Dromer C, Velly JF, et al. Expanding wire stents in benign tracheobronchial disease: indications and complications. Ann Thorac Surg: 1992; 54: 937–940.

Neville WE, Hamouda F, Anderson J, et al. Replacement of the intrathoracic trachea and both stem bronchi with a molded silastic prosthesis. J Thorac Cardiovasc Surg 1972; 63: 569–576.

Orlowski TM. Palliative intubation of tracheo bronchial tree. J Thorac Cardiovasc Surg 1987; 94: 343–348.

Simonds AK, Irving JD, Clarke SW, et al. Use of expandable metal stents in the treatment of bronchial obstruction. Thorax 1989; 44: 680–681.

Strecker EP, Liermann D, Barth KH, et al. Expandable tubular stents for treatment of arterial occlusive disease: Experimental and clinical results. Radiology 1990; 175: 87–102.

Westeby S, Jackson JW, Pearson FG. Bifurcated silicone rubber stent for relief of: tracheo-bronchial obstruction. J Thorac Cardiovasc Surg 1982; 83: 414–417.

CHAPTER II.3

Mediastinal surgery

K. Moghissi

1. General topography

The mediastinum extends vertically from the thoracic inlet to the diaphragm and from one mediastinal pleura to the other transversally. The anterior and posterior walls of the mediastinum are the sternum and the vertebral column respectively. It contains important structures, some of which require room for expansion. This is provided for by mobile lateral walls and loose connective tissue binding the various structures. Although this arrangement is essential to the functioning of the heart and to the distensible oesophagus during deglutition, it also favours the spread of infection which can run through the space and within its various planes. A horizontal line passing from the second costal cartilages to the lower border of the 4th thoracic vertebra divides the mediastinum into the superior mediastinum above and inferior mediastinum below (Fig. 1).

The inferior mediastinum is further subdivided into three compartments by the heart and pericardium: in front is the anterior mediastinum, behind is the posterior mediastinum, and between is the middle mediastinum. There are some important points about the mediastinum and its divisions which are surgically relevant:

The division of the mediastinum into compartments, though empirical, is convenient for topographical classification of mediastinal lesions. It is also of diagnostic value as many tumours and cysts occupy a definite anatomical position within a specific mediastinal compartment.

The pre-vertebral fascia extends from the neck into the superior mediastinum and is attached over the 4th thoracic vertebra. A neck infection behind the fascia spreads down to the front of the 4th thoracic vertebra where it is limited by the lower attachment of the fascia.

The pre-tracheal fascia extends from the neck to the superior mediastinum where it is attached to the fibrous connective tissue of the arch of the aorta. Infection in front of the pre-tracheal fascia opens into the anterior mediastinum.

Between the pre-tracheal and the pre-vertebral fascia, the neck spaces communicate with the superior and posterior mediastinum. A purulent collection in front of the prevertebral fascia can thus track down from the neck to the superior and posterior mediastinum.

2. Diagnostic methods in mediastinal lesions

2.1. Symptoms

Many mediastinal lesions are asymptomatic; pain, dyspnoea, or palpitation may occasionally be present but are not specific to mediastinal pathology. Compressive syndrome of great vessels, trachea or oesophagus is observed in certain tumours.

2.2. Imaging

Radiological investigations provide cardinal diagnostic indices. Tumours and cysts have a definite anatomical position within the compartments of the mediastinum (Fig. 2). Therefore, plain postero-anterior and lateral view chest radiograph give an indication of the possible pathology and the most appropriate investigations to be undertaken. Computerised tomography (CT) of the thorax and/or magnetic resonance imaging (MRI) are usually required to outline the pathology. It is relevant to note that, on a standard postero-anterior chest radiograph, a mediastinal abnormality may not be identified, as many of the mediastinal structures and organs possess similar density and overlap each other. Nevertheless,

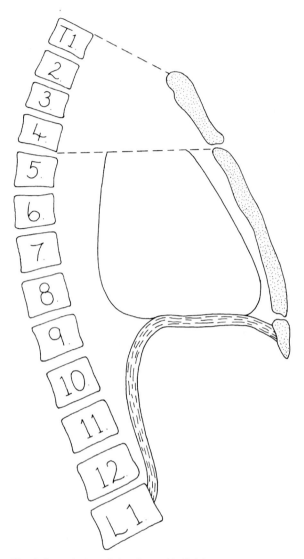

Fig. 1. Lateral view of the chest with division to compartments of the mediastinum.

both CT scan and MRI may have to be undertaken; imaging investigations are complimentary and not competitively exclusive.

- Ultrasonography, either transcutaneous or transoesophageal are important additional investigations in specific pathological situations. Two outstanding areas of their contribution are in the diagnosis of cardiac abnormalities and of mediastinal fluid collection. Transcutaneous ultrasound is extremely useful in the identification of mediastinal, pericardial and loculated pleural fluid collection, as well as in guiding of needle aspiration and tube or catheter drainage to the appropriate site. Transoesophageal ultrasound is now used to evaluate cardiac and aortic lesions and to monitor the effectiveness of the surgical repair of anomalies.

- Isotope scanning with the use of radionuclide Iodine-131 has a definite place in thyroid pathology and 99m-TC is useful in displaying the distribution of the blood supply of an organ under investigation.

2.3. Endoscopy

Bronchoscopy, oesophagoscopy, mediastinoscopy (mediastinotomy) and pleuroscopy are of considerable value in confirming the diagnosis of mediastinal pathology and may provide biopsy material.

With this range of investigatory methods the clinician has to consider:

(a) Which investigations are likely to be most helpful in a given situation,

(b) At what stage to submit a patient to more invasive types of tests such as mediastinotomy and/ or surgical exploration. The latter must always be planned with the double aims of exploration and total excision when this can be undertaken.

2.3.1. Standard cervical mediastinoscopy

Mediastinoscopy (Fig. 3) allows visual and digital exploration of the anterior/superior mediastinum as well as the possibility of obtaining lymph node biopsies. The procedure is of particular value in the diagnosis of hilar or mediastinal lymphadenopathy. The indications for mediastinoscopy are as follows:

- In otherwise undiagnosed mediastinal lymphadenopathy such as Hodgkin's disease.
- In the diagnosis of intrathoracic and pulmonary disease such as sarcoidosis and tuberculosis.
- In bronchial carcinoma:
  - When the diagnosis is in doubt,

plain X-ray (PA and lateral view) would indicate the anatomical position and narrow down the nature of the lesion and the choice of investigations which it would be most useful to follow.

- CT scanning has an important diagnostic role in mediastinal pathology as it can eliminate the difficulty of interpretation related to overlying structures. The use of linear tomography has lessened since the advent of CT but it still has a place in the demonstration of tracheal stenosis.

- MRI has become an invaluable diagnostic tool, particularly in the demonstration of neck structures through to the thoracic inlet and the superior mediastinum. In a number of mediastinal pathologies,

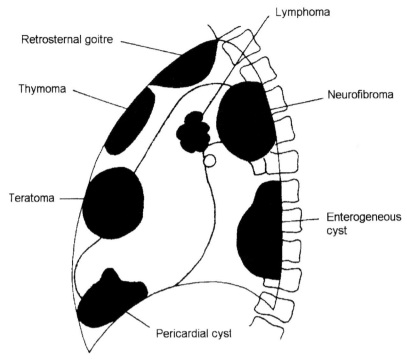

Fig. 2. Topography of the pathological lesions within the mediastinal compartments.

– When operability is in question on account of superior mediastinal lymphatic node involvement,
– In the staging process.

2.3.2. Procedure

Mediastinoscopy is carried out under general anaesthesia, with controlled ventilation, in order to minimise the risk of sudden movement which can occur by coughing or variation of breathing which might disturb the manoeuvre.

• Position of the patient: The patient is placed supine on the table, with the head extended and shoulders supported on a sandbag or inflatable bag. If the table is tilted, foot downwards, facilitating the procedure.

• Cleaning and towelling. The neck and upper part of the chest are cleaned with an antiseptic solution. Drapes, two small and one large, may be sufficient to border the surgical field. Alternatively, a large towel with an appropriate hole in its upper quarter can be used to cover the patient, except for a triangular area bordered by the lower border of the mandible above, the anterior border of the sternomatoid muscles laterally and the upper part of the sternum (exposing the suprasternal notch) inferiorly.

• A 2 to 3 cm incision is made transversely just above the suprasternal notch.

• The paratracheal muscles are separated medially and retracted on each side laterally to expose the trachea. The pretracheal fascia is divided transversely, small veins are coagulated and the inferior thyroid veins are retracted laterally.

• A finger is introduced behind the pretracheal fascia to bluntly dissect the pretracheal space and a tunnel is made between the trachea and the manubrium of the sternum (behind the innominate artery) to accommodate the mediastinoscope. Finger exploration will be useful for palpation of paratracheal lymphadenopathy or other abnormalities and is an essential part of the procedure.

• The mediastinoscope is now introduced in place of the finger in the prepared tunnel. Paratracheal, subcarinal and superior hilar glands can be dissected using the crocodile jaw forceps and small swabs. If there are small bleeding points these should be coagulated using electrocautery, or packed with a swab for a minute or so to clear the field before restarting the dissection. Care should be taken to avoid injury to the left recurrent laryngeal nerve on the left lateral aspect of the trachea.

• A sample of tissue can be obtained by taking a biopsy from pathological lymph nodes. Alterna-

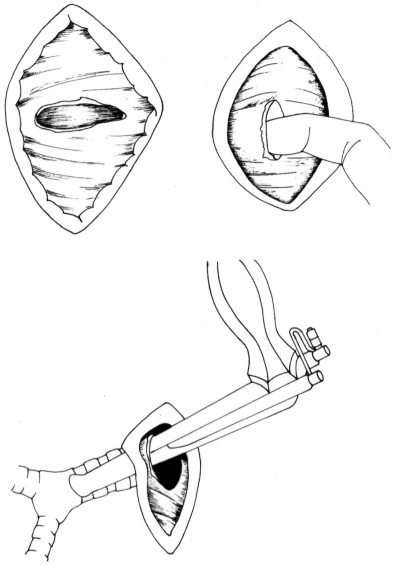

Fig. 3. Diagram illustrating mediatinoscopy procedure. Patient in supine position, head is on the right-hand side of the diagram. Top left: skin incision and splitting of pre-tracheal muscles; top right: finger exploration of the pre-tracheal space down to the mediastinum; bottom: the instrument is introduced into the superior mediastinal space.

tively, the whole gland (if this can be identified) is dissected out for histological examination. Inexperienced operators may aspirate the proposed site of the biopsy (using a long needle and syringe), ensuring first that the structure under vision is not a blood vessel.

- On completion of the examination, the instrument is withdrawn, the pretracheal muscles are approximated using 2 or 3 absorbable stitches and the subcutaneous tissue of the neck is closed. Finally, clips are applied to the skin or subcutical skin closure method is used.

Mediastinoscopy aftercare. One or two hours following operation, chest X-ray should be carried out and regular nursing observations made half-hourly for three to four hours after the procedure. Particular attention should be paid to breathing (stridor due to pressure see below). In uncomplicated cases the patient is discharged a few hours later. Skin clips are removed four days later in the outpatient clinic, when applicable.

Complications of mediastinoscopy. In experienced hands, mediastinoscopy usually has no mortality or morbidity. However, it is important to be aware of the occasional complications which occur in order to inform the patient and to be able to deal with them.

- Haemorrhage: Acute haemorrhage at the time of operation is usually due to inadvertent injury to a major vessel such as the azygos vein or pulmonary artery during biopsy. Very rarely the innominate artery may be injured. The area should be packed with swabs to temporarily control the haemorrhage. An appropriate thoracotomy is then carried out to repair the damaged vessel.
- Pneumothorax: This may be diagnosed at the time of the operation or may be diagnosed post-operatively when the patient is X-rayed. In either case the pleura is drained.
- Surgical subcutaneous emphysema: The patient's chest should be X-rayed. If there is pneumothorax the pleura is drained; if there is no pneumothorax, the patient is observed and again X-rayed if the emphysema does not resolve.
- Dyspnoea and stridor: These are rare complications caused by pressure from a haematoma over and around the trachea. The wound (subcutaneous and pretracheal layer) is opened and the pressure symptoms relieved by evacuation of the haematoma.
- Injury to the recurrent laryngeal nerve: This may occur occasionally during biopsy.

2.3.3. Anterior mediastinoscopy
The field of vision of cervical mediastinoscopy does not allow visualisation of a mass or lymph nodes located in the aorto-pulmonary window. If biopsies are required from such nodes, anterior mediastinoscopy is a convenient alternative or adjunct to cervical mediastinoscopy.

2.3.4. Procedure
- With the patient in supine position and under general anaesthesia and endotracheal intubation, the left hemithorax is cleaned and prepared using appropriate towels.
- A three to four cm incision is made over the left 2nd intercostal space near the costo-chondral junction.
- Pectoralis muscles are divided in the direction of their fibres and retracted to reach the intercostal muscles, which are, in turn, divided above the upper border of the third rib. Entry to the mediastinal pleura may be avoided by blunt dissection and retraction laterally.

- The mediastinoscope, thoracoscope or bronchoscope can then be introduced into the chest and blunt dissection undertaken to reach the desired structure under vision. Once the biopsy sample is obtained the wound is repaired by approximation of muscles (usually only the pectoralis). If the pleura has been opened, a small catheter is left through the incision into the chest and the muscular layer is approximated around it. When the lung is expanded by the anaesthetist using sustained positive pressure, the catheter can be withdrawn and the skin incision closed.
- Chest radiograph should be taken before the patient is discharged a few hours later.

2.3.5. Mediastinotomy
In the strict sense of the word, this term means surgical opening of the mediastinum but in its practical application it signifies a limited opening made for diagnostic biopsies or for the purpose of draining the mediastinum. Therefore, mediastinotomy needs to be differentiated from the surgical approach to the mediastinum for excision of lesions.

Cervical mediastinotomy. This is indicated for drainage of purulent collection in the superior mediastinum, such as that resulting from a perforation of the cervical oesophagus. The patient is placed in the supine position with the head rotated away from the intended side of the drainage (the author prefers to use the right side of the neck). A three to four cm incision is made in the lower part of the neck transversely or along the anterior border of the sternomastoid muscles. The anterior border of the muscle is retracted posteriorly and the omohyoid muscle is divided to expose the carotid sheath. The inferior thyroid vessels may need dividing in order to retract the carotid sheath posterolaterally. The deep cervical fascia is reached and incised in order to enter into the retro-oesophageal space which extends down to the mediastinum.

Posterior mediastinotomy. In the majority of cases of cervical oesophageal perforation, the pleural cavity is also involved and there is usually a purulent pleural effusion in addition to the mediastinal collection. In this case, the drainage of the posterior mediastinum is carried out using a transpleural approach which permits mediastinal mediastinotomy as well as pleural drainage. This approach is more appropriate than either cervical mediastinotomy or extrapleural low posterior mediastinotomy together with separate pleural drainage. The site of fluid collection can be identified by ultrasonic imaging.

When posterior mediastinotomy alone is intended, a small portion of an appropriate rib which is most dependent to the site of fluid collection is excised following a vertical paravertebral skin incision and division of the fibres of latissimus dorsi. A finger is introduced to reach the extrapleural collection of pus, which is first aspirated using a wide bore needle and syringe for confirmation of the site and depth from the surface of the collection.

In transpleural drainage of the posterior mediastinum, a limited posterolateral thoracotomy is made (see thoracotomies) and the mediastinal pleura between the aorta and the oesophagus is incised. One or two drains are inserted in the mediastinum and the pleural space is also drained via a basal chest tube. All drains are connected to an underwater sealed system.

Anterior mediastinotomy. This procedure is usually undertaken for diagnostic purposes of histologically unidentified hilar mass, hilar lymphadenopathy or biopsy of mediastinal glands which are beyond the reach of cervical mediastinoscopy.

With the patient in a supine position an incision is made over the 3rd costal cartilage of the relevant side. The bed of the resected costal cartilage is incised and the pleura gently moved back by blunt dissection to gain access to the pathological glands (previously located by an antero-posterior and lateral view chest radiograph). Digital exploration, followed by biopsy of glands, is carried out. In some cases it may be possible to achieve a larger opening by inserting a small self-retaining retractor (such as the Sellor's combined approximator and rib spreader, Fig. 4 in chapter I.4) to incise the mediastinal pleura and to carry out lung biopsy if required. Insertion of a thoracoscope or bronchoscope through the opening provides additional scope for exploration. At the conclusion of the procedure the wound is closed without a drain if the pleura has not been entered; otherwise a small chest drain is inserted through the site. In all cases the drain is connected to an underwater sealed drainage system.

3. Mediastinal infections — mediastinitis

Mediastinal infections and inflammations are serious conditions with a high rate of mortality if not recognised and treated appropriately in an early stage of evolution. This is particularly the case in the necrotizing type.

3.1. Posterior mediastinitis

This is a serious condition particularly when, as is commonly the case, it follows perforation or anastomotic leak of the oesophagus. Perforation of the oesophagus may be instrumental, spontaneous or through ingestion of a penetrating foreign body. Posterior mediastinitis may also result from thoracic trauma, directly through a penetrating injury or, rarely, indirectly through the rupture of the oesophagus by blunt traumatic injury.

A variety of organisms (gram-positive and gram-negative) as well as anaerobes are usually present.

3.2. Anterior mediastinitis:

Currently the commonest cause of anterior mediastinitis is associated with heart surgery (see also sternal infection, section 6 in chapter II.6). The organisms involved are usually a mixture of aerobic and anaerobic bacteria and gram-negative bacilli. In recent years the methicillin resistant staphylococci aureus (MRSA) organism has become an inevitable assailant particularly in those cases treated by long periods of inappropriate antimicrobial therapy and/or inadequate management.

The rapidity with which infection spreads in the mediastinum is explainable on the basis of the anatomical arrangement of the mediastinum and its fascial spaces.

The general symptoms and signs of mediastinitis are those of serious infection with hyperpyrexia, tachycardia, tachypnoea, acute chest pain and leucocytosis. In addition, more specific signs and symptoms related to the cause of the mediastinitis are present. In mediastinitis following oesophageal perforation, the clinical history and presentation are indicative of the source of the infection. In addition, subcutaneous emphysema and gas in the tissue spaces of the neck and mediastinum are evident radiologically. In the case of mediastinitis following sternotomy, the wound often displays evidence of inflammation and discharge.

3.3. Note on descending necrotizing mediastinitis

This is referred to specifically as acute mediastinitis which occurs as a complication of primary oropharyngeal infection, spreading to neck spaces and then tracking down into the mediastinal spaces. In many cases, diagnosis is made when the infection is far advanced. In the majority of cases, the source of

infection is usually odontogenic or peritonsillar abscesses (Ludwig angina). In addition to symptoms and signs of local and general infection, at presentation there are also manifestations of respiratory and hemodynamic distress signalling bacteriemia and septicaemia. Diagnosis is confirmed by computerised tomography of the neck and thorax showing collection of fluid and/or gas in the cervical and mediastinal tissue spaces. Apart from an appropriate anti-microbial agent it is essential to carry out adequate drainage which consists of:
– Bilateral transverse cervicotomies,
– Debridement of necrotic tissue,
– Leaving open of the wound for healing by second intention,
– Mediastinal drainage,
– Pleural drainage if necessary.

The choice of approach for mediastinal drainage depends on the site of the collection.

3.4. Idiopathic Mediastinal Fibrosis (Chronic Fibrous Mediastinitis)

This is a condition in which the loose connective tissues of the mediastinum are involved in a widespread fibrosis and become hard and constricting. In places, the fibrosis can be discrete and tumour-like.

The aetiology of the condition is obscure. Tuberculosis and syphilis were once thought to be the cause of the disease but lack of evidence has led to the disregarding of this hypothesis. The association of mediastinal fibrosis in some patients with other fibrosing diseases, such as retroperitoneal fibrosis, has led some to suggest a common or related aetiology but the causes of many of these conditions are equally uncertain. It has been suggested that mediastinal fibrosis may be due to an exaggerated response to respiratory infection in some patients with a tendency to develop excessive fibrosis (e.g. mediastinal fibrosis). The most important symptoms and signs are related to SVC obstruction which may be relieved surgically.

3.5. Management of mediastinitis/mediastinal infection

Early diagnosis is imperative in order to introduce appropriate treatment, to check the spread of infection and to prevent septicaemic events. The principle of treatment consists of:
• Identification of the source of infection and the infected space/spaces within the mediastinal compartment and thoracic cavity.
• Drainage of the mediastinum and communicating pleural spaces.
• Cleaning the infected spaces of debris and necrotic material.
• Lavage of the space with appropriate antiseptic (e.g. 1/5000 dilution of aqueous solution of chlorhexidine).
• Provision of adequate parenteral/enteral nutritional support to cope with hypercatabolic state — if there is oesophageal perforation or leak, an efficient delivery of nutrition should be planned.
• Administration of broad spectrum antibiotics to cover a range of aerobic and anaerobic organisms — antibiotic policy should be reviewed in the light of microbiological study of infected material.
• Treatment of the source of infection at an appropriate time (see perforation of the oesophagus and repair of sternal wounds and dehiscence following cardiac surgery).

4. Superior mediastinal/superior vena caval syndrome

This is a serious and distressing condition (Fig. 4) caused by obstruction of the superior vena cava (SVC) resulting in raised venous pressure in the territory of its tributaries and interference with return blood flow to the head. Characteristically, there is engorgement of the veins in the upper part of the body with many visible and dilated veins over the anterior chest wall. There is also oedema of the upper limbs, neck, face and heart. In severe cases cyanosis and complex neuro-cerebral symptoms with headache and dizziness develop, which can culminate in coma and patient's death. The aetiology of SVC is presented in Table 1.

In over 80% of cases, the cause is the invasion of the superior vena cava by bronchial carcinoma, especially small cell type, or from extrinsic compression of the vein by enlarged and malignant mediastinal lymphadenopathy. Other, both malignant and benign mediastinal tumours, are responsible for superior mediastinal syndrome in the remaining 20% of cases. In many patients the obstruction of SVC occurs gradually, due to the insidious evolution of bronchial carcinoma of the right upper lobe. Occasionally there is a super added thrombosis of the left innominate (brachio-cephalic vein) which imposes an added burden on the venous return with an acute clinical presentation as a result.

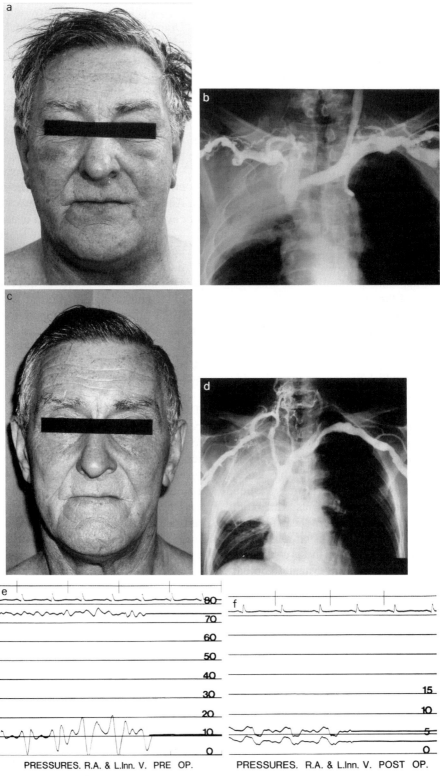

Fig. 4. (a) Face of a patient with superior mediastinal syndrome, (b) venogram of the patient showing almost complete obstruction of the superior vena cava with distended veins, (c) the face of the same patient the day following the operation of innominate to right atrial bypass graft, (d) venogram of the patient after operation showing the bypass graft, (e) pressure recording for demonstrating the gradient across left innominate vein (L.inn.V) above [70 mmHg] and right atrium (R.A.) below [10 mmHg] before the bypass operation, (f) pressure gradient across L.inn.V and R.A. following the bypass operation. Note abolition of the gradient.

Table 1

Aetiology of Superior Vena Caval (SVC) obstruction

Malignant tumours	Benign tumours	Granulomas	Miscellaneous
• Bronchogenic Carcinoma (80%)	• Mediastinal Goitre	• Histoplasmosis	• Mediastinal fibrosis
• Thymoma	• Teratomas	• Tuberculosis	• Trauma
• Germ cell tumours	• Bronchial cysts		• Thrombosis
• Lymphomas			• Cardiac tamponade

4.1. Management of superior vena caval syndrome

General clinical examination is carried out along standard lines, with particular attention being paid to the cardiovascular system. In some cases, it may be difficult to differentiate between high venous pressure arising from the obstructive lesion of the SVC and that caused by constrictive pericarditis. The respiratory system likewise must be thoroughly examined. Wheeze, dyspnoea and chest pains are amongst the common respiratory symptoms in patients with SVC obstruction caused by lung cancer.

- *Radiological examination:* Chest radiograph usually demonstrates pulmonary or mediastinal lesions. In a small percentage of patients with SVC obstruction, the chest radiograph may be interpreted as being normal. Contrast enhanced CT of the thorax or MRI usually establishes the diagnosis and often the cause. Venography outlines the anatomic detail as well as demonstrating the adequacy of collaterals. This procedure is particularly helpful in acute onset cases when the possibility of surgery is being considered (Dyet and Moghissi, 1980). In the great majority of cases a right upper lobe tumour is found with extrinsic obstruction of the SVC by mediastinal glands or by invading tumour.
- *Bronchoscopy:* Shows direct or indirect evidence of tumour affecting the carina or, in many cases, the right main bronchus. An important point about bronchoscopy is that in some cases of SVC obstruction there is so much oedema and venous engorgement that the procedure cannot be tolerated by the patient, who may develop serious respiratory embarrassment. When the procedure is carried out, tissue diagnosis via bronchoscopy can be obtained in no more than 50% of cases. In some cases cytology may be helpful to establish diagnosis.
- *Mediastinoscopy and gland biopsy:* In the presence of major venous engorgement and high ve-

nous pressure, mediastinoscopy may be hazardous and contraindicated, not only because of the risk of haemorrhage during the procedure, but also because of aggravation of mediastinal obstructive syndrome.
- *Needle biopsy:* Percutaneous CT/ultrasound guided needle biopsy technique is, in many cases of SVC obstruction, the only method which can provide a sample for biopsy purposes. The risk of bleeding should be borne in mind.

Tissue diagnosis may, at times, be difficult as there are a limited number of investigations which can provide biopsy material and of these many are either contraindicated or will not provide suitable samples for histological examination. Effort should, however, be made to obtain a cytological diagnosis if suitable histological material cannot be obtained. When neither histological nor cytological diagnosis is available and treatment is a matter of urgency other investigatory techniques, such as CT scan or MRI, should be used in an attempt to establish diagnosis in order to commence treatment.

4.2. Treatment

The treatment of SVC syndrome depends largely on the aetiology and topography of the obstruction. When superior vena caval syndrome is caused by bronchial carcinoma, usually the tumour is oncologically inoperable and often it is surgically unresectable.

The treatment for the majority of cases consists of chemo/radiotherapy and supportive drugs, particularly diuretics. Such treatment reduces the bulk of the tumour and permits development of collaterals which provide a bypass channel for venous return to the heart.
- Sometimes excision of the tumour and lung and resection and reconstruction of SVC with/without grafting is possible. This is particularly the case in patients whose obstruction is not acute or severe and who have been given pre-operative adjunct

chemo/radiotherapy and who have responded to such treatment.

- Placement of intravascular stent into the stenosed superior vena cava relieves the obstructive symptoms and allows the patient to tolerate chemo/radiotherapy better.
- SVC bypass operation: left innominate vein to right atrial graft operation to bypass obstructed SVC (Avasthi and Moghissi, 1977; Moghissi, 1985) was once the only method to provide rapid relief of symptoms. Since the introduction of intravascular stents, the indications for such bypass grafting are limited. However, this author believes SVC bypass graft has a place in some cases. These are acute on chronic cases indicating super added blood clot in left or right innominate vein (8 to 10% of cases) or long segment obstruction affecting the SVC above and below the azygos vein. It is important to note that in malignant SVC obstruction, adjuvant chemo/radiotherapy is an integral part of the management when stent/bypass is used.

5. Mediastinal emphysema (pneumomediastinum)

The causes of mediastinal emphysema (air in the mediastinal space) are:

- Rupture of the bronchus,
- Perforation of the oesophagus,
- Penetrating injuries,
- Spontaneous rupture of an emphysematous bulla, bleb and/or air cyst of the lung into the mediastinal space.

In the case of air escaping from the lung through a rupture of the alveoli or an emphysematous bulla, the mediastinal emphysema may be spontaneous or may follow strain such as coughing or sneezing. In these cases, the air reaches the mediastinum via the perivascular sheath of the pulmonary vessels. Due to the particular anatomical arrangements of the mediastinal and neck spaces, air can appear in the neck as subcutaneous surgical emphysema.

5.1. Clinical presentation

Occasionally mediastinal emphysema is asymptomatic and discovered incidentally. In the majority of cases the clinical presentation is related to the primary cause (e.g. rupture of the oesophagus/trauma). In patients with spontaneous emphysema due to rupture of an emphysematous bulla attached to the mediastinal pleura and caused by coughing, pneumothorax is often present together with pain in the chest. In the absence of pneumothorax the pneumomediastinum may not be symptomatic. Examination of the neck often demonstrates the presence of surgical subcutaneous emphysema. Auscultation may reveal coarse crepitant sounds over the mediastinum (Hamman's signs). Chest radiograph and CT of thorax demonstrate gas in the mediastinal spaces and neck tissues. Contrast study of the oesophagus and tracheobronchoscopy should be performed as appropriate to establish the aetiology.

5.2. Treatment of mediastinal emphysema

In the absence of rupture or perforation of the aero-digestive tract, pneumomediastinum does not usually cause any cardiovascular disturbance; mediastinal pressure has to rise considerably to interfere with the venous return. Nevertheless, in the rare patient with gross mediastinal pressure, there may be neck vein engorgement, dyspnoea and cyanosis.

In cases uncomplicated by pneumothorax, conservative symptomatic treatment will usually suffice. If surgical subcutaneous emphysema is disturbing, one or two 1.5 to 2 cm incisions are made on the chest wall and a catheter inserted under the skin to allow escape of air. Also, in severe cases of pneumomediastinum with superior vena caval compression, bilateral tube thoracostomies to relieve the mediastinal pressure and prevent tension pneumothorax should relieve symptoms. When pneumo-mediastinum is accompanied by pneumothorax, tube drainage of the appropriate pleural space will suffice.

6. Haemomediastinum

Haemorrhage into the mediastinal space is usually post-traumatic (blunt or penetrating injuries) or follows cardiac surgery. In the former the rupture of a major vessel, notably the aorta, requires urgent attention (see thoracic injuries). In those cases which follow cardiac operation, continuous bleeding, excessive drainage or impending cardiac tamponade are the presenting features. Other operations concerned with the mediastinal structure may also be the cause of haemorrhage originating from intercostal arteries. In these cases, inadequate drainage will cause haemomediastinum even when the mediastinal pleura is opened and the pleural cavity is drained. This is particularly relevant to thoracic oesophagectomies.

References and further reading

Ashmann FR. A reassessment of the clinical implication of the superior vena cava syndrome. J Clin Oncol 1984; 2: 961–969.

Avasthi RB, Moghissi K. Malignant obstruction of the superior vena cava and its palliation. J Thorac Cardiovasc Surg 1977; 74: 244–248.

Brook I, Frazier EH. Microbiology of Mediastinitus. Arch Intern Med 1996; 156: 333–336.

Carlens E. Mediastinoscopy: A method for inspection and tissue biopsy in the superior mediastinum. Chest 1959; 36: 343–352.

Cordero L, Torre W, Freire D. Descending necrotizing mediastinitis and respiratory distress syndrome treated by aggressive surgical treatment. J Cardiovasc Surg 1996; 37: 87–88.

Dillemans B, Deneff G, Verschakelen J, Decramer M. Value of computed tomography and mediastinoscopy in pre-operative evaluation of mediastinal nodes in non small cell lung cancer. Eur J Cardiothorac Surg 1994; 8: 37–42.

Dyet JF, Moghissi K. Role of venography in assessing patients with superior vena caval obstruction caused by carcinoma for bypass operation. Thorax 1980; 35: 628–630.

Elia S, Cecere C, Giampaglia F, Ferrante G. Mediastinoscopy vs anterior mediastinotomy in the diagnosis of mediastinal lymphome; a randomised trial. Eur J Cardiothorac Surg 1992; 6: 361–365.

Foster ED, Munro DD, Dpobel ARC. Mediastinoscopy: A review of anatomical relationship and complications. Ann Thorac Surg 1972; 13: 273–286.

Laing AD, Thomson KR, Vrazas JL. Stenting in malignant and benign vena caval obstruction. Australas Radiol 1998; 42(4): 313–317.

Landreau RJ, Hazelrigg SR, Mack M,J et al. Thoracoscopic mediastinal lymph node sampling useful for mediastinal lymph node stations inaccessible by cervical mediastinoscopy. J Thorac Cardiovasc Surg 1993; 56: 92–96.

Luke WP, Pearson FG, Todd TRJ, Patterson GA, Cooper JD. Prospective evaluation of mediastinoscopy for assessment of carcinoma of the lung. J Thorac Cardiovasc Surg 1986; 91: 53–56.

Marty–Ane CH, Alauzen M, Alric P, Serres–Cousine O, Mary H. Descending necrotizing mediastinitis. Advantage with thoracotomy. J Thorac Cardiovasc Surg 1994: 107: 55–61.

Moghissi K. Superior vena caval syndrome. In: Delaure and Eschapasse (eds.), Lung Cancer: International Trends in General Thoracic Surgery. Philadelphia: WB Saunders, 1985; pp. 146–153.

Moncada R, Warpeha R, Pickleman J, Spak M, et al. Mediastinitis from odontogenic and deep cervical infection. Anatomic pathways of propagation. Chest 1978; 73: 497–500.

Olsen PS, Stentoft P, Ellefsen B, et al. Re-medistinoscopy in the assessment of resectability of lung cancer. Eur J Cardiothorac Surg 1997; 11: 661–663.

Papalia E, Rena O, Oliaro A, Cavallo A, Giobbe R, Casadio C, Maggi G, Mancuso M. Descending necrotising mediastinitis: surgical management. Eur J Cardiothorac Surg 2001; 20: 739–742.

Porte H, Metois D, Finzi L, Lebuffe G, et al. Superior vena cava syndrome of malignant origin: Which surgical procedure for which diagnosis? Eur J Cardiothorac Surg 2000; 17: 384–388.

Rendina EA, Venuta F, DeGiacomo T, Franioni F, Ricci L. Comparative merit of thoracoscopy, mediastinoscopy and mediastinotomy for mediastinal biopsy. Ann Thorac Surg 1994; 57: 992–995.

Rieger R, Schrenk P, Woisetschlager R, et al. Video thoracoscopy for the management of mediastinal mass lesion. Surg Endosc 1996; 10: 715–717.

Sancho LM, Minamoto H, Fernandez A, Sennes LU, Jatene FB. Descending necrotizing mediastinitis — a retrospective surgical experience. Eur J Cardiothorac Surg 1999; 16(2): 200–205.

Shah R, Sabanathan S, Lowe RA. Stenting in malignant obstruction of superior vena cava. J Thorac Cardiovasc Surg 1996; 112: 335–340.

Yim CD, Sane SS, Bjarnason H. Superior vena cava stenting. Radiol Clin North Am 2000; 38(2): 409–424.

K. Moghissi, J.A.C. Thorpe and F. Ciulli (Eds.)
Moghissi's Essentials of Thoracic and Cardiac Surgery

CHAPTER II.4

Mediastinal tumours and cysts

P. Fuentes and P. Thomas

1. Introduction

In this chapter, mediastinal lesions presenting as a mass are described. The word mass is used to mean either a tumour or a cyst. Tumour, without qualification, is used to denote a mass of tissue irrespective of its malignant, benign or inflammatory nature. In this context, tumour and mass are used synonymously. When tumour is used to mean a neoplasm, its nature will be indicated by the prefix malignant or benign. The term cyst is employed to signify a mass containing fluid or gas. A cystic tumour is a neoplasm which has central necrosis, fluid or gas.

Mediastinal masses are a diverse and heterogeneous group of lesions whose clinical features are dominated by signs and symptoms of compression or invasion of their neighbouring structure. At times there are extra-thoracic neurological (e.g. myasthenia) and/or hormonal (e.g. thyroid, parathyroid) manifestations which draw attention to their existence.

2. Anatomical consideration

The anatomy of mediastinal spaces and their respective contents have been previously described (chapter II.3). The mediastinum as a whole, and its subdivisions, have three anatomical characteristics relevant to the physio-pathology of their lesions as follows:
- Narrow and confined spaces provide little room for the expansion of volume occupying lesions. This explains early obstructive syndrome in expanding mediastinal masses.
- An extensive network of lymphatics and embryological remnants can easily become the seat of primary and metastatic tumours.

- There is a definite relationship between the tumour origin and its topographical location within the mediastinal compartment (see Fig. 2 in chapter II.3).

3. Clinical features of mediastinal masses

3.1. Many patients with mediastinal tumours or cysts can be asymptomatic (Fig. 1)

In some, clinical features relate to pressure effects on mediastinal structures. Occasionally however, general and extra-thoracic manifestations dominate clinical presentation.

Asymptomatic patients: In more than half of cases, it is radiology which allows the diagnosis of mediastinal pathology of an otherwise asymptomatic patient.

3.2. Pressure effects

There are a variety of presentations as follows:

3.2.1. Tracheo-bronchial compression
When the tracheo-bronchial tree is affected predominantly, dyspnoea, irritating cough and occasionally haemoptysis will be present.

3.2.2. Superior vena caval syndrome
This denotes compression of the major mediastinal venous system or superior vena cava itself with development of collateral venous circulation, oedema of the neck and face and cyanosis of the upper part of the body (see Superior Vena Caval syndrome, section 4 in chapter II.3).

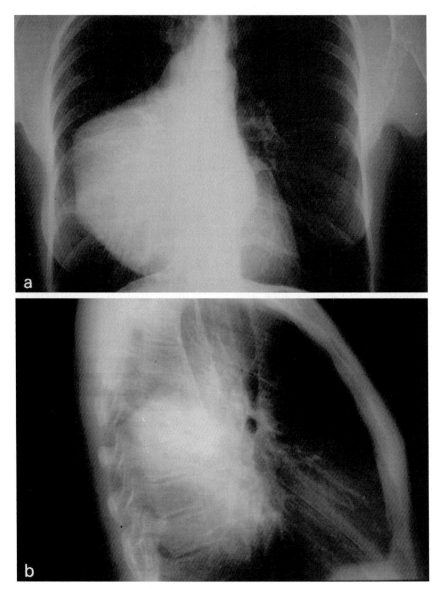

Fig. 1. Chest radiograph of an asymptomatic young female with a large posterior mediastinal tumour: (a) antero-posterior view, (b) lateral view.

3.2.3. Inferior vena caval syndrome

This is less common than its SVC counterpart. It is associated with painful hepatomegaly, collateral venous circulation of the abdomen, oedema of the lower part of the body and ascites.

3.2.4. Pain symptomology

This is characterised by retro-sternal angina-like pain and intercostal and cervico-brachial neuralgia.

3.2.5. Neurological syndromes

These are often due to invasion rather than compression of the nerves. Recurrent laryngeal nerve involvement results in husky bi-tonal voice or complete aphonia. Phrenic nerve involvement will produce diaphragmatic paralysis and elevation of the related dome of the diaphragm. Invasion of sympathetic nerves manifests as Horner's Syndrome. A neurogenic tumour with extension into the spine will cause spinal cord and associated neurological manifestations.

3.2.6. Oesophageal compression

This is uncommon and manifests as progressive dysphagia. Tracheo-oesophageal fistula with associated symptoms may occasionally be present.

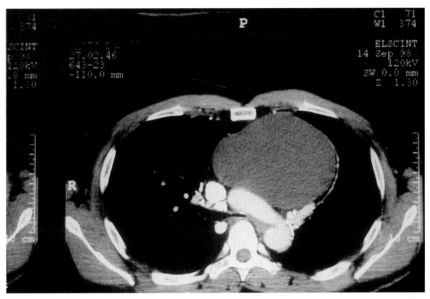

Fig. 2. CT scan of the thorax showing cystic mass in the anterior mediastinum with marked mediastinal shift and compression of the aortic arch and adjacent organs.

3.3. General and extra thoracic effects

3.3.1. Effects on general condition
Deterioration in general health may be the only manifestation of a mediastinal tumour. This could be in the form of pyrexia, asthenia or weight loss.

3.3.2. Extra thoracic symptoms
At times these draw attention to mediastinal tumour, e.g. myasthenia gravis in the case of thymic tumour and thyroid dysfunction in the case of retrosternal goitre.

4. Diagnostic methods

4.1. Imaging

This has been previously described (see imaging techniques, and diagnostic methods in mediastinal pathology, chapter II.3).

CT scan (Fig. 2) and MRI (Fig. 3) of the thorax allows accurate indicative topography of the lesion and its relationship with neighbouring structures.

4.2. Endoscopy

Tracheobronchoscopy and oesophagoscopy demonstrates involvement or compression of the airway or upper alimentary tract. Both procedures are essential in the diagnosis of mediastinal pathology.

Mediastinoscopy and thoracoscopy have a key role in obtaining biopsy samples

4.3. Biological method

Tumour markers are particularly important in the diagnosis of mediastinal tumours and also serve as prognostic indicators as well as monitoring the progress of treatment. Examples of these are auto-antibodies in thymoma, hormones level measurement, serum and urinary metabolites in neurogenic tumours and Beta-hCG (Beta-human chorionic gonadotrophin) and Alfa Feto Protein in hetero plastic disembryoma.

5. Aetiological diagnosis and topography

Aetiological diagnosis of mediastinal tumours is often difficult and, in practice, it is the topography of the lesion within the mediastinal space which tends to determine the origin.

According to their topography mediastinal tumours are described under (see also Table 1):
5.1 Anterior mediastinal tumours
5.2 Middle mediastinal tumours
5.3 Inferior mediastinal tumours

5.1. Anterior Mediastinal Tumours

Anterior mediastinal tumours are distributed into:

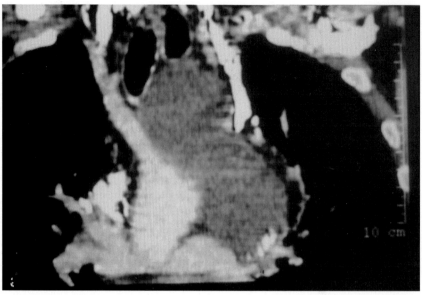

Fig. 3. Multi-planar imaging of a mediastinal tumour infiltrating the left side of the aortic arch, the trachea and upper oesophagus.

Table 1

Topography of cysts and tumors within the mediastinal spaces

Anterior mediastinum	Middle mediastinum	Posterior mediastinum
• Intrathoracic goitres	• Lymphadenopathies/ lymphatic masses – Lymphomas	• Neurogenic tumours
• Thymic tumours	– Lymph node metastases – Tuberculous	
• Lymphomas • Germ cell tumours	– Sarcoid glands	
• Pleuro-peritoneal cysts	• Cysts – Bronchogenic	

- Superior groups
- Middle groups
- Inferior groups

5.1.1. Superior group consists of thyroid tumours and lymphoid tumours
- Thyroid tumours
- Lymphoid tumours

Thyroid tumours. Intrathoracic (substernal/retrosternal) goitres are the most important tumours in the superior part of the anterior mediastinum and represent 15–20% of all mediastinal neoplasia. The condition predominantly affects women (70% of cases). Intrathoracic goitres are mainly of two types:
- Those extending from the neck down to the chest,

so-called "plunging goitres" which form 95% of all cases.
- Ectopic mediastinal goitres represent 5% of cases and frequently co-exist with the "plunging" variety.

Pathologically thoracic thyroid tumours are colloid goitres, essentially adenomas. Exceptionally, they can be inflammatory thyroiditis and rarely (5% of cases) cancer.

Clinical features: It is rare for cases to remain totally asymptomatic. The majority of patients present with compressive syndrome resulting from the expanding tumour mass, particularly affecting the airways. An acute airway obstruction can occur leading to serious respiratory embarrassment and may lead to asphyxiation with fatal consequences. This event is usually precipitated by haemorrhage within the tumour mass. In many instances the presence of cervical goitre and more rarely, the symptoms and signs of thyroid dysfunction, will point to the diagnosis.

The standard chest radiograph will show a mass in the antero-superior compartment of the thorax and associated features related to compressive signs. In 10–20% of cases, thyroid mass may demonstrate calcification. Computed tomography (CT) reveals continuity of the mediastinal mass with the cervical thyroid in "plunging goitres". Images can be enhanced by contrast medium. Thyroid scintigraphy using radioactive iodine (131 or 133) is not particularly useful in cases of thoracic thyroid tumours because of poor concentration of the isotope in these goitres.

Laryngo-tracheoscopy is an important investigation which should be carried out in all cases in order to demonstrate the possible existence of recurrent laryngeal nerve palsy or any tracheal involvement.

The treatment for retro-sternal goitre is surgical resection. In malignant cases, this necessitates excision of the tumour and all involved surrounding structures; this may include a segment of the trachea and superior vena cava. Such an extensive operative procedure is, however, justified by good long-term results.

Lymphoid tumours. Especially lymphomas, can present as a variety of lesions from the root of the neck down to the superior, anterior and middle mediastinum.

Malignant lymphoma are relatively rare tumours and envelop two groups of conditions: Hodgkin's lymphomas (Hodgkin's disease) and non-Hodgkin's lymphomas with an incidence of 3/100,000 and 15/100,000 of population respectively. Nevertheless, 20% of anterior mediastinal masses in adults and 50% of those in infants are lymphatic tumours.

Hodgkin's disease affects young adults preferentially and is histologically characterised by Reed-Sternberg cells. Due to the efficacy of chemo/radiotherapy the disease is now attended by a good prognosis.

Non-Hodgkin's lymphoma covers a wide spectrum and a heterogenous group of tumours both from the histological point of view as well as the age of the patient. The condition affects all ages.

The aetiology of lymphomas is poorly understood. Genetic factors, acquired human immuno deficiencies (immuno-suppressive medication after organ transplantation and acquired immuno deficiency syndrome (AIDS), some viral conditions (Epstein Barr HTLV) and exposure to certain toxins (pesticide, solvents, paints) appear to play a role in their genesis.

Recent developments in immunology, cytogenetics and molecular genetics have established clonal origins of the disease. The understanding and the characterisation of genomic events will assist both diagnosis and treatment.

5.1.2. The middle group of anterior mediastinal tumours are comprised of:
- Thymic tumours.
- Germ cell tumours.
- Parathyroid tumours.
- Chemodectoma.

Table 2

Classification of thymic tumor according to Masoaka

Stage I	Macroscopic encapsulation (complete) and no microscopic invasion
Stage II	Macroscopic invasion into mediastinal fat or pleura or microscopic invasion into capsule
Stage III	Macroscopic invasion into pericardium, great vessels or lung
Stage IVa	Pericardial or pleural dissemination
Stage IVb	Lymphatic or haematogenous metastases

Thymomas. These originate from the epithelial cell component of the thymus and affect all age groups and both sexes in equal proportion. The malignancy of thymomas cannot be based on histological criteria alone except in about 10% of cases. In more than 30% of cases, the tumour is locally invasive to such an extent that surgical excision becomes quasi-impossible. Prognostic indicators are commonly based on criteria proposed by Masoaka (Table 2). Newer prognostic indicators consider morphological criteria and immuno-histochemistry. Some 40% of thymomas are associated with immunological disorders, of which Myasthenia Gravis heads the list. In these, besides clinical signs and electro-myographic changes, identification of antibody anticeptors to acetylcholin is helpful in diagnosis. The goal after surgical resection is to reduce or totally eliminate all cholinergic medication after 48 to 72 hours.

When a thymoma is associated with myasthenia cholinergic medication is best reduced, or even discontinued, 48 to 72 hours prior to surgery. In severe cases plasmapheresis should be undertaken in the week before surgery (3 sessions). Thymomas may be associated with other conditions. The most important of which are erythroblastopenia, hypogamaglaebulinaemia, disseminated lupus erythematosis and rheumatoid polymyositis.

Germ cell tumours (GCT). Germ cell tumours represent 10% of all mediastinal tumours and 20% of neoplasms in the anterior mediastinum. These tumours originate from cells of gonocytes and represent an early anomaly of embryogenesis with development of tumours whose tissue types are foreign to those found normally in the thorax. Their location in the anterior mediastinum is a remarkably constant. They have a variable evolution, often benign but sometimes extremely invasive. Common germ cell tumours are:
- Teratomas.

- Seminomas.
- Malignant non-seminomatous teratoma (NST).

Teratomas: Teratomas are the commonest germ cell tumours. They are composed of at least two of the three embryonic differentiated layers, (endoderm, mesoderm and ectoderm). Teratomas may be composed of mature, immature or mixed cell population.

Mature teratomas are commonly symptomatic with irritating cough, dyspnoea and chest pain. In the course of their evolution, sooner or later they produce signs of mediastinal, pleural or bronchial involvement. Further complication includes development of fistulae into the bronchial tree, pericardium and blood vessels.

Radiologically they appear as a heterogenous cystic mass with calcification. Histology is characterised by the presence of a calcified capsule with diverse tissue content such as bone, cartilage, pancreatic and muscle tissue. The finding of hair and teeth in some explain the term dermoid cyst referred to cystic teratomas.

In summary, teratomas are polymorphic, containing a number of different tissues, one of which may undergo malignant degeneration in 10% of cases. Their treatment consists of surgical resection and, as a rule, they do not recur after complete resection.

Seminomas: Seminomas are malignant tumours which affect young male adults. At an early stage they are asymptomatic and diagnosis is made when the tumour becomes a large mass with signs and symptoms of mediastinal obstruction. At presentation, the patient's general condition is good despite the fact that in about 50% of cases the tumour is unresectable. The levels of tumour markers AFP (alpha feto protein) or Beta-hCG (Beta-human chorionic gonadotrophin) are not raised in seminomas unless the tumour contains a non-seminomatous component. Serum LDH (lactic dehydrogenase) level is, however, often raised. This may give the false impression of lymphoma.

The basic treatment of seminoma is surgical excision followed by chemo/radiotherapy. Even after complete surgical excision there is frequently tumour recurrence but long-term results are generally favourable. Incomplete response to chemo/radiotherapy may result in persistence of tumour cells within the residual fibrous tissue. This is best excised when at all possible.

Malignant non-seminomatomous teratomas: Malignant non-seminomatomous teratomas (NST) are less common than seminomas but equally affect young male adults. They include, embryonic carcinomas, chorionic carcinoma, terato carcinoma, tumours of endodermal sinus and miscellaneous mixed teratomas. NST's are often highly malignant. They are locally aggressive with early lymph node involvement and distant metastases and the possible existence of gynaecomastia. The general condition of the patient is frequently affected and blood profiles may resemble that of leukaemia. Serum LDH is raised in over 90% of cases and high levels of tumour markers Beta-hCG and AFP are diagnostic even when histology is unproven. These tumours are radio-resistant and their treatment consists of multi-drug chemotherapy with platinum compounds followed, after two to three months, by resection of the residual tumour. The prognosis is poor but a 40% long-term survival may be obtained by an aggressive therapeutic approach.

Parathyroid adenoma. These are tumours of ectopic parathyroid glands in the mediastinum and are discovered in the course of the mediastinal search for a "missing" gland of the neck when the biological profile is suggestive of hyperparathyroidsm. Presentation as a mediastinal tumour is exceptional.

Chemodectomas. These are extremely rare and develop from para-aortic chemoreceptor tissues. They are often asymptomatic and are slow growing and benign.

5.1.3. Inferior group of anterior mediastinal tumours
Pleuro-pericardial (pericardial spring water) cyst. This cyst results from failure of fusion of one of the lachnar cavities with others forming the pericardium. Characteristically, it is situated at the anterior costophrenic angle adjacent to the pericardium and diaphragm. Most are in the right chest and are unilocular. The cyst is diagnosed by plain chest radiography and characteristic image on CT scan of the thorax. Treatment is by excision of the cyst accessed by mini-thoracotomy or VATS technique.

Cystic Lymphangioma (cystic hygromas) (lymphangio iomatous cysts). These are benign lesions which can be found along the whole length of the anterior mediastinum from the neck to the diaphragm (Figs. 4 and 5). They are commonly seen in children, often in association with a similar cyst in the axillary of the cervical region. At times, complete resection of the cyst may not be possible because of its anatomical location and its attachment to important structures. In this case, an incomplete excision will have to be

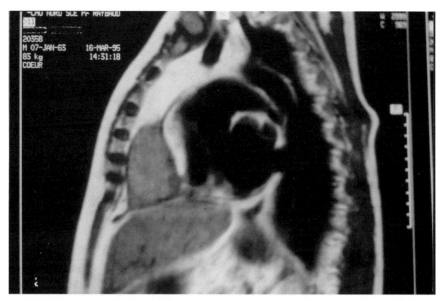

Fig. 4. MRI of the thorax showing a tumor in the lower and anterior mediastinum compressing the heart.

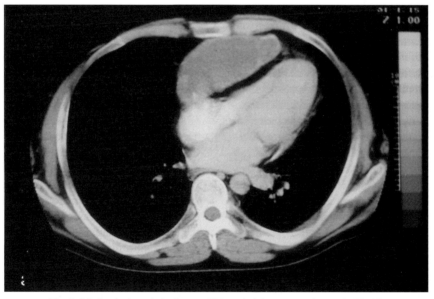

Fig. 5. Mediastinal cystic hydroma: CT scan of the same patient as in Fig. 4.

carried out. This can be complicated by chylothorax. A point about their surgical resection is that care should be taken to ligate the afferrent and efferent lymphatic vessels.

5.2. Middle mediastinal tumours

5.2.1. Mediastinal lymphatic masses
The middle mediastinum is endowed with a rich network of lymph nodes which are important in the pathology of masses of this space. These comprise:

Lymph node neoplasms which are
- Hodgkin's and Non-Hodgkin's lymphomas (which have been described previously).
- Secondary metastatic lymphadenitis of lung cancer (Fig. 6).
- Secondary metastatic mediastinal lymphadenitis from tumours of the abdominal viscera.
- Lymph node enlargement in conjunction with leukaemia, especially chronic lymphoid leukaemia or acute lymphoblastic leukaemia.

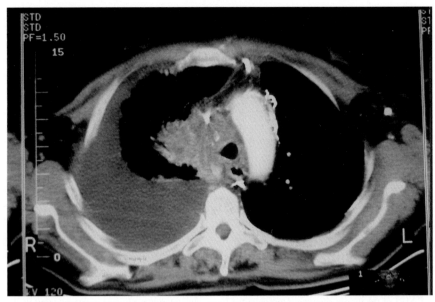

Fig. 6. Infiltrating metastatic adenopathies causing superior vena caval syndrome.

Sarcoidosis. Mediastinal lymph node involvement represents an important mode of presentation in sarcoid. The lesion is characterised by the presence of lymphoid tissue, epitheloid and giant cells but without caseiation or necrosis. The prognosis is good despite episodes of exacerbation. These episodes respond to steroid treatment. In some instances the disease leads to progressive respiratory failure.

Infective lymphadenopathies. These accompany bacterial viral parasitic and mycotic infections.
- Tuberculous lymphadenitis is a specific example of this subgroup showing a typical granulomatous lesion.
- Syphillitic lymphadenitis is now almost extinct.

Miscellaneous lymphadenitis. This is lymph node enlargement seen in individuals affected by immunodeficiency diseases (e.g. AIDS) where there is a development of systemic infection by candida toxoplasmosis and some viral lesions, e.g. cytomegalovirus and Epstein-Barr.

Hyperplastic lymphoid pseudo tumours. Under this terminology are classed a group of diverse conditions amongst which are enlarged lymph nodes of silicosis, rheumatoid polyarthritis, disseminated lupus erythemectosis and amyloid.

5.2.2. Middle mediastinal tumours/cysts other than lymphatic masses

Bronchogenic cysts. This is the commonest of the mediastinal cystic lesions and represents some 6% of the whole of mediastinal masses. It results from an anomaly of segmentation of the primary intestinal tube into respiratory and digestive tube buds. This origin explains the topography of these lesions in the proximity of, and in contact with, the tracheo-bronchial tree. Histologically the cyst is lined by ciliated epithelium and contains mucus. The cyst may remain asymptomatic for a considerable time but with its enlargement comes respiratory system symptoms of cough, pain, haemoptysis and signs of mediastinal obstruction. Presentation as acute respiratory distress and asphyxiation in the newborn is also a possibility.

Treatment of bronchogenic cyst is surgical resection. This can be difficult due to inflammatory changes in and around the cysts and because of the anatomical relationship with the pericardium, great vessels, tracheo-bronchial tree and oesophagus. A wide exposure is often necessary in order to achieve complete excision. At times, a small portion of the wall may have to be left behind. This remnant should be cauterised to minimise the risk of recurrence.

5.3. Posterior mediastinal masses

5.3.1. Neurogenic tumours

Neurogenic tumours represent one-quarter of mediastinal neoplasms and are dominant amongst pathological conditions of the posterior mediastinum. They develop from the sympathetic chain, nerve roots and rami communicans and are generally situated in the paravertebral gutter; 90% are in the superior compartment of the posterior mediastinum. In addition to the mass, radiological investigation may show bony changes in the ribs and vertebra, particularly in children. The finding of widened intra-vertebral foramina can be indicative of a dumb-bell type of tumour. CT scan will indicate the tumour mass and contrast enhancement can provide more precision regarding anatomical position and topography.

It is particularly important to precisely outline the relationship of the tumour with the vertebral foramina and spinal cord in order to plan an appropriate neurosurgical operative approach. It is usually necessary to perform MRI and/or myelography separately or in combination. A further problem concerned with neurogenic tumours emanates from their anatomical relationship with Adamkiewicz arteries. It is important to demonstrate accurately the origins of these arteries which are subject to individual variations to such an extent as to necessitate arteriography of spinal cord arteries.

Neurogenic tumours may originate from nerve sheaths or nerve cells. Malignant neurogenic tumours are found in children more often than in adults: 50% and 20% respectively.

Nerve sheath tumours.
- Schwannoma/Neurinoma: These form 50% of neurogenic mediastinal tumours. They are principally seen in adults over the age of 40 and only exceptionally in children. The incidence of the tumour is equal in males and females and they are discovered by chance in the course of routine radiograph though large tumours may produce chest pain or parasthesia.
- Neuro fibromas: These tumours affect young adults and are usually multiple; they rarely present as a single lesion. Patients with neurofibromas should be investigated fully for possible associated Von Reckinghausen disease; this condition must be considered when the "café au lait" lesions are present. No malignant changes occur in a neurofibroma when it is a single lesion though the risk is significant in multiple neurofibromas.

Nerve cell tumours.
- Neuro blastoma is a malignant tumour, generally of the adrenal gland, originating from a sympathetic ganglion. In more than 85% of cases the tumour is seen in the paediatric population and only exceptionally in adults. Evolution of the tumour is one of malignancy with a poor prognosis.
- Ganglio neuroma: This is an encapsulated benign tumour which arises from sympathetic ganglia.
- Ganglio neuro blastoma: This is a tumour with an intermediate grade of malignancy between neuro blastoma and para ganglioma. The tumour is situated around, and in contact with, the arch of the aorta or the heart. It develops from the autonomic nervous system. The constituent cells of this tumour contain neuro sensory granules which store catecholamines. The tumour itself can be a non-functioning, slow-growing neoplasm in which case its surgical excision is attended by long survival benefit. By virtue of its anatomical relationship complete surgical excision may, at times, be difficult.
- Pheochromocytoma is a functioning type of para-ganglioma which is rarely found in the mediastinum. The tumour secretes catecholamines (adrenaline and noradrenaline) which provokes attacks of paroxysmal hypertension. An abnormally high level in urine of metabolites of catecholamines (vane-mandelic acid) is found in patients with pheochyromocytomas. Histologically, the tumour is often benign and is sometimes found within the complex of familial polyendo crinopathy or Von Hippel–Lindeau disease.
- Neuro epitheliomas – Askin's tumours: These tumours occur in children and young adults. Their histopathology is controversial. They develop in the paravertebral gutter and involve the ribs. There is no catecholamine secretion. Their treatment is multimodal including surgery and chemotherapy. The prognosis is poor.

5.3.2. Other posterior mediastinal tumours

This group of mediastinal masses are much less common than neurogenic tumours and comprises:
- Para-oesophageal cysts.
- Meningeal cysts.
- Retro-vascular goitres.
- Hydatid cysts.

Para-oesophageal cysts (oesophageal duplication). These cysts represent about 1% of mediastinal tumours. They are derived from the primitive intestinal bud which fails to communicate with the lumen of the gut. They can be present along the whole length of the oesophagus but most often (60%) at its lower end. They are frequently associated with deformities of the cervico-thoracic spine.

Para-oesophageal cysts may be symptomatic in children but they are a chance finding in adults, sometimes being discovered abruptly by infective complication and/or haemorrhage occurring in the cysts causing dysphagia by extrinsic compression or producing haematemesis and/or haemoptysis.

Malignant degeneration of the cysts is possible. Radiological diagnosis may not be possible because of the difficulty of differentation from haematoma or intra-mural tumour. Endoscopic examination eliminates endoluminal pathology and intraluminal echography can confirm the peri-oesophageal location and nature of the cyst and its content.

Treatment of para-oesophageal cyst is surgical resection. This can, at times, be difficult due to inflammatory changes of the wall of the cyst. Post-surgical follow-up is important as a number of patients may develop post-operative gastro-oesophageal reflux symptoms.

Meningeal cyst. Congenital meningeal cysts are an exceptional finding in the mediastinum. Their diagnosis is by myelograph coupled with CT.

Posterior retro-vascular goitres. This tumour usually arises from the right lobe of the thyroid behind the major vessels. It can however arise in the left thyroid lobe but in its descent from the neck crosses behind the vessels to the right.

Hydatid cyst of the mediastinum. Mediastinal hydatid cysts are exceptional outside the geographical area where hydatidosis is endemic. They can expand in the mediastinum and present with obstruction of the vena cava or spinal cord syndromes.

6. Treatment strategy of mediastinal tumours/masses

Surgical resection alone usually suffices to treat benign and inflammatory masses and is also the treatment of choice for all malignant mediastinal tumours. In patients with incomplete resection the residual tumour is treated by chemo/radiotherapy. Unresectable cases are also given chemo/radiotherapy with the aim of downgrading the tumour allowing resectional surgery.

Surgical access: as a general rule a wide exposure is required to approach the tumour, some of which may extend and cross over different mediastinal spaces. Obviously surgical access will have to take account of the location of the lesion.

6.1. Anterior and antero-superior mediastinal tumours

These are approached through a cervical incision extended over the chest with manubrial or total sternal split, if needed.

6.1.1. Note on surgical treatment of thymomas
Thymomas often have an unpredictable evolution. Some appear histologically benign and are locally non-invasive but they reoccur after resection. Others look malignant but are attended by long survival. Many authors suggest adjunct chemo/radiotherapy to surgical resection.

Surgical resection is the treatment of choice based on the following principles:
- Median sternotomy incision.
- Wide exposure.
- Excision of thymus gland in its totality including the normal portion of the gland.
- Resection of all tissue which appears to be involved, such as pericardium and pulmonary parenchyma.
- Resection of large vascular trunk, e.g. innominate veins/superior vena cava, if at all possible.
- Excision of pleural infiltration.

The presence of myasthenia is not a contraindication for surgical resection.

6.1.2. Note on the treatment of lymphomas
Malignant lymphomas are treated essentially by radio/chemotherapy. Bone marrow transplantation allows an aggressive protocol of extensive therapy to be undertaken and will counteract marrow aplasia. It is important to have precise histological diagnosis of the type of lymphoma in order to apply the most specific therapy. This necessitates an appropriate sized sample of tissue for biopsy which can only be obtained surgically and not endoscopically in the majority of cases.

The roles of surgery in lymphomas are:
- Provision of an appropriate biopsy.
- Excision of residual tumour after chemotherapy/radiotherapy.
- Reduction of the mass of tumour if exploratory thoracotomy is undertaken, particularly if frozen

section histology cannot, with precision, provide histology of the explored lesion. This is even more relevant if the tumour cannot be excised totally. Note that even after successful chemo/radiotherapy there is a place for surgical excision of the remnant scar tissue which may contain neoplastic cells which would initiate recurrence of the tumour. Whilst MRI and other imaging techniques, such as scintigraphy, will outline the extent of the scar, surgical ablation is the only method to eliminate, with safety, the potential of residual tumour.

6.2. Tumours of middle and posterior mediastinum

These are approached through a thoracotomy incision.

6.3. Cervical region through root of neck to thorax

Tumours extending from the cervical region through the root of the neck to the thorax are accessed via an equally extended incision such as cervico-thoracic, clamshell or hemiclamshell (see thoracic incisions, chapter I.4).

6.4. VATS

The role of VATS in the surgical resection of mediastinal tumours is being currently assessed. At this time, the method should be used in selected, uncomplicated and benign lesions.

The above general plan of treatment applies to all mediastinal masses. There are, however, details related to thymomas and malignant lymphomas which need special consideration.

References and further reading

Aktogu S, Yuncu G, Halicolar H, Ermete S, Buduneli T. Bronchogenic cysts: clinicopathological presentation and treatment. Eur Respir J 1996; 9: 2017–2021.

Brisse H, Paacquement H, Burdairon E, Plancher C, Neuenschwander S. Outcome of residual mediastinal masses of thoracic lymphomas in children: impact on management and radiological follow up strategy. Pediatr Radiol 1998; 28: 444–450.

Fuentes P, Leude E, Ruiz C, Borigoni L, Thomas P, Giudicelli R, Gastaud JA, Morati N. Treatment of lymphomas. A report of 67 cases. Eur J Cardiothorac Surg 1992; 6: 180–187.

Giudicelli R, Pellet W, Fuentes P, Heurte P, Barthelemy A. Reboud E. Ganger to spinal cord arterial vascularisation during surgery for neurogenic tumours of the posterior mediastinum. Ann Chir 1991; 45: 692–694.

Kolomainen D, Hurley PR, Ebbs SR. Esophageal duplication cyst: case report and review of the literature. Dis Esophagus 1998; 11: 62–65.

Masaoka A, Monden Y, Makahara K, Tanioka T. follow up study of thymomas with special reference to their clinical stages. Cancer 1981; 48: 2485–2492.

McKeithan TW. Molecular biology of non-Hodgkins lymphomas. Semin Oncol 1990; 17: 30–42.

Moran CA, Suster S. Primary germ cell tumours of the mediastinum: I. Analysis of 322 cases with special emphasis on teratomatous lesions and a proposal for histopathologic classification and clinical staging. Cancer 1997; 80: 681–690.

Moran CA, Suster S, Przygodzki RM, Koss MN. Primary germ cell tumours of the mediastinum: II. Mediastinal seminomas — a clinicopathologic and immunohistochemical study of 120 cases. Cancer 1997; 80: 691–698.

Moran CA, Suster S, Koss MN. Primary germ cell tumours of the mediastinum: III. Yolk sac tumour, embryonal carcinoma, choriocarcinoma and combined nonteratomatous germ cell tumours of the mediastinum — a clinicopathologic and immunohistochemical study of 64 cases. Cancer 1997; 80: 699–707.

Strollo DC, de Rosado–Christenson ML, Jett JR. Primary mediastinal tumours: part II. Tumours of the middle and posterior mediastinum. Chest 1997; 112: 1344–1357.

Vadasz P, Kotsis L. Surgical aspects of 175 mediastinal goiters. Eur J Cardiothorac Surg 1998; 14: 393–397.

K. Moghissi, J.A.C. Thorpe and F. Ciulli (Eds.)
Moghissi's Essentials of Thoracic and Cardiac Surgery

CHAPTER II.5

Anterior chest wall deformities

K. Moghissi

Anterior chest wall deformities form a heterogenous group of conditions, all of which alter the "normal" appearance of the chest. Some of these cause important psychological and/or physiological derangement and many will need surgical correction. They may be described under two headings:

- Deformities without bony defects:
  These deformities are concerned with abnormal configuration of the sternum and ribs including costal cartilages but without any bone defects. They are exemplified by pectus excavatus and pectus carinatum.
- Deformities with bony defects of the chest wall:
  Examples of these are Poland syndrome and cleft sternum with/without ectopia cordis.

1. Chest deformities without bony defects

Commonest amongst these are:

- Pectus excavatum (syn: funnel chest, thorax en entonnoir) (Fig. 1).
- Pectus carinatum (pigeon chest, sternal prominence, thorax en carene (Fig. 2).

These are the two extremes of a range of deformities which affect the sternum and costal cartilages. They have many similarities and, in principle, the technique of their operative repair is the same; they can be described and discussed together highlighting the differences where applicable.

A typical pectus excavatum is a depression in the sternum which may involve the whole of the sternal body from the level of the 2nd costal cartilage down to, and including, the costal margin.

In a typical pectus carinatum (pigeon chest) the sternum is prominently convex. The name carinatum (hull of a ship) is apt because it indicates the characteristic shape of the sternum in this condition.

Pectus excavatum is more commonly encountered than pectus carinatum and in some cases a mixture of carinatum and excavatum, each affecting one part of the sternum, can be seen. Both excavatum and carinatum deformities appear to have the same aetiology, which has been the subject of much debate. Many textbooks have placed these conditions under

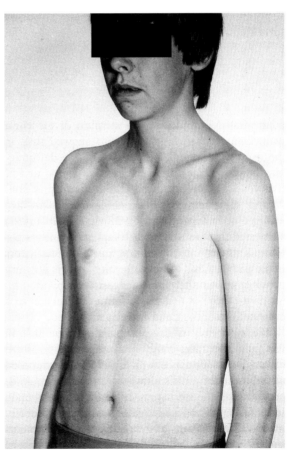

Fig. 1. Pectus excavatum.

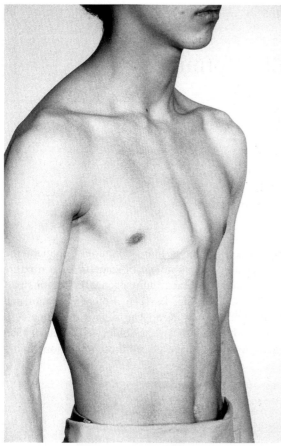

Fig. 2. Pectus carinatum.

congenital deformities of the sternum or the chest wall. One series (Moghissi, 1964) showed that, in the majority of patients in the series, the deformity was noticed not at birth but at or after the age of five years. It appears that if the deformity is congenital, the effects become manifest at a later age and not at birth. Brodkin (1953) and Chin (1957) suggested that the pull of the diaphragm and its abnormal fibrous anterior portion are the basic factors in the pathogenesis of the deformity. This is not very convincing. An alternative suggestion supported by Mullard (1967) is that the deformity is related to a defect of osteogensis and cartillagensis

We subscribe to this view and believe that in this condition there may be an abnormality of the cartilaginous substance which, when superimposed with respiratory difficulties of infancy or childhood, causes the sternum to be drawn inwards upon forcible inspiration and develop sternocostal deformities. Many patients have had respiratory problems such as serious chest infection or respiratory distress, during their infancy. The condition is, most probably,

not hereditary, but familial and it is not uncommon to find several members of the same family or their descendants presenting with the condition (Shamberger et al., 1988).

1.1. Clinical presentation

The majority of patients consult their family doctor and seek specialist advice on cosmetic grounds; as many males as females are psychologically affected by these deformities. In females, a sense of shyness prevents socialising. The young lady illustrated in Fig. 3a and Fig. 3b was in considerable psychological distress, she was withdrawn and disinterested in socialising prior to surgery. Soon after the operation she became the 'belle of the ball' and a year later she was led to the altar.

Some patients have associated cardio/respiratory symptoms, which may or may not disappear following operation, improvement being attributed to the correction of the deformity. The author's opinion is that the deformity is not responsible for the symptoms, except in some children, but it may be associated with respiratory or cardiovascular system conditions causing symptoms on their own account.

1.2. Associated abnormalities

The following associated abnormalities have been recorded in patients with chest deformities, predominantly pectus excavatum:

1.2.1. Scoliosis and spinal deformity
These are present in some 20% of patients with pectus excavatum. It is also present in some patients with carinatum and/or mixed deformities. Both their presence and their incidence depend on the type of chest deformity and the age at which the patient is referred.

1.2.2. Mitral valve prolapse
Clinical or subclinical (echocardiographic evidence) cases of mitral valve prolapse are reported by a number of authors in as many as 30 to 40% of patients, particularly those with pectus excavatum.

1.2.3. Functional and physiological cardio-respiratory deficiency
This may be present in some cases of chest deformities. This cardiac and respiratory impairment is subtle and difficult to substantiate objectively or to correlate with the severity of deformity. Reports

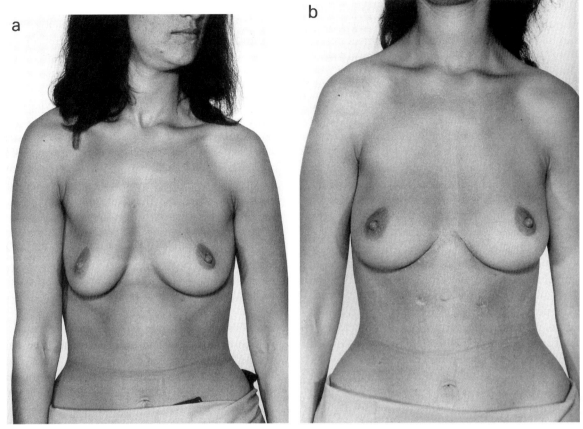

Fig. 3. (a) A young female patient with high non-symmetrical pectus excavatum (note the lower sternal prominence). (b) The same patient one year after surgery with >90% improvement of the deformity.

suggest reduced exercise tolerance and inappropriate cardiac output response to exercise in some of the patients with severe chest deformities.

1.3. Indications for surgery

The primary indications for surgery are psychological and cosmetic and the importance of neither should be underestimated. Beside the cosmetic reasons there is also some evidence to show that the deformity is progressive and will promote spinal deformity. Hence operative correction is indicated to halt the continuation of the process and the development of further deformities such as those of the spine.

1.4. Investigation and preparation for operation

Apart from routine investigation and preparation for surgery, special attention is paid to precise recording of the type and extent of the deformity by clinical photography and radiography of the chest. Associ-

ated cardio-respiratory and coincidental anomalies are recorded and investigated. Repeat clinical photography gives a pictorial record of the progress of the deformity and the surgical results after operation.

1.5. Operation

The basic principle of all operations for sternal deformities is to excise the deformed costal cartilages bilaterally, to detach the lower sternum from the rectus abdominis and the diaphragmatic muscle fibres and to reshape the sternum. Ravitch's (1949) technique was devised on this basis and many surgeons have their own additions to the technique.

1.5.1. Exposure and incision
The patient is placed in a straight supine position with the arms symmetrically placed. The lower neck, anterior chest and abdomen are painted with antiseptic solution. Surgical towels are placed so as to expose the whole of the anterior aspect of the chest and the upper abdomen from the suprasternal

notch down to the umbilicus vertically and from one mid-axillary line to another horizontally. This is necessary in order to make cosmetic assessment during the operation and for placement of pleural drains if required.

The incision may be bilateral transverse submammary or midline vertically over the sternum. The author prefers the former which is attended by better cosmetic results. The skin flap with its subcutaneous fat and pectoralis major and minor is reflected on either side of the incision, the aim being to expose the deformed sternum and costal cartilages. For the lower cartilages, this means their detachment from the rectus abdominis muscles.

Care should be taken not to devitalise skin. This is the only chest operation in which the author does not use electrocoagulation. Warm packs are used to protect the muscle and oozing tissues and blood vessels are tied with catgut.

The perichondrium of the individual rib is peeled off from the underlying cartilages and sub-perichondrial excision of the full length of the deformed cartilages is made. Some surgeons excise the deformed cartilages as well as the perichondrium but the author preserves these. The sternum is freed after all deformed cartilages are excised and the perichondrium and intercostal muscles are divided near the sternum to provide better freedom of the lower part of the bone which, in some cases, is held down by these structures. The xiphisternal joint is transsected (or the process is excised altogether) to further free the sternum which can now be lifted up.

A suitable position of the sternum is then achieved by transverse osteotomy. In many symmetrical deformities, this is the only osteotomy which is required. In some cases, the sternum is so deformed that multiple osteotomies have to carried out. A few stitches are placed to approximate the edges of the sternal osteotomy to ensure correct positioning. Fixation of the sternum in the corrected position is maintained in different ways by different operators. Ravitch advised fixation by placing a wedge of the patient's ribs in the posterior osteotomy; others, including the author, support the correction by placing a stainless steel flat bar or strut under the sternum. The bar is fixed onto the front of a rib on both sides by a stitch. Alternatively, one end of the bar is fixed to the anterior aspect of a rib on one side by a stitch. The other end, after passing behind the sternum, is placed in the marrow of a rib in the opposite side. This is only possible with the use of a tapering bar.

Once the bony correction is completed and supported, the pectoralis muscles are stitched together in the midline. This may not be possible over all areas of the sternum, but the subcutaneous fat and skin are closed in two layers. The use of absorbable stitches and subcutical skin closure gives a better cosmetic result. We place at least one drain in the mediastinum and one in each of the pleural spaces if they have been entered. The drains are connected to an underwater sealed system without suction and removed 24 hours later. The patient is mobilised the day following operation and discharged home eight to ten days later. Some surgeons will discharge the patient earlier than eight post-operative days. This can safely be undertaken providing that arrangements for physiotherapy can be made in order to maintain correct posture.

1.6. Results and complications

There should be no mortality in cases without severe associated abnormalities and none have been reported in large published series.

Major complications of surgical repair are rare. Nevertheless minor complications are not uncommon. These are:

- Pneumothorax or haemothorax. Pneumothorax, when present, is usually noted on the post-operative chest radiography on the second or third post-operative day. This will require aspiration or tube thoracostomy. Haemothorax, if present, requires tube drainage connected to an underwater sealed system.
- Wound complications such as subcutaneous haematoma, dehiscence and sepsis usually relate to an area of the lower part of the sternum.
- Displacement of the metallic sternal support, when such is used, can be serious. It can penetrate the heart and cause cardiac injury. In case of displacement the support should be removed.
- Pericardial effusion: this is usually minor. Only rarely is it important enough to require tamponade. Monitoring of the patient should be carried out and if there are signs of pericardial effusion, appropriate investigation should be undertaken and the pericardium aspirated or drained.

1.6.1. Cosmetic results
In simple, uncomplicated and symmetrical deformities the results are generally good. Pectus carinatum gives a better result than pectus excavatum. Patients without spinal deformity will also have better results.

However, there is an overall recurrence of between 5 to 10% of cases after five years.

2. Chest deformities with bony defects

2.1. Poland syndrome

In 1841 Alfred Poland reported on a case in which there was absence of pectoralis major and minor together with hyperplasia of the breast and syndactyly. The original description did not mention sternal and rib deformities. In the course of time, additional abnormalities, including those of the sternum and ribs, were observed. At present, Poland syndrome is viewed as a spectrum of abnormalities which may or may not include pectus excavatum/carinatum. The excavatum, when present, is on the side of the pectoralis muscle and breast deficiencies.

Involvement of the chest surgeon concerns the repair of chest and sternocostal deformities as described in correction of pectus excavatum and pectus carinatum. The total repair of the deformity may also include breast augmentation and implantation. These repairs/reconstructions need a multidisciplinary approach requiring the participation of a plastic and reconstructive surgeon as well as the thoracic surgeon.

2.2. Sternal defects/sternal cleft

A number of deformities result from failure of ventral fusion of the sternal bar during the intrauterine development of the sternum and body wall, thus producing sternal cleft with or without ectopia-cordis. In the case of sternal cleft with no ectopia-cordis the pericardium and intra-thoracic viscera are intact and in their normal position. The repair of sternal cleft should be undertaken as early as possible after birth in order to achieve direct primary closure without prosthesis or the need for procedures which would involve chondrotomy and/or costal cartilage lengthening.

3. General scheme of management of candidates for surgical repair of chest deformities

- Record symptoms and reason for referral indicating patients desire for surgical repair.
- Carry out clinical examination and clearly note the extent of sternal, rib and spinal involvement; indicate the type of deformity and any associated abnormalities.
- Arrange clinical photography.

- Routine laboratory examination.
- ECG and pulmonary function test.
- Chest radiography (antero-posterior and lateral view) and CT scan of thorax.
- Carry out additional investigation in cases with associated abnormalities and defects.
- Thorough counselling of patients and the family (or parents in case of a child) of the plan of the operation, its objective, risks and possible complications and record of same in the case notes.

References and further reading

Brodkin SH. Pectus excavatum. Surgical indications and time of operation. Pediatrics 1953; 11: 582.

Chin EF. Surgery of funnel chest and congenital sternal prominence. Br J Surg 1957; 44: 360–363.

Dalrymple–Hay MJR, Calver A, Lea RA, et al. Migration of pectus excavatum bar into the left ventricle. Eur J Cardiothorac Surg 1997; 12: 507–509.

Eastridge CE, Prather JR, Hughes FA, Young JM, McCoughan JJ. Actinomycosis: a 24 year experience. Southern Med J 1972; 65(7): 839–843.

Haller JA Jr. Complication of surgery for pectus excavatum. Chest Surg Clin N Am 2000; 10: 415–426, ix.

Hsich MJ, Liu HP, Chang JP. Thoracic actinomycosis. Chest 1993; 104(2): 366–370.

Kabiri H, Lahlou K, Achir A, et al. Les Aspergillomes pulmonair. Resultat du traitement chirurgical: à propos d'une series de 206 ca. Chirurgie 1999; 124: 655–660.

Kroll SS, Walsh G, Ryan B, King RC. Risks and benefits of using Marlex mesh in chest wall reconstruction. Ann Plast Surg 1993; 31: 303–306.

Lacquet LK. Congenital deformities of the anterior chest wall. In: Grillo HC, Eschapasse H (Eds.), International Trends in general thoracic surgery (Vol. 2), Major challenges. Philadelphia: WB Saunders, 1987; pp. 328–337.

Loop FD, Lytle BW, Cosgrove DM, et al. Sternal wound complication after isolated coronary artery bypass grafting: early and late mortality, morbidity and cost of care. Ann Thorac Surg 1990; 49: 179–187.

Martini N, Huvos AG, Burt ME, Heelan RT, Bains MS, McCormack PM, Rusch VW, Weber M, Downey RJ, Ginsberg RJ. Predictors of survival in malignant tumours of the sternum. J Thorac Cardiovasc Surg 1996; 111: 96–106.

Moghissi K. Long term results of surgical correction of pectus excavatum and sternal prominence. Thorax 1964; 19: 350–354.

Morshuis WJ, Folgering HT, Baretsz TO, et al. Exercise cardiorespiratory function before and one year after operation for pectus excavatum. J Thorac Cardiovasc Surg 1994; 107: 1403–1409.

Mullard KS. Observation on the aetiology of pectus excavatum and other chest deformities and a method of recording them. Br J Surg 1967; 54: 115–120.

Pairolero PC, Arnold PG. Management of recalatrant median sternotomy wounds. J Thorac Cardiovasc Surg 1984; 88: 357–364.

Poland A. Deficiency of the pectoralis muscle. Guys Hospital Rep 1841; 6: 191–193.

Ravitch MM. Operative treatment of pectus excavatum. Ann
Surg 1949; 129: 429–444.

Ravitch MM. Congenital deformities of the chest wall and their
operative correction. Philadelphia: WB Saunders, 1977.

Robicsek F. Surgical treatment of pectus carinatum. Chest Surg
Clin N Am 2000; 10: 357–376.

Shamberger RC, Welch KJ. Surgical repair of pectus excavatum.
J Paed Surg 1988; 23: 615–622.

K. Moghissi, J.A.C. Thorpe and F. Ciulli (Eds.)
Moghissi's Essentials of Thoracic and Cardiac Surgery

CHAPTER II.6

Infection and inflammation of the chest wall

K. Moghissi

1. Introduction

Primary inflammatory conditions of the chest wall, which are now rare, were of considerable importance some 50 years ago. With the exception of fungal and tuberculous abscesses, which are still occasionally encountered, other chest wall infections such as syphilis are practically unheard of, at least in the western world and developed countries. One of the characteristics of these abscesses is that they may appear in the chest wall far away from the site of their origin.

2. Sepsis of the chest wall

Septic wounds of the chest wall may arise from a number of sources:
- An untreated empyema may discharge on the surface of the skin (empyema necessitatis).
- There may be a discharging wound of the chest after successful control of pleural infection by rib resection and drainage; this can be due to osteomyelitis and sequestration of the rib end.
- Thoracotomy wound sepsis is now uncommon particularly in non infected elective operations.
- Suppurative chondritis can occur following a penetrating wound and infection of the cartilage. Alternatively, the condition occurs as a complication of the thoraco-abdominal incision. The purulent infection and the resulting sinus can persist for weeks with demoralising effects. The cartilage, track and necrotic tissues at the source, need excising. This is often the only method which brings about complete healing.

3. Osteomyelitis of the ribs in children

- This deserves a mention because it can manifest as a febrile condition, with pain in the chest and a radiological appearance of extrapleural haematoma. The bone itself will be normal looking at the onset of symptoms but a week or ten days later, the rib will show changes detectable radiologically. Aspiration of pus and the administration of antibiotics will control the infection.

4. Tuberculosis of the chest wall

This presents as a cold abscess which is often the result of caseating tuberculous lymphadenitis of nodes which are situated around the neck of the ribs or lymph nodes related to the internal mammary vessels. The infection from the posterior group of glands tracks down and forward through the intercostal space and the covering muscles to emerge below the pectoralis muscles. Infection from the anterior group of glands arises near the costal cartilages. Administration of anti-tuberculous drugs, together with aspiration, usually checks the infection. The continuation of infection despite treatment is an indication for the surgical excision of the glands, together with the track and the abscess cavity. Tuberculous infection in other parts should be suspected and searched for but as a rule the disease will be limited to the chest wall alone.

5. Actinomycosis of the chest wall

This is usually the manifestation of deep-seated infection. Unlike tuberculosis aspiration alone will not be able to bring about healing. Sometimes the infection is limited and can be treated conservatively by administration of antibiotic and drainage of purulent material. At times surgical excision becomes necessary.

6. Sternal infection

6.1. Common causes

At the present time, the commonest cause of sternal infection is the surgical sternotomy most commonly used in heart surgery. This may be associated with, or result from, anterior mediastinal infection. In some cases the infection is limited to a segment of sternum with sequestration and sinus formation. In other cases, sternotomy wounds break partially or completely causing an outpouring of the purulent material. Apart from the presence of infection, sternal dehiscence will have a considerable influence on the normal respiratory mechanics and requires urgent repair. Median sternotomy disruption and infection are serious complications with significant morbidity and mortality. Its incidence is reported to be between 0.3–5% with mortality of 14–47%.

When sternal wound sepsis is accompanied with mediastinal infection, an aggressive policy should be adopted. The principles of treatment are:

- Exposure of anterior mediastinum by re-opening of sternal wound.
- Debridement or cleaning of the area using an antiseptic solution (e.g. aqueous solution of chlorhexidine/providine iodine).
- Administration of appropriate antibiotics based on mircobiological testing and sensitivity.
- Closure of wound with adequate drainage of the anterior mediastinal space.
- Frequent irrigation of wound and anterior mediastinum with antiseptic solution.

More limited infection with sinus formation and sequestration needs exploration and removal of sequestrum followed by drainage. In severe cases of osteomyelitis and infection of the anterior mediastinal space, muscle flap transposition or pedicle transplant of the greater omentum are used to bring about complete healing.

6.2. Tuberculosis

Tuberculosis infection of the sternum is now rare in Europe. In some cases, the condition may cause a serious problem when the skin becomes secondarily infected and resistant to conservative treatment.

7. Bornholm's disease (epidemic pleurodynia) [1]

This is not in reality a disease, but a syndrome characterised by the following:
- Pain in the chest accentuated by breathing.
- Pyrexia of varying degree.
- Headache, vomiting and sometimes shivering.

The white cell count and the appearance of the chest radiograph is normal.

The condition has an epidemic tendency during the warmer months amongst children and young adults and has an incubation period of two to five days. Symptoms disappear spontaneously in two or three days and the diagnosis is made by exclusion. There is no treatment except symptomatic measures and reassurance.

8. Tietze's disease (syn: Tietze's Syndrome, costeochondritis, thoracochondralgia)

This condition is characterised by:
- Pain and tenderness with swelling of one of more upper costal cartilages (there are no local inflammatory signs nor are there any manifestations of respiratory diseases).
- Occasionally swelling alone is present without pain.

Symptoms disappear in one to ten weeks but residual swelling may remain longer or even permanently.

The diagnosis is made by exclusion of other causes of swelling of the chest wall. No specific treatment is required but local infiltration with local anaesthetic and hydrocortisone once or twice will reassure the patient and alleviate symptoms.

9. Chondral dislocation and osteoarthritis (slipping ribs)

Each of the true ribs has a separate chondrosternal joint. These can be the seat of osteoathritis, causing pain and clicking joints. The treatment in the first instance consists of infiltration of local anaesthetics and hydrocortisone. In resistant and troublesome cases excisional surgery may have to be considered.

---

[1] Bornholm's disease was described by Sylvest (1934), a Danish doctor, when holidaying on the island of Bornholm, where his two sons developed the condition. It was also described by W.N. Pickles (1933) of Yorkshire. Infection by Coxsackie B virus appears to be the causative agent.

References and further reading

Barnea Y, Cohen M, Giladi M, et al. Abdominal recovery after laparotomy and omental transposition into a grossly contaminated median sternotomy wound. Ann Plast Surg 2000; 45: 15–18.

Belcher P, McLean N, Breach N, et al. Omental transfer in acute and chronic sternotomy wound breakdown. Thorac Cardiovasc Surg 1990; 38: 186–191.

Castello JR, Centella T, Garro L, et al. Muscle flap reconstruction for the treatment of major sternal wound infections after cardiac surgery: a 10-year analysis. Scand J Plast Reconstr Surg Hand Surg 1999; 33: 17–24.

El Oakley RM, Wright JE. Postoperative mediastinitis: classification and management. Ann Thorac Surg 1996; 61: 1030–1036.

Lindsey JT. A retrospective analysis of 48 infected sternal wound closures: delayed closure decreases wound complications. Plast Reconstr Surg 2002; 109: 1882–1885.

Losanoff JE, Richman BW, Jones JW. Disruption and infection of median sternotomy: a comprehensive review. Eur J Cardiothorac Surg 2002; 21: 831–839.

Moor EV, Neuman RA, Weinberg A, et al. Transposition of the great omentum for infected sternotomy wounds in cardiac surgery. Report of 16 cases and review of published reports. Scand J Plast Reconstr Surg Hand Surg 1999; 33: 25–29.

Nakano N, Miyauchi K, Suzuki H, et al. Large chest wall abscess due to microaerophilic streptococcus. Eur J Cardiothorac Surg 2002; 21: 925.

Paik HC, Chung KY, Kang JH, et al. Surgical treatment of tuberculous cold abscess of the chest wall. Yonsei Med J 2002; 43: 309–314.

Pickles WN. Bornholm Disease: an account of a Yorkshire outbreak. Br Med J 1933; 2: 817–819.

Satta J, Lahtinen J, Raisanen L, et al. Options for the management of post-sternotomy mediastinitis. Scand Cardiovasc J 1998; 32: 29–32.

Sylvest E. Epidemic Myalgia (English translation). Oxford University Press, 1934.

Tammelin A, Hanbraeus A, Stahle E. Mediastinitis after cardiac surgery: improvement of bacteriological diagnosis by use of multiple tissue samples and strain typing. J Clin Microbiol 2002; 40: 2936–2941.

K. Moghissi, J.A.C. Thorpe and F. Ciulli (Eds.)
Moghissi's Essentials of Thoracic and Cardiac Surgery
© 2003 Elsevier Science B.V. All rights reserved

CHAPTER II.7

Thoracic outlet syndrome (TOS)

K. Moghissi

1. Introduction

This term refers to a set of symptoms and signs resulting from compression of the brachial plexus and sub-clavian vessels (neuro-vascular bundle) at the thoracic outlet.

The key to TOS is the understanding of the anatomical relationship between the neurovascular bundle and the musculo-skeletal structure, notably the scalenus anterior muscle and the first rib, at the root of the neck.

2. Anatomy (Fig. 1)

At the root of the neck, the neurovascular bundle (brachial plexus and subclavian vessels) traverses the

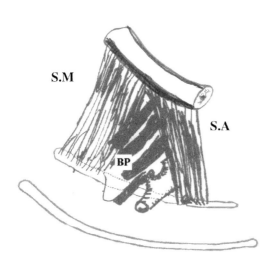

SCALENE TRIANGLE

Fig. 1. Scalene triangle. SA = scalenus anterior muscle, SM = scalenus medius muscle, BP = brachial plexus.

cervico-axillary canal. The entrance of the canal, which is the area between the clavicle above, and the first rib below, is divided into two compartments by insertion of the scalenus anterior into the scalene tubercle of the first rib. The most medial is the costo-clavicular space proper, bounded by the clavicle above, and the first rib below, costo-clavicular ligament antero medially and scalenus medius posteriorly. This space is crossed by brachial plexus and sub clavian vessels (both artery and vein). The more postero-lateral compartment is the scalene triangle. This triangle (space) has the clavicle above, the first rib below, scalenus anterior in front and scalenus medius posteriorly. The triangle is traversed by brachial plexus and sub-clavian artery but not the vein. The scalene triangle is the most important site of compression and the majority of cases of TOS result from structural abnormalities of this area.

Note on brachial plexus:

The plexus is formed by the anterior primary rami of C5, C6, C7, C8 and Th1 spinal nerve roots. It consists of trunks, cords and nerves. The anterior primary rami of C5 and C6 join to form the upper trunk. The C7 anterior primary ramus from the middle trunk and C8 and Th1 anterior primary rami join to form the lower trunk. The trunks divide into an anterior and a posterior division. The anterior divisions of upper and middle trunk join to form the lateral cord, the anterior division of the lower trunk forms the medial cord. All the posterior divisions of the trunks (upper, middle and lower trunks) join to form the posterior cord.

Important nerves derived from cords are:

1. *Lateral cord: Median nerve (root C5–C6, C7) and muscular cutaneous nerve*
2. *Medial cord: Ulnar nerve (roots C8 Th1)*
3. *Posterior cord: Radial (roots C5 to Th1)*

3. Clinical manifestation

TOS predominantly affects females aged between 20 and 50 years. The symptoms and signs may be classified into three groups, accordingly three types of TOS are described.

- Neurogenic type: which relates to compression of brachial plexus elements and in which neurological symptoms and signs predominate.
- Vascular type where the manifestations are predominantly vascular.
- Mixed type: both vascular and neurological signs and symptoms are present with one or the other being more predominant.

The majority of cases are in fact of mixed type.

3.1. Neurogenic TOS

This is the commonest form accounting for between 90 to 95% of all cases. Pain, paraesthesia and muscular weakness are the usual features. Typically, the presentation is pain in the shoulder, arm and forearm. It is often within the territory supplied by the ulnar nerve derived from lower trunk C8 and Th1 roots, which includes medial aspects of the arm and hand, the fifth finger and the lateral aspect of the middle finger. The pain may be initiated by physical exercise or with the arm in abduction during sleep or strenuous exercise. Hyperesthesia in the territory of the ulnar nerve and muscular atrophy in the hypothenar is usually present.

Whilst the ulnar nerve derived from the lower trunk and medial cord of the brachial plexus is the usual involved nerve, other nerves derived from the upper trunk and lateral cord of the plexus can also be affected. This is particularly the case when cervical rib is the cause.

In some cases, the pain distribution is such that it mimics angina pectoris (pseudo angina) with its distribution across the anterior chest wall.

3.2. Vascular compression

This is characterised by coldness and cyanosis of the hand and finger and vascular ischaemic pain on exertion. In 8 to 10% of cases, unilateral Raynaud's phenomenon can be present. These signs can be precipitated by raising the arm in a hyper-abduction position. Typically, some movement such as turning the head or lifting heavy objects may cause pain and blanching and cyanosis of the fingers followed by redness and reactive hyperaemia.

These manifestations may be the precursor of serious and more drastic vascular events related to thrombosis, established stenosis and/or aneurysm of the subclavian artery resulting in ulceration and gangrene of the fingers.

At times, palpation over the para scapular area reveals pulsation of post stenotic dilatation and aneurysm of the subclavian artery.

Manifestations of venous compression in acute cases are discoloration of the affected part and peripheral venous engorgement. These changes herald phlebothrombosis. In more chronic instances, there develop a network of venous collaterals.

3.3. Mixed type

In this form, both neurological and vascular features are evident in differing proportions.

4. Aetiology

The clinical manifestations are as a consequence of compression of the neuro vascular bundle which, in turn, can be caused by a number of factors. Most of these are concerned with congenital anomalies or anatomical abnormalities. Amongst these are:

4.1. Cervical rib

Although the cervical rib can be asymptomatic in many individuals, in some it is the cause of TOS. Rudimentary incomplete cervical rib with a fibrous band continuing and attached to the first rib will have the same effect.

Abnormality of scalene muscles and other factors affect the width of inter-scalene triangle.

4.2. Trauma

Neck trauma is an important cause in neurogenic type of TOS. This is particularly the case in 'whiplash' accidents involving hyperextension of the neck. In other cases, fracture of the first rib or the clavicle may be the cause. In some instances, occupational sustained trauma in individuals whose occupation involves long spells of hyperextension of the neck will be the cause of TOS.

4.3. Fibrous band

Such a band displaces the neurovascular bundle and exerts compression.

5. Diagnosis

History and clinical examination plays an essential part in the diagnosis of TOS. In most cases specific investigation is useful to exclude other conditions or associated diagnosis. Neurological examination is intended to reveal sensory or motor deficits with their segmental distribution. Various manoeuvres are employed to enhance and display pain and its root.

- The vascular component of TOS concerns subclavian vessels and their branches which affect the circulation in the upper limb.
  Radial pulse and its volume in dynamic state and different position of the arm is monitored. Loss or reduction in volume is an indication of TOS.
- Adson's test is based on loss of radial pulse when the scalene muscles, that is scalenus anterior and scalenus medius, are tightened thus reducing the width of the scalene triangle space. The patient takes a deep breath and holds it whilst the neck is extended and rotated towards the affected side. The radial pulse disappears or its volume substantially reduces.
- Hyperabduction test: 90 degree abduction of the arm in extreme rotation produces symptoms of pain and loss (or reduction) of pulse in the affected extremity.
- Tinels test: pressure over the scalene muscles in the supraclavicular area produces a radiating pain or paraesthesia in the ipsilateral upper extremity.

5.1. Specific investigations/tests

5.1.1. Neurophysiological tests
These are useful in differential diagnosis.
- Electromyography (EMG) tests the motor function and is usually normal in TOS.
- Nerve conduction velocity of the ulnar, median, radial and musculo cutaneous nerves can be measured and gives important information. The velocity is measured across the outlet, around the elbow and in the forearm. Decreased velocity across the outlet is consistent with TOS.

5.1.2. Vascular investigations
Clinical observation and examination is usually sufficient to determine vascular TOS. However, Doppler examination is useful to record some postural changes of the flow in the arterial system. It can also show the site of arterial occlusion, post-stenotic dilatation and/or mural thrombosis.

Vascular laboratory studies are useful in con-firming the diagnosis but, per se, without clinical findings, are not of diagnostic significance.

5.1.3. Arteriography
Opinion is divided on the use of arteriography as a routine procedure. I believe arteriography is indicated in some cases to eliminate associated arterial anomalies. Indications of arteriography include the presence of a paraclavicular pulsating mass suspect of being an aneurysm and absence of the radial pulse. Coronary angiography is also indicated in cases where there is difficulty of differential diagnosis or when there is an associated myocardial ischemia. Venography is indicated in venous obstruction.

5.2. Radiology

Chest radiography is essential to eliminate intrathoracic conditions with symptomology akin to TOS.
- Cervical spinal X-ray will detect vertebral abnormalities, cervical rib and first rib anomalies.
- CT scan of the thorax is necessary to exclude superior sulcus (Pancoast) tumour and lesions in the root of the neck and thoracic outlets.
- Magnetic resonance imaging (MRI) can be of assistance for differential diagnosis of TOS and conditions such as herniated disk. MRI alone cannot establish the diagnosis of TOS and its normality does not exclude the existence of TOS.

6. Surgical exploration

Having reviewed the range of diagnostic and investigatory methods it should be acknowledged that, in a small number of cases, no pathology can be detected. In some such cases surgical exploration is justified.

7. Treatment

7.1. Conservative treatment

This consists of physiotherapy and pain relieving medication. Physiotherapy regimens such as neck stretching and shoulder girdle strengthening exercises are helpful and beneficial to some patients. These, together with appropriate analgesic medication and sedatives, will reduce pain and relieve muscle spasms. Smoking should be stopped. It is doubtful if true neurogenic TOS will respond to such conservative measures other than temporarily. In the vascular form of TOS, patients should be monitored carefully since complications can have serious consequences (thrombosis with subsequent gangrene of fingers).

7.2. Surgical treatment

This consists of decompression of neurovascular bundles and involves correct diagnosis of the cause of compression. The indications for surgical treatment are failure of conservative treatment to relieve symptoms and signs of impending vascular ischaemic complications.

Choice of operation: A number of operations have been advocated to relieve compression on the neurovascular bundle. These may be described under three headings:

7.2.1. Intervention on soft tissue

This is exemplified by sclenectomy in which the scalene muscles are divided thus relieving the compression within the inter-scalene space.

- Anterior and middle sclenectomy: in this operation, the scalene triangle is exposed through a supraclavicular incision (see scalene node biopsy, section 2.5.1 in chapter I.2). Scalenus anterior muscle is divided near its insertion to the scalene tubercle. The scalenus medius is then exposed and divided near to its cephalic end. Care should be taken to identify the content of the Scalenus triangle and avoid injury to neuro vascular structures.

7.2.2. Excision of cervical rib

When a cervical rib is the cause of compression, the operation should be focused on excision of that anomaly. It is important to recall that there are various forms of cervical ribs: complete cervical rib, complete cervical rib joining the first rib, incomplete rib and rudimentary rib with a band joining the first rib. In a complete cervical rib which joins the first rib, often the supernumerary rib needs excision as well as the first rib.

Cervical rib resection: the operation is carried out through a supraclavicular transverse incision some 3 to 4 cm above the clavicle about 2 to 3 cm from the midline. The incision is carried laterally for 6 to 8 cm. The cervical rib is found within the scalenus medius muscle.

7.2.3. First rib resection

Complete excision of the first rib is now the standard operation for cases other than those caused by a cervical rib. The operation may be carried out via a

posterior thoracoplasty incision, an anterior route or transaxillary access method. Whichever approach is used, it is important to free the first rib and divide the scalene muscles which form the walls of scalene triangle space.

- Thoracoplasty approach: In this approach the first rib is accessed posteriorly. The patient is placed in lateral position and a vertical paravertebral incision is made along the vertebral border of scapula then in continuation over the line of the rib. The first rib is identified and freed completely using a periosteum elevator. This approach has the advantage of allowing a good view of the bundles. Since the popularity and ease of the transaxillary approach posterior thoracoplasty incision is used mostly for recurrent cases and in those patients whose first rib had not been removed in its entirety at previous operation for this condition.

- Transaxillary approach: the patient is placed in the lateral position with the arm elevated. The position can be maintained during the operation by attaching the forearm to a frame over the head of the table and protected by a soft cushion and padding. An 8 to 10 cm incision is made in the axilla. Exposure can be improved by mobilisation of the anterior border of latissimus dorsi which is the posterior edge of the wound. The first rib is reached after division of scalenus medius and scalenus anterior. The rib is freed from fibrous and muscular mass and is then excised totally from its costovertebral to costochondral joint.

- Other approaches: The first rib may be approached by supra-clavicular, infra-clavicular or combined incisions.

Results of operation. First rib resection has a success rate of up to 80%, although some authors suggest similar results following sclenectomy, particularly when it is coupled with supraclavicular first rib resection (Sanders et al., 1989). However, this view has been contested by others (MacKinnon et al., 1995).

8. Complications

- Neurological complications: These are the most serious and can occur following hyper-abduction at operation. Injury of Th1 (first thoracic) nerve root may occur due to stretching or surgical mishap (cutting). Phrenic nerve injury results in diaphragmental paralysis.

- Accidental entry to the pleural space will result in pneumothorax and collapse of the lung. This can be dealt with by drainage of the pleural space.

- Haemorrhage: Intra-operative accidental injury to subclavian vessels should be detected and repaired. Post-operative ooze of blood (haematoma) in the extra pleural space needs evacuation and haemothorax requires drainage. In the latter case, the patient is monitored since exploration may be necessary if the drainage continues. The patient should be monitored in order to initiate appropriate further management.

References and further reading

Caldwell JW, Crane CR, Krusen EM. Nerve conduction studies in the diagnosis of the thoracic outlet syndrome. South Med J 1971; 64: 210–212.

Clagett OT. Presidential address, Research and Prosearch. J Thorac Cardiovasc Surg 1962; 44: 153–166.

Coletta JM, Murry JD, Reeve TR, et al. Vascular thoracic outlet syndrome. Successful outcome with multimodal therapy. Cardiovasc Surg 2001; 9: 11–15.

Kashyap VS, Ahn SS, Machleder HI. Thoracic outlet neurovascular compression approaches to anatomic decompression and their limitations. Semin Vasc Surg 1998; 11(2): 116–122.

Mackinnon S, Patterson GA, Urschel HC Jr. Thoracic Outlet Syndrome. In: Pearson FG, Deslauriers J, Ginsberg RJ, et al. (Eds.), Thoracic Surgery. New York: Churchill Livingstone 1995; pp. 1211–1235.

Redenback DM, Neleiy B. Comparative study of structures comprising the thoracic outlet in 250 human cadavers and 72 surgical cases of thoracic outlet syndrome. Eur J Cardiothorac Surg 1998; 13: 353–360.

Remy Jardin M, Remy J, Masson P, et al. CT angiography of thoracic outlet syndrome; evaluation of protocols for the detection of arterial stenosis. J Comput Assist Tomogr 2000; 24(3); 349–361.

Roos DB. Transaxillary approach for first rib resection to relieve thoracic outlet syndrome. Ann Surg 1966; 163: 354–355.

Sanders RJ, Pearce WH. The treatment of thoracic outlet syndrome: a comparison of different operations. J Vasc Surg 1989; 10: 626–634.

Urschel HC Jr. The history of surgery for thoracic outlet syndrome. Chest Surg Clin N Am 2000; 10(1): 183–188.

Urschel HC Jr, Razzukk MA, Wood RE, Paulson DL. Objective diagnosis (ulnar nerve conduction velocity) and current therapy of the thoracic outlet syndrome. Ann Thorac Surg 1971; 12: 608–609.

K. Moghissi, J.A.C. Thorpe and F. Ciulli (Eds.)
Moghissi's Essentials of Thoracic and Cardiac Surgery
© 2003 Elsevier Science B.V. All rights reserved

CHAPTER II.8

Chest wall tumours

A. Mearns

1. Benign tumours

The majority of chest wall tumours are benign and cartilaginous in origin.

1.1. Chondromas

Chondromas are often asymptomatic and present as a swelling at the anterior end of the ribs. CT and MRI are needed in a number of cases to diagnose them. Malignant degeneration of chondromatous tumours is rare.

1.2. Fibrous dysplasia

Although often described amongst neoplasms, the condition is not true neoplasia but a developmental abnormality of ribs in which the medullary cavity is filled with fibrous tissue and random formation of poor trabecule. The commonest site is the posterior aspect of a rib near its angle. The presentation is one of a painless lytic lesion, at times with bone expansion.

1.3. Other conditions

A number of other benign tumours or tumour-like conditions affect the musculoskeletal wall of the thorax. They present as a swelling of chest wall. These are:
- Eosinophilic granuloma.
- Chondroma.
- Osteochondroma.
- Desmoid tumour.
- All soft tissue benign tumours.

1.4. Lipoma

Lipoma of the chest wall requires a special mention since, by their characteristic radiolucency, they can be diagnosed radiologically, notably by CT scanning. Also, although they usually develop extrapleurally they may have extension and have an intrathoracic component.

1.5. Management

In all benign tumours, surgical resection is undertaken. Excision biopsy should be tried for lesions less than 3 cm in all diameters. Larger lesions should have incisional biopsy with later clearance including the biopsy site and planned reconstruction if needed.

2. Malignant chest wall tumour

Primary malignant chest wall tumours are rare and often diagnosed late when they are in an advanced stage of their development since patients may prevaricate as to the importance of the symptoms. At presentation, pain and swelling are common and such symptoms need careful assessment to improve the diagnostic rate. More florid but less common symptoms are rarely missed. Pleural effusion, symptoms related to brachial plexus and spinal compression are readily apparent. At times, the lesion may be detected incidentally at chest X-ray. Imaging will begin with chest radiography and include CT scan; increasingly, MRI is being used particularly to assess spinal involvement.

2.1. Malignant primary tumours

Important malignant primary chest wall neoplasms are:

- Chondrosarcoma: This is said to be the commonest malignant primary chest wall neoplasm. It presents usually as a circumscribed mass; differential diagnosis between this lesion and benign osteochondroma is difficult. Large lesions, greater than 4 cm, are considered to be malignant.
- Fibrosarcomas are also common amongst malignant chest wall neoplasms. Radiologically, these tumours may show areas of necrosis and calcification. On the whole, their presentation gives no indication of their identity.
- Plasmacytomas are the commonest of sternal tumours. There is a relationship between multiple (systemic) myeloma and plasmacytoma. The latter can be the first manifestation of the former.
- Ewing's sarcoma principally occurs in children but it may also be seen in adults. It presents as cystic or expansive tumour of the ribs and clavicle.
- Osteogenic sarcoma.
- Askin's tumour, a neoplasm, first described by Askin, is a highly malignant tumour which, like Ewing's sarcoma, is grouped amongst primary neuroectodermal tumours (PNET).

3. The management of primary malignant chest wall tumours

3.1. Resection

Resection should be undertaken whenever possible. Modern prostheses and multimodality therapy have improved the outcomes in primary chest wall tumours. High cure rates are now to be expected in Ewing's sarcoma. Extensive areas of chest wall may be resected for chondrosarcoma with little or no loss of breathing capacity.

3.2. Chondrosarcoma

Chondrosarcoma grows locally and may become a large growth (Figs. 1a and 1b). Frequently it recurs because of inadequate clearance. The only difficulty with resection in these patients is involvement of the vertebral body. However, operative resection is the only effective treatment. Recently, mesenchymal chondrosarcoma has been identified; this is an aggressive form which metastasises early and carries a poor prognosis. This variant may account for some deaths in earlier series, particularly if metastases have been identified.

3.3. Ewing's sarcoma

Ewing's sarcoma is best managed by initial incisional biopsy and then planned resection followed by local radiotherapy and chemotherapy.

3.4. Plasmacytoma

This is the commonest primary tumour of the sternum. Solitary plasmacytoma of the chest wall is treated by wide local excision followed by thorough supervision. Chemotherapy is introduced on evidence of systemic disease.

3.5. Rarer tumours

Rarer tumours such as Askin's tumour and Desmoid tumour are treated also by wide excision and reconstruction of chest wall.

4. General principles of surgical treatment

4.1. General

The fixed points of the chest wall are the lower sternum and tranverse processes of the vertebrae. Reconstruction must maintain the connections of the lower sternum otherwise there will be pain and limitation of movement. The patient can manage without the manubrium and upper part of the sternum although most find prosthesis reassuring. Clavicles should not be fixed to the prosthesis as the mobility of the scapula may be impaired and the fixation may well break. The clavicles may be removed or partially resected with impunity. The scapula covers large defects posteriorly but defects down to the sixth or seventh rib posteriorly will allow the scapula to bind at its lower pole where it may fall into the defect, A prosthesis will prevent this. If the prosthesis is attached to the transverse processes of the vertebrae the chest wall movement will be restricted. One should try to avoid this by leaving a gap between the edge of the plate and the transverse processes; The plate will then move with the ribs. Local resection of parts of, and even complete, vertebral bodies have been attempted with the spine's integrity being maintained with metal plates and rods.

4.2. Prostheses

Prosthesis are usually mesh, either heavy and single layer or a sandwich of two layers of lighter mesh,

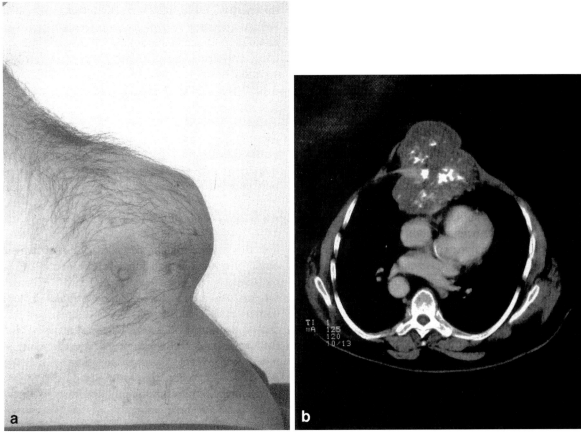

Fig. 1. A patient with chondrosarcoma of anterior chest wall that had been ignored for more than 10 years and was now massive and involving the sternum. This man had poliomyelitis and was confined to a wheelchair and therefore was not suitable for a major resection involving the lower sternal area as he was dependent on his upper limb girdle for mobility. The illustrations show: (a) the size with thinning of the skin over the tumour and the biopsy site through healthy skin, (b) CT scan shows the pre-operative extent of this tumour which is probably larger in its intrathoracic portion than its extrathoracic presentation. Because of the need for stability of the lower sternal area in order for his upper limb girdle to function, this tumour was only subject to volume reduction and the tumour was taken flush with the chest wall.

with a plate of meythyl methacrylate moulded to shape between.

4.3. Approach

The planned approach must include optimal imaging and prior histology. For small tumours excision biopsy is recommend to avoid implantation recurrence. For larger tumours, the initial biopsy must be planned so that the skin incision may be excised en bloc with the resected chest wall mass. All tissues involved beneath the chest wall such as thymus, lung, pericardium and pleura should form part of the en-bloc mass excision. For rib tumours, wide resection includes at least the rib above and below plus a four centimetre margin along the line of the rib because of possible intramedullary and periosteal

extension. The tumour is widely excised with frozen section sampling of the resection margin if needed and then the reconstruction is undertaken. The pre-operative planning should include identifying soft tissues for transposition; muscle, latissimus dorsi or pectoralis major, omentum or a myocutaneous flap based on axillary blood supply to latissimus dorsi. Direct cover of prosthetic material with skin alone has a high complication rate. If there is any infective component, omentum is probably the tissue of choice.

4.4. Summary

The value of prosthetic reconstruction is that the integrity of chest wall function is maintained and the patient is able to breathe spontaneously. Perioperative mortality should be low. The use of paravertebral extrapleural local analgesia provides good pain relief and suppresses the stress response, adding to the quality of outcome in these major reconstructions.

5. Survival after excision of a chest wall tumour

Survival after chest wall reconstruction has improved steadily over the last thirty years. The indicators for survival are adequacy of resection and histological grading. There is no adjuvant therapy for chondrosarcoma. Solitary plasmacytoma fully excised survives well in the absence of its expression as systemic disease. There are a few five year survivors in the latter group although chemotherapy is indicated. Periodic screening and long term follow up is required.

With wide surgical excision, irradiation to the tumour bed and adjuvant chemotherapy Ewing's sarcoma of rib is demonstrating the same improved prognosis as the long bone tumour. Askin's tumour is rare but genetically akin to Ewing's sarcoma. The recorded cases are few and the tumour is best linked with Ewing's sarcoma for informed management.

Desmoid tumours are not classically malignant but tend to recur locally. Therefore, the principles of wide excision with reconstruction as necessary is the correct approach.

6. Malignant secondary chest wall tumours

6.1. Carcinoma of the lung

Carcinoma of the lung invades the chest wall by direct invasion. Since the development of more sophisticated imaging techniques, a greater number of such invasions is diagnosed. Of importance are superior sulcus and diaphragmatic involvement by lung cancer. In this respect, CT and MRI scans are very important in defining involvement of the chest wall. Simple extra-pleural clearance is not adequate: en-bloc resection with chest wall is more effective.

6.2. Breast cancer

Breast cancer is somewhat different in that the chest involvement follows excision; that is recurrence in the chest wall, ribs and even penetration to the pleura are not uncommon as part of local recurrence. With combination chemotherapy and hormone therapy, chest wall excision and reconstruction with prosthesis and latissimus dorsi flap, is effective.

6.3. Mesothelioma

Mesothelioma commonly invades the chest wall and causes great pain. There is no effective treatment. Palliative care with DXT and effective pain relief may help but life expectancy at this stage is poor.

6.4. Others

The ribs are commonly the site for metastases particularly from prostate, thyroid and bronchus. Local radiotherapy for pain relief is the best we can offer for local management combined with systemic therapy appropriate to the primary tumour. It is commonly necessary to biopsy such metastases when they present singly or late in the course of the primary tumour management.

References and further reading

Burt M, Fulton M, Wessner-Dunlap S, Karpeh M, Huvos AG, Bains MS, Martini N, McCormack PM, Rusch VW, Ginsberg RJ. Primary bony and cartilaginous sarcomas of chest wall: results of therapy. Ann Thorac Surg 1992; 54: 226–232.

Burt M, Karpeh M, Ukoha O, Bains MS, McCormach PM, Rusch VW, Ginsberg RJ, Martini N. Medical tumours of the chest wall: solitary plasmacytoma and Ewings sarcoma. J Thorac Cardiovasc Surg 1993; 105: 89–96.

Mansour KA, Anderson TM, Hester TR. Sternal resection and reconstruction. Ann Thorac Surg 1993; 55: 838–843.

McFee MK, Pairolero PC, Bergstralh EJ, Piehler JL, Unni KK, McLeod RA, Bernatz PE, Payne WS. Chondrosarcoma of the chest wall: factors affecting survival. Ann Thorac Surg 1985; 40: 535–541.

Pairolero PC, Arnold PG. Chest wall tumours: experience with 100 consecutive patients. J Thorac Cardiovasc Surg 1985; 90: 367–372.

Sabanathan S, Shah R, Mearns AJ. Surgical treatment of primary chest wall tumours. Eur J Cardiothorac Surg 1997: 11: 1011–1016.

CHAPTER II.9

The diaphragm

K. Moghissi

1. Anatomy

The diaphragm is a musculotendinous structure which separates the thorax from the abdominal cavity (Fig. 1). It has a central tendon, to the periphery of which are attached muscle fibres arising from the lumbar vertebrae, sternum and lower ribs. The muscle fibres take their origin from the upper lumbar vertebrae and the medial and lateral arcuate ligaments; laterally they arise from the lower six costal cartilages and anteriorly from the back of the xiphisternum. From these origins, all fibres converge towards the central tendon into which they are inserted. The posterior fibres form the crura of the diaphragm, these have special surgical roles with respect to the lower oesophagus as it passes from the chest to the abdomen.

There are three major openings in the diaphragm allowing the passage of structures from the chest to the abdomen:

- Aortic opening: This is behind the diaphragm opposite the 12th thoracic vertebra and provides a passage for the aorta, azygos vein and thoracic duct.
- Vena caval opening: This is situated in the right leaf of the central tendon opposite the 8th thoracic vertebra. The opening allows the passage of the inferior vena cava and the right phrenic nerve.
- Oesophageal opening (oesophageal hiatus of the diaphragm or simply the hiatus): This is at the level of the 10th thoracic vertebra and provides a passage for the oesophagus, the vagi and the oesophageal branches of gastric vessels.

The phrenic nerve supplies the diaphragm giving motor supply to the muscles of the dome. The crura are supplied by spinal nerves. The sensory supply is from the phrenic and intercostal nerves.

The diaphragm is essentially a respiratory muscle; however, the crura surrounding the oesophagus have a possible role in the lower oesophageal sphincteric action.

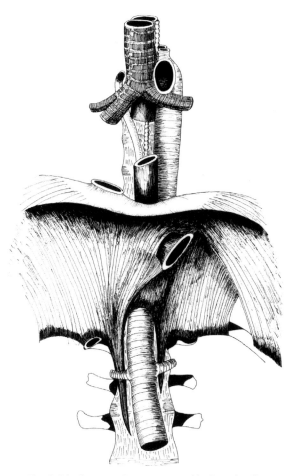

Fig. 1. Diaphragm and arrangement of its "openings".

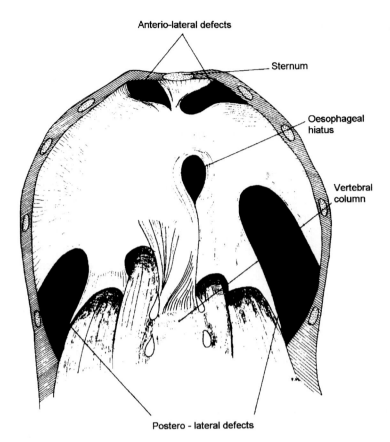

Fig. 2. Topography of congenital defect of the diaphragm.

The diaphragm is developed between weeks eight through ten of intra-uterine life from the fusion of several components, notably the following:

- Septum transversum: This mesodermal septum forms the central tendon and the anterior part of the diaphragm, it grows posteriorly to meet the dorsal mesentery.
- Dorsal mesentery of the foregut: This is joined by muscle fibres to form the crura and the postero-central part of the diaphragm and fuses with the septum transversum anteriorly.
- Cervical myotomes: These migrate down and fuse to the septum transversum and the dorsal mesentery of the foregut. The fusion of the above mentioned structures complete the separation of the thorax and abdomen except in two areas on the postero-lateral part of the diaphragm (pleuroperitoneal canals) these are then closed by:
- Pleuroperitoneal membrane: One on each side which completes the partition of the thorax from the abdomen.

2. Congenital diaphragmatic hernias

Protrusion of abdominal content through a congenital defect is the basis of these hernias. Figure 2 shows common congenital defects and the corresponding hernias. It is reported that diaphragmatic hernias occur in one in 2000 births and that they are collectively responsible for 8% of congenital malformations causing death during the first few days of life (Butler and Claireaux, 1962). Associated with congenital hernias are two other anomalies which have important bearing on the design of surgical repair and its outcome. Incomplete rotation or malrotation of the gut which, if unrecognised at the time of surgery, may lead to post-operative intestinal obstruction. Also pulmonary hypoplasia with failure of normal lung expansion following the reduction and repair which leaves a residual pleural space.

The common congenital hernias of the diaphragm are as follows:

- A large hernia through absent diaphragmatic dome or absent hemidiaphragm.

- Postero-lateral diaphragmatic hernia (known as Bochdalek hernia), due to the absence of the pleurperitoneal membrane.
- Subcostosternal (retrosternal, Morgagni) hernia due to congenital defect in the anterior portion of the diaphragm.
- Congenital hiatal hernia from lack of development in the portion of the diaphragm around the hiatus.

2.1. Congenital absence of the hemidiaphragm

Complete absence of the diaphragm is extremely rare, as is absence of the hemidriaphragm or the dome. The defect allows a large portion of the upper abdominal viscera to be placed in the chest. The abnormality is discovered at birth or soon after as a respiratory distress syndrome. Chest radiograph is usually diagnostic.

2.1.1. Management

One of the first steps is to introduce a nasogastric tube to deflate the stomach and relieve the intrathoracic tension which is the cause of distress. Supportive measures are then applied according to needs, i.e. oxygen and in some cases, endotracheal intubation and positive pressure ventilation until operative reduction of the hernia is undertaken. Endotracheal intubation, if required, should be carried out by an experienced operator. Intubation of those neonates with distress syndrome can be very difficult. Also intubation of the oesophagus followed by assisted ventilation will have the consequence of further increasing the intrathoracic tension with fatal outcome.

The repair of hernias due to congenital absence of hemidiaphragm is difficult and can be attended by a high mortality. Associated anomalies of pulmonary and intra-abdominal viscera add further complications and risk factors. In the absence of other anomalies the repair can be carried out via the abdominal or thoracic route. The abdominal approach has the advantage that possible anomalies of the intra-abdominal viscera can be assessed and corrected. The repair and reconstruction of the diaphragm using prostheses is however difficult. The thoracic route provides an easier way for the repair and reconstruction but has the added difficulty of the possibility that the herniated intra-abdominal viscera may not be repositioned easily into the abdomen. In both approaches, there is the possibility that the peritoneal cavity may not accommodate a large herniated portion and the abdomen cannot be closed. In this event, following the repair, the peritoneum is first sutured to the abdominal wall muscles then, after undermining, the skin is closed by subcutaneous and cutaneous sutures only to produce a ventral hernia which may be repaired at a later date.

2.2. Posterolateral (Bochdalek) hernia

This hernia results from the lack of separation of the thoracic and abdominal cavities due to persistence of the pleuroperitoneal canal (see section 1 above). The defect is in the posterolateral portion of the diaphragm, usually in the region of the 10th to 11th rib. Bochdalek hernia is the commonest congenital diaphragmatic hernia and predominantly affects the left side. The hernia is usually diagnosed during childhood.

The presenting features may be repeated pulmonary infection or acute intermittent pain and vomiting, though many cases are discovered by incidental chest radiograph. The presence of bowel sounds on auscultation of the chest may draw attention to the existence of the hernia. Chest radiograph and other radiological investigations establish the diagnosis.

2.2.1. Management

In acute situations such as the presence of respiratory problems or intestinal obstruction, decompression by nasogastric tube aspiration is undertaken and biochemical abnormalities are corrected before urgent surgical operation is undertaken. Repair should also be undertaken in uncomplicated cases. In the rare right-sided hernia, right thoracotomy is the usual approach. For the repair of left-sided hernia, the thoracic or abdominal approach may be used. Consideration should be given to the mode of presentation and the age of the patient. In uncomplicated hernias, the thoracic approach is preferable as this not only provides good exposure but also facilitates reduction, if necessary, by incising the diaphragmatic edges of the defect. Also, repair and reconstruction of the defect following the reduction of the hernia is easily achieved through the chest. In acute obstructive symptoms in infancy, the abdominal approach may be considered as the preferred route of access as there may be associated intra-abdominal anomalies requiring surgical attention.

2.3. Substernocostal (Morgagni) hernia

A hernia occurring through a congenital retrosternal defect was first described by Morgagni in 1769. It has received many names, of which substernocostal appears the most appropriate. There are several varieties of these hernias: unilateral, bilateral or truly substernal. Many are asymptomatic and are discovered incidentally at routine chest radiograph. Others may present as pain in the upper abdomen and the chest during adolescence or even at an older age. Occasionally, the hernia is complicated by intestinal obstruction. Clinical examination in uncomplicated cases is unrevealing and radiological investigations are generally not diagnostic. Induction of pneumonoperitoneum, in adults, followed by upper abdominal/lower chest X-ray may be helpful in demonstrating the upper abdominal viscera protruding into the chest surrounded by gas shadow. Barium swallow studies will be helpful when a portion of the gastrointenstinal tract is included in the hernia.

2.3.1. Surgical management

In the rare event of obstruction, the pre-operative preparation of the patient is similar to that of intestinal obstruction. Surgical repair may be via thoracotomy or laparotomy, depending on the site and extent of the opening. Most of these hernias can easily be reduced through a subcostal incision. There is usually a sac which can be excised. The edges of the diaphragm are then stitched to the chest wall (sternum or costal cartilages). When the defect is more one-sided, a thoracic approach (with the patient in the anterior oblique position) is an easy route but closure of the defect may not be easy.

The author's preferred approach for an extensive and complicated hernia is through an abdomino-mediastinal approach. An upper midline abdominal incision is extended upwards over the sternum, the lower part of which is divided. Good exposure is thus obtained, allowing reduction of the hernia even in the presence of intra-thoracic adhesions. Furthermore, this approach facilitates the repair of the defect (Moghissi, 1981).

3. General presentation and clinical features of diaphagmatic hernias

3.1. Presentation

3.1.1. Presentation as an acute respiratory symptom

Large congenital hernias such as those resulting from the absence of a hemidiaphragm constitute an acute respiratory emergency in neonates and are an important cause of perinatal mortality. Left-sided hernias are more common than right. The stomach and most of the upper abdominal viscera will find

their way into the left chest. Exactly how much and which structures will be displaced into the chest is governed by the presence or absence of a peritoneal sac. When a sac is present, both the extent of the hernia and the herniated structures will be limited.

In large hernias, dyspnoea is pronounced and the presence of intra-abdominal viscera in the left chest displaces the heart and mediastinum to the right simulating dextrocardia. When smaller postero-lateral hernias are present, respiratory symptoms are less apparent.

3.1.2. Presentation as intermittent pain

In young children with small to moderate congenital hernias, pain may be intermittent and the only presenting feature. A congenital paraoesophageal hernia may contain large portions of the stomach which has rotated on its horizontal axis in the chest. The volvulus of the stomach behind the heart causes obstruction and acute chest pain resembling cardiac ischaemic pain. When the hernia is temporarily and/or spontaneously reduced, the true cause of the acute pain and distress of the child remain undiagnosed.

3.1.3. Acute intestinal obstruction

Acute intestinal obstruction due to volvulus may, in some cases, be the presenting feature of diaphragmatic hernia. This mode of presentation often occurs in adults. Occasionally vomiting and haematemesis accompany or precede the signs of obstruction.

3.1.4. Asymptomatic

Some congenital hernias remain completely asymptomatic and are found in the course of chest radiography.

3.2. Physical signs

Auscultation may indicate the presence of bowel sounds high in the chest. The following case is an interesting illustration of the clinical presentation of a congenital diaphragmatic hernia.

A boy aged five years had been noticed to have intermittent attacks of acute pain and screaming, particularly at night, since birth. The cries were attributed to "wind" and when the child was attended to and taken out of his cot the cries would stop. The general practitioner had examined the child on several occasions but had found no abnormal physical signs. One night the child was seized with pain which lasted for half an hour. The practitioner who saw the child found bowel sounds in the left chest on auscultation and sent him to hospital as an emergency. When the child was seen at the hospital he was calm but on account of the general practitioner's findings, diagnosis of the diaphragmatic hernia was made; chest radiograph and examination confirmed the presence of a congenital hernia of the Bochdalek type. This was repaired and the child recovered and has remained well to date into adult life.

4. General notes on operative technique for diaphragmatic hernias

4.1. Trans-thoracic approach

The patient is placed in the lateral position and thoracotomy is carried out through the 8th or 9th intercostal space. The lung is retracted upwards. The hernia and its contents are identified and reduced into the abdomen. The reduction is facilitated by appropriate enlargement of the opening. Repositioning of the spleen into the abdomen (if within the hernia) needs particular care and gentleness to avoid injury. Attention should also be paid to the untwisting of the stomach or bowels which may become entangled with omental adhesions. The defect is then closed directly or by using a Teflon prosthesis sewn to the edges of the defect with uninterrupted continuous sutures using non-absorbable materials.

4.2. Trans-abdominal approach

A left or right subcostal incision is made with the patient in a slightly oblique position (20–30° tilt). The incision provides good exposure by retraction of the left lobe of the liver. Traction of the intestine easily reduces the hernia but repositioning of the spleen into the abdomen may present difficulties.

The closure of the defect is undertaken following reduction of the contents of the hernia. Some surgeons prefer a combination of subcostal and thoracotomy incisions (i.e. two separate incisions). In some neonates this may become necessary but in adults it is not usually required.

References and further reading

Beresford MW, Shaw NJ. Outcome of congenital diaphragmatic hernia. Paediatric Pulmonol 2000; 30: 249–256.

Butler N, Claireaux AE. Congenital diaphragmatic hernia as a cause of peri-natal mortality. Lancet 1962; 1: 659–663.

Langer JC. Congenital diaphragmatic hernia. Chest Surg Clin N Am 1998; 8: 295–314.

Moghissi K. Operation for the repair of obstructed substernocostal (Morgagni) hernia. Thorax 1981; 36(5): 392–304.

Naunheim KS. Adult presentation of unusual diaphragmatic hernia. Chest Surg Clin N Am 1998; 8: 359–369.

Tsang TM, Tam PK, Dudley NF, Steven J. Diaphragmatic agenesis as a distinct clinical entity. J Paediat Surg 1995; 30: 16–18.

SECTION III

The Oesophagus

K. Moghissi, J.A.C. Thorpe and F. Ciulli (Eds.)
Moghissi's Essentials of Thoracic and Cardiac Surgery

CHAPTER III.1

The oesophagus

K. Moghissi

1. Surgical anatomy

The oesophagus is a hollow muscular tube lined with stratified squamous epithelium extending from the pharynx to the stomach, a length of 25 cm in an adult. Beginning in the neck behind the cricoid cartilage opposite the 6th cervical vertebrae, it descends in front of the vertebral column, passing through the whole length of the neck and thorax to enter the abdomen through the hiatus of the diaphragm, level with the 10th thoracic vertebra. After a short distance in the abdomen, the oesophagus joins the stomach. The oesophago-gastric junction is at the level of the 11th thoracic vertebra.

The oesophagus has three parts: cervical, thoracic and abdominal. The cervical part is in the midline behind the trachea whose posterior non-cartilaginous and muscular wall is separated from the anterior wall of the oesophagus by loose connective tissues; this is convenient for surgical mobilisation. The relationship with the trachea is maintained until its entrance to the thorax, at which point the oesophagus deviates slightly to the left of the midline to pass behind the left main bronchus. In its passage from the neck to the thorax it lies behind the tracheal bifurcation in front of the vertebrae with the arch of the aorta to its left and the parietal pleura of the right pleural cavity and azygos vein to its right.

The thoracic part of the oesophagus is placed in the posterior mediastinum; at first it bears slightly to the right of the midline. Here in the upper thorax it lies between the descending thoracic aorta to its left and the parietal pleura at its right, while the left atrium is in front. Some 4–5 cm above the diaphragm the oesophagus deviates yet again, slightly to the left behind the pericardium. At the hiatus it lies in front of the aorta, touching the parietal pleura on the left side.

The abdominal part of the oesophagus is a 2–3 cm-long tube which begins as it passes through the hiatus in front of the aorta and ends in joining the stomach at the cardia.

The oesophageal tube has 3 relatively narrow segments:
- At the pharyngo-oesophageal junction
- At the point of entry of the oesophagus into the thorax
- At its lower end (cardia)

2. Structure of the oesophagus

The oesophagus has a mucous membrane which is lined with squamous epithelium for most of its extent, except for a short intra-abdominal segment where the lining in this terminal intra-abdominal segment changes for some 2–3 cm to junctional columnar epithelium with a few or no parietal cells.

Beneath the epithelium there is a submucosal layer which, though thin, is strong and is made up of connective areolar and vascular tissues with few smooth muscle fibres. The mucosa and submucosal layers contain superficial and deep mucous glands. It also contains the Meissner's plexus of nerves. Outside the submucosal layer there is a muscular coat in two layers, an inner circular and the outer longitudinal. In the cervical part, the muscular tissue is predominantly composed of striated (voluntary) fibres. In the thoracic and abdominal portions, the musculature is all of the smooth (involuntary) variety. Between the circular and longitudinal muscle strands lie the intermuscular connective tissues containing the Auerbach's plexus of nerves and vascular network. The thoracic oesophagus is draped by the mediastinal pleura.

2.1. Blood supply, lymphatics and nerves

The oesophagus receives its arterial blood supply from:

(a) Inferior thyroid artery in its cervical portion
(b) Oesophageal branches of the aorta, for the thoracic portion
(c) Inferior phrenic and left gastric arteries for the lower parts of the oesophagus including the abdominal portion.

The venous drainage follows the arterial supply. There is a rich submucosal venous plexus which joins to form larger vertical veins. These veins are inter-communicating and drain into the cervical veins, azygos venous system, left gastric vein and the portal system of veins. Thus, there is a communication between the systemic and portal veins which is important both in the production of varices (in the event of portal hypertension) as well as for the provision of a channel for dissemination of malignant diseases. The presence of perforating branches from submucosal veins to the azygos system of veins is responsible for the lack of extension of the oesophageal varices proximal to the lower half of the oesophagus.

Lymphatic drainage of the oesophagus follows the venous and arterial supply. There is a rich submucosal lymphatic channel running longitudinally which then drains via the perforating branches into the cervical, mediastinal and coeliac groups of lymph nodes.

Nerve supply of the oesophagus is through the sympathetic and parasympathetic nerves. The parasympathetic supply is via the vagi. The recurrent laryngeal nerves supply the cervical oesophagus. The vagi form a plexus around the thoracic oesophagus which joins towards the hiatus to form two major trunks. The left nerve becomes anterior and the right posterior; they lie on the corresponding surfaces of the stomach. The thoracic sympathetic chain of the splanchnic nerves and branches of the coeliac sympathetic plexus join to give the sympathetic supply to the oesophagus.

3. Specific anatomical features of the pharyngo-oesophageal and oesophago-gastric junction

3.1. Pharyngo-oesophageal junction

The pharynx extends from the base of the skull to the pharyngo-oesophageal junction. The cavity of the pharynx is related anteriorly to the nasal cavity, the mouth, and the larynx; hence the terms nasopharynx, oropharynx, and laryngo-pharynx. The pharyngo-oesophageal junction is guarded by the circular fibre of the inferior constrictor, the cricopharyngeus muscle, which during swallowing relaxes to allow entry of the bolus into the oesophagus proper. Although the anatomical arrangement of the cricopharyngeus lends itself to the sphincteric function, some studies (Zaino et al., 1970) have suggested the possible existence of an intrinsic sphincter at the pharyngo-oesophageal junction in addition to the cricopharyngeus muscle.

3.2. Gastro-oesophageal junction and the anatomy of the hiatus (Figs. 1a and 1b)

The anatomical arrangement of the hiatus is intimately related to the lower oesophagus and the gastro-oesophageal junction. It is therefore fitting to consider them together.

The hiatus is a slightly left-sided opening. Apart from minor variations, the hiatal muscle arises from the right crus of the diaphragm. The peritoneal reflection near the hiatus consists of the two layers of the lesser omentum which separate to enclose the oesophagus and then join to form the gastrosplenic ligament. The oesophagus is held in the hiatus by a fascia, the phreno-oesophageal ligaments described by Allison (1951). According to Hayward (1961), there are two layers of phreno-oesophageal ligaments, the lower layer being the continuation of the fascia transversalis of the abdomen. The ligament passes from below the diaphragm and is inserted by a series of digitations into the oesophageal adventitia some 2 cm above the oesophago-gastric junction. It is toughest anteriorly and on the left, where the hiatus opens into the general peritoneal cavity. The upper layer of the phreno-oesophageal ligament is the continuation of the endothoracic fascia and covers the thoracic surface of the hiatal muscles. The margin of the hiatus blends with the oesophageal adventitia.

Anatomical features of the oesophago-gastric junction must be considered under two headings:

3.2.1 Anatomical gastro-oesophageal junction
3.2.2 Surgical gastro-oesophageal junction

3.2.1. Anatomical gastro-oesophageal junction
The true anatomical gastro-oesophageal junction is situated below the diaphragm where the oesophagus ends and projects into the stomach. The portion of the oesophagus lined by squamous epithelium, how-

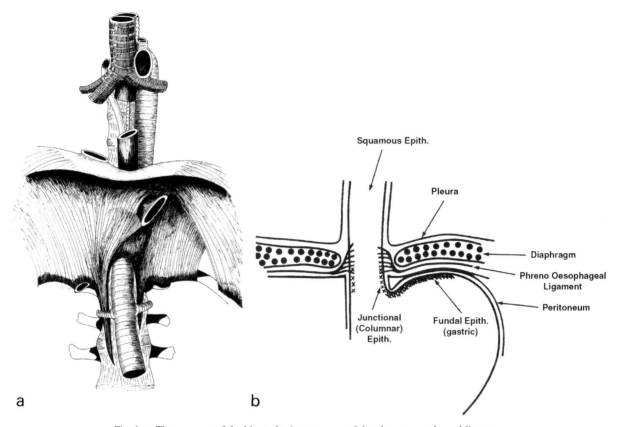

Fig. 1. a: The anatomy of the hiatus. b: Arrangement of the phreno-oesophageal ligament.

ever, does not extend that far down. It stops at about the level of the entry of the oesophagus into the hiatus or the insertion of the phreno-oesophageal ligament. Below this level the abdominal oesophagus (about 2–3 cm) is lined by junctional columnar epithelium.

3.2.2. Surgical gastro-oesophageal junction

The surgical gastro-oesophageal junction is some 2 cm above the anatomical junction and is where the thoracic and abdominal oesophagus meet. It is embraced by structures around the hiatus. In cases of sliding hernias and peri-oesophagitis it can be recognised when viewed from the thoracic cavity by the site of insertion of the phreno-oesophageal ligament. The latter is an important surgical landmark because:

(a) It indicates approximately the level of the junctional mucosa.

(b) A sliding hiatal hernia may be considered as being reduced when the phreno-oesophageal ligament is below the diaphragm.

(c) The ligament is the only tangible structure which can indicate the degree of shortening in ac-

quired short oesophagus, resulting from reflux oesophagitis and stricture associated with hiatal hernia (chapter III.8).

The distance between the site of the insertion of the ligament to the oesophagus and the hiatus is indicative of the scale of shortening as, in the normal, the two are apparently at the same level, i.e. the site of attachment of the ligament to the oesophagus is level with the diaphragmatic hiatus.

At or about the hiatus, the lower oesophagus assumes sphincteric function, acting as a one-way valve. It relaxes to allow entry of the bolus into the stomach but prevents its regurgitation back into the oesophagus. Traditionally, this region has been called 'the cardia' but as Hayward (1961) points out, there is no clear definition of the cardia. In anatomical terms the cardia is probably the lowest 2 cm of the lower oesophagus. In physiological terms the sphincteric portion of the lower oesophagus is more extensive than that (between 3–5 cm in length), as demonstrated by manometric and pressure recording studies.

References

Allison PR. Reflux oesophagitis, sliding hiatal hernia and anatomy of the repair. Surg Gynec Obstet 1951; 92: 419–431.

Hayward, J. The lower end of the oesophagus. Thorax 1961; 16: 36–41.

Zaino C, Jacobsen JG, Lepow H et al. The pharyngo-oesophageal sphincter. Springfield, Illinois, USA: Charles C Thomas, 1970.

CHAPTER III.2

Manifestation and investigation of oesophageal diseases

K. Moghissi

1. Introduction

In the absence of an effective screening programme, patients with oesophageal conditions are discovered by the clinical manifestations of the disease. These are of considerable importance to general practitioners and specialists alike.

2. Symptoms and signs of oesophageal diseases

2.1. Pain

Pain of oesophageal origin can be felt over a wide area of the chest along the segmental dermatomes of C8 to TH10. It is suggested that sensory fibres are carried via sympathetic nerve endings found in the oesophageal submucosa. These sensory fibres enter the spinal cord through the dorsal root. They eventually joint the spinothalamic tract. This arrangement is responsible for:

(a) The oesophageal pain being felt on the skin dermatomes.
(b) The lack of precision in the definition of oesophageal pain due to overlap with pain arising from other viscera, but sharing the same dermatomes.

Inflammation, distension or contraction (spasm) of the oesophagus creates pain which is, at times, indistinguishable from cardiac ischaemic pain. However, oesophageal pain can be of a different modality and intensity and is typically but not always associated with swallowing.

2.2. Heartburn (Pyrosis)

This is an unpleasant and distressing substernal burning sensation. It is the hallmark of gastro-oesopha-

geal reflux and typically is experienced in the supine position or when the individual bends down. The contact of acid with the mucosa appears to be the responsible stimulus and the sensation is usually relieved by ingestion of alkalis.

2.3. Dysphagia

Difficulty in swallowing or painful swallowing is an important manifestation of oesophageal diseases. It is important to note the severity and duration of dysphagia. The severity of dysphagia may be graded as follows (Moghissi et al., 1977):

Grade 0   No dysphagia
Grade I   Dysphagia to solid food (meat, fish)
Grade II   Dysphagia to semi-solid food (mince)
Grade III Dysphagia to purée and soft food (mashed potato with gravy)
Grade IV   Dysphagia to liquid

Mechanical obstruction, severe inflammation or ulceration and motility disturbances are the most important causes of dysphagia. The seriousness of dysphagia due to cancer of the oesophagus, together with its poor prognosis, should remind every general practitioner and specialist to consider every dysphagic patient above the age of 40 years, without any obvious cause (e.g. foreign body) as a possible carcinoma case unless otherwise disproved. This statement may appear too categoric, but it is justified when viewed in the light of the consequence of alternative policies.

2.4. Vomiting — regurgitation

In true vomiting the content of the stomach is brought up. In regurgitation, the bolus may go down the oesophagus and remain stagnant in its obstructed and distended lower end, before being brought up. This can occur in cases of large pharyngeal pouches or achalasia of the cardia.

2.5. Observation on weight/weight loss

Weight loss occurs typically in dysphagic patients with carcinoma of the oesophagus. It also occurs, rarely, in patients with longstanding benign oesophageal strictures and those with a particular aversion to food. Hiatal hernia patients are usually obese or overweight.

2.6. Hiccup

A number of patients in an early stage of their obstructive oesophageal disease develop hiccup.

2.7. Anaemia

Some patients with gastro-oesophageal reflux are anaemic, even in the absence of a demonstrable oesophageal ulcer.

2.8. Haematemesis

Patients with oesophageal varices or ulcers may develop haematemesis as the presenting clinical manifestation of their condition. Some chronic ulcers can bleed acutely and profusely. These are usually either penetrating oesophageal ulcers which can erode the aorta, or gastric ulcers which develop in the herniated stomach (hiatal hernia).

2.9. Malnutrition

This is characteristic of cancer of the oesophagus. The mechanism of malnutrition is three-fold:
(a) Dysphagia and lack of food intake.
(b) Metabolic disturbance caused by the cancer, particularly with multiple liver secondaries.
(c) Lack of appetite which is associated with cancer.

2.10. Respiratory symptoms

Some patients with oesophageal disease are brought to notice because of respiratory tract symptoms. It is not unusual for a patient with achalasia of the cardia to present with repeated chest infection, or for a hiatal hernia patient to present with bronchospasm or nocturnal cough.

3. Investigations of oesophageal diseases

3.1. Clinical investigations

History-taking is an important part of investigation of patients with oesophageal diseases and must not be ignored in favour of radiological and laboratory tests alone. In many patients dysphagia can be interpreted as vomiting. Some patients will not admit to or notice the gradual onset of dysphagia because they adapt by taking increasingly softer consistency food or even liquid. Proper history taking can differentiate and clarify symptoms.

3.2. General laboratory examination

Blood count and biochemical profile are routine laboratory investigations. Their normality does not contribute much to the diagnosis but their abnormality may be significant enough to be of diagnostic help (e.g. anaemia caused by occult bleeding in patients with hiatal hernia).

3.3. Radiology

3.3.1. Chest radiograph
A plain chest radiograph may give a clue to the diagnosis of the oesophageal condition; large mediastinal shadowing due to a dilated oesophagus or a pericardiac 'shadow' in a para-oesophageal hernia are typical examples. In many other conditions, however, the chest radiograph can be completely normal.

3.3.2. Barium examination
Barium swallow examination is a mandatory investigation in all oesophageal diseases. Liquid, semi-solid and barium sandwich are used as appropriate and can indicate the type, location and severity of an obstructive lesion. Video recording has, in addition, the advantage of providing an overall dynamic picture of the pattern of swallowing and the motor activity of the oesophagus. This can be reviewed and studied repeatedly.

3.4. Physiological studies

The function of the oesophagus is to propel the food bolus from the mouth, by the act of swallowing, into the stomach. It therefore follows that dysfunction of the oesophagus will affect the swallowing mechanism. Mechanical obstruction of the oesophagus and the resulting dysphagia can be diagnosed by radiological technique. Motor disorders of the oesophagus produce dysphagia without mechanical obstruction. Swallowing and the pattern of oesophageal motility can be visualised by videoradiography and, more objectively, studied by manometry.

3.5. Oesophagoscopy

Oesophagoscopy is the visual examination and inspection of the oesophagus with a light-carrying instrument, the oesophagoscope. This simple description of oesophagoscopy does not, however, convey its full uses, which may be described as follows:

• Diagnostic:
  The mucosal surface of the oesophagus is examined macroscopically and biopsy material is obtained.
• Therapeutic: This is carried out for the purpose of:
  – Extraction of a foreign body lodged in the oesophagus (see chapter III.5).
  – Dilatation of oesophageal stricture
  – Control of bleeding varices
  – Endoscopic intubation and stent placement
  – Laser therapy

Broadly there are two types of oesophagoscope: rigid and flexible fibre optic instruments. Table 1 presents the characteristics and specific indication of each.

3.5.1. Oesophagoscopy with the rigid instrument
A typical rigid oesophagoscope used in the United Kingdom is the Negus or modified Negus instrument (Fig. 1). It is a graduated light-carrying hollow tube through which the lumen of the oesophagus is examined directly. All modern instruments have fibre optic light. Accessory pieces of equipment are:
– Biopsy forceps
– Foreign body remover and various grasping forceps
– Telescopes with magnification

Preparation for oesophagoscopy using the rigid instrument. The examination is carried out under general anaesthesia and endotracheal intubation with the cuff inflated. This is mandatory when there is evidence of longstanding oesophageal obstruction or in cases of oesophageal stagnation such as achalasia (mega-oesophagus). In such cases it is advisable to admit the patient a day or two beforehand in order to clean debris from the oesophagus. This is required to:

(a) Prevent tracheal aspiration of the oesophageal contents during anaesthesia before the endotracheal tube is inserted.
(b) Ensure a clear view of the oesophageal mucosa.

A golden rule is not to use an oesophagoscope on patients without prior barium swallow studies, except for the removal of a foreign body in the oesophagus. In these cases a chest X-ray should be taken beforehand. That this rule has been eroded by some who carry out a great number of 'screening' endoscopies is understandable, considering the high percentage amongst these who may not require any further investigations. This, however, should not apply to patients with obstructive symptoms, nor to those who will have to undergo barium study examination as part of their investigations. Having treated many instrumental oesophageal perforations referred from other centres, the author's view on this subject is adherence to the rule as stated above.

Table 1

Characteristics of rigid and flexible oesophagoscope

	Characteristics and criteria	Rigid oesophagoscope	Flexible oesophagoscope
(1)	General anaesthesia	Usually required	Usually not required
(2)	Passage of instrument	More difficult	Less difficult
(3)	Viewing	Direct	Indirect
(4)	Diagnostic 'spectrum'	Good	Good
(5)	Assessment of extent of carcinoma	Good	Good except for pharyngo-oesophageal junction
(6)	Stricture dilatation	Excellent	Generally not as good for long strictures
(7)	Foreign body extraction	Excellent	Not suitable (possible)
(8)	Examination of patient with deformed and fixed neck	Not suitable (possible)	Good
(9)	Examination of upper stomach	Possible (but unsatisfactory)	Easy
(10)	Examination of stomach and upper intestinal tract	Not possible	Excellent

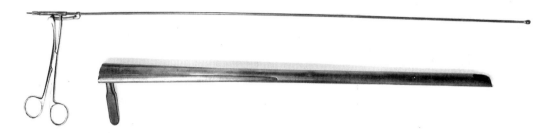

Fig. 1. A typical rigid oesophagoscope, with biopsy forceps above.

Technique of oesophagoscopy.

Step 1: With the patient in supine position, the head is flexed using a pillow or the headpiece of the operating table. A towel is placed around the head and over the eyes of the patient to safeguard against injuries. A pad of gauze is then placed over the upper lip and teeth for protection. The mouth is opened and the oesophagoscope inserted as near to the midline as possible (the endotracheal tube should be positioned to the left of the mouth). The direction of the instrument at this stage is vertical (downwards), with its bevelled edged anterior. The visual field shows from the front backwards and consists of the tongue, the tip of the epiglottis and then the hard and soft palate with the uvula in between.

Step 2: When the instrument is advanced further in a vertical and posterior direction, the upper part of the laryngopharynx is reached. This is recognisable by the visual field showing the aryepiglottic folds surrounding the endotracheal tube. Laterally on each side the pyriform fossa and posteriorly the pharyngeal wall can be seen.

The oesophagoscope is advanced further to view the posterosuperior border of the larynx (anterosuperior border of the laryngopharynx) which is formed by the arytenoids and the interarytenoid folds; posteriorly is the pharynx. The bevelled edge of the instrument is inserted behind the arytenoids, lifting them and the larynx forwards. This brings into view the opening of the oesophagus; this is the ring of the cricopharyngeus, part of the inferior constrictor muscles covered by the mucous membrane.

Step 3: The oesophagoscope is introduced into the oesophageal lumen by advancing it through the cricopharyngeus in a forward and near 40° horizontal direction. In doing so it is important to:

(a) Take care not to let the tip of the instrument press against the posterior pharyngeal wall which is in contact with the prominent body of the 7th cer-

vical vertebra. In addition, in elderly or arthritic patients, osteophytes can project further bony prominences towards the back of the pharynx. The compression of the thin posterior wall of the pharynx between the instrument and the spine can cause injuries and accounts for some instrumental ruptures at this level.

(b) Be absolutely certain to see the inlet of the oesophagus before advancing the instrument.

Step 4: When the oesophagoscope has entered into the cervical oesophagus proper, the patient's head is extended by placing a pillow under the shoulders or by adjusting the head extension section of the table. Suction of the oesophageal contents is then carried out before proceeding to further advance the instrument into the lumen, which is straightforward, provided there are no obstructions. At the diaphragmatic opening (the cardia) it is often necessary to slightly elevate the upper abdominal region so that the instrument can be introduced into the stomach.

3.5.2. Endoscopic anatomy of the oesophagus

The normal anatomical narrowings of the oesophagus are not particularly noticeable at oesophagoscopy. The level of a lesion within the oesophagus may be estimated in two ways:

- By the position of the lesion in relation to some of the structures within the chest, such as the arch of the aorta, whose anatomical situations are fixed and well-known.
- By the level of the lesion down the oesophagus, as indicated by the graduation of the oesophagoscope, from the incisor teeth or the upper alveolus, bearing in mind that in an adult the pharyngo-oesophageal junction (cricopharyngeal ring) is situated at about 15 cm and the cardia (gastro-oesophageal junction) is placed at 40 cm, both from the upper alveolus.

The length of an average adult oesophagus being about 25 cm, a lesion which is seen through the oesophagoscope to be at 27–28 cm is in fact situated in the mid-oesophagus (i.e. 12–13 cm below the oesophageal inlet which is at 15 cm). This point corresponds to the level of the arch of the aorta at the boundary of the superior and inferior (posterior) mediastinum.

It must, however, be realised that the length of the oesophagus is subject to variation according to the height of the individual. The total oesophagoscopic length of the oesophagus in an individual can be estimated by measuring the distance between the upper alveolus and xiphoid process of the sternum when the patient is in supine oesophagoscopy position with the neck extended.

When the endoscopic level of a lesion from the alveolus is set against the length of the oesophagus, as estimated by the above method, the relative position of the lesion for the individual under examination can be surmised.

To the naked eye, the normal oesophageal mucosa appears smooth in texture and white with a tinge of pink in colour. The gastric mucosa with its columnar epithelium is less smooth and more pink than the oesophageal mucosa.

The following observations should be made and noted on the oesophagoscopy report:

- The operator's name.
- The anaesthetist's name.
- Ease or difficulty of the procedure.
- Pharyngeal pathology.

- Oesophageal mucosal lesions with particular reference to:
  - Macroscopic appearance of the lesion.
  - The level of the lesion within the oesophagus and its extent.
  - The number and location of biopsy samples.
  - Endoscopic diagnosis of the lesion.
- In cases of oesophagitis, the following additional notes are relevant:
  (a) The level at which oesophagitis starts.
  (b) The severity of oesophagitis using accepted scale (Table 1 in chapter III.6).
  (c) Ulcer present/not present.
- In cases of tumour, the following additional notes are relevant:
  (a) The extent of tumour expansion in the lumen.
  (b) The area at which tumour arises from the circumference of the oesophagus and the degree of obstruction that it causes.
  (c) Biopsies should be taken from a representative sample and also from healthy looking mucosa at the margin of the lesion.
- Oesophago-gastric mucosal junction level.
- Oesophageal length assessed by external measurement from mouth to xiphoid process.

3.5.3. Flexible fibre optic oesophagoscopy
Instrument. The instrument (Fig. 2) consists of a flexible tube which incorporates light-fibre bundles as well as an optic system. Additional channels are provided for the introduction of biopsy forceps and for suction. The proximal (ocular) end has a focusing

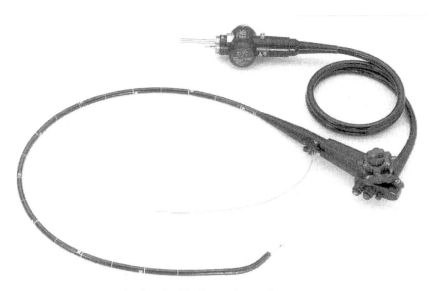

Fig. 2. A flexible fibre optic oesophagoscope.

adjustment, one inlet point for the forceps channel, an opening allowing controlled suction and another inlet and channel for flushing and for allowing air to be blown into the oesophagus. The oesophagoscope has its light source, biopsy forceps, a range of grasping and other devices for interventional oesophagoscopy as well as a range of optional accessories such as a teaching attachment, camera, screen and video recording equipment.

Technique. This is generally carried out under topical anaesthesia but, in some nervous individuals and when other endoscopic examinations such as bronchoscopy have to be undertaken, the procedure is best carried out under general anaesthesia.

For topical anaesthesia each endoscopic unit uses its own combination of drugs consisting of a mucosal surface spray of Lignocaine (4–20%) to anaesthetise the back of the tongue, laryngo-pharynx and pharynx, and an intravenous sedative/hypnotic such as Midazolam (benzodiazepine) with/without Atropine.

The initial introduction of the instrument is performed with the patient either sitting or lying on his/her left side. The passage of the instrument through the pharynx is controlled either visually through the instrument or by palpation using the left index finger (or index and middle fingers) as a guide. In either case, attention is paid to clearly identifying structures and the oesophageal entrance before advancing the instrument further forward. The distal end of the instrument at this point is slightly curved forward. The introduction into the oesophagus is helped by the patient swallowing, or by injecting a small amount of air through the scope. The passage through the cricopharyngeal ring is the most important part of the oesophagoscopy. Oesophageal perforation in flexible fibre optic oesophagoscopy occurs generally at this level. The author's experience in dealing with the many oesophageal perforations referred to him compels him to say that those who state that there are no oesophageal perforations when a flexible fibre optic instrument is used, are those whose perforations have been dealt with by others. Once the instrument is clearly placed into the oesophagus, the position of the distal end is returned to the midline and adjusted accordingly. The oesophagoscope is then advanced into the oesophagus. The rule is to see first and then to advance. The instrument is introduced easily into the stomach which is also examined.

The findings are recorded as previously described when using the rigid instrument.

3.5.4. Contraindications for oesophagoscopy
There are very few contraindications for oesophagoscopy.

Rigid oesophagoscope should be considered as contraindicated:
- In patients not fit for general anaesthesia.
- In patients with anatomical abnormalities of the pharynx and severe neck osteoarthritis or spinal deformities.

In such circumstances the flexible instrument must be used under topical anaesthesia. However, the flexible instrument gives neither the same type of information nor the full range of functions afforded by the rigid instrument. Table 1 summarises some of the characteristics of oesophagoscopy using rigid and fibreoptic instruments. Oesophageal surgery departments must have both types of equipment and use either or both instruments as appropriate, since in some cases the two instruments are complementary to each other.

3.5.5. Complications of oesophagoscopy
Perforation. The most important and by far the most serious complication of oesophagoscopy is perforation. Knowing the potential fatal outcome in a high percentage of patients with oesophageal perforation caused by instrumentation, one is astonished to find that in some hospitals, the task of oesophagoscopy, for removal of a foreign body in particular, is assigned to inexperienced oesophagoscopists. The most common cause of this complication is technical ineptitude; this is not to say that accidental perforation does not occur in expert hands, but its incidence will be lower when it is performed by an experienced operator. The most important factor relating to fatality following perforation is the failure of early recognition of the accident and lack of appropriate emergency treatment. Perforations will be dealt with in detail later (chapter III.11).

Bleeding. In its severe form this can occur in cases of oesophageal varices. Minor bleeding can follow oesophageal biopsies, particularly from a chronic ulcer.

Bronchospasm. This can occur with aspiration of oesophageal contents into the trachea. Patients should have bronchoscopic clearance of the bronchial tree in addition to administration of a bronchodilator.

Pulmonary collapse and infection. This occurs rarely and is also caused by tracheal inspiration of the oesophageal contents.

3.5.6. Oesophagoscopy after-care

The patient is examined clinically and radiologically before allowing food intake. Clinically, particular attention is paid to possible surgical subcutaneous emphysema, and pain in the neck, back and epigastric regions. Postero–anterior chest and lateral neck radiographs are taken 2–3 hours after the oesophagoscopy. This we believe to be mandatory after oesophagoscopy and dilatation or following foreign body extraction. If there is no air in the soft tissues of the neck, mediastinum or pleural space, then the patient is allowed to take food and drink.

If perforation is suspected, all food and fluids are withheld and further investigations are undertaken (see perforation of the oesophagus, chapter III.11).

Reference and further reading

Moghissi K, Hornshaw J, Teasdale PR, Dawes EA. Enteral nutrition in carcinoma of the oesophagus treated by surgery: nitrogen balance and clinical studies. Br J Surg 1977; 64: 125–128.

CHAPTER III.3

Oesophageal function tests

J.A.C. Thorpe

1. Introduction

In 1883, Kronecker and Meltzer were the first to investigate the swallowing mechanism using oesophageal balloons. However, it was not until the 1950s that Ingelfinger and Code were able to provide more insight into oesophageal function using transducer probes. Today, more reliable microtransducer and pH probe technology has revolutionised the assessment of normal and abnormal oesophageal function.

Before discussing the pathological aspects of pharyngeal and oesophageal motility disorders, it is important to have a fundamental knowledge of normal physiology and the modern clinical techniques now adopted for the diagnosis of disorders of motility.

1.1. The swallowing mechanism

The swallowing mechanism is very complex. It involves an *oropharyngeal stage*, which lasts for one second and involves:

- elevation and retraction of the soft palate with nasopharyngeal closure
- upper oesophageal sphincter opening
- laryngeal closure
- tongue loading
- tongue pulsion
- pharyngeal clearance

This is followed by an *oesophageal stage* where the bolus is transmitted to the stomach with orderly unidirectional peristalsis and coordinated relaxation of the lower oesophageal sphincter. The volume and consistency of the bolus affect the timing. The innervation, neuromuscular physiology and medullary control mechanisms are complex and still incompletely understood. The current model is described in Fig. 1.

1.2. Clinical assessment and investigations

1.2.1. Clinical assessment
A good clinical history and examination is invaluable in the assessment of pharyngeal and oesophageal motility disorders. The three clinical presentations are:
- Heartburn
- Dysphagia/Odynophagia
- Chest pain

Gastro-oesophageal reflux disease (GORD) is often concomitant with oesophageal motility disorders and should also be considered. Dysphagia should not be confused with a globus sensation, i.e. the feeling of a lump in the throat.

There are many causes of pharyngo-oesophageal dysphagia, including: webs, strictures, carcinoma, extrinsic masses and denervation motility disturbance, e.g. scleroderma (failed peristalsis), or excessive/abnormal peristalsis (hypercontractile oesophagus), e.g. diffuse oesophageal spasm, nutcracker oesophagus.

1.2.2. Investigations
The following investigations will be necessary in most cases and their importance will be discussed in context with the individual motility disorder. Oropharyngeal and oesophageal disorders will be discussed separately.
- Record weight and dietary intake
- Haematological/biochemical profile
- Barium swallow/video barium
- Fibre optic oesophagoscopy/endoscopic ultrasound
- Pharyngo-oesophageal manometry
- Twenty-four hour ambulatory pH monitoring

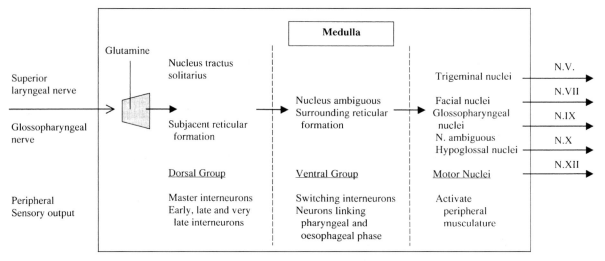

Fig. 1. Current model of central control pathways of swallowing

1.3. Oesophageal manometry

Manometric investigation is mandatory in most cases of dysphagia and essential prior to antireflux surgery or motility surgery. It is also a useful tool in evaluating the results of surgery.

Several recording techniques are used. The most accurate technique incorporates the use of multilumen catheters with small external diameter linked to a hydraulic capillary infusion system, e.g. the Andorfer pump. This low-flow perfusion technique is very reliable and gives reproducible results. Technically the procedure requires some expertise and is used mainly for research. Modern microtransducer catheters are now very reliable though more expensive. They have the advantage of simplicity and ease of use and are well tolerated by patients because of their small diameter.

1.3.1. Technique

The catheter assembly is passed through the nose with topical anaesthesia and the patient is encouraged to swallow small amounts of fluid through a straw. Once the transducers are in the stomach, a positive pressure wave is obtained on inspiration or on palpation of the abdomen. A 1 cm station pull-through is then carried out. At the region of the hiatus, a high-pressure zone (HPZ) is encountered, which at its lower end represents the diaphragm and at its upper end the lower oesophageal sphincter (LOS), which on wet or dry swallow should relax completely to baseline pressure (0–5 mmHg) (Fig. 2). Impaired relaxation is a feature of achalasia.

The catheter bundle is then pulled back slowly at 1 cm intervals and peristaltic function assessed in the oesophageal body. The upper oesophageal sphincter is then located and resting pressure and the relaxation response assessed. With a transducer in the pharynx, pharyngo-oesophageal coordination can be assessed but interpretation of the responses in this area requires experience.

1.4. pH testing

This is an integral part of upper GI tract investigation and is usually combined with manometry. Once the HPZ is located at manometry or by X-ray localisation (usually unnecessary), the pH probe is placed 5 cm above the HPZ/LOS. The probe is usually calibrated to acid and alkaline pH and a reference electrode is placed on the skin. The probe is then connected to an ambulatory digital monitor and the patient sent home for 24 hours. The patient makes an accurate record/diary of eating habits, posture, medication and symptoms and a marker button can be pressed when the patient has significant symptoms. A computer analysis is then made and the 24-hour pH recording analysed.

It is important to appreciate the computer criteria for the programme as these can differ. The pH recording is usually based on DeMeester's criteria and specific scores obtained. A reflux episode is defined as pH 4 or less. The normal pH in the oesophagus is pH 7. The computer analyses the total duration of pH <4, the total number of episodes and the duration of the longest episode. A result of pH <4 for a pe-

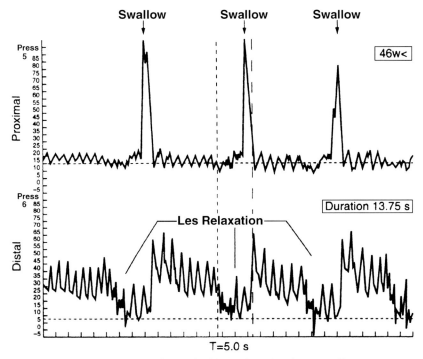

Fig. 2. Manometry of normal LOS showing relaxation on swallow

riod >4% of the 24-hour period studied is considered pathological.

Other types of pH probe can be used to assess bile reflux in special circumstances, e.g. post-gastrectomy.

2. Oropharyngeal dysphagia (Table 1)

2.1. Causes

High dysphagia can be caused by structural or propulsive abnormalities. Structural abnormalities may arise from trauma, radiation, surgery, tumour, caustic injury and congenital and acquired deformities. Propulsive abnormalities can result from dysfunction of intrinsic musculature, peripheral nerves or central nervous system.

2.2. Management

Fortunately, oropharyngeal dysphagia is relatively uncommon but it does pose a serious management problem. It is rarely amenable to specific therapy. Dysphagia secondary to Parkinson's disease and myasthenia gravis often improves with medical therapy. However, therapy for most of these disorders is structured around the management of nutritional and aspiration complications.

Clinical evaluation should include a video contrast swallow together with pharyngeal and upper oesophageal manometry if possible to assess which aspect of the swallow mechanism is abnormal. Tech-

Table 1

Aetiology of oropharyngeal dysphagia

Anatomic:
– Postcricoid web
– Vertebral osteophyte
– Hypopharyngeal diverticulum/cricopharyngeal bar
– Tumour/surgical resection
– Radiotherapy/vagal damage

Neurologic:
– Cerebrovascular accident
– Poliomyelitis
– Amyotrophic lateral sclerosis
– Parkinson's disease
– Cerebral palsy
– Intracerebral/medullary tumour

Motor:
– Oculopharyngeal muscular dystrophy
– Myotonic dystrophy
– Myasthenia gravis
– Tardive dyskinesia and dystonia

Other:
– Xerostomia (oral dryness)

nically, however, manometry may be difficult to perform and to interpret accurately in these patients.

A nasal voice or nasal regurgitation suggests paresis of the soft palate. Inadequate bolus formation may be a consequence of tongue weakness; aspiration suggests impaired laryngeal elevation. Excess salivation may require cholinergic-type drugs and absence of salivation may necessitate lubricants or artificial saliva, which are now available.

Different feeding tactics, e.g. using a straw or an infant feeder, and postural compensation can maintain oral intake of food. Physiotherapy and speech therapy are important in rehabilitating the stroke patient and a dietitian should monitor nutritional progress. Failure to maintain an adequate intake orally is an indication for fine-bore nasogastric feeding, a percutaneous endoscopic gastrotomy tube (PEG) or a fine-bore feeding jejunostomy.

Aspiration may require aggressive nasotracheal toilet, mini-tracheostomy or formal tracheostomy if severe.

Occasionally oesophageal dilatation or cricopharyngeal myotomy can be effective in some patients with a hypertensive or abnormally relaxing UOS and hypopharyngeal diverticulum.

3. Oesophageal motility disorders

3.1. Presentation

Motility disorders affecting the body of the oesophagus usually present with symptoms of altered diet, dysphagia, odynophagia, chest pain and often heartburn and indigestion. Symptoms are usually chronic but may be acute. Chest pain can readily mimic an acute anginal attack or myocardial infarction. Up to 60% of patients with non-cardiac chest pain (NCCP) have an oesophageal disorder. The history is very important, with particular reference to diet, e.g. intolerance of fluids rather than solids would indicate achalasia.

3.2. Investigation

Dysphagia is a serious symptom and should always be investigated. Routine investigations should include:
- barium swallow/video barium
- endoscopy
- manometry
- ambulatory pH monitoring.

Other investigations which may be of value include:

Table 2

Oesophageal motility disorders

Disorder	Radiology	Manometry	pH test/other
Achalasia	Bird's beak/rat-tail appearance at cardia	Normal-high LOS pressure, non-relaxing on swallow Synchronous spastic activity in oesophageal body	Not associated with reflux pH may be positive after myotomy
Diffuse oesophageal spasm	Spastic activity Reflux Corkscrew appearance Diverticulae	Normal/high spastic waves Occasional normal peristalsis Normal LOS	pH occasionally positive Muscle hypertrophy EUS
Hypertensive LOS	Impaired oesophageal clearance	LOS pressure >45 mmHg May have impaired relaxation	Usually negative pH test
Reflux/spasm	Reflux Spastic activity Hiatus hernia	Peristalsis normal Low-pressure LOS Occasional spastic wave forms	
Nutcracker	Spasm	Hypertensive peristalsis Normal-high pressure LOS May see impaired relaxation	Usually negative pH test Muscle hypertrophy on EUS
Scleroderma	Reflux Impaired oesophageal and gastric clearance	No peristalsis Flat trace Absence of LOS	pH positive

LOS = lower oesophageal sphincter; EUS = endoscopic ultrasound.
Non-specific oesophageal motility disorders (NSOMD) — these are a distinct manometric group that do not fulfil the above criteria. They have impaired clearance with low-pressure swallow activity and occasional spastic activity. Non-transmitted swallows >30%.

- ambulatory manometry
- Bernstein acid perfusion test
- edrophonium stimulation test for NCCP
- balloon dilatation sensitivity test
- endoscopic ultrasound
- oesophageal mucosal potential difference
- cerebral evoked response.

Table 2 provides a summary of the expected findings in various conditions.

3.3. Management of oesophageal motility disorders

The majority of oesophageal motility disorders can largely be treated conservatively with reassurance, medication and occasional dilatation. The patient with persistent symptoms will need careful evaluation, as inappropriate surgery to the oesophagus could result in lifelong problems with swallowing.

It is imperative that prior to embarking on surgery, full investigations are carried especially to exclude carcinoma of the cardia, which may present as a pseudoachalasia.

Isosorbide dinitrate is of some use in DOS, and anticholinergics, e.g. hyoscine or propantheline, may be used to reduce peristalsis. However, there have been no controlled trials of their efficacy. Calcium channel blockers, e.g. nifedipine and diltiazem, are occasionally effective in reducing spastic activity and non-cardiac chest pain. If there is evidence of gastro-oesophageal reflux, antacids/proton pump inhibitors are useful. Where there is evidence of low sphincter pressure and impaired oesophageal clear-ance, metoclopramide is a useful drug, which also improves gastric emptying.

Temporary subjective relief can be obtained by bouginage or balloon dilatation of the oesophagus in spastic disorders.

For patients with intractable symptoms and failed medication/dilatation, surgery may be indicated. This should be performed in a unit with expertise in the management of the oesophagus. It may be necessary to perform oesophagomyotomy (partial/complete) with the addition of an antireflux procedure, e.g. Belsey Mk IV repair, if there is documented gastro-oesophageal reflux.

It is important not to perform an overtight repair in the presence of impaired oesophageal motility, as dysphagia may well be worse post-operatively. Where diverticulae are present, there is often an underlying motility disorder, e.g. DOS, and a myotomy should be added to the diverticulectomy.

In achalasia, balloon dilatation is preferred for the older patient, but for the younger patient, a Heller myotomy is recommended. This can be performed by a laparoscopic, thoracoscopic or minithoracotomy approach.

The results of surgery appear to be superior to balloon dilatation.

Reference and further reading

Castell DO. The esophagus (2nd ed.). Boston: Little, Brown, 1995.

K. Moghissi, J.A.C. Thorpe and F. Ciulli (Eds.)
Moghissi's Essentials of Thoracic and Cardiac Surgery
© 2003 Elsevier Science B.V. All rights reserved

CHAPTER III.4

Congenital oesophageal atresia and tracheo–oesophageal fistula (TOF)

K. Moghissi

1. Introduction

This refers to a variety of congenital defects resulting from the misdirection of the original foregut tube or the lack of its separation into oesophagus and trachea. There are several variants of oesophageal atresia. In the commonest type the upper oesophagus has a blind end and the lower portion opens into the trachea, thereby establishing a tracheo-oesophageal fistula. The variants are illustrated in Fig. 1.

2. Diagnosis

The existence of the condition is frequently suspected before birth because of the frequent association of oesophageal atresia and hydramnios. The typical clinical presentation is that the newborn baby cannot swallow saliva, which collects in the mouth and causes respiratory difficulties. Any attempt at feeding produces an accumulation of fluid which spills into the lungs and produces cyanosis and acute respiratory distress. The respiratory difficulties become more pronounced when, due to gastric distension and the existence of tracheo-oesophageal fistula, the gastric content is aspirated into the airways. Untreated, the newborn will present with severe respiratory distress syndrome resulting in death. The diagnosis is made by the above clinical findings and confirmed by the impossibility of passing a nasogastric catheter into the stomach. For this purpose it is best to use a fairly large catheter in the oesophagus which indicates on X-ray its radio-opaque tip being arrested in the upper oesophagus, together with gas-filled stomach and small bowel. A few drops of radio-opaque contrast solution in the nasogastric

catheter will outline the blind pouch (Fig. 2). Care must be taken not to spill the opaque medium into the trachea. It is also important to make resuscitation equipment available when investigations are in process. It is estimated that about 50% of all cases of oesophageal atresia have associated congenital abnormalities related to cardiovascular, gastro-intestinal and other systems.

3. Management of oesophageal atresia and TOF

Surgery is the only treatment and consists of a one-stage operation to close the tracheo-oesophageal fistulous communications and to reconstruct the oesophagus by end-to-end anastomosis. Swift peri-operative preparations are necessary in order to carry out the surgical operation in the best possible circumstances.

- Continuous production of saliva and its inhalation creates a dangerous situation. Aspiration of the upper pouch via a nasopharyngeal catheter is carried out to prevent inhalation of the pool of saliva.
- The baby is nursed in a head down position in the oxygen cot to assist postural drainage.
- Prophylactic antibiotic (penicillin) and intramuscular injection of an appropriate dose of vitamin K is recommended.
- One stage repair is preferable for all except high--risk cases (e.g. pulmonary infection), those associated with other abnormalities which need more urgent correction and infants requiring improvement of their condition to withstand the operation.
- Most important of all, the operation should be undertaken by a paediatric surgeon trained in oesophageal techniques or thoracic surgeon and a team

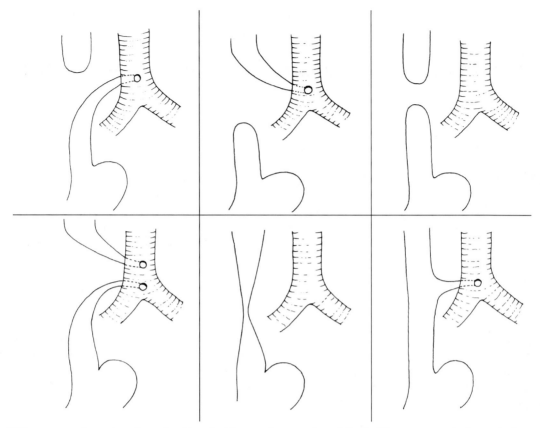

Fig. 1. Different types of oesophageal atresia with and without tracheo-oesophageal fistula. The commonest is the one in the upper left picture.

used to operating on babies with experience in oesophageal atresia.

3.1. Timing of the operation

The operation is undertaken as soon as the infant's condition is judged to have been stabilised and thorough evaluation of associated lesions such as vertebral defect, anorectal malformation and congenital heart conditions have been made.

3.2. The operation

A variety of techniques may be used. The standard technique will be described below.

3.2.1. The primary anastomosis

A right thoracotomy is carried out through the 4th intercostal space; in these infants a short 5–6 cm skin incision and muscle-sparing approach is generally adequate. The mediastinum and the oesophageal bed is approached by incising the mediastinal pleura. The azygos vein is divided between ligatures. The distal segment of the oesophagus is identified and followed upwards. Communication with the lower trachea or the right main bronchus is usually by a still narrower channel. This is divided and its tracheal side is sutured using interrupted 4/0 non-absorbable sutures. Two 4/0 stay sutures are applied on each corner of the oesophageal end of the fistulous opening. Some mobilisation of the distal oesophagus is necessary but the utmost care should be exercised to preserve the vascular supply. A small catheter is introduced through this opening of the oesophagus into the stomach. Gentle suction empties air and some fluid with deflation of the stomach. The proximal segment is next identified. This is much larger and at times appears as a dimple in the fatty tissues of the upper posterior mediastinum. The identification is facilitated by the introduction of a catheter from the nose or mouth. In the majority of cases the proximal segment easily reaches the distal segment without tension, particularly after separation from the trachea of its fibrous connection. The bulbous upper segment is then incised in its most dependent part and anastomosed with the distal segment. It is important to

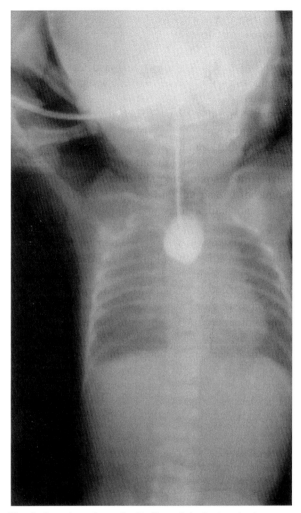

Fig. 2. Oesophageal atresia. Pooling of the barium in the upper segment.

resect the fistulous end of the distal segment, for a further 2–3 mm, in order to achieve a wider and better vascularised anastomosis. The anastomosis is performed with one layer of interrupted sutures using 4/0 non-absorbable sutures mounted on a fine atraumatic needle. The stitches should take all the thickness of the oesophagus on both segments. It is helpful to apply 3–4 stitches before tying, during which the segments are gently approximated. Before completion of the anastomosis, a fine nasogastric tube is introduced. The chest is closed with a fine drain in the pleural space.

3.2.2. Two stage operation (Figs. 3a, 3b and 3c)

In approximately 10% of cases of atresia the two oesophageal segments may not reach to allow the primary anastomosis to be performed. In such cases

the fistulous opening is dealt with as described for the one-stage operation through a right thoracotomy. The distal oesophagus is closed by fine sutures and the chest closed. The patient is then placed in a supine position. A cervical oesophagostomy (left side) and gastrostomy is performed. The infant is then discharged from hospital and fed for 12–18 months through the gastrostomy. During this time, fluids and food are also given by mouth to encourage coordination of swallowing. The second stage of the operation is undertaken 12–18 months after the first stage, with the aim of reconstructing the oesophagus. This involves colonic interposition (oesophago-coloplasty according to Waterston's method) between the cervical and the lower oesophagus just above the gastro-oesophageal junction (Waterston et al., 1962).

- Post-operatively parenteral and enteral (gastrostomy) feeding is continued until resumption of oral intake.

Post-operative care. The infant is nursed in an incubator. The author uses an intravenous infusion for 24 hours, then tube feeding for a further 3 days before feeding by mouth on the 4th to 5th day. Prevention of aspiration, pneumonitis and chest infection should be the major concerns in the post-operative period. Overhydration is lethal; it is better to err on the side of underhydration (the volume of fluid required is about 70–75 ml/kg body weight/24 hours).

3.3. Notes on the results of the operation for oesophageal atresia

The results of surgery depend principally upon early diagnosis and the experience of the surgical team. The best results are achieved in centres familiar with oesophageal surgery and experienced in dealing with such cases. The number of cases is small, probably no more than one in every 6000–8000 births, and therefore a centre dealing with one million inhabitants might encounter one or two cases per year. Apart from prompt diagnosis, referral to a centre with expertise is essential if a good chance of survival is to be expected.

Waterston et al. (1962) at Great Ormond Street Hospital in London treated 218 infants with 109 (50%) surviving — 85% of the survivors were amongst the 'common type atresia' and their survival was dependent on their birth weight. In low risk cases 36 of the 38 infants survived. Koop and associates (1974) reported a survival rate of 66% in 134 patients; 44 infants amongst these were full term

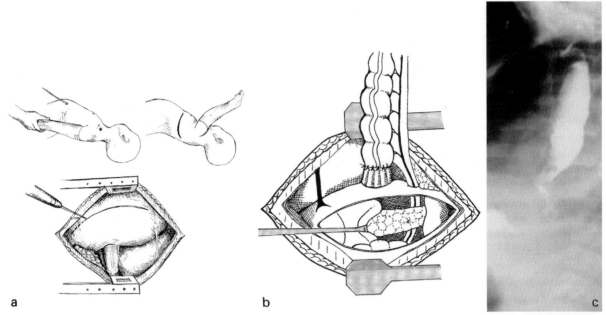

Fig. 3. (a) Diagram depicting two-stage operation of colon interposition for oesophageal atresia. Top left: Cervical oesophagostomy and gastrostomy (TOF has been dealt with). Top right: Left thoracotomy incision. Bottom: Left thoracotomy findings. The lower oesophageal remnant and the diaphragmatic incision with diathermy. (b) Shows diagram of colon interposition between cervical oesophagostomy (not shown) and the oesophageal remnant (shown). (c) Barium contrast study of the patient 6 years after the operation of colon interposition.

and without associated pulmonary infection or other anomalies. All these survived the operation. Boyle and Foker (1994) had no mortality in 60 selected infants treated by primary repair. Current mortality is about 11% (Deurloo et al., 2002).

Problems of atresia with a long gap

Whilst the primary repair is the aim in all cases, a long gap, usually in excess of 2 cm, will create anastomic tension with a risk of anastomosis disruption. It is important to note that, apart from the gap itself, a number of other factors such as existence of double fistula and high localisation of the fistula can be determinant of anastomic tension. A variety of manoeuvres such as circular myotomy (Livaditis et al., 1972) and bouginage of the upper pouch to achieve elongation, mobilisation of stomach effectively creating a hernia (Marujo et al., 1991) have been advocated to allow repair without the use of substitute in order to reduce tension on the suture line and the anastomosis. Of these, circular myotomy appears simpler and has the advantage of being feasible at the time of intended primary repair should there be doubt about the anastomosis.

According to Boyle and Foker (1994), primary repair can be carried out in most, if not all, cases even when there is apparent anastomatic tension. However, primary repair in such cases carries a risk

of gastro-oesophageal reflux and subsequent stricture formation.

When primary repair is not feasible, a two-stage operation is usually required, i.e. exteriorisation in the neck (oesophagostomy) of the proximal segment, closure of fistula and feeding gastrostomy are initially carried out followed by coloplasty later (12–18 months after).

References and further reading

Alexander F, Johanningman J, Martin LW. Staged repair improves outcome of high-risk premature infant with esophageal atresia and tracheoesophageal fistula. J Paediatr Surg 1993; 28: 151–154.

Bax KM, Der Zee DC. Feasibility of thoracoscopic repair of oesophageal atresia with distal fistula. J Paediatr Surg 2002; 37: 192–196.

Boyle EM, Foker JE. Primary repair of ultra long gap esophageal atresia: Results without a lengthening procedure. Ann Thorac Surg 1994; 57: 576–579.

Chittmittrapap S, Spitz L, Kiely EM, et al. Oesophageal atresia and associated anomalies. Arch Dis Child 1989; 64: 364–368.

Deurloo JA, Ekkelkamp S, Schoorl M, et al. Esophageal atresia: historical evaluation of management and results in 371 patients. Ann Thorac Surg 2002; 73: 267–272.

Kimura K, Nishijima E, Tsugawa C, Collins DL, Lazar EL, Stylianos S, Sandler A, Soper RT. Multistaged extrathoracic esophageal elongation procedure for long gap esophageal atresia: experience with 12 patients. J Pediatr Surg 2001; 36: 1725–1727.

Koop CE, Schnaufer L, Broennie AM. Esophageal atresia and tracheoesophageal fistula: Supportive measurers that affect survival. Pediatrics 1974; 54: 558–564.

Lessin MS, Wesselhoeft CW, Luks FI, DeLuca FG. Primary repair of long-gap esophageal atresia by mobilisation of the distal esophagus. Eur J Pediatr Surg 1999; 9: 369–372.

Livaditis A, Radberg L, Odensjo G. Esophageal end-to-end anastomosis: Reduction of anastomotic tension by circular myotomy. Scand J Thorac Cardiovasc Surg 1972; 6: 206–214.

Marujo WC, Tannuri U, Maksoud JG. Total gastric transposi-

tion: an alternative to esophageal replacement in children. J Paediatr Surg 1991; 26: 676–681.

Moghissi K, Hornshaw J, Teasdale P, Dawes EA. Parenteral nutrition in carcinoma of the oesophagus treated by surgery: Nitrogen balance and clinical studies. Brit J Surg 1977; 64: 125–128.

Rejjal A. Congenital anomalies associated with oesophageal atresia. Am J Perinatal 1999; 16: 239–244.

Waterston DJ, Bonham-Carter RE, Aberdeen E. Oesophageal atresia tracheoesophageal fistula: A study of survival in 218 infants. Lancet 1962; 1: 819–822.

K. Moghissi, J.A.C. Thorpe and F. Ciulli (Eds.)
Moghissi's Essentials of Thoracic and Cardiac Surgery
© 2003 Elsevier Science B.V. All rights reserved

CHAPTER III.5

Foreign bodies in the oesophagus

K. Moghissi

1. Introduction

A variety of blunt or sharp objects can be retained in the oesophagus following their accidental or intentional ingestion. A blunt object has to be relatively large to lodge in the oesophagus unless there is a pre-existing pathology. The existence of such pathology must be considered in all cases where a small object (less than about 2 cm) or a food bolus is found impacted in the oesophagus.

The subsets of population at an increased risk of foreign body ingestion are: children (particularly those below the age of 2), psychiatric patients, and elderly individuals with badly-fitting dental prosthesis.

Amongst blunt objects, coins head the list of frequency of occurrence of ingestion, especially in children. The most common culprits amongst sharp objects are bones of fish, chicken and other animals.

The nature of ingested foreign body varies with geography, cultural characteristics and customs of a population.

The location of impaction of a foreign body usually corresponds to the site of the relative anatomical constriction of the oesophagus which are:
- Pharyngo-oesophageal junction.
- At the point where the oesophagus enters the thorax and is compressed by the aortic arch and the left main bronchus.
- In the lower part of the oesophagus just above or at the oesophago-gastric junction (level with oesophageal sphincter).

An overall majority (60–70%) of impacted foreign bodies (FB) are usually found in the cervical oesophagus.

2. Diagnosis

A retained foreign body in the oesophagus needs to be diagnosed and treated early if potentially life-threatening complications are to be avoided. Diagnosis relies on the triad of history and clinical examination, radiology and endoscopy.

2.1. Clinical history and examination

Precise history-taking is of paramount importance as, in the majority of adult patients, this leads to diagnosis as well as establishing the nature of the foreign body. In some psychiatric patients the clinical history is unhelpful and in children the accidental foreign body ingestion may have passed unnoticed. Patients are usually symptomatic and common presenting complaints are:
- sensation of choking
- pain or discomfort on swallowing
- dysphagia and vomiting
- excessive salivation with/without blood staining

In children, symptoms may be absent but, when present, include:
- refusal to take food
- vomiting and excessive salivation

In the absence of complications such as perforation, clinical examination may be unrevealing except in those with coexisting pathology affecting anatomical integrity or physiological function of the oesophagus.

2.2. Radiology

Radiology contributes in locating the site and nature of the foreign body within the oesophagus when objects happen to be radio-opaque. Plain antero-pos-

References and further reading

Al-Qudah A, Daradkeh S, Abu-Khalaf M. Esophageal foreign bodies. Eur J Cardiothorac Surg 1998; 13: 494–498.

Athanassiadi K, Gerazounis M, Metaxas, et al. Management of oesophageal foreign bodies: a retrospective review of 400 cases. Eur J Cardiothorac Surg 2002; 21: 653–656.

Blair SR, Graeber GM, Cruzzavala JL et al. Current management of esophageal impactions. Chest 1993; 104: 1205–1209.

Campbell JB, Condon VR. Catheter removal of blunt esophageal foreign bodies in children. Pediatr Radiol 1989; 19: 361–365.

Erbs J, Babbitt DP. Foreign bodies in the alimentary tract of infants and children. Appl Ther 1965; 1103–1109.

Hawkins DB. Removal of blunt foreign bodies from the oesophagus. Ann Otol Rhinol Laryngol 1990; 99: 935–940.

Jackson CL. Foreign bodies in the esophagus. Am J Surg 1957; 93: 308–312.

Jackson RM, Hawkins DB. Coins in the esophagus. What is the best management? Int J Pediatr Otorminolaryngol 1986; 12: 127–135.

Lam HC, Woo JK, Van Hasselt CA. Management of ingested foreign bodies: a retrospective review of 5240 patients. J Laryngol 2001; 115: 954–957.

Lyons MF, Tscuchida AM. Foreign bodies of the gastrointestinal tract. Med Clin N Am 1993; 5: 1101–1114.

Moghissi K. Editorial comment. Eur J Cardiothorac Surg 1998; 13: 499.

Nandi P, Ong GB. Foreign bodies in the esophagus: Review of 2394 cases. Br J Surg 1978; 65: 5–9.

CHAPTER III.6

Gastro–oesophageal reflux and hiatal hernia

K. Moghissi

1. Introduction

The basic function of the oesophagus is to deliver food into the stomach. The stomach may be considered as a reservoir which receives a great volume of food intermittently but disposes of its contents slowly over a period of time. Competence of the gastro-oesophageal junction is a necessity since otherwise, reflux of the stomach content will occur. The common association of sliding hiatal hernia and gastro-oesophageal reflux compels these to be considered together.

In 1996 the International Society for Diseases of the Oesophagus (ISDE) formed a sub-committee (Matthews, 1996) to present a classification for hiatal hernia and gastro-oesophageal reflux. The committee considered that in hiatal hernia/reflux complex, the principal components that may be abnormal relate to: anatomy (A), function (F), and pathology (P).

Anatomy: relates to contrast study (barium swallow) and presence/absence of hiatal hernia.

Function: relates to acid reflux as demonstrated by 24 hours pH study.

Pathology: relates to the findings at endoscopy.

The classification has a designated scale for each parameter: A, F and P (Table 1).

Any discussion on gastro-oesophageal reflux necessitates a review of the factors which are involved in the normal anti-reflux mechanism.

These are:

1.1. Lower oesophageal sphincter (LOS)

This is a physiological rather than an anatomical entity. With manometry, an area of the lower oesophagus 3–5 cm long can be demonstrated to have tone when at rest. In response to swallowing, the sphincter opens to let the food enter the stomach; it then closes the lumen preventing reflux. The lower oesophageal sphincter must be considered as the primary and fundamental factor preventing gastro-oesophageal reflux. Other factors which are described in the vast literature and briefly discussed below, should be put in their perspective of a secondary role.

1.2. Angle of implantation

This is the oesophago-gastric junctional angle. Alteration of the angle in a sliding hiatal hernia may be a contributory factor to the creation of reflux.

Table 1

A proposed classification for hiatal hernia and gastro-oesophageal reflux: H.R. Matthews (on behalf of ISDE sub-committee), 1996

A = Anatomy	0 = No hernia
	1 = Small intermittent sliding hiatal hernia
	2 = Constant (irreducible) hiatal hernia
	3 = Mixed/Para-oesophageal hernia
F = Function	0 = Normal acid exposure
	(pH < 4 for up to 3.9% of recording time)
	1 = Increased acid exposure
	(pH < 4 for 4–7.9% of recording time)
	2 = Increased acid exposure
	(pH < 4 for 8–19.9% of recording time)
	3 = Increased acid exposure
	(pH < 4 for 20% or more of recording time)
P = Pathology [a]	0 = No macroscopic mucosal abnormality
	1 = Isolated or non-confluent erosive lesion of the mucosa
	2 = Circumferential or confluent erosive lesions in the mucosa
	3 = Chronic lesions involving the wall of the oesophagus, stricture, short oesophagus or penetrating ulcer

[a] Based on barium endoscopy or operative findings.

1.3. Flap valve

In the interior of the oesophago-gastric junction, this is created, partly at least, because of the angle of implantation and is a further factor in the anti-reflux mechanism.

1.4. Structure of the hiatus and the phreno-oesophageal ligament

Disregarding minor variations (well documented by Allison (1951), Collis et al. (1954) and Hayward (1961)), the hiatal muscle is derived mainly from the right crus of the diaphragm with the addition of some fibres from the left crus. The crural muscle encircles the oesophagus. This, together with the attachment of the peritoneum and the phreno-oesophageal ligament, produces a pinchcock effect on the oesophagus which holds the lower oesophagus closed and provides its competence.

1.5. Effect of the intra-abdominal pressure on the lower oesophagus

Basically this theory suggests that the intrathoracic negative pressure is transmitted to the lumen of the oesophagus. However, the intraluminal pressure of the abdominal portion of the oesophagus is under the influence of the negative intrathoracic pressure, but its outside is surrounded by higher intra-abdominal

pressure. The differential pressure across the wall of the lower oesophagus may be responsible for its competence.

1.6. Chemical and hormonal influence

There is evidence to suggest that the LOS function is influenced by hormones and chemicals (Giles et al., 1969; Castell and Levine, 1971; McGuigan, 1973).

What emerges from exhaustive literature on the subject of competence of the gastro-oesophageal junction can be summarised as follows:
(a) No individual factor appears to be sufficient to produce anti-reflux mechanism without the support of others. The most significant factor, however, is the inherent tone of the LOS.
(b) The causes of reflux may be different in different individuals and may be multifactorial.

2. Hiatal hernia

Hiatal hernias should be discussed under two separate headings. First, they can be regarded simply as the protrusion of an intra-abdominal viscus, usually the stomach, through the oesophageal hiatus of the diaphragm. Secondly, the sliding variety of hiatal hernia is so very commonly associated with gastro-oesophageal reflux that it should be considered quite separate from other hiatal hernias, because its surgical treatment should provide an anti-reflux mechanism. It is therefore important to distinguish the types of hiatal hernia and to discuss them separately.

Hiatal hernia may be subdivided into three types:
2.1. Sliding hiatal hernia (Fig. 1): In this type the gastro-oesophageal junction, normally below the diaphragm, ascends from its position to enter the chest. In an early stage the hernia is reducible and thereafter the junction can be brought down under the diaphragm later to become fixed.
2.2. Para-oesophageal hiatal hernia (Fig. 2): In this type of hernia the lower end of the oesophagus and the gastro-oesophageal junction remain in their normal anatomical positions but a large portion of the stomach with its peritoneal covering protrudes into the chest through an enlarged hiatus. The stomach often rotates (volvulus) and progressively migrates behind the heart and to the right chest.
2.3. Mixed type of hernia: In this type of hernia the components of both the sliding and the

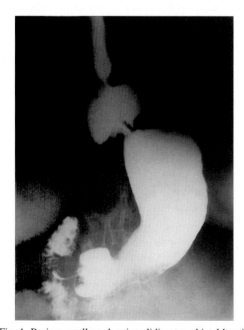

Fig. 1. Barium swallow showing sliding type hiatal hernia

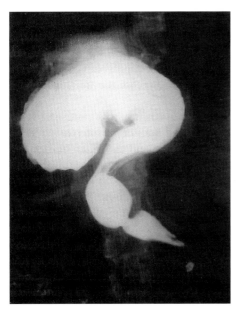

Fig. 2. Barium swallow showing para-oesophageal hernia. Notice the volvulus of the stomach.

para-oesophageal hernias are found: that is, the lower part of the oesophagus slips up some distance above the hiatus and at the same time the peritoneal covered stomach moves into an enlarged hiatus.

For practical purposes the discussion should concentrate on the sliding and para-oesophageal hernias, as mixed hernias should be treated like sliding or para-oesophageal hernias depending on their clinical and pathological behaviour (i.e. the presence of reflux).

2.1. Sliding hiatal hernia

Sliding hiatal hernia is one of the most common conditions encountered in medical practice. How common the condition really is in the general population is difficult to assess as in many instances the hernia remains asymptomatic. In practice gastro-oesophageal reflux is frequently associated with a sliding hiatal hernia and, conversely, the hernia is often associated with reflux.

The consequence of reflux is oesophagitis. Allison (1951) showed that what was important in hiatal hernia was the associated gastro-oesophageal reflux; Barrett (1950) suggested the term reflux oesophagitis for oesophageal inflammatory changes which occur as a result of reflux. The precise nature of the chemicals which cause oesophagitis is not known but acid is probably the most important component.

Like any other inflammation, reflux oesophagitis has its sequelae. It can resolve when the effect of the stimulus (in this case reflux) ceases but it may progress into a chronic inflammation with fibrous scarring or ulceration. Fibrous scarring is responsible for stricture formation and scarring of the oesophagus. In some cases, reflux oesophagitis affects not only the oesophageal wall but also peri-oesophageal tissues including the mediastinal pleura. The resulting fibrous tissue formation in and around the longitudinal muscles of the oesophagus produce contraction and shortening. In effect, the result of shortening is the ascent of the gastro-oesophageal junction to higher than its original level. The shortening may therefore be defined as an (irreducible) elevation of the phreno-oesophageal ligament above the oesophageal hiatus of the diaphragm. Shortening and the stricture often occur together but, when the inflammatory changes predominantly affect the oesophageal lumen, stricture is more prominent. At other times the pathology involves the mural and peri-oesophageal tissues and the result is shortening.

2.1.1. Clinical presentation

The main symptoms of patients with sliding hiatal hernia and gastro-oesophageal reflux relates to oesophagitis.

- Heartburn: This sensation starts in the epigastric region and propagates retrosternally upwards, usually not beyond the sternal angle. It is a combination of burning and discomfort rather than a sharp pain. Heartburn is the manifestation of acid reflux and oesophagitis.
- Pain: This can be located retrosternally or in the back; it may be dull or sharp and spasmodic. There appears to be no direct relationship between pain and the oesophagitis and its severity. Therefore, pain may be more of a spasm or muscular contraction.
- Flatulence and Eructation: Over production and disposal of 'wind' seems to be a particular characteristic of many patients with hiatal hernia. Occasionally a patient will 'belch' almost constantly. It is suggested that flatulence is largely due to aerophagy.

The author recalls a considerably obese patient of 90 kg whose complaint, besides heartburn and vomiting, was mainly incessant belching, which was embarrassing to her and others to a degree that she had become a recluse. Naturally many physicians and surgeons tried to reduce her weight and treat her symptoms but with no measure of success. A psychiatrist added his expertise to that of the other physicians without a hope. Reluctantly the repair of her hernia was undertaken with prompt relief of the belching, though not entirely of the flatulence which required a measure of dieting.

- Dysphagia: Even without a stricture, dysphagia can be present. The causes of dysphagia without a stricture is muscular spasm and motility disturbances of the oesophagus.
- Nausea and vomiting: Nausea can be present at any time. Vomiting, when present, occurs at the end of a meal.

2.1.2. Diagnosis

Of the investigatory methods at our disposal, radiology is concerned with the anatomical demonstration of hernia, whereas manometric and pH studies will indicate the decrease in the lower oesophageal sphincter pressure and the gastro-oesophageal reflux, respectively (see chapter III.3). Oesophagoscopy (oesophago-gastroscopy) is essential, not only to assess objective evidence of oesophagitis and its severity, but also to discover ulceration as well as to exclude neoplasms. A biopsy is usually undertaken from the abnormal mucosa and from the gastro-oesophageal mucosal junction.

2.1.3. Treatment

Broadly the treatment falls within:
- Conservative management
- Surgical treatment

Conservative management. Hiatal hernia without symptoms of gastro-oesophageal reflux needs no treatment. Symptomatic hernias are treated by measures which aim at reducing the reflux and/or changing the ingredients of gastric juice in such a way as to diminish its effects on oesophageal mucosa.

Reduction of weight in an overweight patient will help to reduce the hernia and its symptoms of reflux. The author does not believe that the loss of weight improves symptoms but the weight reduction diet may be also responsible for symptomatic relief.

Reflux, which commonly occurs in these patients at night, can be reduced or prevented by raising the head of the bed on blocks or by using several pillows to achieve the 'uncomfortable' position of almost sitting up in bed. Patients are asked not to wear a tight belt or corset.

There is controversy about diet, particularly with regard to fibre; some patients, particularly during symptomatic episodes, cannot tolerate fibre whilst others can. Chocolate and fatty food should be avoided. Alcohol and tobacco consumption should be eliminated as both reduce the lower oesophageal sphincter pressure and provoke gastro-oesophageal reflux. Cigarettes increase the frequency of acid reflux.

Medication: Antacids and antispasmodics are both helpful: the former by increasing the pH of the refluxing juices and the latter by removing the painful effect of the spasm produced by the reflux.

H_2 receptor antagonists reduce basal nocturnal and stimulated acid secretion. They thus reduce oesophagitis and assist healing of oesophageal ulcer.

Proton pump inhibitors (Omeprazol) inhibit gastric parietal cell H^+, K^+ and ATPase. The latter is the final step in gastric acid secretion and, therefore, inhibits both basal and stimulated gastric acid secretions.

Prokinetic agents such as metoclopramide (Maxolon) are helpful in some cases. They appear to reduce reflux by enhancing gastric emptying, increasing sphincteric pressure and oesophageal acid clearance.

Drugs which enhance reflux or produce mucosal injury should be avoided or be prescribed in their enteric coated form. In this respect non-steroid anti-inflammatory drugs such as Aspirin are important since they are in common use. Whenever possible their oral intake should be avoided.

Surgical treatment. Surgical treatment of sliding hiatal hernia means repair of the hernia together with an anti-reflux mechanism which should be an integral part of the repair. Patients are selected for repair on the basis of symptoms related to the complications of gastro-oesophageal reflux. Those patients suffering from severe reflux without a demonstrable hernia will still need anti-reflux operation when there is objective evidence of gastro-oesophageal reflux (at this moment in time, from pH and motility studies) It must, however, be emphasised that although the various investigatory methods provide us with evidence of gastro-oesophageal reflux and help us plan the most appropriate operation, the surgical procedure is carried out on the basis of 'symptoms' and not on 'evidence' of reflux alone without symptoms.

In general, it is now accepted that symptoms of gastro-oesophageal reflux may be temporary or intermittent and a period of medical and conservative treatment (antacids and antispasmodics, avoidance of alcohol and smoking together with a weight-losing diet) should be tried. If this proves unsuccessful, surgery is then undertaken. Some of the criteria for selection of patients for surgery are:

- Patients who have received medical treatment for the last 6 months without symptomatic relief.
- Patients who on endoscopic examination are shown not to have benefited from conservative treatment and are still presenting with severe oesophagitis.
- Patients with an ulcer not healing by medical treatment and presenting with haematemesis.
- Patients who have suffered intermittently but present with a developing stricture.
- Patients with a lesion suspected to be a neoplasm together with a hiatal hernia.

2.1.4. Methods of repair

It has been said that there are as many methods for repair of hiatal hernia [1] as there are surgeons and the conclusion which is drawn from this is that no method is perfect. The statement is, of course, no more than an aphorism and, in reality, there are principally a few main methods of repair carried out by a great number of surgeons, each of whom adds variations to already established methods.

The objectives of an operation for gastro-oesophageal reflux associated with sliding hiatal hernia should be:

- Control of reflux requiring repositioning 2–3 cm of the lower oesophagus (intra-abdominal portion of the oesophagus) in the abdominal cavity.
- Creating of anti-reflux valvular mechanism.
- Repair of hiatal hernia and tightening of the oesophageal hiatus by approximation of the two components of the right crus of the diaphragm posteriorly.

Historically Allison (1951) was the first in the modern era of thoracic surgery to draw attention to the lower oesophagus, hiatal hernia and the anatomy of repair. Allison's method of repair of hiatal hernia and control of reflux was mainly based on positioning a length of the lower oesophagus below the diaphragm and tightening the enlarged hiatal opening.. The recognition of the lower thoracic oesophagus was crucial and the site of the insertion of phreno-oesophageal membrane (ligament) to the

oesophagus was taken as the landmark of boundary between the thoracic oesophagus (above) and abdominal oesophagus (below) it. Allison also regarded the tightening of the hiatus as an important step of the operation both in regard to control of reflux and prevention of recurrence of the hernia.

Almost simultaneous to the development and evolution of Allison type of repair, other anti-reflux methods were being designed, notably by Nissen (1956), and later by Belsey (1977), and Toupet (1963).

Three methods of repair of hiatal hernia will be described. No attempt is made to compare their results since no clear evidence based on trial is available and those who have attempted randomised trial cannot profess to be proficient in equal measure in all of the methods. However, the results of each operation individually as per published literature will be recorded.

Allison repair (Fig. 3). This operation (and its variance) was the commonest operative method in many centres in the 1950s and 1960s for repair of all types of hiatal hernia but is now scarcely performed. This author believes its use and, particularly, its misuse for inappropriate cases has been partially responsible for its elimination from the repertoire of contemporary surgeons. The operation is an anatomical repair and, as such, its anti-reflux effects have been uncertain. The Allison method encompasses steps which form essential parts of other operations (Nissen, Belsey). These particularly apply to oesophageal exposure and mobilisation and hiatal crural approximation. The author believes that the Allison type of repair is still justifiable for simple hernias without reflux (i.e. para-oesophageal/rolling type) and in the absence of shortening.

The author believes that its use is rationally justifiable in simple para-oesophageal hernias with no evidence of gastro-oesophageal reflux, no shortening and no other abnormality. Under these circumstances the operation can be carried out with minimum disturbance and is particularly useful in the elderly.

The operation may be described under three major steps:

- Exposure and mobilisation of the oesophagus and hernia
- Reduction of the hernia
- Repair

Exposure and mobilisation of the oesophagus and hernia: The operation is carried out through a left postero-lateral thoracotomy. The thoracic cavity is usually entered through the 7th intercostal space

---

[1] In recent years there has been an array of publications concerned with laparoscopic (and thoracoscopic) repair of both sliding and para-oesophageal hiatal hernia. Such 'mini access' procedures in experienced hands are attended by good results but the long-term results need evaluation.

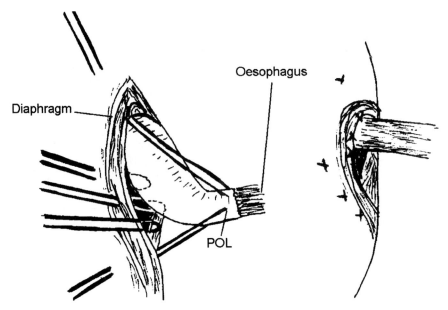

Fig. 3. Allison's repair of hiatal hernia (Left). The sutures are inserted into the phreno-oesophageal ligament (POL) and the diaphragm. (Right) The hernia is now reduced and the crura approximated.

stripping the upper periosteum of the 8th rib. The lower part of the oesophagus is mobilised (see section 3 in chapter III.17). A sling is passed around the oesophagus and held up by an assistant. This helps further mobilisation of the oesophagus which should be carried out from the hiatus up to the arch of the aorta. There are a few oesophageal vessels, two or three in number which need to be tied off and divided. Attention is now focused on clearing the hiatus and the phreno-oesophageal ligament from the fibro-fatty tissue surrounding the oesophagus; the aim is to identify the phreno-oesophageal ligament and to divide its attachment to the hiatal border but to see it clearly attached to the oesophagus.

Reduction of the hernia: This is achieved firstly by suturing the phreno-oesophageal ligament and the surrounding fibrous tissue around the lower oesophagus to the under-surface of the diaphragm (see below) about 1cm from the hiatal margin. One way to do this is to pick up the phreno-oesophageal ligament with double-ended needle sutures, pass both ends through the hiatus and then bringing both needles out through the diaphragm and the hiatal border to be tied on its thoracic aspect. In this way the phreno-oesophageal ligament is stitched to the under-surface of the diaphragm. The reduction is helped by making a 2–3 cm incision in the diaphragmatic dome avoiding the phrenic nerve then introducing the tip of the sling (which encircles the oesophagus) through the hiatus in front of the oesophagus and recovering it (i.e. by

picking up the two ends of the sling) through the diaphragmatic incision.

Repair: The aim is to identify the two limbs of the crural muscle and approximate them to tighten the hiatus around the oesophagus. For this, usually two stitches are required well inserted into the crural muscles. Both the identification of the crural limbs and the stitching are made easier if:

(a) The assistant pulls gently downwards and forwards on the sling around the oesophagus (which is now passed via the hiatus and is brought out through the diaphragmatic incision referred to above).

(b) The index and ring fingers of the left hand are introduced through the hiatus, posterior to the oesophagus, into the abdomen lifting up the right component of the crural muscle.

When these stitches are inserted the hernia-reducing stitches (see reduction of hernia above) are tightly tied and the hernia is thus reduced and the phreno-oesophageal ligament is fixed to the border of the hiatus. The crural stitches are then tied to approximate the two limbs of the crura without creating a narrow hiatus. The objective is to allow room for the tip of the index finger to be accommodated between the oesophagus and the hiatus posteriorly. Some surgeons (including the author) in addition fix the lower oesophagus to the border of the hiatus with 4–5 stitches. The small diaphragmatic incision is now repaired by

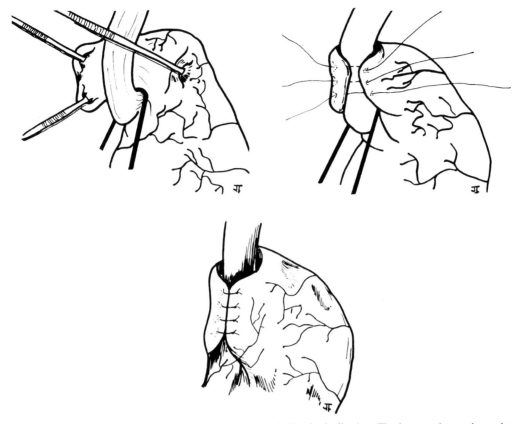

Fig. 4. Nissen type repair of hiatal hernia (from left to right). Steps in the fundoplication. The bottom picture shows the completed fundoplication.

a mattress stitch and oversewn by a second running stitch. The chest wound is then closed with a drain in the pleural space connected to an underwater sealed drainage system.

Operation of total fundoplication (Nissen type operation) (Fig. 4). We are careful to avoid calling the operation of total fundoplication Nissen's fundoplication, as it is now clear that those who regularly perform this procedure (including the author with experience of just over 600 fundoplications), all exploit the principle of Nissen's fundoplication but with added variations.

The principle of the method is to create a well, or a flutter valve, by wrapping the fundus of the stomach totally (360 degrees) around the lower oesophagus under the diaphragm. To do justice to the founder of the total fundoplication, his method of operation will be described first. The author's variation of the method of total fundoplication is then described.

- Nissen's fundoplication: The abdominal approach
  This approach was used by Nissen for hiatal

hernia with gastro-oesophageal reflux but uncomplicated by shortening of the oesophagus or other associated conditions such as oesophageal ulcers and cardiospasm. The abdominal cavity is entered by a left subcostal incision. The intra-abdominal position of the oesophagus is exposed after transverse incising of the peritoneal fold covering the gastro-oesophageal junction. This can be achieved by retraction of the spleen and the left lobe of the liver to right and left respectively after division of the left triangular ligament. The aim is to encircle the lower oesophagus first by a finger then by a sling; the upper part of the gastrosplenic and gastrohepatic ligaments with enclosed vessels have to be divided. The sling is pulled downwards and with the right hand fingers the fundus is passed behind the oesophagus to the left towards the liver (the lesser curvature) side. In this way the posterior wall of the fundus passes from the left to the right behind the oesophagus.

A series of 3–4 sutures are now placed, stitching together from left to right the anterior wall of the fundus, the anterior surface of the oesophagus (not entering the mucosa or the anterior vagus nerve), and the posterior wall of the fundus (which is now facing anteriorly and to the right followed its passage behind the oesophagus). The first (top) stitch is inserted as high as possible, followed by the remaining 2–3 stitches at about 1 cm intervals. The lower stitches may not be able to pick up the oesophageal wall. These stitches when tied unite the anterior and posterior wall of the gastric fundus, creating the total plication around the oesophagus. In order to avoid too tight a plication, a large bougie (such as size 48 F mercury Maloney bougie) may be introduced into the stomach prior to approximating fundoplication stitches. The bougie is removed and the abdominal wall is then closed.

- Nissen's transthoracic fundoplication

The pleural cavity is entered through the 7th or 8th intercostal space. The pulmonary ligament is divided and the oesophagus encircled by a sling. The sling is pulled forward to expose the posterior part of the hiatus which is cleaned of fibro-fatty tissue. The hiatus is widened and the gastro-oesophageal junction and fundus of the stomach are exposed; the parietal peritoneum is opened to gain a better access and the fundus is brought up into the chest through the hiatus. This may involve ligation and division of the uppermost short gastric vessels. The fundoplication is carried out in the same manner as in the abdominal approach. The edges of the hiatus are then anchored to the fundus (which itself is around the oesophagus) by interrupted sutures. The chest is closed with a drain in the pleural space.

Moghissi modification of Nissen total fundoplication. The operation carried out by the author is based on Nissen's total fundoplication with the following modifications.

- The approach is through the left posterolateral thoracotomy with the patient in the right lateral position. The pleura is entered usually through the 7th intercostal space by stripping the peritoneum of the upper border of the 8th rib.
- The oesophagus is encircled by a sling and is fully mobilised up to the aortic arch. Nissen's original operation does not insist on this point, which allows reduction of the hernia and lower oesophagus to below the diaphragm in cases of moderate oesophageal shortening.
- The hiatus is cleared from all the fibro-fatty tissues, taking care not to damage the vagus nerves.
- The fundus of the stomach is mobilised through the abdomen via phreno-laparotomy. For this the

diaphragm is incised circumferentially and peripherally, avoiding damage to the phrenic nerve branches.

- The fundus of the stomach is mobilised by ligating and dividing the uppermost portion of the gastrosplenic omentum and its enclosed blood vessels. The upper portion of the gastrohepatic omentum is dealt with likewise.
- Two fingers of the left hand are introduced through the abdomen into the hiatus to lift up the peritoneum and the phreno-oesophageal ligament (POL) on the lateral aspect of the oesophagus. This brings into prominence the phreno-oesophageal ligament and allows the dissection of all the hiatal attachments of the oesophagus. The fundus of the stomach is brought up through the hiatus into the chest. As the lesser curvature side has also been mobilised, the fundus and part of the body of the stomach can be brought into the chest with ease.
- The total fundoplication is now carried out. This is achieved in the following fashion:

The fundus is grasped by the right hand and passed posterior to the oesophagus and picked up by Babcock tissue forceps at the anterolateral aspect (ventral aspect) of the oesophagus, which is thus encircling half of its circumference. Another pair of Babcock forceps is applied to the part of the fundus which is still on the lateral aspect of the oesophagus.

The fundoplication stitches (3–4) are now inserted: the uppermost takes on the left side (a) of the fundus, then passes through the POL and finally the right side (b) of the fundus. The successive stitches pass through the two sides of the fundus and pick up the oesophageal muscle below the POL or the upper part of the oesophago-gastric junction at its lesser curvature side. Care should be taken not to enter the mucosa. These fundal stitches are tied: care should be taken not to produce too tight a fundoplication. The right amount of tightening is when the tip of the index finger can be introduced between the encircling fundus and the oesophagus. The upper border of the fundus is now anchored to the oesophageal muscle by a few interrupted stitches (3/0 silk).

Note: the total length of the fundoplication is about 3–3.5 cm. The plication should be fairly loose. This may be gauged and guided by a Maloney bougie size 46–48 in the oesophagus after passage of which there should be no space between the plication and the lower oesophagus. The lower end of the oesophagus surrounded by the fundus is now reduced below the diaphragm. This is easily achieved by introducing the two ends of the original sling around the oesophagus into the hiatus from the chest side and picking the tips from the abdominal side of the hiatus via phrenolaparotomy. Then the two ends of the sling are passed through a small additional diaphragmatic incision.

Following reduction of the hernia (i.e. the oesophago-fundul complex) the pull on the sling exposes the 'V' shaped two limbs of the crural muscles posteriorly which are approximated by 2–3 stitches. These stitches are tied not too tightly and should allow the tip of the index finger to be accommodated between the edge of the hiatus (anteromedially) and the oesophagus.

- Finally the lower oesophageal muscle is anchored to the border of the hiatus from above (chest side) and/or from below (diaphragmatic side).

- The diaphragmatic incision is closed in two layers and the chest closed with a drain in the thoracic cavity connected to an underwater sealed drainage system.

My modification of Nissen's fundoplication has the following features:
- Access to the abdomen through the diaphragm
- Good mobilisation of the oesophagus
- The first plication stitch includes the phreno-oesophageal ligament to provide more secure plication
- The crura approximation reducing the hiatal size
- The lower oesophagus is anchored to the border of hiatus.

Mark IV Belsey repair (Fig. 5). This operation is carried out through a left posterolateral thoracotomy with the patient in the right lateral position. The approach is via the 6th intercostal space. The oesophagus is first mobilised fully to below the aortic arch and the hiatus is cleared from areolar fibro-fatty tissue by sharp dissection. This involves division of 1–2 oesophageal vessels notably posterolaterally. Attention is paid not to damage the vagus nerves. Abdominal entry is made anteromedially where this can be carried out by incising the phreno-oesophageal ligament. Deep to this structure 1–2 short gastric ves-

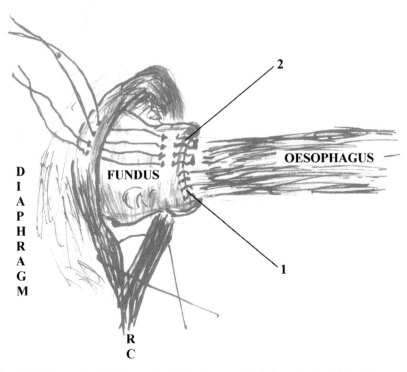

Fig. 5. Diagram of Belsey Mark IV repair of hiatal hernia. 1: The first row of stitches already tied. 2: The second row of stitches are inserted but not yet tied. One of the crural stitches is shown.

sels will have to be tied off and divided. The two components of the right crus which surrounds the oesophagus (oesophageal hiatus) are now identified and cleared. The approximation of the two components between which the hiatal hernia occurs is an important part of the operation. This is achieved by 3–5 stitches picking up the crural muscles posteriorly. These sutures are intended to convert the posterior V-shaped gap part of the hiatus into a narrower Y shape. These stitches are not tied at this stage.

The fundus of the stomach is now brought up to the chest anteriorly through the hiatus to wrap around two thirds of the circumference of the oesophagus antero-laterally (260–270 degrees) and attached to the oesophagus by two rows of mattress stitches using non-absorbable sutures. The first row approximates the stomach to the oesophagus 1–1.5 cm above the cardia. The second row of sutures wraps the stomach a further 1–1.5 cm above the first row of sutures. This row of stitches incorporates the antero-lateral border of the hiatus. Thus each stitch passes through the lower oesophagus, the sero-muscular coating of the stomach and the crus of the diaphragm. Each row will have 3–5 sutures.

Belsey emphasised the importance of these stitches and makes the point that when they are tied, they approximate without tissue strangulation. Effectively, the first row of sutures creates partial fundoplication and the second row of stitches, when tied, maintains the fundoplication below the diaphragm. The crural approximating stitches are tied to narrow the gap between the two components of the right crus. Once these stitches are tied to the hiatus, admit the tip of the index finger behind the oesophagus.

2.2. Para-oesophageal hiatal hernia (rolling hernia)

2.2.1. Introduction
In this type of hernia, the gastro-oesophageal junction remains in its normal position but a variable portion of the stomach protrudes through the hiatus into the chest. In the author's surgically treated cases, 80% of patients with para-oesophageal hernia are female, the majority of whom over the age of 70 years.

2.2.2. Anatomical features
The salient anatomical features of para-oesophageal hernia are as follows:
- The herniated stomach enters the chest along and in front of the lower end of the oesophagus which itself retains its usual anatomical position.

- The hernia always possesses a peritoneal sac which often is adherent to the base of the left lung and the mediastinal pleurae.
- As a consequence of the differential pressure between the abdomen and the thoracic cavities, the hernia tends to enlarge progressively. In the course of time the whole of the stomach is herniated in the chest, the greater curvature lying uppermost. Occasionally spleen omentum, transverse colon and even small bowel migrate in the chest. In some cases the whole of the stomach enters the thorax, in which case the cardia and pylorus are positioned side-by-side. In this situation the stomach is twisted and placed upside down in the chest behind the heart and overlapping its right and left borders.
- There are also varying degrees of volvulus of the stomach with the serious risk of obstruction, strangulation and bleeding.

2.2.3. Clinical features and diagnosis
In many instances a large para-oesophageal hernia presents with such mild symptoms that it escapes investigation and discovery. In these the condition is found incidentally in the course of chest radiography showing the stomach as a retrocardiac gas and fluid containing mass (shadow) in the chest. It is, however, rare to find a para-oesophageal hernia which is truly asymptomatic. In effect, even in asymptomatic cases, patients would admit to some discomfort or pain which they have considered as unimportant.

In some cases the symptoms are severe enough for the patient to seek medical advice. Unlikely sliding hiatal hernia, heartburn and gastro-oesophageal reflux are absent in 'pure' para-oesophageal hernias. Nevertheless:
- Some patients have a mixed type hernia and the 'sliding element' with its gastro-oesophageal reflux remains overshadowed by the observation of the stomach bulge on the X-ray film.
- Intermittent vomiting and pain are often present in these symptomatic hernias, even in the absence of obstruction.

The common symptoms of para-oesophageal hernia are:
- Anaemia
- Intermittent upper abdominal discomfort and pain, with or without vomiting
- Dyspnoea due to space-occupying stomach in the chest
- Pseudo-anginal attacks.

Rarely, acute haemorrhage is the presenting symptom and, in such cases, a gastric ulcer is usually present. In some cases sudden attacks of pain and vomiting accompanied by shock can mimic myocardial infarction to such an extent that the sufferer finds themselves in a coronary care unit. These signs denote an acute obstruction or impending strangulation.

The diagnosis of para-oesophageal hernia is made radiologically. A plain chest radiograph indicates a fluid and gas containing shadow behind the heart. Barium swallow confirms the diagnosis. Oesophagoscopy should always be carried out to exclude associated pathology.

2.2.4. Treatment

There is no medical treatment for the condition except for symptomatic relief of pain and correction of anaemia.

In acute cases with signs of obstruction, decompression of the stomach by aspiration through a nasogastric tube is undertaken in order to reduce the distension of the thoracic stomach and prevent strangulation. Intravenous fluid is given and blood electrolytes checked and abnormalities corrected. Other supportive measures are applied as the case requires. Following a short preparation, surgical operation should be undertaken to reduce the hernia. In some cases, this will be an emergency when strangulation is present. In chronic symptomatic and even asymptomatic cases, surgical treatment should be considered because of the potential risk of complications, (provided that the patient is suitable for operation). Advanced age is not a contraindication to surgery, particularly in patients with symptoms interfering with quality of life.

The operation may be carried out by abdominal or thoracic approach. Thoracic approach has the advantage of good exposure of volvulated stomach and the intra-thoracic adhesions of the sac. Abdominal access is less traumatic and is more advantageous to those with poor respiratory reserve.

The aim of surgery in para-oesophageal hernia (without gastro-oesophageal reflux) is:
- Reduction of the hernia
- Repair of the defect

In the absence of reflux, the provision of anti-reflux mechanism, which is the mandatory requirement in treatment of sliding hiatal hernia, is not needed.

In abdominal approach, an upper laparotomy is performed. The entire stomach may be in the chest and only pylorus and duodenum will be seen in proximity of the hiatus. The reduction of hernia involves division of some adhesions and 'de-twisting' of the stomach. Attention should be paid to identify the lower oesophagus early in the course of reduction of hernia to avoid injury. The surgeon should also keep in mind that intra-thoracic adhesions and injury to the lung caused by blunt dissection can result in post-operative complications.

Following reduction of the hernia and excision of the peritoneal sac, the oesophageal hiatus is closed anterior to the oesophagus by interrupted non-absorbable sutures. The lesser curvature is then sutured posteriorly to the muscle of the right crus of the diaphragm.

The trans-thoracic operation is indicated in most cases except for those with cardio-respiratory deficiency. The approach is particularly suitable for those who may have large hernia with evidence of ulceration and intra-thoracic adhesion.

The operation consists of a left (limited) postero-lateral thoracotomy through the 7th intercostal space. At entry to the chest, the sac with its contents is seen to protrude through a large hiatal defect. The sac is opened and excised, adhesions are divided and the correct anatomical position of the stomach (volvolus) is ensured. This may involve excision of some omentum attaching the greater curvature to the sac maintaining the volvolus. The hernia is then reduced and the opening (hiatus) is repaired by approximating the crural muscle thus closing the hiatal gap. The muscular component may be thin and, at times, require reinforcement (by pericardium/thin Teflon felt) so that the approximating stitches hold without tearing the muscle. The phreno-oesophageal ligament (membrane) is then anchored by stitches to the border of the neo-hiatus and the chest is closed with a basal underwater sealed drain left in the pleural space.

References and further reading

Allen MS. Open repair of hiatus hernia: Thoracic approach. Chest Surg Clin N Am 1998; 8(2): 431–440.

Allison PR. Peptic ulcer of the oesophagus. J Thorac Surg 1946; 15: 308–317.

Allison PR. Reflux oesophagitis sliding hiatal hernia and the anatomy of repair. Surg Gynecol Obstet 1951; 92: 419–431.

Allison PR. Peptic oesophagitis and oesophageal stricture. Lancet 1970; 25: 199–202.

Allison PR. Hiatus hernia: a 20 year retrospective survey. Ann Surg 1973; 178: 273–276.

Barrett NR. Chronic peptic ulcer of the oesophagus and oesophagitis. Br J Surg 1950; 38: 175–182.

Baue AE, Belsey RH. The treatment of sliding hiatus hernia and reflux oesophagitis by the Mark IV technique. Surgery 1967;

62: 396–406.

Belsey RHR. Hiatus hernia. Modern trends in gastroenterology. London: Butterworth, 1952.

Belsey RHR. Mark IV repair of hiatal hernia by the trans-thoracic approach. World J Surg 1977; 1: 475–481.

Carlson MA, Condon RE, Ludwig KA, Schulte WJ. Management of intrathoracic stomach with polypropylene mesh prosthesis reinforced transabdominal hiatus hernia repair. J Am Coll Surg 1998; 187(3): 227–230.

Castell DO, Levine SM. Lower oesophageal sphincter response to gastric alkalinisation: a new mechanism for treatment of heartburn with antacids. Ann Intern Med 1971; 223–227.

Collis JL, Kelly JD, Wile AM. Anatomy of the crura of the diaphragm and the surgery of hiatus hernia. Thorax 1954; 9: 175–189.

DeMeester TR, Bonavina L, Albertucci N. Nissen fundoplication for gastro-oesophageal reflux disease. Evaluation of primary report in 100 consecutive patients. Ann Surg 1986; 204: 9–20.

Edye MB, Canin-Endres J, Gattorno F, Salky BA. Durability of laparoscopic repair or paraoeosphageal hernia. Ann Surg 1998; 228(4): 528–535.

Ellis FH Jr, Gregg JA. Fundoplication for gastro-oesophageal reflux: A comparison of pre-operative and early post-operative manometric findings. Chest 1972; 62: 142–145.

Ellis FH Jr, Crozier RE. Reflux control by Fundoplication: a clinical and manometric assessment of Nissen operation. Ann Thorac Surg 1984; 38: 387–392.

Ellis FH Jr, Crozier RE. Reflux control by fundoplication. Ann Thorac Surg 1992; 54: 1231–1235.

Geha AS, Massad MG, Snow NJ, Baue AE. A 32 year experience in 100 patients with giant paraoeosphaeal hernia: The case for abdominal approach and selective antireflux repair. Surgery 2000; 128: 623–630.

Giles GR, Mason MC, Humphries C. Action of gastrin on lower oesophageal sphincter in man. Gut 1969; 10: 730–734.

Hayward J. The lower end of the oesophagus. Thorax 1961; 16: 36–41.

Hayward J. The phreno-oesophageal ligament in hiatal hernia. Thorax 1961; 16: 41–45.

Hayward J. The treatment of fibrous stricture of the oesophagus associated with hiatal hernia. Thorax 1961; 16: 45–55.

Kitchin LI, Castell DO. Rationale and efficacy of conservative therapy for gastro-oesophageal reflux disease. Arch Intern Med 1991; 151: 448–454.

Kahrilas PJ. Cigarette smoking and gastro-oesophageal reflux disease. Gasteroenterol Clin North Am 1990; 19: 217.

Kahrilas PJ. The role of hiatus hernia in GERD. Yale J Biol Med 1999; 72: 101–111.

Matthews HR (on behalf of ISDE sub-committee). A proposed classification for hiatal hernia and gastroesophageal reflux. Dis Esophagus 1996; 9: 1–3.

McGuigan JE. Consequences of excess herniae secretions in digestive disease. Mayo Clin Proc 1973; 48: 634–636.

Moghissi K. Modification of Nissen total fundoplication. In: Moghissi K, Essentials of Thoracic and Cardiac Surgery. London: Heinemann, 1986; pp. 232–233.

Nissen R. Eine einfache Operation zur Beeinflussung der Refluxösophagitis. Schweiz Med Wochenschr 1956; 86: 590–592.

Oddsdottir M. Paraesophageal hernia. Surg Clin North Am 2000; 80(4): 1243–1252.

Skinner DB, Belsey RHR. Surgical management of oesophageal reflux with hiatus hernia. J Thorac Cardiovasc Surg 1968; 53: 33–54.

Toupet A. Technique d'oesophago-gastroplastie avec phréno-gastropexie appliquée dans la cure radicale des hernies hiatales et comme complément de l'opération de Heller dans les cardiospasmes. Mem Acad Chir (Paris) 1963; 89: 384–389.

Van den Berg M, Scheltinga MR, Eijsbouts QA, Cuesta MA. Elective laparoscopic repair of type II paraoesophageal hernias. Ann Surg 1998; 228(4): 623–624.

Vollan G, Stangeland L, Soreide JA, et al. Long term results after Nissen fundoplication and Belsey Mark IV operation in patients with reflux oesophagitis and stricture. Eur J Surg 1992; 158: 357–360.

Zaino C, Jacobsen JG, Lepow H, et al. The pharyngo-oesophageal sphincter. Springfield, Illinois: Charles C Thomas, 1970.

Zaniotto G, Anselmino M, Costantini M, Boccu C, Ancona E. Laparoscopic treatment of gastro-esophageal reflux disease: Indications results. Int Surg 1995; 80(4): 380–385.

K. Moghissi, J.A.C. Thorpe and F. Ciulli (Eds.)
Moghissi's Essentials of Thoracic and Cardiac Surgery
© 2003 Elsevier Science B.V. All rights reserved

CHAPTER III.7

Lower oesophagus lined by columnar epithelium (Barrett's oesophagus)

K. Moghissi

1. Historical background

In 1950, in the course of discussion on oesophagitis and oesophageal ulcers, Barrett drew attention to congenital short oesophagus. He believed this condition to be due to a developmental anomaly in which the distal oesophagus is malformed by a tubular intrathoracic stomach. This externally resembles the oesophagus but is internally like the stomach, covered by gastric type mucosa with columnar epithelium. Allison and Johnstone (1953) showed convincingly that Barrett's tubular intra-thoracic stomach was in fact the oesophagus itself lined by gastric mucous membrane. By 1957 Barrett altered his original views and adopted Allison and Johnstone's suggestion. This culminated in the publishing of his observations on "the lower oesophagus lined by columnar epithelium" and definition of the characteristics of the condition which has become known as Barrett's Oesophagus. It is important to acknowledge firstly Allison's contribution to this condition, and secondly, to recognise that almost simultaneously the condition was described by Lortat–Jacob (1957).

It is useful to recall some of these characteristics. Barrett (1957) said, "When the lower oesophagus is found to be lined by columnar cells the abnormally placed mucous membrane extends upwards from the oesophago-gastric junction in a continuous, unbroken sheet." This deformity is not associated with or complicated by other anatomic changes, that is:

1. The external appearances and the muscular anatomy of the stomach and the oesophagus are normal.
2. There is no anatomical change in the mediastinum.

3. The blood supply from the aortic segmental arteries and the left gastric artery is normal.
4. The crus of the diaphragm and the peritoneal reflections in the neighbourhood of the hiatus are normal.

Figure 1a illustrates this point. It is important to compare the situation of a tubular stomach (acquired short oesophagus) which can appear as lower oesophagus lined by columnar epithelium. The difference relates to the insertion of phreno-oesophageal ligament (POL) which, in this case, is not in the region of the hiatus (Fig. 1b).

Development of the fibre optic instrument and the expansion of endoscopy by gastroenterologists have influenced the definition of Barrett's oesophagus and have added a new dimension to the frequency of its diagnosis.

2. Definition

Ever since Barrett's original description, its definition has been the subject of debate with regard to the length of metaplastic mucosa and histological subtype, i.e. intestinal metaplasia or glandular epithelium.

At present the generally agreed definition of Barrett's oesophagus is that of a condition in which the distal 3 cm or more of the oesophagus is covered by columnar epithelium. There would be no problem in adopting this simple definition, which appears at first sight satisfactory, provided that the lower oesophagus and gastro-oesophageal junction could be easily identified at endoscopy. This is not always the case. Furthermore, in his original description Barrett referred to the oesophagus as a whole, in all

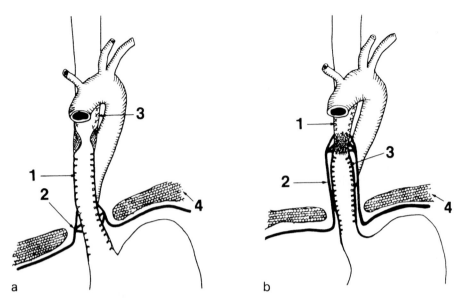

Fig. 1. (a) Diagram illustrating Barrett's and Allison's concept of the lower oesophagus lined by columnar epithelium (Barett's oeso-phagus). (b) Diagram of acquired short oesophagus: 1. Columnar mucosa; 2. Phreno-oesophageal ligament; 3. Squamous epithelium; 4. Diaphragmatic muscle of the hiatus.

its structural components, and not exclusively to the mucosa upon which the endoscopic redefinition is based. Whilst there is confusion and controversy regarding Barrett's oesophagus and its definition there should be no doubt about the facts that:

- Barrett's oesophagus as per the criteria originally laid down by Barrett does exist.
- The endoscopic diagnosis of the oesophago-gastric junction at endoscopy is neither easy nor accurate and the recovery of columnar epithelium in biopsy material from an area thought by the endoscopist to be oesophagus does not necessarily equate with the diagnosis of Barrett's columnar epithelial lined oesophagus.
- Even if the oesophago-gastric junction can be surmised with the use of such techniques as manometric studies, the demonstration of columnar epithelium in the lower oesophagus does not entitle us to an automatic diagnosis of Barrett's oesophagus, since information about the rest of the oesophagus (musculature, vascular supply and hiatus) cannot be obtained at endoscopy.

These points are made in the hope that it will be appreciated that there is a difference between true Barrett's oesophagus and the condition termed as such by endoscopists, which may not fulfill the criteria laid down by Barrett.

The crux of the matter is that true Barrett's oesophagus remains an anatomical entity; the present concept is an endoscopic one, advanced mainly by

endoscopists, since most of the present-day diagnosis of Barrett's oesophagus is made at oesophagoscopy by the endoscopist.

3. Aetiology

The aetiology of Barrett's columnar epithelial lined oesophagus has been the subject of controversy since Barrett's original reports. It was initially thought that the condition was congenital but general opinion, backed by strong evidence, suggests that the condition is not congenital but is caused by gastro-oesophageal reflux. In fact there is universal belief that Columnar Epithelial Lined Oesophagus (C.E.L.O.) is a manifestation of reflux disease where the normal squamous epithelium becomes replaced, after erosion, by columnar epithelium. In some cases, however, this general rule does not hold true.

Examples of this are columnar epithelium found high in the oesophagus of children and occasional cases in adults where the whole of the oesophagus is covered by columnar epithelium without any evidence of oesophagitis. In these we believe that congenital aetiology cannot be ruled out. It may be that there are in fact two types of C.E.L.O. The first is in the majority of cases where C.E.L.O. is acquired and is a consequence of gastro-oesophageal reflux. In these the oesophageal wall other than the mucosa may or may not be affected; at its worst there is stricture and muscular shortening. The second type is the true Barrett's oesophagus in which columnar epithelium lines an otherwise normal oesophagus. Some of these cases are possibly congenital in origin.

4. Clinical manifestations in uncomplicated cases

The condition may be asymptomatic and indeed true incidence of the condition in the general population is unknown. One post-mortem study suggests 2% of the adult population has Barrett's mucosa (Cameron et al., 1990). When symptomatic the presentation is akin to that of gastro-oesophageal reflux disease (see chapter III.6). There is, however, predominance of male over female in Barrett's oesophagus which also affects younger patients. In the presence of complications (see below) dysphagia, loss of weight, pain and bleeding may become the presenting symptoms.

4.1. Treatment of uncomplicated cases

Treatment of uncomplicated cases has been subject to considerable debate, principally because of the possibility of malignant degenerative changes in some patients with metaplastic columnar mucosa. The rational therapy appears to be that which is directed toward supression/elimination of gastro-oesophageal reflux and high gastric acid output. An anti-reflux operation will deal with the symptoms but will achieve mucosal conversion to the original squamous epithelium in less than 50% of cases. Non-operative treatment including proton pump inhibitor medications, photodynamic or NdYAG laser therapy cannot achieve long-lasting success. The reason is that ablation of columnar epithelium alone, in the absence of an anti-reflux mechanism, will not eliminate the factors responsible for the reflux which caused development of the lesion. Therefore, these patients need some sort of endoscopic supervision programme.

5. Complications of columnar epithelial lined (Barrett's) oesophagus

The presence of columnar epithelium in the lower oesophagus may be asymptomatic but can be associated with three types of complication which were recorded by Barrett and subsequently confirmed by others. These are:
- Stricture formation
- Penetrating ulcer
- Neoplastic changes

5.1. Oesophageal stricture

Strictures of the oesophagus associated with C.E.L.O. have the following characteristics:
- They are a consequence of reflux and are usually formed at the junction between the squamous and the newly formed metaplastic columnar mucosa of the oesophagus. This was referred to by Barrett (1957) and Allison (1970) and shown to be the case by meticulous intra operative study (Moghissi, 1979; Moghissi and Goebells, 1990).
- They are usually high in the oesophagus, sometimes as high as the aortic arch and higher than the original oesophago-gastric epithelial junction (Figs. 2a and 2b). It must be emphasised that it has been demonstrated by anatomo-pathological studies that not all high oesophageal strictures are formed in C.E.L.O. or Barrett's oesophagus. The key to the differential diagnosis between a simple reflux stricture associated with acquired short oesophagus and a stricture in Barrett's oesophagus is that in the latter both the lower oesophageal sphincter and phreno-oesophageal ligaments are at, or near, the oesophageal hiatus of the diaphragm whereas in the former both sphincter and phreno-oesophageal ligaments are higher than the hiatus and near the level of the stricture itself (Moghissi and Goebells, 1990; Moghissi, 1992).

5.2. Penetrating ulcer

It was observation of an oesophageal ulcer, which prompted Barrett and afterwards Allison and Johnstone to formulate the concept of C.E.L.O. Allison referred to these ulcers as Barrett's ulcer. Characteristically these are deep, penetrating ulcers within the columnar epithelium of the oesophagus, which tend to perforate and cause profuse haemorrhage. Barrett's ulcer is usually resistant to medical management or conservative operation. Surgical resection and reconstruction is usually required.

5.3. Neoplasia

In his original description Barrett (1957) referred to neoplasia developing with C.E.L.O. (Fig. 3). He stated that, if the columnar cell growth is discovered at the level of the arch of the aorta, the usual explanation is that the patient has developed a columnar cell cancer de novo in columnar oesophageal mucosa.

The subject of adeno-carcinoma arising from C.E.L.O. has attracted much attention in recent years.

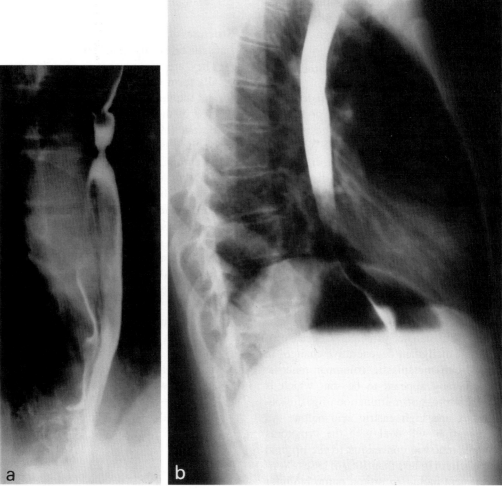

Fig. 2. (a) Barium swallow of an 18 year old patient with typical Barrett's stricture. (b) The same patient following operation of dilatation and total fundoplication one year later.

Its prevalence has been recorded by some to be about 10% (Naef and Ozzello, 1975) but others consider this risk to be much lower (Spechler et al., 1984). There appears to be a gradual increase both in the number of cases of Barrett's oesophagus and the rate of adeno-carcinoma arising from it. There also seems to be a tendency to attribute every adeno-carcinoma within the oesophagus to be the result of Barrett's oesophagus. However, neither the true incidence of adeno-carcinoma in C.E.L.O. nor the nature of the relationship between the two conditions can be clearly assessed since the incidence of C.E.L.O. in the general population is unknown and much of the published material has been based on inadequate anatomo-pathological study. It is generally agreed that there is higher risk of cancer development in patients with C.E.L.O. but such risk has to be evaluated not only in the terms of num-

ber and percentage but in relation to the length of time it has taken for the cancer to develop since the initial diagnosis of C.E.L.O. Also the presence of adeno-carcinoma in the mid thoracic oesophagus is not necessarily evidence of its having developed from C.E.L.O although there is a high probability of that being the case. In a comprehensive anatomopathological study of 58 patients with adeno-carcinoma of the mid-thoracic oesophagus undergoing resection, 11 (19%) were found to have the tumour in the midst of normal columnar (Barrett's oesophagus) (Moghissi and Papiri, 1992). In the remaining, the cancer was an extension from gastric adeno-carcinoma, including some of which were within a hiatal hernia. In another study (Moghissi et al., 1993) of over 400 patients with complications of gastro-oesophageal reflux with/without Barrett's oesophagus followed for a period of 2–20 years (mean 11.5 years) the inci-

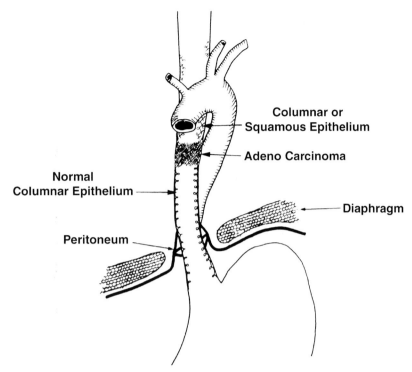

Fig. 3. Diagram illustrating Barrett's adeno-carcinoma.

dence of cancer arising from Barrett's oesophagus was 15–20 times higher than those without Barrett's mucosa.

There is now a general acceptance that the development of cancer from metaplastic columnar epithelium is a staged process beginning with low-grade dysplasia going through moderate-to-severe dysplasia and then to carcinoma in situ and invasive cancer. Nevertheless, it is important to note that:

- Some 40–50% of cases of severe dysplasia are, in fact, true adeno-carcinoma (DeMeester et al., 1991; Heitmiller et al., 1996). This corresponds with my personal experience.
- Grading of dysplasia in its mild-to-moderate state suffers from inter-observer variation.
- Not all dysplastic changes will become carcinoma and there is no way of identifying which patients with dysplasia will/will not develop carcinoma.

At the present time it is prudent to state that there is possibly a higher risk of cancer development in patients with C.E.L.O. than in the general population and that epithelial dysplasia in a biopsy specimen requires either surgical consideration or careful supervision of the patient according to the severity of the dysplasia. However, one recent study dismisses the value of surveillance except in those with higher risks (intestinal metaplasia and those with stricture

and ulcer) (McDonald et al., 2000). Our practice is to surgically explore patients with high grade dysplasia and atypical cells and to carry out frozen section at the time of operation. Should this prove to be negative we carry out an anti-reflux procedure. If the frozen section demonstrates high grade dysplasia and/or suspicion of adenocarcinoma we proceed to resection. This practice is based on personal experience that in some resected specimens, severe dysplasia of the mucosa, with atypical cells at pre-operative biopsy, was associated with invasive adenocarcinoma at operation. Also, we have observed that dysplasia on biopsy sample may coexist with adenocarcinoma that is not recognisable by endoscopic inspection of the mucosa. Recently we have employed photodynamic therapy for high grade dysplasia/carcinoma in situ when patients were considered as unsuitable or high risk for operative resection.

6. Summary of management of Barrett's oesophagus

In the absence of stricture, ulcer and neoplastic changes the treatment is similar to that of gastro-oesophageal reflex disease. In intractable cases these reflux symptoms are relieved by effective anti-reflux operation.

By definition, the stricture in true Barrett's oeso-phagus is high in position and generally attended by no abnormality of the oesophageal wall (other than the mucosa) or the hiatus. Experience indicates that even in chronic cases all such patients can be offered conservative operation of dilatation of stricture cou-pled with an anti-reflux procedure and that the gas-tro-oesophageal junction can always be brought down under the diaphragm, i.e. no acquired shortening.

Barrett's chronic and penetrating ulcer is often attended by oesophageal wall destruction for which the treatment of radical surgical resection and recon-struction becomes mandatory.

Patients with neoplastic degeneration require the usual consideration of oesophageal cancer treatment, with surgical resection when possible, as the primary choice. It is important that the tumour, dysplasia and all of the metaplastic mucosal zone is resected.

There remains a group of patients with C.E.L.O. and epithelial dysplasia at biopsy specimen. We be-lieve high-grade dysplasia is an instance of carci-noma in situ and should be treated as such with resection. Low-grade dysplasia requires endoscopic supervision even after anti-reflux operation. The role of photodynamic therapy (PDT) is yet to be defined. At the present time, PDT should be reserved for pa-tients unsuitable for surgical operation or those with low-grade dysplasia in whom PDT may be coupled with medication and/or anti reflux surgery. Supervi-sion and re-treatment in such cases is necessary.

Note on molecular genetic and biomarkers in Barrett's oesophagus.

Efforts have been made, through many studies, to identify genetic alterations in Barrett's oesophagus and the progression to adenocarcinoma. The princi-pal genetic changes appear to be loss of $p16$ gene expression, loss of $p53$ expression (by mutilation and deletion), increase in cyclin D1 expression, the induction of aneuploidy, and the losses of Rb, DCC and APC chromosomal loci (Jenkins et al., 2002). At present there is no biomarker to allow the predic-tion of which patients with Barrett's metaplasia will progress to cancer; the monitoring of molecular and genetic events will assist clinicians in planning more effective follow-up of these patients.

References and further reading

Alder RH. The lower oesophagus lined by columnar epithelium. J Thorac Cardiovasc Surg 1963; 45: 13–34.

Allison PR. Peptic oesophagitis and oesophageal strictures. Lancet 1970; 11: 199–201.

Allison PR, Johnstone AS. The oesophagus lined with gastric mucous membrane. Thorax 1953; 8: 87–101.

Barr H, Shepherd NA, Dix A, Roberts DJH et al. Eradication of high grade dysplasia in Columnar lined (Barrett's) oesopha-gus by photodynamic therapy with endogenously generated protoporphyma ix. Lancet 1996; 348: 584–585.

Barrett JR. Chronic peptic ulcer of the oesophagus and oe-sophagitis. Br J Surg 1950; 38: 175–182.

Barrett JR. The lower oesophagus lined by columnar epithelium. Surgery 1957; 41: 881–894.

Bremner CG, Hamilton DG. Barrett's oesophagus controversial aspects. In: DeMeester TR, Skinner DB (Eds.). Oesophageal disorders, pathophysiology and therapy. New York: Raven Press, 1985; pp. 233–239.

Bremner CG, Lynch VP, Ellis FH Jr. Barrett's oesophagus, con-genital or acquired? An experimental study of oesophageal mucosal regeneration in dog. Surgery 1970; 28: 209–216.

Cameron AJ, Ott BJ, Payne WS. Barrett's oesophagus: incidence of adeno carcinoma and long term follow up. N Eng J Med 1985; 313: 857–859.

Cameron AJ, Zinniteister AR, Ballard DJ, Carey JA. Prevalence of columnar lined Barretts oesophagus: Comparison of pop-ulation based clinical and autopsy findings. Gastroenterology 1990; 99: 918–922.

Dahms BB, Rothstein FC. Barrett's oesophagus a consequence of chronic gastro-oesophageal reflux. Gastroenterology. 1984; 86: 318–323.

DeMeester TR, Attwood SEA, Smyrk T, et al. Surgical therapy in Barrett's oesophagus. Am J Surg 1991; 161: 97–100.

DeMeester TR. Surgical therapy for Barrett's oesophagus: pre-vention, protection and excision. Dis Esophagus 2002; 15: 109–116.

Ferguson MK, Waunheim KS. Resection for Barrett's mucosa with high grade dysplasia implication for prophylastic photo dynamic therapy. J Thorac Cardiovasc Surg 1997; 114: 824–830.

Hayward J. The lower end of the oesophagus. Thorax 1961; 16: 36–41.

Hayward J. The Phreno oesophagael ligament in hiatal hernia repair. Thorax 1961; 16: 41–45.

Heitmiller RF, Redmond M, Hamilton SR. Barrett's oesophagus with high grade dysplasia. An indication for prophylactic esophagectomy. Ann Surg 1996; 224: 66–71.

Hennessy PTJ. Barrett's oesophagus. Br J Surg 1985; 72: 336–340.

Jenkins GJ, Doak SH, Parry JM, et al. Genetic pathways involved in the progression of Barrett's metaplasia to adenocarcinoma. Br J Surg 2002; 89: 824–837.

Laukka MA, Wang KK. Initial results using low dose photo dynamic therapy in the treatment of Barrett's oesophagus. Gastro-intestinal Endoscopy 1995; 42: 59–63.

Lee RG. Dysplasia in Barrett's oesophagus: a clinico-pathologi-cal study of 6 patients. Am J Surg Path 1985; 9: 845.

Lortat-Jacob JL. Endo brachyesophage. Ann Chir 1957; 11: 1247–1254.

McDonald CE, Wicks AC, Playford RJ. Final results from 10 years cohorts of patients undergoing surveillance for Barrett's oesophagus: Observational study. BMJ 2000; 321: 1252–1255.

Moghissi K. Conservative surgery in reflux stricture of the oeso-phagus with hiatal hernia. Br J Surg 1979; 66: 221–225.

Moghissi K. Barrett's oesophagus: does it exist, is it congenital? In: Seiwert JR, Holscher AM, Diseases of the oesophagus. New York: Springer Verlag, 1988; pp. 537–539.

Moghissi K. The enigma of Barrett's oesophagus: putting the record straight. Eur J Cardiothorac Surg. 1991; 5: 13–16.

Moghissi K, Goebells P. Relevance of anatomo-pathology of high oesophageal strictures to the design of surgical treatment. Eur J Cardiothorac Surg 1990; 4: 91–96.

Moghissi K. Definition of adeno carcinoma arising in columnar epithelial lined oesophagus (Barrett's adeno carcinoma). Dis Esophagus 1992; 5: 37–43.

Moghissi K, Papiri N. A clinical pathological study of the origin of adeno carcinoma of the mid thoracic oesophagus and the results of surgical resection. Chirurgie 1992; 79: 935–937.

Moghissi K, Sharpe DAC, Pender D. Adeno carcinoma and Barrett's oesophagus: a clinico-pathological study. Eur J Cardiothorac Surg 1993; 7: 126–132.

Monier P, Fontolliet C, Savary M, Ollyo JB. Barrett's oesophagus or columnar epithelium of the lower oesophagus. Ballieres Clinical Gastroenterology 1987; 1: 4.

Naef AP, Ozzello L. Columnar lined lower oesophagus: an acquired lesion with malignant predisposition. J Thorac Cardiovasc Surg 1975; 70: 826–835.

Overholt BF, Panjehpour M. Barrett's Oesophagus, Photo dynamic therapy for ablation of dysplasia reduction of specialised mucosa and treatment of superficial oesophageal cancer. Gastro intestinal Endoscopy 1995; 42: 64–70.

Overholt BF, Panjehpour M, Photodynamic therapy for Barrett's esophagus: clinical update. Am J Gastroenterol 1996; 91: 1719–1723.

Reid BJ, Lewin K, Van De Venter C et al. Barrett's oesophagus: high-grade dysplasia and intramucosal carcinoma detected by endoscopic biopsy surveillance. Gastroenterology 1986; 90: 601.

Ribet M, Mensier E, Pruvot FR. Barrett's oesophagus and adeno carcinoma. Eur J Cardiothorac Surg 1987; 1: 29–32.

Sjogren RW Jr, Johnson LF. Barrett's oesophagus: a review. Am J Med 1983; 74: 313–321.

Skinner DB, Walther BNC, Riddell RW, Schmidt H, Sascone E, DeMeester RT. Barrett's oesophagus comparison of benign and malignant cases. Ann Surg 1983; 198: 544–565.

Spechler SJ, Robbins AH, Rubins HB, Vincent ME, Heeren P, Doos W G, Colton T, Schimmell CM. Adeno carcinoma and Barrett's oesophagus: an overrated risk? Gastroenterology 1984; 87: 927–933.

Spechler SJ, Goyal RK. Barrett's oesophagus. N Eng J Med 1986; 6: 362–371.

Spechler SJ, Goyal RK. The columnar lined intestinal metaplasia and Barrett. Gastroenterology 1996; 110: 614–621.

Wijnhoven BP, Tilanus HW, Dinjens WN. Molecular biology of Barrett's adenocarcinoma. Ann Surg 2001; 233: 322–337.

Wolf BS, Marshak RH, Som ML. Peptic oesophagitis and peptic ulceration of the oesophagus. Am J Roentgenol 1958; 79: 741–759.

Wolfsen HC, Woodward TA, Raimondo M. Photodynamic therapy for dysplastic Barrett's esophagus and early esophageal adenocarcinoma. Mayo Clin Proc 2002; 77: 1176–1181.

K. Moghissi, J.A.C. Thorpe and F. Ciulli (Eds.)
Moghissi's Essentials of Thoracic and Cardiac Surgery
© 2003 Elsevier Science B.V. All rights reserved

CHAPTER III.8

Surgery of reflux stricture

K. Moghissi

1. Introduction

The term reflux stricture is used to describe oesophageal stenosis which follows reflux oesophagitis.

The terminology used here and which was adopted by the author over twenty years ago (Moghissi, 1979) appears to have been originated by Barrett (1950) who introduced 'reflux oesophagitis' as a variety of oesophagitis caused by reflux. Allison (1951, 1970) described reflux oesophagitis with stricture. Nevertheless, the term peptic stricture is still used by some in place of reflux stricture.

The pathogenesis of reflux has been discussed previously (chapter III.6).

2. Clinical presentation

Dysphagia is the outstanding symptom, typically in a patient who has suffered from symptoms of reflux. It is an interesting observation that symptoms of heartburn and pain in a patient with gastro-oesophageal reflux associated with hiatal hernia tend to disappear when the stricture is formed. However, dysphagia coinciding with or appearing in patients who still suffer from reflux symptoms is most probably caused by neoplasm.

Loss of weight is not a common feature in this type of stricture.

Anaemia and pain may be present, particularly if there is a chronic ulcer at or about the stricture. Other symptoms may also be present, e.g. pneumonitis related to the severity of dysphagia.

3. Investigation of reflux stricture

- Clinical history and examination help to exclude other pathologies.
- Chest radiograph and barium swallow are of obvious importance to show the pathology of the mediastinum and the characteristics of the stricture.
- Physiological studies: By the time a stricture has formed, it may be argued that manometric and pH studies will be irrelevant but at times reflux stricture can be associated with other motor dysfunction of the oesophagus. In the majority of cases, however, the physiological studies are not mandatory provided other investigations indicate the type of stricture.

3.1. Endoscopy

Oesophagoscopy should be carried out in all cases of stricture to exclude neoplasm and to gain endoscopic information of the type of lesion. It is a mistake to rely entirely on a report of barium contrast studies for 'diagnosis' of dysphagia, considering that coincidental existence of hiatal hernia with carcinoma is frequently observed and carcinoma developing in a chronic stricture is also a possibility (Moghissi, 1977).

However, in cases of dysphagia, oesophagoscopy should be carried out following barium contrast study and not preceding it. Also, in our view, oesophagoscopy in these cases should be carried out by the treating surgeon with the view to obtaining the following information which is of practical importance:
(a) Level of stricture from the upper alveolus,
(b) Severity of the stricture (tight, firm, soft),
(c) Presence of ulcer, granulation tissue, and inflammation at or about the stricture,
(d) Level of stricture with respect to the length of the patient's oesophagus (section 3.5.2 in chapter III.2).

In all oesophagoscopic examinations for stricture, a biopsy above, at, and if possible, below the lesion are taken, as a reflux stricture is usually at the squamocolumnar epithelial junction, a point of importance in the aetiological diagnosis of strictures. Also, coexistence of carcinoma is a possibility.

4. Management of patients with reflux stricture

Reflux oesophagitis being the precursor of stricture formation, prophylactic surgery of anti-reflux operation is indicated in patients with severe oesophagitis who have not responded to conservative medical treatment. When stricture is already present, a tailored treatment option should be adopted.

The last 30 years have seen fundamental change in our attitude towards treatment of reflux stricture of the oesophagus. Prior to the 1960s the tendency was to treat patients with stricture either with repeated dilatation or with resection and reconstruction. Towards the 1970s a shift occurred towards conservative operations.

The management of patients with reflux stricture may be considered under the following principle headings:

(4.1) Dilatation of the stricture — bouginage
(4.2) Permanent intubation
(4.3) Conservative surgical operation
  • Antireflux operation alone.
  • Dilatation of stricture coupled with anti-reflux procedure.
  • Roux-en-y duodenal diversion.
(4.4) Resection of the stenotic lesion followed by reconstruction of the alimentary tract.

4.1. Dilatation of the stricture

Some gastroenterologists and a few practising surgeons are of the opinion that the majority of oesophageal strictures yield to dilatation. They will therefore recommend this modality of treatment. In the author's experience, it is neither desirable nor indicated to propose dilatation as a definitive and sole modality of treatment, except for a small number of patients with a defined indication. The reasons are that:

• Dilatation alone is not a permanent solution to the stricture problem for as long as gastro-oesophageal reflux remains unchecked since it perpetuates reflux and recurrence of the stricture.
• In patients undergoing frequent and repeated dilatation, the stricture tends to recur, often at a higher level than the original one.
• Repeated dilatation can be attended by perforation

of the oesophagus. The incidence of this varies according to the skill of the operator and the method used. Nevertheless, in larger series of stricture treated by dilatation the perforation rate is significant.
• Neoplastic degeneration can occur in some chronic cases of reflux stricture (Moghissi, 1977).

It is important to realise that repeated dilatation constitutes the only avenue of treatment for some patients. In my own series of 465 patients with reflux stricture, 58 (12.5%) received repeated dilatation as the sole form of treatment because of poor general condition, cardiac or respiratory failure and disabling disease.

The success of oesophageal dilatation is variably reported as being between 70 to 88% though often the criteria of success has been based on the avoidance of surgical operation and not on quality of swallowing. These results must therefore be interpreted with some scepticism.

For dilatation of a stricture to be effective, it needs to be coupled with surgical or pharmacological control of reflux. The choice of medication is dependent on several factors such as the nature of reflux, the number and duration of reflux episodes per day and motility of the oesophagus. The question arises as to the optimal stage at which a patient who is undergoing treatment by dilatation should be considered for surgery. Opinion varies except in the case of the elderly, disabled and patients unsuitable for operation. In other patients, generally after 2 or 3 dilatations and appropriate medication, if the stricture persists, the patient should be offered surgical treatment. Hill et al. (1970) have shown that significantly better results can be obtained after anti-reflux operation in patients operated early in the course of their disease, having undergone fewer dilatations, than in those having had multiple dilatations pre-operatively. This observation accords with my own experience.

4.1.1. Technique of dilatation
The choice of bougies depends on the individual's experience. Discussion of the superiority of one particular method of dilating a stricture over another cannot hope to be rational since an operator (surgeon or physician) generally favours the method with which he/she is most familiar.

When a rigid open-ended oesophagoscope is employed under general anaesthesia, mercury loaded bougies such as Hurst or Maloney are preferable to the rigid gum-elastic variety, since the former adapts

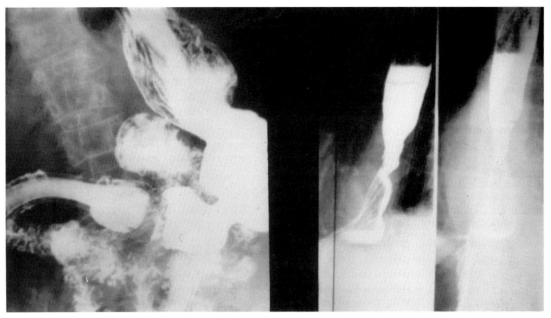

Fig. 1. Left: migration of indwelling oesophageal tube into the duodenum causing pyloric obstruction 6 months after its placement. Right: recurrence of oesophageal stricture.

to the tortuosity of the oesophagus and the distorted passage created by the stenotic lesion. Dilatation in conjunction with a flexible instrument necessitates the use of a guide wire, to which is threaded the Eder-Puestow dilating system or Celestin bougies. Our preference is to use a rigid instrument and Maloney bougies of increasing diameter to 56 F.G. although in some cases we employ the Eder-Puestow System of dilators.

4.2. Permanent intubation/stent

Using an indwelling oesophageal tube or stent in benign strictures should be avoided, except in exceptional circumstances, since the long term morbidity and complications of tubes/stents outweigh their usefulness for the following reasons:
- Tubes or stents tend to work loose from benign strictures after a time and become dislodged. The stricture will then return, as illustrated in one of a number of cases (Fig. 1) referred to the author from other departments.
- Tubes or stents have no anti-reflux mechanism and, in the recumbent position, the intubated patient will have free reflux of gastric content into the oesophagus.
- Some tubes or stents have a tendency to perforate the oesophagus.
- All prosthetic tubes or stents are prone to block-

age requiring frequent attention. This is particularly the case in some mentally impaired individuals.

4.3. Conservative surgery

This refers to surgical methods which aim at relief of the obstruction and prevention of recurrence of stenosis without the major surgery of resection.

4.3.1. Anti-reflux operations alone
An anti-reflux operation alone can occasionally bring about resolution of the stricture when the stenosis is not tight or firm and involves a short segment. It is, however, doubtful if a tight fibrotic stricture which hardly allows the passage of a bougie can be resolved by anti-reflux operation alone.

4.3.2. Dilatation of stricture combined with antireflux
These operations basically have two components:
(a) Relief of the obstruction which is achieved by dilatation of the stricture or its incision,
(b) An effective anti-reflux procedure.

The author believes that the prerequisite of this type of simple conservative surgery is the absence of acquired shortening of the oesophagus.

Based on this principle, many conservative surgi-

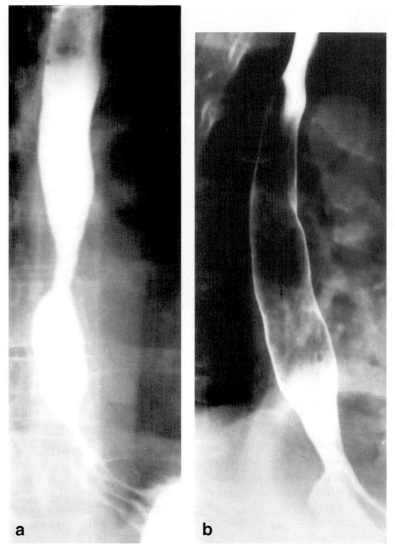

Fig. 2. Mild stricture associated with a reducible hernia. (a) Before and (b) after conservative operation of dilatation and total fundoplication.

cal methods have been developed (Hayward, 1961; Herrington et al., 1975 and Moghissi, 1979).

In 1961, Hayward showed that stricture associated with hiatal hernia can be effectively treated by peri-operative dilatation of the stricture combined with an Allison type of hiatal hernia repair (Fig. 3 in chapter III.6). Subsequently, a number of authors have used different techniques of dilatation coupled with a variety of anti-reflux procedures.

Dilatation of the stricture is carried out either pre-operatively or intra-operatively. The latter is a safer method in tight and fibrotic strictures since it has the added advantage that the suitability of the case for conservative method can be tested at operation. Once dilatation is satisfactorily achieved,

the anti-reflux procedure is carried out. The author's preference is to carry out a modification of Nissen's classical total fundoplication (see section 2.1.4 in chapter III.6).

In a mild to moderate stricture, pre-operative endoscopic dilatation followed by anti-reflux procedure is usually suffice (Figs. 2a and 2b).

In tight strictures, the author favours transgastric retrograde dilatation. A carefully placed gastrotomy is performed through which digital exploration of the stenotic lesion is first carried out. Biopsy is then taken for frozen section histological examination to exclude malignancy before transgastric retrograde bouginage is performed using Hegar's (metallic) bougies of increasing diameter, passed by one hand

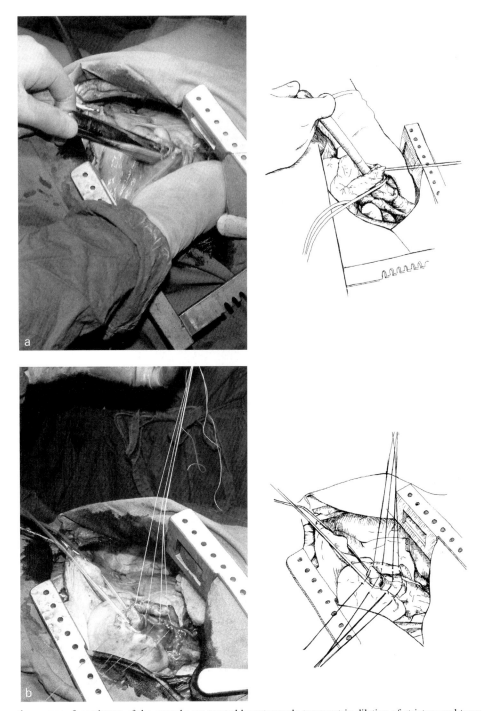

Fig. 3. Conservative surgery for stricture of the oesophagus treated by retrograde transgastric dilation of stricture and trans-thoracic total fundoplication. (a) Transgastric retrograde dilation using Hegar dilators (note thoraco-phreno laparotomy access). (b) Fundoplication stitches being inserted (photo and diagram). (Fig. 3 is continued overleaf.)

through the gastrotomy, whilst the lower oesophagus which has been mobilised, is held firmly in the other hand. In this way a controlled and guided dilatation can safely be performed (Figs. 3a through 3c).

The choice of anti-reflux operation after suitable dilatation depends on a number of factors:
• Personal preference and experience of the surgeon.

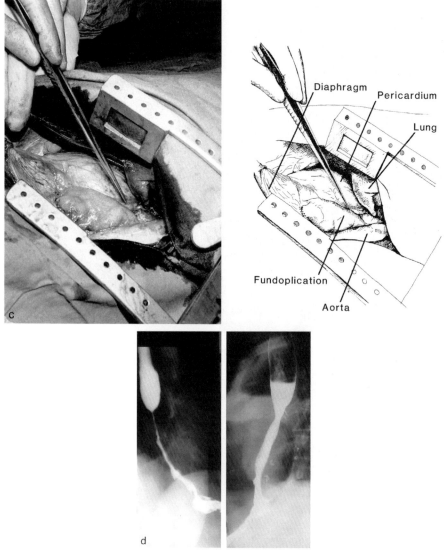

Fig. 3 (continued). (c) Total fundoplication is completed. Note in this case the stricture was associated with acquired short oesophagus. Therefore, the fundoplication is left in the mediastinum (photograph and diagram). (d) Pre-operative (left) and post-operative (right) Barium swallow of the patient with stricture associated with acquired short oesophagus (eight years later).

- Anatomo-pathology of the oesophagus with particular reference to the degree of shortening.
- Previous oesophageal and/or gastro-intestinal operation.

The author's preference is to carry out total fundoplication (modified Nissen type operation, section 2.1.4 in chapter III.6). Some other surgeons have used Collis gastroplasty added to by Nissen or Belsey type fundoplication with/without dilatation of stricture (Pearson et al., 1976; Orringer et al., 1978; Alexiou et al., 1999).

4.3.3. Roux-en-y duodenal diversion

This operation may be classified amongst conservative surgical methods in the sense that it neither interferes with the stricture nor surgically with the oesophagus. As the name implies, the operation consists of creation of a duodenal diversion which is achieved by interruption of gastro-duodenal continuity, establishment of a side-to-end gastro-jejunostomy which forms one of the limbs of the Y and an end-to-side jejuno-jejunal anastomosis forming the second limb of the Y. An anterectomy and sometimes vagotomy is added to the basic diversion operation. The operation has been shown to be successful

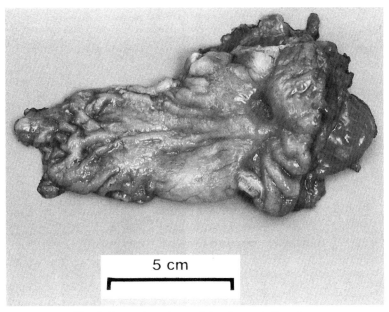

Fig. 4. Resected specimen of chronic penetrating ulcer.

in some patients with intractable reflux and particularly when there is evidence that bile is a major component of the refluxing fluid.

4.3.4. Contra-indications for conservative surgery in reflux stricture

Whilst conservative operation can be offered to most patients with reflux stricture requiring surgery, there are contra indications to such operations:

- Patients with fibrotic and severe undilatable stricture and/or those with long-standing penetrating ulcer.
- Patients with multiple previous oesophageal operation.
- Those who have had gastric resection.
- When there is a great degree of oesophageal shortening.
- When there is suspected malignancy.

4.3.5. Conservative surgery in strictures associated with short oesophagus

Acquired short oesophagus is an anatomo-pathological and surgical entity which may be defined as a fixed and irreversible elevation of the gastro-oesophageal junction above the oesophageal hiatus (Moghissi, 1983). By definition, those conservative surgical methods which require the reduction of the associated hiatal hernia, i.e. repositioning of the gastro-oesophageal junction under the diaphragm, cannot hope to succeed in treating strictures associated

with short oesophagus. Following Collis' (1961) introduction of the operation of gastroplasty, an effective lengthening of the oesophagus can be achieved by tubularisation of the stomach. However, gastroplasty alone will not produce an anti-reflux mechanism. When combined with a Belsey (Pearson et al., 1971) or Nissen (Orringer et al., 1978) type anti-reflux fundoplication procedure, gastroplasty appears to achieve successful results in patients with stricture associated with acquired short oesophagus.

Another approach to the treatment of this type of stricture is to carry out the operation of intra-thoracic fundoplication. The author's modification of the Nissen intrathoracic fundoplication, practised for the last 20 years, has proved successful. Initially the method was assessed in 45 patients with severe stricture associated with short oesophagus (Moghissi, 1983). 83% of patients had no recurrence of stricture or symptoms of gastro-oesophageal reflux for a follow-up period of 1 to 10 years (mean 6.8 years, Fig. 3d). The objective of intrathoracic fundoplication is to construct an effective Nissen-type 360° fundoplication after intra-operative dilation. Since the lower oesophagus, which is surrounded by the fundus of the stomach, cannot be placed under the diaphragm because of the shortening, it is left in the mediastinum. The operation is carried out through the left chest with the diaphagramatic incision placed peripherally to gain access to the abdomen. For the intra-thoracic total fundoplication to be successful

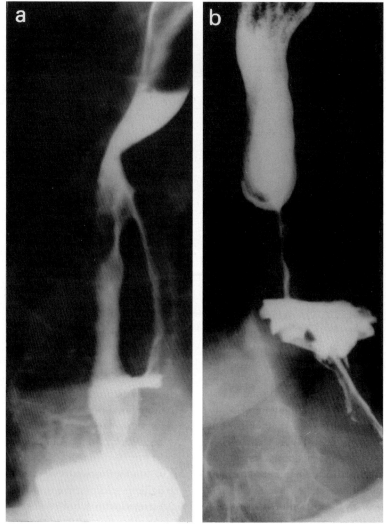

Fig. 5. (a) Barium swallow of a patient with severe high oesophageal stricture and short oesophagus. (b) Same patient five years after partial oesophagectomy and high oesophagogastric anastomoses with no dysphagia.

in reflux stricture with short oesophagus, it requires certain provisos:

- Effective intra-operative dilatation of the stricture is required.
- Care should be taken not to devascularise the gastric fundus.
- The top of the fundoplication wrap should be stitched to the phreno-oesophageal ligament (POL) which should be clearly identified and is usually stretched and situated 4–8 cm above the hiatus.
- Effort should be made to construct a tubular, rather than bulky, fundoplication in order that this may be placed predominantly in the posterior mediastinum and not in the left chest.

- The vagi (nerves) should be preserved and if they are injured or not clearly identified a pyloroplasty will be required.

4.4. Excisional surgery

This method is based on resection of the stricture and part of the oesophagus and reconstruction of the upper alimentary tract using a substitute. Over the past 30 years, there has been a considerable shift of opinion from an excisional policy in reflux stricture in favour of conservative operation, but there are still occasions in which radical surgery needs to be applied.

The present indications for excisional surgery are:

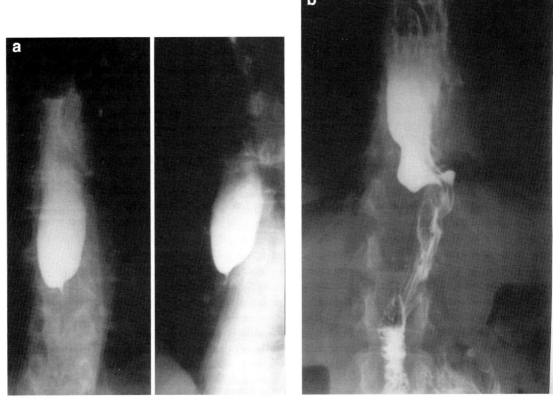

Fig. 6. (a) Barium swallow of an 80 year old woman with very severe stricture of the oesphagus. (b) Post-operative barium swallow of the same patient eight years later. The patient was treated by oesophagectomy through a left thoracotomy with a short segment of oesphagectomy and oesophago-gastric anastomosis. The patient survived to the age of 91 years with no problems.

- Failure of conservative operation and recurrence of the stricture.
- Patients with multiple previous (often two or three) operations for gastro-oesophageal reflux disease.
- Patients with chronic penetrating ulcer (Fig. 4) and previous history of acute haemotemesis.
- Cases in which neoplasia cannot be definitely ruled out and when even intra-operative frozen section histology is indecisive for malignancy.

There are principally three methods of reconstruction of the upper alimentary tract following resection of the oesophagus. These methods relate to the use of three different oesophageal substitutes:
- Stomach tube.
- Isolated jejunal loop: jejunal interposition.
- Colonic tube: colonic interposition.

When the stomach is used, the oesophageal excision is followed by an oesophago-gastric anastomosis. Reconstruction with jejunal and colonic tubes involve isolation and interpostion of the jejunal/colonic segment with its vascular transplant between remnant oesophagus and stomach.

4.4.1. Resection and reconstruction with use of the stomach

This can be carried out in two ways (Figs. 5a and 5b):

(a) In high stricture, an extensive resection and high anastomosis will be required. The operation is carried out as a two-stage procedure which is undertaken sequentially.

In the first stage, with the patient in supine position, a laparotomy is carried out and the stomach mobilised. All gastric vessels are tied off and divided except for the right gastro-epiploeic and its arcade along the greater curvature which is carefully preserved. The abdomen is closed after enlargement of the oesophageal hiatus.

In the second stage of the operation, a right thoracotomy is carried out. The oesophagus is mobilised, the stomach is drawn through the hiatus into the chest and the segment of the diseased oesophagus excised. An appropriate gastric tube is then fashioned and an end-to-side oesophago-gastric anastomosis is performed. This operation was originally advocated by Lewis (1946) for mid-thoracic oesophageal cancer. It has been extensively used for oesophageal stricture with proven long lasting results. Figure 6 shows the case of a young patient in whom the operation was used 21 years ago after two previous anti-reflux operations. She has had no problems with the upper alimentary tract since that time.

(b) Limited resection of the oesophagus. The author carries this out through a left thoracotomy with incision of the diaphragm (phrenotomy) to gain access to the upper abdominal viscera. My operation is a modification of that designed by V.C. Thompson (1945) for lower thoracic oesophageal cancer. The stomach is mobilised partially through the abdomen (accessed via peripheral and circumfrential diaphragmatic incision) and partially through the enlarged hiatus and is pulled into the chest through the latter. The segment of the oesophagus, together with the stricture, is resected and an end-to-side oesophago-gastric anastomosis is performed. This operation is not recommended for young patients since control of reflux is difficult and recurrence

of the stricture is inevitable in the long-term. In elderly patients, results are good with relatively low mortality and morbidity. Figures 6a and 6b shows the case of an 80-year-old lady with severe fibrotic stricture who survived for 9 years with good quality of life and good swallowing. She died, aged 91, of heart failure.

It is important to place the stomach in the mediastinum and not in the left chest. This is best achieved by carefully choosing the site of anastomosis. It is also possible to fashion at least partial fundoplication around the anastomosis. The mortality of this operation is less than 3%.

• Jejunal interposition

This operation (Fig. 7) has not received much favour in recent years. It was introduced and used extensively by Allison (1957) and Brain (1967). The experience of Allison indicates good long-term results for this operation in cases of reflux stricture. This has also been our personal experience in a limited number of cases operated between 1970 and 1988. Our indication has been for patients with failed operations for stricture. The overall mortality

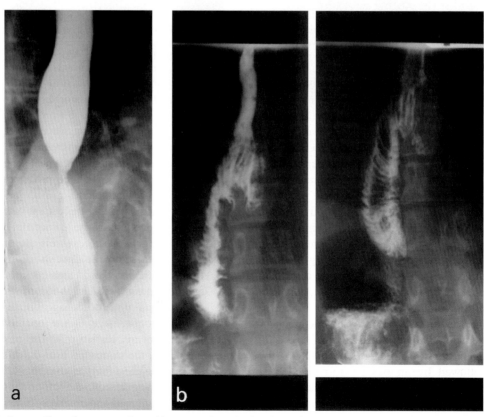

Fig. 7. (a) Barium swallow of a young patient with an oesophageal stricture requiring frequent dilation. (b) Barium swallow of the same patient ten years after resection and jejunal interposition.

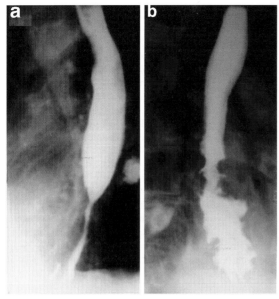

Fig. 8. (a) Barium swallow of a patient with a severe stricture who has had two previous hiatal hernia operations. (b) Barium swallow of the same patient five years after oesophagectomy with colonic interposition/reconstruction. The patient was alive and well at the last follow-up eleven years after operation.

in cases of reflux stricture with excellent long-term results. The left thoracophrenolaparotomy approach is ideal and provides a good exposure for coloplasty of the lower oesophagus. The left half of the transverse colon with its arcade supplied by the ascending branch of the left colic artery is isolated and is used as a substitute. After resection of oesophagus with its stricture, the isolated portion of the colon is divided, passed through the hiatus and placed in the chest isoperistaltically. An end-to-end oesophago-colonic and an end-to-side cologastric anastomosis establishes the continuity of the upper alimentary tract. A colo-colic anastomosis (left half of the transverse colon to the upper part of the descending colon) is then performed to complete the operation. The overall mortality of the operation is 4.8–6.9% and long-term results are generally good, particularly in those with short segment oesophagectomy (Jaysingham et al., 1999). These results are reproducible as has been shown by other authors (Moghissi, 1983; Thomas et al., 1997). In the author's series of 495 oesophageal strictures over a period of 22 years, there have been 42 colonic replacements with a mortality of 4.7% with good functional results.

in our series of 48 patients was two (just over 4%). Long-term functional results remain excellent for a follow up of between 4 and 22 years.

The operation is performed through a left thoraco-phreno-laparotomy and/or occasionally using a standard thoraco-laparotomy approach (section 2.2 in chapter III.17). An appropriate length of loop of jejunum, usually the second loop, is isolated with its blood supply which is carefully preserved. The loop is divided proximally and distally after the oesophagus is mobilised and the intended portion to be replaced is measured. The oesophago-gastric junction is divided and the stomach end is sutured. The loop of the jejunum with its vascular pedicle is then transplanted isoperistaltically to the chest through the hiatus after resection of the diseased portion of the oesophagus. The proximal end of the loop is anastomosed end-on with the divided end of the oesophagus. The distal end of the loop is then anastomosed to the stomach, thus bridging the gap produced by the resected oesophagus. A jejuno-jejunostomy then completes the operation.

• Colonic interposition (Fig. 8)

The colon as a substitute was first employed at the turn of the century, but its use was pioneered and popularised by Belsey who demonstrated a relatively easy approach to the problem of coloplasty

References and further reading

Alexiou C, Salama FD, Begg D. Comparison of long term results of total fundoplication gastroplasty and Belsey mark IV anti-reflux operation in relation to the severity of oesophagitis. Eur J Cardiothorac Surg 1999; 15: 620–626.

Allison PR. Reflux oesophagitis, sliding hiatal hernia and the anatomy of repair. Surgery Gynecol Obst 1951; 92: 419–431.

Allison PR. Peptic oesophagitis and oesophageal stricture. Lancet 1970; 2: 199–202.

Allison PR. Peptic ulcer of the oesophagus. Thorax 1948; 3: 20–42.

Allison PR, Wooler GN, Gunning AJ. Oesophago-jejunal gastrostomy. J Thorac Surg 1957; 33: 738–748.

Barrett NR. Chronic peptic ulcer of the oesophagus and oesophagitis. Br J Surg 1950; 38: 175–182.

Beggs FD, Salama FD, Knowles KR. Management of benign oesophageal stricture by total fundoplication gastroplasty. J R Coll Edin 1995; 40: 305–307.

Belsey RHR. Reconstruction of the oesophagus with left colon. J Thorac Cardiovasc 1965; 49: 33–55.

Brain RHF. The place for jejunal transplantation in the treatment of simple stricture of the oesophagus. Ann R Coll Surg Eng 1967; 40: 100–118.

Collis LJ. Gastroplasty. Thorax 1961; 6: 197–206.

Hayward J. The treatment of fibrous stricture of the oesophagus associated with hiatal hernia. Thorax 1961; 16: 45–55.

Herrington LL, Wright RS, Edwards WH. Conservative surgical treatment of reflux oesophagitis and oesophageal stricture. Ann Surg 1975; 181: 552–566.

Hill LD, Gelfand M, Bauermeister D. Simplified management

of reflux oesophagitis with stricture. Ann Surg 1970; 172: 638–651.

Jaysingham K, Lerut T, Belsey RHR. Functional and mechanical sequalae of colon interposition for benign oesophageal stricture. Eur J Cardiothorac Surg 1999; 15: 327–332.

Lewis I. The surgical treatment of carcinoma of the oesophagus. Br J Surg 1946; 34: 18–31.

Moghissi K. Carcinoma of cardia and thoracic-oesophagus co-existing with and following sliding hiatal hernia and peptic stricture. Thorax 1977; 32: 342–347.

Moghissi K. Conservative surgery for reflux oesophagitis with stricture: A comparison between two methods (summary). Thorax 1978; 33: 130.

Moghissi K. Le traitement des stenoses peptique de l'oesophage: À propos de 200 cas. Chirurgie 1979; 105: 161–170.

Moghissi K. Conservative surgery in reflux stricture of the oesophagus associated with hiatal hernia. Br J Surg 1979; 66: 221–225.

Moghissi K. Intrathoracic fundoplication for reflux stricture associated with short oesophagus. Thorax 1983; 38: 36–40.

Moghissi K, Goebells P. Relevance of antamo-pathology of high oesophageal strictures to the design of surgical treatment. Eur J Cardiothorac Surg 1990; 4: 91–96.

Nissen R. Eine einfache Operation zur Beeinflussung der Reflux-ösophagitis. Schweiz Med Wochenschr 1956; 86: 590–592.

Orringer MB, Sloan H. Combined Collis–Nissen reconstruction of the oesophago-gastric junction. Ann Thorac Surg 1978; 25: 16–21.

Pearson FG, Henderson RD. Long term follow up of peptic strictures managed by dilatation, modified Collis gastroplasty and Belsey hiatus hernia repair. Surgery 1976; 80: 396–404.

Pearson FG, Langer B, Henderson RD. Gastroplasty and Belsey hiatus hernia repair. An operation for the management of peptic stricture with acquired short oesophagus. J Thorac Cardiovasc Surg 1971; 61: 50–63.

Thomas P, Fuentes P, Guidicelli R, Rebound E. Colon interposition for oesophageal replacement: Current indications and long term function. Ann Thorac Surg 1997; 64; 757–764.

Thompson VC. Carcinoma of the oesophagus, resection and oesophago-gastrectomy. Br J Surg 1945; 32: 377–380.

K. Moghissi, J.A.C. Thorpe and F. Ciulli (Eds.)
Moghissi's Essentials of Thoracic and Cardiac Surgery

CHAPTER III.9

Corrosive injuries/chemical burn of the oesophagus

K. Moghissi

1. Introduction

Corrosive injuries of the oesophagus occur following accidental or intentional ingestion of acid or alkaline substances.

Amongst acids are sulphuric and hydrochloric acids which are usually contained in batteries; the majority of substances used for household cleaning and bleaches for drainage and toilets are alkaline.

Both acids and alkalines, when ingested, produce burn of the upper digestive tract, inflammation and necrosis of the mucosa followed by ulceration. The immediate effects depend on the concentration and potency of the ingested substance.

Local lesions may vary from upper alimentary tract inflammation to severe ulceration and perforation. In addition, the upper respiratory airway may become involved. General effects also vary and in severe cases, shock and cardio-respiratory failure may be present.

2. Initial evaluation and management

History taking is important and provides a guide to identification of the nature of the ingested substance. Physical examination is essential to evaluate the condition of the patient at presentation and to initiate emergency measures.

- Identification of injurious agent by history taking is important.
- An initial evaluation should be made of the general condition of the patient, the cardiorespiratory state and, as far as possible, the extent of the local lesion.
- First aid and initial management in all but trivial cases entails establishment of intravenous infusion, administration of antibiotic and analgesia.

- A neck and chest radiograph (anterior and lateral views) is taken. Additional imaging investigations may be necessary depending on clinical findings.
- An initial oro-pharyngo-oesophagoscopy is arranged. The timing and even the necessity of this endoscopy have been the subject of debate.

The author prefers to carry out endoscopy as soon as the patient's condition is sufficiently stable to allow examination under general anaesthetic. He also believes, at least for the oro-pharyngeal inspection, that an open-ended rigid instrument is preferable as this allows direct vision. Bronchoscopic examination should also be undertaken at the same time. Expertise is needed to perform endoscopy skilfully and with minimum trauma. The point of importance is to eliminate the need for an emergency surgical operation if there is no perforation or to identify the possible perforation and its location. It should be emphasised that occasionally the extent of the injury only becomes apparent a few days after ingestion. This is particularly the case for oesophago-airway fistula. Therefore, close surveillance of the patient is required even if their initial condition is good.

There is no need for repeat oesophagoscopy until 4–6 weeks later when reassessment becomes necessary. In severe cases, a gastrostomy should be established for nutrition and oral diet introduced only with gradual increase in consistency during the course of 2–6 weeks, depending on the severity of oesophageal wall damage.

Administration of steroid in the initial course is controversial and debatable. The author does not use steroid nor recommend it in the initial stage of management in those patients with multiple perforations and/or in rare cases of complete necrosis of the oesophagus. Total excision of thoracic oesophagus and staged reconstruction (section 7.3 in chapter III.17)

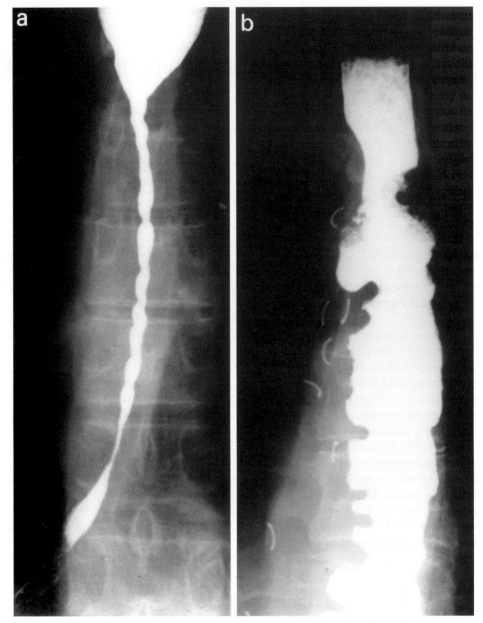

Fig. 1. (a) Barium swallow of a middle-aged patient who, twenty years previously, had accidentally swallowed caustic material. He was originally treated by dilation; this was followed by gastrostomy which was in situ for 15 years. (b) Long segment colonic substitute was used for reconstruction. Barium swallow five years post-operative.

may become necessary. Some surgeons prefer resection and reconstruction even at an early stage (Gossot et al., 1987).

3. Further management

Oesophageal stricture is the usual sequelae of corrosive injuries. This can present in many forms. In some cases, the stricture is mild and requires only one or two dilatations using mercury filled (Maloney type) bougies, which are capable of negotiating distorted passages. In some cases the stricture is firm, tight and elongated. Surprisingly, some of these also yield to dilatation.

Rarely, stricture requires resection and replacement of the oesophagus using a substitute.

However, in the author's experience, many cases will respond to repeated dilatation and only excep-

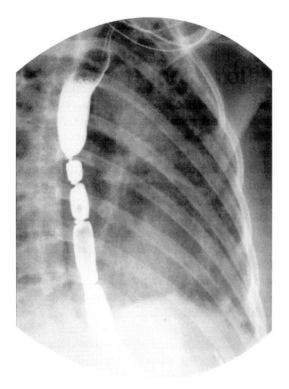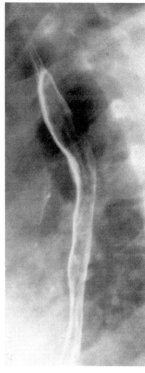

Fig. 2. (a) Barium swallow of a young woman who developed a series of strictures in the oesophagus producing a string of beads-like picture. The patient had four dilations over a one-year period with complete cure of dysphagia. (b) Barium swallow of same patient showing normal transit post-treatment.

tionally is replacement needed. The choice of substitute depends on topography and extent of the stricture. Colonic interposition is usually attended by long-standing good results (Figs. 1a and 1b, Figs. 2a and 2b).

References and further reading

Bapa RS, Bakhshi GD, Kantaria CV, et al. Self-bouginage: long-term relief of corrosive oesophageal stricture. Indian J Gastroenterol 2001; 20: 180–182.

Broto J, Asensio M, Jorro CS et al. Conservative treatment of caustic esophageal injuries in children: 20 years of experience. Paed Surg Int 1999; 15: 323–325.

Chernousov AF, Bogopolskii PN. Bouginage of oesophagus in critical burn strictures. Moskow, Khirurgiia (Mosk) 1998; 10: 25–29.

Choi RS, Killehei CW, Lund DP, Healy GB, et al. Esophageal replacement in children who have caustic pharyngo-oesophageal strictures. J Pediatr Surg 1997; 32: 1083–1087.

Gossot D, Sarfati E, Celerier M. Traitement des brulures graves du tractus digestif supérieur par oesogastrectomy à thorax fermé. Ann Chirurgie 1987; 41: 581–585.

Luostarinen M, Isolauric J. Esophageal perforation and caustic injury: Approach to instrumental perforations of the esophagus. Dis Esophagus 1997; 10: 86–89.

Tseng YL, Wo MH, Lin MY, Lai WW. Outcome of acid ingestion related to aspiration pneumonia. Eur J Cardiothorac Surg 2002; 21: 638–643.

Vereczkei A, Varga G, Poto L, Havarth OP. Management of corrosive injuries of the oesophagus. Acta Chir Hung 1999; 38: 119–122.

CHAPTER III.10

Miscellaneous oesophageal obstruction

K. Moghissi

1. Oesophageal webs and rings

Webs and rings are a fibrous membrane like a 'diaphragm,' projecting into the lumen of the oesophagus producing an effective obstructive lesion. Apart from occasional reflux stricture, which presents as a ring-like stenosis with little inflammation or ulceration, there are two types of membranous webs.

1.1. Cervical web and Plummer–Vinson (Paterson–Kelly) syndrome

This is a thin shelf-like membrane projecting into the lumen of the pharnygo-oesophageal junction. It predominantly affects women and the main symptom is dysphagia. The latter may be associated with glossitis and anaemia in which case the term 'Plummer–Vinson' (or 'Paterson–Kelly') syndrome is applied. Of importance is that contrast medium examination may fail to show the existence of the web but careful endoscopy (particularly using the rigid oesophagoscope) will demonstrate it.

Treatment is oesophagoscopy and dilatation, which effectively breaks the membrane though this may have to be repeated. Alternatively NdYAG laser may be used to incise (evaporate) the membrane. Anaemia and nutritional deficiencies, when present, should be corrected.

1.2. Lower oesophageal web (Schatzki's ring) or lower oesophageal ring

This is a circular membrane at the lower end of the oesophagus at, or near, the oesophageal hiatus of the diaphragm. It often is associated with a sliding hiatal hernia and at endoscopic examination will appear as a thin (1 to 2 mm) membrane attached circumferentially to the oesophageal mucosa at the squamo-columnar epithelial junction.

The main symptom is dysphagia. The web is often recognised radiologically as an annular indentation or a ring of construction (Fig. 1). Since its description by Ingelfinger and Kramer (1953) and then by Schatzki and Gray (1953), the condition has been known as Schatzki's ring. The aetiology of the condition is not well understood. Gastro-oesophageal reflux has been implicated by some as the possible cause but pathologically, the membrane seems to be unlike that of a reflux structure. Diagnosis of the condition is made radiologically and sometimes endoscopically. Both investigations may however fail to show the web which can be found at operation after gastrotomy and retrograde finger exploration.

When patients are symptomatic and the web has been demonstrated endoscopically, the opening can be dilated. Surgical treatment involving excision may be necessary at times, in which case, it is coupled with an antireflux procedure.

2. Extrinsic obstructions of the oesophagus

This a group of heterogeneous conditions which cause obstruction by extrinsic compression of the oesophagus with/without invasion of its wall.

- Extrinsic pressure by tumour
  Neoplasms affecting cervical and mediastinal structures in the immediate vicinity of the oesophagus can compress or infiltrate it and cause dysphagia.
  The commonest amongst these tumours is lung cancer and/or its satellite lymphadenopathies. The patient may initially consult his doctor because of dysphagia. Investigation will usually reveal the primary diagnosis. Treatment of secondary oesopha-

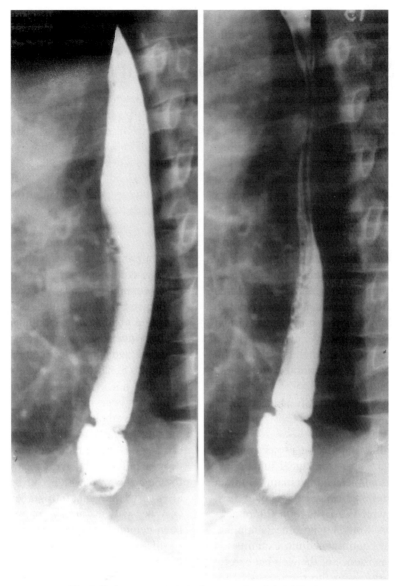

Fig. 1. Barium contrast study demonstrating Schatzki's ring.

geal involvement by a tumour may be difficult. Radiotherapy, intubation or oesophageal bypass operation are possibilities which may be considered in order to overcome dysphagia.

• Extrinsic pressure by vascular anomalies
Congenital anomalies of the aortic arch such as aortic ring or an aberrant subclavian artery may cause dysphagia (dysphagia lusoria). Also, aneurysm of the arch and descending aorta may, at times, cause external pressure. An enlarged left atrium is also said to cause oesophageal obstruction because of its close relationship to the oesophagus. Nevertheless, there are many instances in which a patient with a greatly increased (giant) left atrium has no difficulty of food ingestion. In these cases, dysphagia may be more related to oesophagitis and stricture caused by cardiovascular drugs which temporarily become impacted in the oesophagus rather than left atrial enlargement.

3. Post-operative oesophageal stricture

This is a group of aetiologically heterogeneous oesophageal lesions which occur following diverse operations on the oesophagus or other parts of the alimentary tract.

3.1. Post-oesophagectomy stricture

- Stenotic lesions early after operation are usually due to:
  - inadequate anastomotic channel,
  - Excess granulation tissue/over healing at the site of anastomosis and scarring.
- Strictures which appear 2 or 3 months (or later) after resection and reconstruction are due to:
  - reflux into the oesophageal remnant followed by inflammatory scarring,
  - recurrence of tumour in the oesophagus.

3.2. Stricture following anti-reflux operation

A number of factors may be responsible for occurrence of such a stricture:
- Stenosis associated with poor surgical technique such as constriction by fundoplication and too tight a hiatal repair.
- Stricture associated with recurrence of gastro-oesophageal reflux and subsequent stenosis.
- Stricture following vagotomy and pyloroplasty: temporary dysphagia after this procedure is not infrequent. However, persistent dysphagia is accompanied by a demonstrable stenotic segment at the level of hiatus and 2 to 3 cm below in the abdominal portion of the oesophagus. The cause of such stricture is not clear; trauma to the lower end of the oesophagus and gastro-oesophageal reflux are two possible factors.

3.3. Stricture following other surgery

Stenotic lesions of the oesophagus may follow operations other than those on the oesophagus especially on the alimentary canal. Several factors may be responsible for their formation; the most important appear to be:
- Gastro-oesophageal reflux and stricture.
- Naso-gastric tube causing inflammatory stricture.

- Medication in tablet form which may temporarily lodge in the oesophagus; high on this list are potassium tablets given in conjunction with diuretics.

4. Drug-induced oesophagitis and stricture

There are a number of medications in tablet form which may cause oesophagitis and subsequent ulceration and stricture if they are lodged, for any length of time, in the oesophagus. Most important amongst these tablets are potassium preparations given to patients in conjunction with diuretics. Such preparations, in patients with gastro-oesophageal reflux with spasm or minor oesophageal obstruction, can lodge in the oesophagus causing severe oesophagitis, ulceration and scarring stricture. Some medication used for arthritis, when given in tablet form, has a similar affect. This has particular implications for elderly patients with osteo-arthritis and a degree of gastro-oesophageal reflux whose medication should be planned with care and reflection.

References and further reading

DeVault KR. Lower esophageal (Schatzki's) ring: pathogenesis, diagnosis and therapy. Dig Dis 1996; 14: 323–329.

Ingelfinger FJ, Kramer P. Dysphagia produced by a contractile ring in the lower oesophagus. Gastroenterology 1953; 23: 419–430.

Jamieson J, Hinder RA, DeMeester TR, Litchfield D, Barlow A, Bailey RT Jr. Analysis of thirty-two patients with Schatzki's ring. Am J Surg 1989; 158: 563–566.

Morris CD, Kanter KR, Miller JI Jr. Late-onset dysphagia lusoria. Ann Thorac Surg 2001; 71: 710–712.

Schatzki R, Gray JE. Dysphagia due to diaphragm-like localised narrowing in the lower oesophagus (lower oesophageal ring). Am J Roentgenol Radiother Nucl Med 1953; 70: 911–923.

Woods RK, Sharp RJ, Holcomb GW 3rd, Snyder CL, Lofland GK, Ashcraft K, Holder TM. Vascular anomalies and tracheoesophageal compression: a single institute's 25 year experience. Ann Thorac Surg 2001; 72: 434–438.

CHAPTER III.11

Perforation of the oesophagus

K. Moghissi

1. Introduction

Rupture of the oesophagus is potentially one of the most lethal oesophageal conditions. Nevertheless, when diagnosed early and treated efficiently it has a favourable outcome in the majority of cases.

2. Terminology

The term perforation of the oesophagus (transmural rupture) is used here to mean a complete rupture of the wall in its full thickness so that there is a fistulous communication between the lumen and the spaces which surround the oesophagus. This fistula will lead to an outpouring of the oesophageal contents.

Incomplete perforation with dissection of the oesophagus is referred to as intramural rupture. The mucosal tear is yet another form of rupture in which there appears to be no real dissection of the wall. Mucosal tearing of the lower oesophagus associated with massive haemorrhage was first described by Mallory and Weiss in 1929 and is now universally known as the Mallory–Weiss syndrome.

3. Complete perforation — rupture of the oesophagus

Post-emetic rupture of the oesophagus was first described by Boerhaave in 1723 (cited in Derbes and Mitchell, 1955). Barrett (1947) reported the first successfully treated case. Such perforations are generally known as spontaneous ruptures. Since the development of endoscopy and oesophageal bougienage there is another important group of oesophageal ruptures caused by oesophagoscopy, this is instrumental perforation of the oesophagus. These two forms of perforation have to be considered separately, not only because of their different aetiology but also because of their pathology and management.

3.1. Aetiology of oesophageal perforation

By far the greatest number of oesophageal perforations are caused by instrumentation. In a review of 511 perforations from the literature (Jones, 1992) 43% of the cases were instrumental and the remaining 57% were due to a variety of causes, consisting of: trauma, spontaneous, intubation and operative injuries, tumour and other miscellaneous aetiology.

4. Instrumental perforations

This type of perforation usually results from:
- The passage of instrument with injury occurring generally at the pharyngo-oesophageal junction or less frequently at the oesophago-gastric junction
- Biopsy forceps injury to the wall during the procedure
- Dilatation of stricture and the false passage of bougies.

The incidence of instrumental perforation varies according to the expertise of the operator, pathology of the oesophagus, the type of instrument used and additional procedures such as bougienage and oesophageal biopsy. There is a higher incidence of rupture with a rigid oesophagoscope than with the flexible instrument. There is also an increased risk of perforation in therapeutic (i.e. bougienage) than in diagnostic oesophagoscopy. The incidence of instrumental perforation is between 0.1 to 0.3%. A survey by the British Society of Gastroenterology (1986) involving nearly 40,000 patients reported an incidence of 0.096%. However, whilst the rate for a simple diagnostic endoscopy was 0.018%, the incidence for

Table 1

Instrumental perforation of the oesophagus: Incidence per site in 38 patients

Location	Number	%
1. Cervical	10	26.3
2. Upper and middle thoracic	10	26.3
3. Lower thoracic	16	42
4. Isolated, abdominal oesophageal perforation	2	5.2

Table 2

The early and later presenting symptoms and signs of oesophageal perforations in 48 patients expressed as a percentage

Symptoms and signs	Cervical perforation		Thoracic perforation	
	Early	Late	Early	Late
Sore throat	100	50	98	33
Pains in neck or chest	100	50	100	38
Dyspnoea	0	0	60	100
Dysphagia	100	100	85	77
Surgical subcutaneous emphysema	50	0	45	0
Cellulitis of the neck	50	100	7	0
Pneumothorax	0	0	60	100
Fever	50	100	50	90
Shock	20	25	7	33

dilatation of stricture in 3% of the patients was 0.9%. In the author's own series (Moghissi, 1988) of 2932 diagnostic and interventional oesophagoscopies, the overall incidence was 0.24%. In this series, 43% of patients had dilatation of stricture. The incidence for diagnostic (including foreign body extraction) and dilatation of stricture was 0.058% and 0.48% respectively.

Perforation can occur at any level of the oesophagus:

• Pharyngo-oesophageal junction/cervical oesophagus: where there may be difficulty in negotiating the pharyngolarynx to enter into the oesophagus proper. The site of such a perforation is usually just above, or in proximity to, the cricopharyngeous ring of the inferior constrictor but the pathological signs are referable to the neck and superior mediastinum (see arrangement of mediastinal spaces).
• Upper and middle thoracic oesophagus: this usually follows extraction of a foreign body or occasionally the forcible passage of the instrument through a distorted oesophagus above a stricture.
• Lower thoracic oesophagus: this usually follows dilatation of a stricture by bougienage or during a biopsy.
• Abdominal oesophagus: this usually occurs together with the perforation of the lower thoracic oesophagus but only rarely as an isolated perforation. The difficulty of negotiating the gastro-oesophageal junction by oesophagoscope, bougie or forcible balloon dilatation, e.g. for achlasia of cardia, is the responsible cause in the majority of cases.

The relative number of perforations in different locations recorded in 38 patients is shown in Table 1.

4.1. Clinical features and diagnosis

The clinical features of perforation of the oesophagus vary according to the location of the perforation and the stage at which the patient is examined, i.e.

the delay between the perforation and the patient's examination (Table 2).

4.1.1. Perforation of the cervical oesophagus

In an early stage (within a few hours) of the accident, the patient experiences pain in the throat and neck. There may be difficulty in swallowing saliva. Examination at this stage reveals surgical subcutaneous emphysema and possibly some induration in the soft tissues of the neck. At a later stage, there

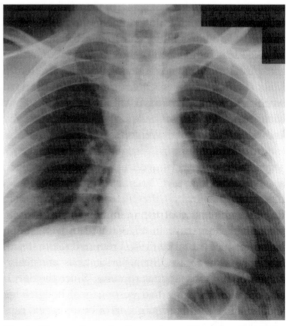

Fig. 1. Chest radiograph of a patient with perforation of the cervical oesophagus. Note the paramediastinal abscess with fluid level — also right pleural reaction (48 hours after perforation).

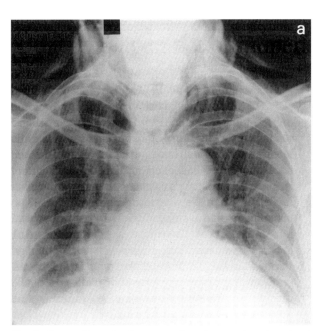
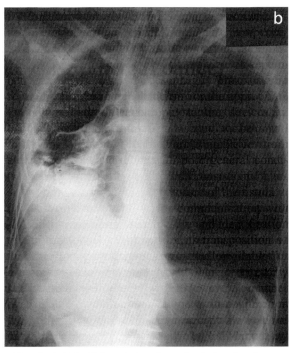

Fig. 2. Chest radiograph of an upper thoracic oesophageal perforation: (a) early (within 12 hours) there is mediastinal and neck space emphysema and right-sided pleural effusion, (b) after 24 hours there is hydro-pneumothorax. The contrast study shows considerable leak and oesophago-mediastino-pleural fistula.

is cellulitis and purulent exudation around the oeso-phagus and in the retro-oesophageal space tracking down into the superior mediastinum. Dysphagia and general signs of infection appear. Chest and lateral neck radiographs usually confirm the diagnosis. In an early stage, air appears in the soft tissues of the neck. At a later stage there is widening of the supe-rior mediastinal shadowing indicating mediastinitis. In addition, a mediastinal abscess with a fluid level or pleural effusion may be present (Fig. 1).

4.1.2. Perforation of the upper thoracic oesophagus
In an early stage, there is pain, dyspnoea and dys-phagia. Examination of the patient reveals surgical emphysema in the supraclavicular regions and the neck. Chest radiograph in the early stage shows me-diastinal emphysema (pneumomediastinum) or may demonstrate a right-sided pneumothorax (Fig. 2). The presence of pneumothorax may not be clini-cally appreciated nor can it be demonstrated on a chest radiograph particularly if the X-ray is an an-tero-posterior view taken in supine position. Even lateral chest X-ray may not show the pneumothorax. Mediastinal emphysema, widening of the space and pleural collection of fluid should be taken as definite indications of oesophageal leak (see mediastinitis).

At a later stage, signs of infection and rapid de-terioration in the general condition of the patient occur. There are clinical and radiological signs of hydro-pneumothorax. After 48 to 72 hours the pa-tient becomes seriously dehydrated and very sick with rapidly developing signs of toxaemia and car-diorespiratory failure.

4.1.3. Perforation of the lower thoracic oesophagus
In an early stage, there is pain in the back (lower chest) and the upper abdomen. Dyspnoea, dysphagia, vomiting and nausea are usually present. Clinical ex-amination reveals surgical subcutaneous emphysema and signs of left-sided pneumothorax. At a later stage, there is a gradual deterioration of the patient's general condition with development of infection, tox-aemia, hydropneumothorax and dehydration culmi-nating in cardiorespiratory failure. Chest radiograph in an early stage indicates pneumomediastinum (pos-sible pneumopericardium) and left-sided pneumoth-orax. At a later stage there is generally a gross left-sided hydro(pyo)pneumothorax with collapse of the lung (Fig. 3).

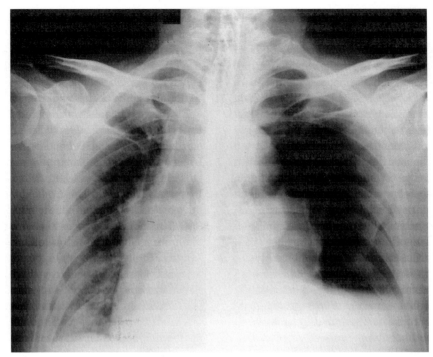

Fig. 3. Chest radiograph of a patient with perforation of lower thoracic oesophagus. Note left-sided hydro-pneumothorax (72 hours after perforation).

4.1.4. Perforation of the intra-hiatal and abdominal oesophagus

In the case of perforation at the extreme lower end of the oesophagus the diagnosis may become particularly difficult. Firstly, there may be few or no clinical signs in the chest and all symptoms in an early stage are referable to the upper abdomen. Acute pain is present in the epigastric region often together with nausea and vomiting. Attempts at drinking cause severe pain. Surgical emphysema, which is usually present in perforations in other parts of the oesophagus, is generally absent or not remarkable. At an early stage, chest and abdominal X-rays may show no detectable abnormalities; later there may be a small pleural reaction.

4.2. Management of instrumental oesophageal perforation

An early diagnosis and treatment of instrumental perforation of the oesophagus is usually attended by a favourable outcome. Late diagnosis is usually attended by high mortality, irrespective of the type of treatment which is undertaken. It is therefore important to examine the patient clinically and radiologically following oesophagoscopy particularly after dilatation of strictures or extraction of a foreign body.

On suspicion of perforation, oral fluid and food intake are withheld and expert advice should be sought.

The factors influencing management of patients with perforations are:

(1) Anatomical site of the perforation
(2) The speed with which the diagnosis is made
(3) Clinical condition of the patient generally and at the time of the diagnosis more specifically
(4) The pre-existing pathology of the oesophagus.

Some general principles are applicable to perforation, irrespective of the anatomical sites or the pathology of the oesophagus. These are briefly outlined under general management. Perforations in different sites and pathology require specific management and, therefore, a separate discussion.

4.2.1. General principles of management of oesophageal perforations

- As soon as the diagnosis is made, oral intake of food and liquid is withdrawn. It must be remembered that even without oral intake, a normal individual secretes in excess of a litre of saliva per day. In a perforation this may collect in the mediastinum or the pleural cavity.
- A central venous catheter is inserted for central venous pressure (CVP) monitoring and intravenous nutritional purposes.

- An intravenously administered antimicrobial regimen consisting of one or more broad-spectrum antibiotics is instituted.
- Determination of the exact site of the perforation is an important point in the management of patients. This is achieved by:
  - Radiological methods using a contrast medium, e.g. Gastrograffin. Acquisition of good films is important; video film of the transit is most useful.
  - Endoscopy is mandatory not only to determine the site of oesophageal perforation but with the objective of visualising the pathology of the oesophagus above and around the area of the perforation. It is imperative that endoscopy is carried out by the surgeon who proposes to undertake the surgical operation which may be required.
  - CT of the thorax which assess the state of the mediastinum (air, fluid) is necessary only in difficult diagnostic cases and when extrusion of a foreign body is suspected.
- Nutritional management: In all perforations intravenous (i.v.) feeding is essential initially. It is, however, mandatory to consider an appropriate route for enteral nutrition in addition in order to switch to this method of feeding when the early hypercatabolic state has subsided but oral feeding may not be possible.
- A naso-gastric tube should be introduced to aspirate saliva. The tube should be placed with the tip above the site of perforation. If gastrostomy is carried out this tube may with care be inserted from the stomach upwards. This principle is the mainstay of *conservative* management. It is applicable to small perforations in an otherwise healthy oesophagus with air/fluid collection confined to a localised area of the neck or mediastinum and no pneumo/hydrothorax.

4.2.2. Specific management of perforation according to the site

Perforation of cervical oesophagus. Perforation in this portion of the oesophagus usually has a good prognosis because it can be diagnosed early. In a series of 38 patients with oesophageal perforations treated (Table 1), 10 patients had cervical oesophageal perforations. All survived using conservative medical treatment with drainage of neck and mediastinal space.

- A central venous catheter is inserted for i.v. feeding.

- The neck space should be drained.
- In some cases of cervical oesophageal perforation, the extravasation appears further down in the oesophagus at the level of the carina into the mediastinum due to dissection of the oesophagus from the neck to the thoracic part of the tube.
- The mediastinum is generally drained via the right chest. The drain should be placed in the retro-oesophageal space. It should be emphasized that the mediastinal drain must be connected to an underwater sealed drainage system. It is necessary to drain the right pleural space as well, if the pleura is entered, or if there is pleural fluid which should be considered as contaminated and septic.
- Feeding gastrostomy (or fine tube jejunostomy) is established in order to carry out enteral feeding after a few days of parenteral nutrition, until healing of the perforation which could take four to ten weeks. Oral feeding may be resumed after three to four weeks. Healing may be encouraged by local endoscopic application of a solution of 20% sodium hydroxide (NaOH) solution only to the site of perforation under vision and if the perforation is small with no stenosis below or around. The drains are removed when there is radiological evidence of healing and there is no further discharge and full expansion of the lungs has been achieved.

Perforation of thoracic oesophagus. The perforation of the thoracic oesophagus is usually more serious than that of the cervical oesophagus. It usually occurs in the course of dilatation of a stricture or following oesophageal biopsy. It is therefore likely that drainage alone will give only temporary benefit or be merely a first step towards the later complete treatment. Furthermore, the repair of perforation of the oesophagus such as that caused by carcinoma or stricture has little chance of success.

A number of therapeutic options are available to treat thoracic oesophageal perforations. The selection of any of the options depends on the circumstances which are usually governed by three factors:

- Time factor: early presentation (24 to 36 hours after the injury) versus late presentation (after 36 hours)
- Location of the perforation: Upper and mid-thoracic oesophagus versus the lower thoracic or pre-hiatal perforations
- Pre- or co-existence of a pathology other than the perforation (e.g. stricture or tumour).

The general principles of treatment are:
- To control the oesophageal leak

– To drain the pleural and mediastinal spaces in order to eliminate sepsis
– Prevention of gastric juice refluxing and leaking through the perforation into the mediastinum
– Prevention of flow of saliva leaking through the perforation into the mediastinum
– Provision of nutritional support
– Provision of ventilatory support.

The above principles can be fulfilled through the following therapeutic possibilities:
• Direct repair of the perforation
• Resection and reconstruction of the oesophagus
  (a) One stage
  (b) Delayed (two stages)
• Diversion and exclusion
• Direct repair.

In early perforations and in the absence of additional oesophageal pathology, this method is successful in the majority of cases. A few practical details are worthy of mention:
– The edges of the perforation should be trimmed before suturing.
– It is important to expose the whole extent of the perforation. For this it might be necessary to incise the muscular layers of the oesophageal wall above and below the visible mucosal opening. It is important to find the mucosal site of the perforation. This can be well above the site of muscular tear.

A right thoracotomy is performed to access the upper and mid-thoracic oesophageal perforation. Left thoracotomy exposes lower pre-hiatal ruptures. Debridement is carried out in all cases. The rupture may be sutured in two layers or, as the author prefers, in one through-and-through layer of interrupted stitches using 3.0 non-absorbable material. Buttressing may be required.

In very early perforations it may not be necessary to protect the suture line. Nevertheless, this will be required in most cases after 24 hours. The author prefers to use intercostal muscle graft in upper and mid-thoracic perforations and omentum in the lower perforations. For those perforations in the lower pre-hiatal region a total fundoplication is the obvious choice (see section 2.1.4 in chapter III.6).
• Excisional surgery
(a) Resection and immediate reconstruction of the oesophagus is carried out in one procedure using the stomach or jejunum as a substitute. This method is suitable for early presentation cases of instrumental perforation where there is an additional oesophageal pathology such as tumour or stricture.

(b) Two stage oesophagectomy and reconstruction
The first stage consists of:
– Oesophagectomy (trans-hiatal or trans-thoracic), the oesophago-gastric junction is stapled/sutured,
– Cervical oesophagostomy to divert saliva,
– Gastrostomy for feeding,
– Drainage of mediastinum and pleural space.

The second stage of the operation is undertaken 4–6 months later and consists of reconstruction of the upper alimentary tract using stomach or colon as a substitute. The indications for this procedure are late presentation of the perforation with or without additional oesophageal pathology.
• Oesophageal exclusion

Oesophageal exclusion can be achieved using a number of techniques. This method is suitable for late presentation of perforation without additional oesophageal pathology and where it is estimated that oesophageal rupture is relatively small. The principle of oesophageal exclusion consists of:
– Diversion of saliva via a cervical oesophagostomy or T-tube in the oesophagus placed above the perforation. In this case the lower limb of the T-tube is blocked and a snare is passed around the oesophagus (and tube) to prevent saliva flowing distally. In cases of lateral oesophagostomy the flow of saliva distal to the stoma should be prevented by small oesophageal tube and suction.
– Gastrostomy for prevention of refluxing juice entering the oesophagus and leaking into the mediastinum
– Jejeunostomy for nutrition
– The mediastinum and the pleura need draining
– Healing is monitored by contrast medium radiography.

5. Spontaneous rupture of the oesophagus

Barrett (1947) was the first to report a case of spontaneous rupture of the oesophagus successfully treated by operation. Typically the rupture occurs after a large meal or following a heavy drinking session and during retching or vomiting. The patient experiences a severe pain in the upper abdomen and lower chest. The pain is accompanied by dyspnoea and shock. Undiagnosed and untreated the patient becomes very ill with toxaemia, dehydration and signs of cardiovascular collapse. Death will follow within a few days.

Almost always the rupture occurs within the last few centimetres of the thoracic oesophagus just above the diaphragm (Fig. 4). Examination of the oesophagus at operation shows a longitudinal tear in-

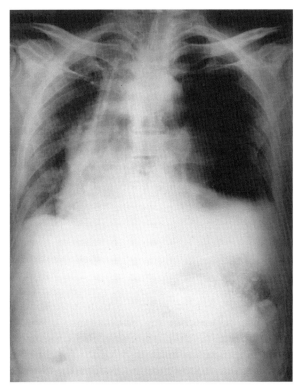

Fig. 4. Chest radiograph of a patient with spontaneous rupture typically involving the lower 5–6 cm of the lower thoracic oesophagus. Hydro-pneumothorax and mediastinal emphysema and fluid collection are seen.

volving all layers of the oesophagus. Within hours of the rupture, there is a considerable oedema, necrosis of the oesophageal wall and pouting of the mucosa. The oesophageal wall looks as though it has been scorched. The intra-abdominal oesophagus is usually unaffected. Mediastinal oedema and necrotizing acute inflammation develop early, and often very quickly, with a great deal of haemorrhagic mediastinitis. The pathological findings and the shattered look of the oesophagus suggest that a sudden and extreme intraluminal pressure is involved in the development of spontaneous rupture.

5.1. Diagnosis

The history and symptoms are at times indistinguishable from that of perforated duodenal or gastric ulcer. In fact, some patients with spontaneous rupture are, in error, submitted to laparotomy. In these, it is only on negative findings that the diagnosis is revised. There are, however, important diagnostic signs which can be easily demonstrated if the patient is carefully examined. These are:

- Pleural effusion
- Surgical subcutaneous emphysema which is usually present and palpable in the neck.

The diagnosis is confirmed radiologically and endoscopically. Plain radiograph of the chest demonstrates hydropneumothorax with corresponding collapse of the lung. It also shows the presence of air in the soft tissue of the neck and mediastinum. Gastrograffin swallow shows the 'track' and the deposition of the dye in the left pleural cavity. It is important to perform oesophagoscopy on these patients in order to eliminate associated oesophageal pathology which can, at times, coexist with spontaneous rupture. This may be done at the time of operative repair.

5.2. Management

After the diagnosis of perforation is established, the first and principle objective is to assess and stabilise the general and biochemical state of the patient.

- After confirmation of hydropneumothorax, drainage of the pleural space is established via an intercostal tube placed at the base of the chest posteriorly or through mid-axillary line.
- A sample of blood is despatched to the laboratory for a full blood count, biochemical profile and emergency blood group and cross match.
- A central venous catheter is inserted for central venous pressure (CVP) measurement which will indicate the hypovolaemic state. The central venous catheter can also be used for intravenous infusion.
- A bladder catheter is inserted to measure the existing urinary output and then to monitor it.
- Drainage of the chest and re-expansion of the lung may provoke a great deal of pain which should be alleviated by suitable analgesics.
- A sample of pleural fluid is despatched to the bacteriology department for identification of organisms, culture and sensitivity to antibiotics.
- Intravenous administration of antibiotic should commence.
- An electrocardiogram is carried out for future reference.

Further management of the patient depends on several factors which include:
(a) The general condition of the patient,
(b) The age of the perforation

It is generally preferable to repair the perforation if at all possible. This is, however, subject to the age of the perforation. Early cases (24 to 36 hours) can be repaired. The repair is carried out through a left thoracotomy and by one layer of through-and-through transverse stitching using non-absorbable material with reinforcement (buttress stitches).

Many surgeons feel that stitching alone may not suffice and with the amount of necrosis and devascularisation which is usually associated with spontaneous rupture, the simple repair of the tear will not hold.

Pericardial and/or muscle grafts have been used by some to reinforce the repair. The author's personal preference is to repair the tear and then to mobilise the fundus of the stomach which is brought up into the chest in order to protect the repair by total fundoplication (see section 2.1.4 in chapter III.6). Alternatively, the lower oesophageal perforation is an ideal indication for a pedicle–omental graft over the suture line. In all cases, thorough toilette of the chest cavity is carried out and the pleural space, as well as the posterior mediastinum, are drained.

6. Intramural spontaneous perforation

The term refers to the mucosal tear resulting in dissection of the oesophagus with creation of a double-barrelled oesophagus. The dominant symptom is retrosternal or epigastric pain and dysphagia, vomiting and haematemesis are often present. In many cases, no predisposing pathology can be evoked. Symptoms may at times resemble myocardial infarction.

Electrocardiogram and chest X-ray are usually unremarkable. Only sometimes is there a small pleural effusion. Barium or Gastrograffin swallow shows a typical diagnostic picture of a double-barrelled oesophagus (Fig. 5; Moghissi and Joyeux, 1977).

6.1. Management

The patient can often be treated conservatively by gastrostomy or parenteral feeding for 7–14 days, according to the severity of the case. Surgical treatment is occasionally required for drainage of the chest and/or perforation when there is doubt about the integrity of the oesophagus.

7. Mallory–Weiss syndrome

This is usually painless upper alimentary tract bleeding which manifests as haematemesis or occasionally melaena. The cause is a localised mucosal tear in the lower oesophagus. Contrast medium radiography is usually unhelpful and the diagnosis is made endoscopically. At times, the latter is also unhelpful and a

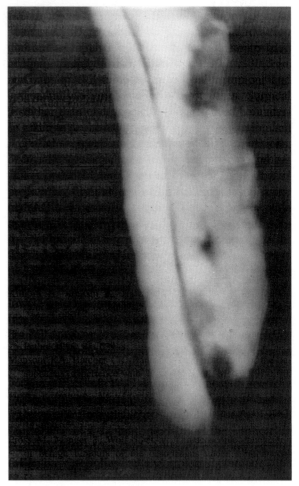

Fig. 5. Barium contrast study showing a typical picture of a double-barrelled oesophagus due to intramural oesophageal perforation.

surgical exploration is the only means of establishing the definite diagnosis.

In some instances the haemorrhage subsides spontaneously and there follows no recurrence of haemorrhage or any symptoms. When the bleeding does not subside, surgical exploration is mandatory. In the absence of any demonstrable oesophageal lesion, an upper abdominal incision and gastrotomy near the oesophagogastric junction provides excellent exposure. Intragastric blood clot is evacuated and the stomach washed with saline solution to demonstrate the site of laceration. The bleeding mucosal tear is repaired with continuous 2.0 absorbable vicryl. Attention is paid not to overlook any other pathology such as a gastric or duodenal ulcer. The gastrostomy and abdominal wound are then repaired, leaving a nasogastric tube in the stomach. Food intake is allowed after a few days.

References and further reading

Barrett NR. Report of a case of spontaneous perforationof the oesophagus successfully treated by operation. Br J Surg 1947; 35: 216–218.

Brinkman WT, Shanewise JS, Clements SD, Mansour KA. Transesophageal echocardiography: not an innocuous procedure. Ann Thorac Surg 2001; 72: 1725–1726.

British Society of Gastroenterology (1986) Memorandum. Endoscopy committee of the British Society of Gastroenterology. J Medical Defence Union 1986; 3: 17–18.

Collins C, Arumugasamy M, Larkin J, Martin S, O'Sullivan GC. Thoracoscopic repair of instrumental perforation of the oesophagus: first report. Ir J Med Sci 2002; 171: 68–70.

Dawson J, Cockel R. Oesophageal perforation at fibre optic gastroscopy. BMJ 1981; 283: 583.

Derbes VL, Mitchell RE Jr. Herman Boerhaave's *Atrocic Nec Descriptiprius, Morbi Historia* (the first translation of the classic case of rupture of the oesophagus, with annotations). Bull Med Libr Assoc 1955; 43: 217–240.

Jones WG, Ginsberg RJ. Oesophageal perforation — a continuing challenge. Ann Thorac Surg 1992; 52: 534–543.

Jougan J, Cantini O, Delcambre F, Miniti A, Velly JF. Esophageal perforation: life-threatening complication of endotracheal intubation. Eur J Cardiothorac Surg 2001; 20: 7–10.

Kerr WF. Spontaneous intramural rupture and intramural haematoma of the oesophagus. Thorax 1980; 35: 890–897.

Mallory GK, Weiss S. Haemorrhage of the cardiac orifice of the stomach due to vomiting. Am J Med Sci 1929; 178: 506–515.

Marks IN, Keet AD. Intramural rupture of the oesophagus. BMJ 1968; 25: 537–538.

Moghissi K. Instrumental perforation of the oesophagus. Br J Hosp Med 1988; 39(3): 231–236.

Moghissi K, Joyeux A. Rupture spontané intramurale de l'oesophage. J Chir 1977; 113(3): 263–267.

Moghissi K, Dietel M, Taylor GA. Oesophageal problems: use of nutritional support. In: Dietel M (ed.), Nutrition in clinical surgery (2nd ed.). Baltimore: Williams and Wilkins 1985; pp. 524–528.

Moghissi K, Pender D. Instrumental perforations of the oesophagus and their management. Thorax 1988; 43: 642–646.

Ohri S, Leikakos T, Pathi V, Townsend I, Fontain W. Primary repair of isaterogenic oesophageal perforation and Boerhaave's syndome. Ann Thorac Surg 1993: 55: 605–606.

Sandrasagra GA, English TAH, Milstein BB. The management and prognosis of oesophageal perforation. Br J Surg 1978; 65: 624–632.

Triggiani E, Belsey R. Oesophageal trauma incidence diagnosis and management. Thorax 1977; 32: 241–249.

Wang N, Razzourk AJ, Safavi A, et al. Delayed primary repair of intrathoracic esophageal perforation: is it safe? J Thorac Cardiovasc Surg 1996; 111: 114–122.

CHAPTER III.12

Motor disorders of the oesophagus

K. Moghissi

1. Introduction — Classification

Under this heading, we describe a group of conditions whose common characteristic is motility disturbance of the oesophagus as demonstrated by manometric study criteria. It is relevant to note that demonstration by manometric examination of abnormal pattern of motility, with no functional impairment or symptoms, is of no clinical significance. Therefore, clinical diagnosis of a motor disorder should not be based solely on abnormal motility pattern.

The usual symptoms associated with motor disorders are dysphagia and/or chest pain. Oesophageal chest pain is, at times, difficult to differentiate from cardiac ischemic pain, not only in intensity but also because they may co-exist. A clear history of onset of pain, its association with dysphagia or exercise and its radiation will facilitate the line of investigations to be pursued first to elucidate the aetiology. Cardiac investigation should always take precedence over oesophageal studies when in doubt.

Oesophageal motor disorders may be rationally grouped by manometric criteria. However, there is no universally accepted manometrically based classification because of difficulties in labelling some abnormal manometric patterns, variation in technique used and interpretation of results. Existing classifications take account of:

- Lower oesophageal sphincter (LOS) pressure and relaxation,
- Pattern of peristaltic activities of the body of the oesophagus with particular reference to:
  - Presence or absence of peristaltic activities,
  - Amplitude of peristaltic waves and contraction and manner of occurrence of contractions (spontaneous versus during swallow),

- Location of contractions and pattern of progression along the oesophagus (coordinated and sequential or otherwise).

Spechler and Castell (2001) have provided a comprehensive classification of functional disorders (Table 1).

For simplicity and ease of description we have classed motor disorder as follows:

- Condition characterised by lack of or inadequate relaxation of LOS including:
  - Achalasia
  - Pseudo-achalasia.
- Spastic disorders of the oesophagus exemplified by:
  - Diffuse oesophageal spasm
  - "Nutcracker" oesophagus.
- Miscellaneous motility disorders:
  - Oesophageal hypocontraction, e.g. disorder of the oesophagus in scleroderma
  - Unclassified non-specific motility disorders.

2. Motor disorder related to inadequate or lack of LOS relaxation

2.1. Achalasia of the cardia

Hurst in 1915 (cited in Ellis and Olsen, 1969) introduced the term achalasia (lack of relaxation) to describe a condition in which the lower oesophageal sphincter fails to relax in advance of an oncoming food bolus which, therefore, stops short of entering normally into the stomach.

Onset of the disease is often insidious with progressive dysphagia as the presenting symptom. Occasionally dysphagia may start suddenly following a psychological upset or strain. Pain is often present

Table 1

Spechler and Castell (2001): 'Functional' classification of oesophageal motility disorders

Achalasia (true disorder)

- Absent distal peristalsis
- Elevated resting LOS (>45 mmHg)
- Incomplete LOS relasation (residual pressure >8 mmHg)
- Elevated baseline oesophageal pressure

Incoordinated motility

- e.g. Diffuse oesophageal spasm
- Simultaneous contractions ≥20%
- Wet swallows
- Intermittent peristalsis
- Repetitive contractions ≥3 peaks
- Prolonged duration contractions >6 seconds
- Retrograde contractions
- Isolated incomplete LOS relation >8 mmHg

Hypercontraction oesophagus

- e.g. Hypertensive peristalsis (nutcracker)
- Increased distal peristaltic amplitude >180 mmHg
- Increased peristaltic duration >6 seconds
- Hypertensive LOS
- Resting LOSP >45 mmHg
- Incomplete LOS relaxation (residual pressure 8 mmHg)

Hypocontracting oesophagus

- Ineffective motility
- Increased non transmitted peristalsis >30%
- Low distal peristaltic amplitude <30 mmHg
- Hypotensive LOS (may be secondary to GOR)
- Resting LOSP 10 mmHg

and regurgitation is characteristic of well-developed cases. Nutritional deficiencies and pulmonary complications may exist in advanced cases.

2.1.1. Diagnosis

Diagnosis is made radiologically and by manometric studies. Barium contrast transit in fully developed cases shows considerable dilatation and elongation of the oesophagus with a string like stenosis of the lower "cardia" region of the organ (Fig. 1a). Video-radiography examination and recording has the advantage of a dynamic image showing both the characteristics of transit through the sphincter and the radiological features of peristaltic waves which can be repeatedly viewed.

Typical manometric features of a well-developed case are:

- Lack or inadequate relaxation of the LOS during wet swallow,
- Reduced or absent peristaltic activities in the body of the oesophagus, particularly at its distal end. It

is to be noted that there is some variation in the peristaltic activities in less well-developed cases

Endoscopy is not diagnostic but should be carried out to exclude neoplasia. This examination in well-developed cases shows considerable dilatation of the oesophagus which contains a large amount of food debris.

2.1.2. Aetio-pathology

The aetiology of primary achalasia is unknown. Anatomo-pathological features in a fully developed case show a dilated, elongated and thick walled tube in the whole of its extent except for the lower 5 to 6 cm. This is remarkably constricted and is straight, more fibrotic and thinner. The mucosa is often folded and presents with inflammatory changes and petechial haemorrhage. Microscopically, a typical achalasia has degeneration of neurones in the oesophageal wall and absence or reduction in a number of ganglion cells in Auerbach's plexus.

2.1.3. Management

Treatment options in achalasia are:

(a) Conservative medical treatment

Antispasmodics are generally ineffective. Reflux symptoms, if present, can be alleviated using anti-secretory drugs. Nitrate and calcium channel blocking drugs can be tried though these provide relief of pain rather than improvement in dysphagia.

(b) Dilatation

Balloon or other types of bougie have superseded the original Hurst mercury bougie. The author's preference is Maloney flexible bougies passed under direct vision. The mechanism by which dilatation is effective is difficult to explain. However, a number of patients respond to treatment which needs to be repeated at intervals. There is risk of perforation and/or subsequent gastro-oesophageal reflux.

(c) Surgery

Oesophageal myotomy (Fig. 1b): In the classical Hellers (1913) operation (cited in Ellis et al., 1958), myotomy is carried out over the constricted area of the oesophagus, incising and sharply dividing the whole of the muscle layer in the area and exposing the mucosa. The myotomy is extended upward to the cone-shaped zone above the constriction and down to the stomach to expose 0.5 to 1 cm of gastric mucosa. Care should be taken not to injure the mucosa. Should this occur, transverse stitching using slow-absorbing sutures will repair the mucosa. Most thoracic surgeons advocate a longer myotomy from the constricted inferior pulmonary vein, a distance of 8 to 10 cm.

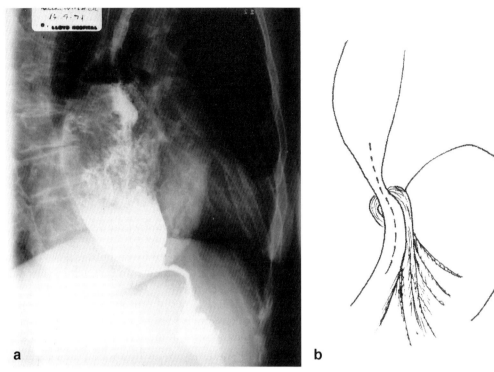

Fig. 1. (a) Barium swallow of a patient with achalasia of the cardia, (b) oesophageal myotomy.

– Laparotomy was originally used for 'classic' myotomy. Left thoracotomy is predominantly used by thoracic surgeons with the patient in right lateral position. Thoracotomy needs to be through 7th or 8th interspace and the limited access, muscle splitting method may be used.

– Laparoscopy and thoracoscopy access have been used in recent years. If extended myotomy is required thoracoscopy or thoracotomy approach should be carried out.

– Oesophagectomy: A selected few patients may need to undergo oesophageal resection and reconstruction for complicated and/or advanced achalasia or where there is suspicion of neoplasia.

– Results of myotomy are good in a high percentage of patients whether the trans-abdominal or trans-thoracic approach is used. Experience shows that uncomplicated cases have better results than those complicated by perforation through previous dilatation or in patients with associated reflux.

It is important that the operative procedure is designed and tailored to the individual patient.

• *Note on additional anti-reflux procedure*

The frequency of post-operative gastro-oesophageal reflux following myotomy in some series has lead to the recommendation that an anti-reflux procedure be carried out at the time of myotomy. In the author's experience this is only desirable when indicated by pre-operative evidence of reflux, and in those with reflux stricture in whom dilatation and anti-reflux procedures are needed.

– Complications of the operation are:
  Haemorrhage (reactionary),
  Pulmonary infection.

2.2. Pseudo-achalasias (syn: Atypical disorders of LOS relaxation)

This is a condition in which a dilated oesophagus is found together with inadequate relaxation and duration of relaxation of LOS. However, in some cases there is a high amplitude oesophageal contraction. Also, unlike primary (typical) achalasia the aetiology is usually identifiable. Dysphagia is the outstanding symptom.

Two examples of the condition are:
• Chagas disease seen in central and South America in which the oesophagus is infected by protozoan parasites *Trypanosoma cruzi*
• Malignancy of the lower oesophagus in the region of the sphincter.

In both of the examples above, manometric studies alone are insufficient to achieve the diagnosis.

3. Spastic oesophagus

3.1. Diffuse oesophageal spasm

Diffuse oesophageal spasm (DOS) is a condition of unknown aetiology clinically characterised by episodes of spontaneous intermittent dysphagia and chest pain during deglutition. Unlike achalasia there are no demonstrable organic lesions in the wall of the oesophagus or abnormalities of the nervous plexus.

Contrast study shows normal transit or a variety of non-specific 'undulations' which radiologists refer to as 'tertiary contractions'. Sometimes a picture of corkscrew oesophagus is produced. There may also be multiple diverticula-like images.

The manometric pattern is generally described as being one of uncoordinated spastic contractions affecting the lower thoracic oesophagus. In more detail, such uncoordinated waves of contraction are characterised as simultaneous, repetitive and high amplitude waves. Richter et al. (1989) suggested that simultaneous contractions induced by wet swallow are the key characteristics of DOS. It is important to note that such simultaneous contractions can be observed at times in some cases with known aetiology such as gastro oesophagus reflex.

3.2. Hypertensive oesophagus (syn: 'nutcracker' oesophagus and oesophageal hypercontraction)

This condition is clinically akin to DOS with chest pain and dysphagia as the principal symptoms but with different manometric characteristics. The motility patterns most frequently reported are high amplitude peristaltic waves in the lower oesophagus which are not diffuse but segmental. The height of the amplitude of contractions has been the subject of debate. Dalton et al. (1988) suggested the amplitude should exceed 180 mmHg whereas Benjamin et al. (1983) put a value of 120 mmHg as a cut-off level for these waves of contraction to be diagnostic of nutcracker oesophagus. The resting pressure of LOS is not usually elevated.

3.2.1. Treatment
Treatment of spastic oesophageal disorders is difficult and essentially symptomatic.

In patients with evidence of reflux, anti-secre-

tionary drugs (H$_2$ antagonists and proton pump inhibitors) should be tried.

- Reassurance, psychotherapy and sedatives or anti-depressants may be useful in some patients with anxiety and depressive tendency in order to alleviate their symptoms.
- Nitrates and calcium channel blockers often succeed in relieving chest pain.
- In selected patients when medication brings no relief extended myotomy is indicated.

4. Miscellaneous motility disorders

4.1. Hypocontraction of the oesophagus

This is exemplified by oesophageal disorder in scleroderma (syn: progressive systemic sclerosis, systemic sclerosis).

Scleroderma is a disorder of connective tissue in which there is an excessive deposition of collagen and fibrous tissue in the skin, alimentary tract and many other organs such as lungs, heart and kidneys. In the case of the oesophagus, fibrosis and vascular obliteration affect oesophageal muscles and the wall generally. The clinical manifestation is dependent on the:
(a) Extent of the disease,
(b) Organs which are predominantly or exclusively involved.

The incidence of oesophageal involvement is variable. In one post-mortem study reported by D'Angelo et al (1969) there was a 74% oesophageal involvement.

4.1.1. Clinical presentation
Compared with the high incidence of oesophageal involvement found in post-mortem cases, the clinical symptomatic oesophageal complication of the disease is much less prevalent. Oesophageal disorders of scleroderma occur mostly in patients with arteriosclerosis and Raynaud's phenomenon.

The patients' symptoms are related to gastro-oesophageal reflux with heartburn and typically, regurgitation of food. Dysphagia, when present, is more attributable to reflux stricture than motility disorder.

Barium swallow studies show a variety of features ranging from normal to the presence of a stricture. In some patients, the oesophagus contour is straight and there is a reduction of peristaltic activities similar to achalasia. Reflux can be demonstrated in symptomatic patients.

Manometric changes are usually seen in the distal two-thirds of the oesophagus. The peristaltic activities are diminished or absent resulting in ineffective oesophageal motility and lack of response to swallow. The sphincteric pressure is usually reduced (hypotensive) but it does relax in response to swallowing.

The basic management is symptomatic and is similar to the treatment of gastro-oesophageal reflux and its complications. Effort should be made to treat the reflux with medication. A surgical antireflux procedure in severely symptomatic patients is indicated with the hope of preventing stricture formation. For those who have already developed stricture, surgical treatment should be considered. Two points regarding surgical treatment of this reflux stricture are relevant. The disease (scleroderma) is progressive and the results of surgery may be subject to the clinical and pathological course of the disease. Also, it is preferable not to excise the stricture but to carry out conservative surgery.

4.2. Miscellaneous non-specific (unclassified) conditions

There are a number of oesophageal motor disorders the manometric pattern of which do not correspond to any of the hitherto named conditions. Some such manometric abnormalities are accompanied by symptoms whilst others are asymptomatic. At the present time, the interpretation of these motor disorders and their correlation with symptoms remains speculative. This is supported by the fact that therapeutic correction in some symptomatic patients does not bring relief of symptoms.

- Hypertensive sphincter: The majority of patients do not have severe symptoms, presumably because the sphincter, in spite of its raised pressure, will relax in response to swallow. Those who have severe symptoms benefit from extended myotomy.
- Corkscrew oesophagus: This is more a radiological description of an oesophageal condition, or even a curiosity, than a clinical entity or disease (Fig. 2). The condition can be asymptomatic or mildly symptomatic. At times it is associated with pain and dysphagia and manometric findings are characteristic of diffuse spasm.

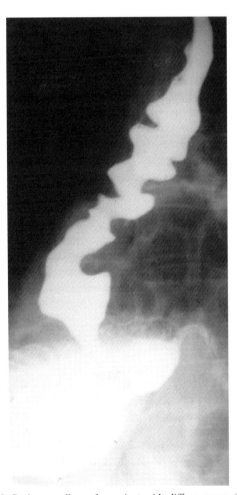

Fig. 2. Barium swallow of a patient with diffuse spasm (corkscrew oesophagus).

References and further reading

Achem SR, Kolts BE, Burton L. Segmental versus diffuse nutcracker esophagus: an intermittent motility pattern. Am J Gastroenterol 1993; 88: 847–851.

Adler DG, Romero Y. Primary esophageal motility disorders. Mayo Clin Proc 2001; 76: 195–200.

Benjamin SB, O'Donnell JK, Hancock J, et al. Prolonged radio nuclide transit in 'nutcracker esophagus'. Dig Dis Sci 1983; 28: 775–779.

Clouse RE, Staino A. Manometric patterns using esophageal body and lower sphincter characteristics. Findings in 103 patients. Dig Dis Sci 1992; 37: 289–296.

Dalton CB, Castell DO, Richter JE. The changing face of the nutcracker esophagus. Am J Gastroenterol 1988; 83: 623–628.

D'Angelo WA, Fries JF, Masi AT, Shulman LE. Pathological observation in systemic schlerosis (scleroderma): A study of 58 autopsy cases and 58 matched controls. Am J Med 1969; 46: 428–440.

Devaney EJ, Lannettoni MD, Orringer MB, et al. Esophagectomy for achalasia: patient selection and clinical experience. Ann Thorac Surg 2001; 72: 854–858.

Ellis F Jr., Olsen EM, Holman CB, et al. Surgical treatment of cardio spasm (Achalasia of the oesophagus). Considerations of aspects of esophago-myotomy. JAMA 1958; 166: 29–36.

Ellis FH Jr., Olsen AM. Achalasia of the oesophagus (Major problems in clinical surgery, Vol. *a*). Philadelphia: WB Saunders, 1969; p. 221.

Finley RJ, Clifton JC, Stewart KC, Graham AJ. Worsley DF. Laparoscopic Heller myotomy improves esophageal emptying and the symptoms of achalasia. Arch Surg 2001; 136: 892–896.

Goldblum JR, Whute RI, Orringer MB, et al. Achalasia: a morphologic study of 42 resected specimens. Am J Physiol 1992; 18: 327–337.

Gonlachanvit S, Fisher RS, Parkman HP. Diagnostic modalities for achalasia. Gastrointest Endosc Clin N Am 2001; 11: 293–310.

Holloway RH, Dodds WJ, Helm JF, et al. Integrity of cholinergic innervation to the lower esophageal sphincter in achalasia. Gastroenterology 1986; 90: 924–929.

Jordan PH Jr. Long term results of esophageal myotomy for achalasia. J Am Coll Surg 2001; 193: 137–145.

Lock G, Holstege A, Lang B, et al. Gastrointestinal manifestations of progressive systemic sclerosis. Am J Gastroenterol 1997; 92: 763–771.

Nguyen NT, Wang P, Follette D. Laparoscopy or thoracoscopy for achalasia. Semin Thorac Cardiovasc Surg 2000; 12: 201–205.

Pasrica PJ, Rai R, Ravich WJ, et al. Botulinum toxin for achalasia: long term outcome and predictors of response. Gastroenterology 1996; 110: 1410–1415.

Reynolds JC, Parkman HP. Achalasia. Gastronterol Clic N Am 1989; 18: 223–255.

Richter JE, Bradley LA, Castell DO. Esophageal chest pain: current controversies in pathogenesis, diagnosis and therapy. Ann Intern Med 1989; 110: 66–78.

Spechler SJ, Castell DO. Classification of oesophageal motility abnormalities. Gut 2001; 49: 145–151.

K. Moghissi, J.A.C. Thorpe and F. Ciulli (Eds.)
Moghissi's Essentials of Thoracic and Cardiac Surgery

Diverticula of the oesophagus

D. Nikzas, K. Moghissi and J.A.C. Thorpe

1. Definition and classification

The term diverticulum is used to describe sacculation other than that caused by a stricture. In some cases the diverticulum is a mere mucosal protrusion through a weakened oesophageal wall. This is referred to as false diverticulum. In others the sacculation involves the complete layers of the wall; this is a true diverticulum. Diverticula may project from the wall at any location of the oesophagus and, rarely, they can present as diffuse mural diverticulosis.

Diverticula may be classified according to their location along the oesophagus, their aetiology and the mechanism of their formation or by the structure of their wall.

1.1. Location

The most common locations are:
- Pharyngo-oesophageal junction (i.e. Zenker's diverticulum — Fig. 1),
- Mid-oesophagus (near left main bronchus — Fig. 2),
- Distal oesophagus, just above the oesophageal hiatus (epiphrenic diverticula).

1.2. Mechanism of development

According to the mechanism of their formation, diverticula are known as:
- Pulsion diverticula — formed by an increase in intraluminal oesophageal pressure
- Traction diverticula — developed as a result of pulling the oesophageal wall from without.

By and large, pharyngo-oesophageal junction and epiphrenic diverticula develop by pulsion mechanism and are a mucosal protrusion through the wall (i.e. false). Mid-oesophageal diverticula are mostly true diverticula and until recently they were thought to develop by traction mechanism, such as that resulting from the pulling by chronic tuberculous lymphadenitis (or histoplasmosis) in the mediastinum. This however is believed only rarely to be the case.

1.3. Aetiology

Aetiological factors involved in the development of diverticula are varied and, to a certain extent, depend on their location.
- In Zenker's diverticulum, the disorder of co-ordination between pharyngeal muscle contraction and the upper oesophageal sphincter relaxation

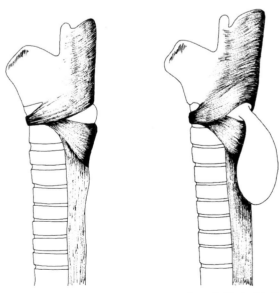

Fig. 1. Diagram showing pharyngo-oesophageal (Zenker's) diverticulum (pharyngeal pouch).

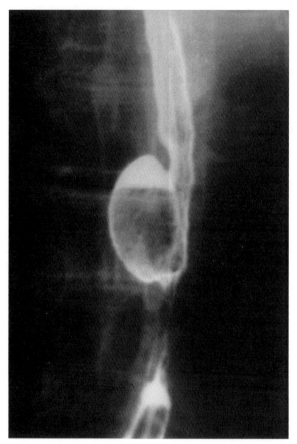

Fig. 2. Contrast study demonstrating mid-oesophageal diverticulum.

during swallowing is a major factor. This leads to the development of a high pressure within the pharynx which forces mucosal protrusion through the Killian dehiscence, an anatomical weakness in the posterior muscular wall of the pharynx between the oblique fibres of the inferior constrictor and the transverse fibres which form the cricopharyngeus ring.

- In the case of mid-oesophageal diverticula, the traction mechanism once suggested is now discarded by many in favour of pulsion mechanism occasioned by oesophageal motility disturbances. Physiological studies using manometric and dynamic contrast swallow methods indicate that diffuse oesophageal spasms, vigorous achlasic and other non-specific oesophageal motility disorders are present in most patients with mid-oesophageal diverticula.
- The aetiology in epiphrenic diverticula, although rarely congenital, is generally attributed to a motor disorder of the lower oesophagus. An ab-

normally high relaxation pressure of the lower oesophageal sphincter with/without gastro-oesophageal reflux is almost always implicated.
- A rare condition of diffuse intramural diverticulosis is said to arise from secondary changes in submucosal oesophageal glands. Such changes occur in consequence of chronic inflammatory processes promoting dilatation of excretory conduits with the development of diverticulosis, which may be segmental or diffuse in extent.

1.4. General investigation of diverticula

- Barium contrast study is a mandatory requirement. Dynamic images obtained by video recording is preferable.
- Endoscopy is necessary in all.
- Motility and pH studies are important additions which can determine the operative or treatment method.

2. Pharyngo-oesophageal junction (syn: Zenker's Diverticulum — pharyngeal pouch)

This is a false diverticulum and consists of mucosal herniation at the pharyngo-oesophageal junction between the oblique and horizontal fibres of the inferior construction muscle of the pharynx (Killian dehiscence: Fig. 1). The condition was first described by Ludlow (1769) but it is Zenker's name which is associated with pharyngeal pouches due to his particular interest and review of the condition in 1874 (Zenker and Von Ziemssen, 1874). The fact that the condition usually occurs in patients over the age of 50 years overrules its congenital aetiology.

Physiological studies indicate that motility disturbances at or about the pharyngo-oesophageal junction are important aetiological factors. The size of the pharyngo-oesophageal diverticulum can vary between a dimple to a large bag which descends behind the oesophagus to reach the root of the neck. Association of pharyngeal pouch with hiatal hernia and gastro-oesophageal reflux is not uncommon, both representing the manifestation of oesophageal motor disorders.

2.1. Clinical features and diagnosis

The condition affects predominantly the male population over the age of 60 years. A number of patients with large diverticula are asymptomatic. The symptoms, when present, are intermittent dysphagia, regurgitation and vomiting of undigested food. Sometimes the prodromal symptoms are dominated by cough, foul smelling sputum and chest infection. At times nutritional deficiencies and loss of weight are predominant symptoms.

Diagnosis is established by contrast study showing the pouch. Video radiography is an important addition to demonstrate rapid sequence of the swallow. Endoscopy is a mandatory requirement, not only to eliminate mucosal anomalies and neoplastic changes but also to remove existing food debris and occasional foreign bodies which can be lodged in the pouch.

It is important to emphasise that:

- Pharyngo-oesophagoscopy needs to be carried out by an expert, preferably using a rigid open-ended instrument,
- Extreme care is required to visualise the pouch and its opening which is found behind the anteriorly situated pharyngo-oesophageal junction opening.

Physiological studies are useful in order to evaluate gastro-oesophageal reflux and motility disturbance. This should be considered as essential in the young and those with clinical incidence of reflux. Such studies become particularly relevant in those who are to be considered for surgical treatment in assisting choice of appropriate treatment method.

2.2. Treatment

There are a number of treatment options. The choice of method depends on many factors which include severity of symptoms, frequency of complication episodes such as chest infections, age and the general condition of the patient. Treatment methods are:

2.2.1. Bouginage

This may be applicable as a temporary measure in those who are being prepared for surgical resection. In this category are those with severe dysphagia and a large pouch with a wide neck. Such patients may have a serious respiratory infection needing treatment prior to operation for these diverticula. Repeated dilatation may also be indicated as a sole therapeutic method in those who are unfit or unsuitable for any operative procedure or when the surgical option is rejected by the patient.

2.2.2. Diverticulectomy/Endoscopic division of oesophago-diverticular wall (Dohlman's procedures)

This consists of endoscopy and division of septum between the pouch and the oesophagus. The muscular septum is divided using diathermy or the appropriate laser. More recently endoscopic stapling devices are used for diverticulectomy.

Diverticulectomy is particularly suitable for frail, elderly patients and those with poor general condition.

2.2.3. Diverticulopexy

The operation consists of exposure and identification of the sac (pouch) followed by its transposition so that the 'fundus' of the sac is turned upside down. The sac is thus suspended and then is fixed by stitches to the prevertebral fascia.

2.2.4. Cricopharyngeal myotomy

This operation can be carried out as the sole modality treatment when the diverticulum is small. It is also performed by many as complimentary to surgical excision of the diverticulum. After exposure of the diverticulum to its neck, the posterior horizontal part of the cricopharyngeus, which lies below the neck of the pouch, is identified and incised vertically. The aim is to divide all muscular strands by carrying the incision down to the mucosa. The incision should cover the whole length of the horizontal fibres and reach the oesophageal muscle proper distally. Myotomy, thus transforms a narrow neck diverticulum to a wide necked one.

2.2.5. Excision of the diverticulum (radical operation)

This consists of exposure of the diverticulum and its excision. Surgical exposure can be obtained by a variety of approaches and incisions. An oblique incision along the anterior border of the sternomastoid muscles gives a generous exposure. On the other hand, horizontal incision over the lower third of the sternomastoid provides a better cosmetic result. In both cases, the incision is deepened and the sternomastoid muscle is retracted laterally and backwards to expose the carotid sheath which in turn is retracted laterally. The omohyoid muscle is divided and the thyroid gland with the larynx are retracted medially. The inferior thyroid artery and the middle thyroid vein may have to be divided between ligatures in order to get better access to the diverticulum, which is found behind the oesophagus itself. Injury to the recurrent laryngeal nerve is avoided. Several methods can be used for the identification of the sac.

The authors recommend packing the pouch through the mouth beforehand with ribbon gauze soaked in an antiseptic solution (aqueous solution of 1/5000 chlorhexidine); this permits the identification and easy dissection of the pouch at operation. Once the pouch is dissected and the neck of the diverticulum is clearly identified the gauze is removed per oral by the anaesthetist who has retained the end clipped outside the mouth. Once the apex of the diverticulum is identified it can be grasped with tissue forceps (such as Allis or Duval forceps). Dissection is continued upwards towards the neck of the diverticulum. The neck of the diverticulum, as it protrudes between the horizontal and oblique fibres of the inferior constrictor, is divided and sewn over. Alternatively a curved clamp applied to the neck of the sac at a right angle to the oesophagus, or a transfixation catgut stitch, achieves the objective. This is then covered over by three or four fine non-absorbable interrupted stitches applied to the musculature of the pharynx and oesophagus. There is no need for a drain in simple cases but when there are adhesions and oozing it is worthwhile inserting a corrugated drain in the peri-oesophageal space before closure of the wound. Feeding is resumed 48 hours after operation and the drain is withdrawn 24 hours after that. The patient is discharged four to five days after the operation.

3. Mid-oesophageal diverticula

These diverticula (Fig. 2) are reported by many as traction diverticula because of their frequent association in the past with tuberculous or other chronic lymphadenitis, They are often accompanied by motility disturbances of the oesophagus. Many cases are asymptomatic. When symptomatic, dysphagia and odynophagia are the usual symptoms. Sometimes the mode of presentation is one of repeated episodes of respiratory infections. Bleeding and oesophago-airway fistula occasionally complicate the condition. Surgical intervention is indicated in symptomatic cases and those presenting with complication. Barium contrast study, oesophagoscopy (sometimes bronchoscopy) and manometric studies are the prerequisite for surgical intervention. Excision of diverticulum is carried out after an appropriate thoracotomy and exposure. Myotomy alone may suffice for patients with motility disorders.

4. Lower oesophageal diverticula (epiphrenic)

In view of their position in the lower 8 to 10 cm of the oesophagus, these pulsion diverticula are referred to as epiphrenic or paradiaphragmatic diverticula. Often asymptomatic, these are usually associated with other oesophageal conditions. In 160 patients reported by Allen and Cladgett (1965), only 66 had no associated lesions and hiatus hernia followed by diffuse oesophageal spasm headed the list of concomitant conditions with 55 and 39 cases respectively. Except for local complications, such as inflammation at or around the diverticula which caused dysphagia and pain, in most instances symptoms are the result of associated conditions. In these, surgical treatment should be undertaken. Diverticulectomy is not advisable because in many instances the disease is the result of motility disturbance of the oesophagus and excision of a pouch is not likely to deal with the motility problem. Also in a high percentage of cases there are associated conditions which should be considered in the plan of treatment. The common practice is long segment oesophageal myotomy with or without diverticulectomy. Preferably, the surgical treatment of associated conditions such as repair of hiatal hernia is also undertaken.

Not everyone sees the necessity for diverticulectomy, except for diverticula with a very narrow neck, and many surgeons (including the authors) believe it to be non-contributory to surgical results and adding to possible complications. However, the treatment of the associated pathology is mandatory and may demand excision of the diverticulum together with part of the oesophagus followed by reconstruction.

References and further reading

Allen TA, Clagett OT. Changing concept in the surgical treatment of pulsion diverticula of the lower oesophagus. J Thorac Cardiovasc Surg 1965; 50: 455–462.

Cook J, Gabb M, Panagopoulos V, et al. Pharyngeal (Zenker) diverticulum is a disorder of upper oesophageal sphincter opening. Gastroenterology 1992: 103: 1229–1231.

Dohlman C, Mattson B. The role of the crico-pharyngeal muscle in cases of hypo-pharyngela diverticula. A cinero-entenograph study. Am J Roentgenol 1939; 81: 561–569.

Ellis FJ Jr., Schlegal JF, Lynch VP et al. Crico-pharyngeal myotomy for pharyngo-oesophageal diverticulum. Ann Surg 1969; 170: 340–349

Ingelfinger FJ, Kramer P. Dysphagia produced by a contractile ring in the lower oesophagus. Gastroenterology 1953; 23: 419–430.

Ludlow A. A case of obstructed deglutition from a perternatural dilation of a bag formed in the pharynx. Observations and enquiries. Society of Physicians London 1769; 3: 85–101.

Mirza S, Dutt SN, Minhas SS, Irving RM. A retrospective review of pharyngeal pouch surgery in 56 patients. Ann R Coll Surg Eng 2002; 84: 247–251.

Omote K, Feussner H, Stein HJ, Ungeheuer A, Siewert JR. Endoscopic stapling diverticulostomy for Zenker's diverticulum. Surg Endosc 1999; 13: 535–538.

Schatzki R, Gray JE. Dysphagia due to diaphragm-like localised narrowing in the lower oesophagus (lower oesophageal ring). Am J Roentgenol, RadioTher Nucl Med 1953; 70: 911–923.

Zenker FA, Von Ziemssen H. Krankheiten des Ösophagus. In: Von Ziemssen H (ed.), Handbuch der speziellen Pathologie und Therapie (vol. 7, part 1 supp). Leipzig: FC Vogel, 1874; pp. 1–208.

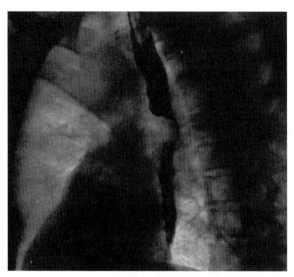

Fig. 1. Barium contrast study of Leiomyoma.

4. Other miscellaneous tumours

A variety of different benign tumours are seen from time-to-time and reported in the literature.

- Neurofibromas are generally submucosal (intramural) and can be totally asymptomatic.
- Schwannomas are more on the external surface of the oesophagus.
- Lipomas are generally small and asymptomatic.
- Hemangiomas are tumour-like malformations. They are submucosal and, as expected, can cause haemorrhage.

- Adenomas of the oesophagus are rare polypoid masses which occur occasionally and develop from metaplastic mucosa. Some appear to have the potential of malignancy.
- Granular cell tumours are a benign tumour and generally asymptomatic in most cases. Surgical rather than endoscopic excision should be undertaken to avoid recurrence.
- Pseudo-tumours are rare tumour-like conditions, usually arising in the lower oesophagus and often pedunculated. Their origin is uncertain but is possibly from ulceration of the lower oesophagus.

References and further reading

Cochet B, Hohl P, Sans M, et al. Asphyxia caused by laryngeal impaction of an esophageal polyp. Arch Otolaryngol 1980; 106: 176–178.

Kimura H, Konishi K, Kawamura T, et al. Smooth muscle tumours of the oesohagus; clincopathological findings in six patients. Dis Esophagus 1999; 12: 77–81.

Lee RG. Adenoma arising in Barrett's oesophagus. Am J Clin Pathol 1986; 85: 629.

Mansour KA, Hatcher CR, Haun CL. Benign tumour of the oesophagus: experience with 20 cases. South Med J 1977; 70: 48.

Plachta A. Benign tumours of the oesophagus: review of the literature and report of 99 cases. Am J Gastroenterol 1962; 38: 639.

Pross M, Manger T, Wolf S, et al. Thoracoscopic enucleation of benign tumours of the oesophagus under simultaneous flexible esophagoscopy. Surg Endosc 2000; 14: 1146–1148.

CHAPTER III.15

Cancer of the oesophagus

A. Lerut and G. Decker

1. Epidemiology

Oesophageal cancer currently ranks ninth in the list of the most common cancers in the world. As it is asymptomatic in its early stages, most cases are diagnosed at an advanced stage when the disease has spread beyond the oesophagus. The overall 5-year survival of oesophageal cancer therefore is only 2–8%. Incidence of oesophageal carcinoma ranges widely according to sex, race, geographical area and socio-economic background. In most countries, oesophageal carcinoma is two to four times more frequent in males than in females. Squamous cell carcinoma is five times as frequent in blacks compared to Caucasians. The annual age-adjusted incidence varies from 5/100,000 in the USA to 12.5/100,000 in some regions of France (Normandy). Endemic areas however exist in China (Linxian province), South Africa (Transkei) or Iran, with incidences up to 139/100,000 in Linxian or 263/100,000 in females from the Caspian Sea littoral of Iran (Waterhouse et al., 1974; Desoubeaux et al., 1999; Pera, 2000).

In many parts of the world, e.g. Germany, Denmark and the former Soviet Union, the incidence of oesophageal carcinoma has been rising, maybe in part due to increased alcohol consumption. In Finland and other countries, however, the incidence and mortality from oesophageal cancer seems to be declining.

Incidence patterns of histological subtypes are also changing. While the incidence of squamous cell carcinoma is stable or even on the decrease in some countries, adenocarcinoma of the oesophagus and gastro-oesophageal junction (GO junction) has had the fastest rising incidence of all carcinomas in the western world during the 1970s and 1980s. Internationally, the incidence of adenocarcinoma of the oesophagus is estimated to have risen by 5–10% per year during the eighties. In Olmsted County (Minnesota, USA) the incidence of oesophageal adenocarcinoma rose from 0.13 for 1935–1971 to 0.74 for 1974–1989 while the incidence of adenocarcinoma of the oesophago-gastric junction rose from 0.25 to 1.34 per 100,000 person-years during the same time period (Pera et al., 1993). In France (Burgundy) the proportion of adenocarcinomas has risen from 5.6% between 1976 and 1987 to 20.1% between 1991 and 1993 (Desoubeaux et al., 1999). In Norway the annual incidence of adenocarcinoma increased by 17% for the male population and 14% for the female population between 1983 and 1992.

In our own institution (Table 1; Lerut, 1998), the proportion of adenocarcinomas amongst all operated carcinomas of the oesophagus and gastro-oesophageal junction rose from 54% in 1991, to 61% between 1992 and 1996 and reached 85% in 1997.

2. Aetiology

Epidemiological studies have identified heavy tobacco and alcohol consumption as the two main risk factors for developing oesophageal squamous cell carcinoma. More than 95% of patients with a squamous cell carcinoma are smokers. The number of cigarettes smoked and the amount of alcohol intake might play a role but their individual causal relationship is hard to demonstrate since these two habits frequently coexist.

Genetic predisposition is unusual but has been illustrated for autosomal dominant keratosis palmaris and plantaris (Tylosis). Ninety-five percent of these patients may develop oesophageal cancer before the age of 65. Nutritional factors may play an important role as deficiencies in vitamins A, B, C and D have been identified in those regions with the highest inci-

Table 1

Histologic type and anatomical site of all carcinomas of the oesophagus and GOJ resected at the University Hospital of Leuven between January 1996 and April 1999 (Lerut, 1998).

	Adenocarcinoma carcinoma	Squamous cell	Other [a]	Total
Cervical oesophagus	0	9	0	9
Upper thoracic oesophagus	0	21	0	21
Mid thoracic oesophagus	9	48	1	58
Lower thoracic oesophagus	99	25	2	126
Gastro-oesophageal junction	95	0	0	95
Total	203	103	3	309

[a] Other: one undifferentiated small cell carcinoma, one melanoma and one adeno-squamous carcinoma

dences of oesophageal cancer. Carotenoids, vitamins C and E and calcium supplements might act as preventives of oesophageal carcinogenesis. A prospective randomised double blind study from Huixian has shown that oral calcium supplementation (600 mg/day) may favor regression of pre-cancerous lesions, which are endemic in that part of China. Nitrosamines derived from nitrites and nitrates in food may further act as important carcinogens while regular consumers of aspirin and other non-steroid anti-inflammatory drugs might benefit from a relative risk reduction (odds ratio from 0.37 for adenocarcinoma to 0.49 for squamous cell carcinoma).

Other risk factors have been involved such as caustic injury, achalasia, oesophageal webs and Plumner–Vinson syndrome. Although there is no definitive evidence, chronic inflammation and prolonged exposure of the oesophagus to potent carcinogens secondary to oesophageal stasis of endoluminal contents seems to be a common mechanism leading to cancer in these conditions.

Chronic inflammation such as in gastro-oesophageal reflux oesophagitis might be another risk factor. A nationwide epidemiological study in Sweden (1995–1997), identified a strong and probably causal relationship between gastro-oesophageal reflux and oesophageal adenocarcinoma (Lagergren et al., 1999). The more frequent, severe and long lasting the symptoms of gastro-oesophageal reflux were, the greater was the risk of adenocarcinoma of the oesophagus (odds ratio 43.5). Such a strong relationship, however, was not identified for adenocarcinoma of the cardia (odds ratio 4.4).

Most adenocarcinomas (20–80%) of the distal oesophagus arise from metaplastic areas of specialized columnar epithelium (Barrett), usually of the intestinal type. Patients presenting with the latter have a 5% risk of developing oesophageal cancer within five years. As this risk is at least fifty times higher compared to a normal population, Barrett's oesophagus certainly requires continuous endoscopic surveillance. The modalities of such an ideal surveillance programme however remain controversial.

3. Pathology

Oesophageal carcinoma results from an accumulation of mutations in different suppressor genes and oncogenes. Multiple chromosomal deletions have been implicated (13q, 5q, 18q, 3p, 9p, 17q). As in many other epithelial tumours, *p*53 mutation results in loss of apoptosis and seems to be an early event in the cascade towards oesophageal carcinoma. Over-expression of *p*53 usually precedes aneuploidy and is a feature of a wide spectrum of pathologic changes from metaplasia to low or high grade dysplasia up to invasive carcinoma, both for adenocarcinoma and squamous cell carcinoma. In Barrett's metaplasia a clear correlation exists between over-expression of *p*53 and malignant degeneration.

The most frequent histological types of oesophageal carcinoma are squamous cell carcinoma and adenocarcinoma (Table 1). Their histological features may be well, moderately or poorly differentiated. Undifferentiated carcinomas (either large or small cell), combined adenosquamous carcinomas, or other malignant neoplasms such as melanomas or sarcomas may occasionally occur in the oesophagus.

Squamous cell carcinoma (SCC) is most frequently localized in the middle third of the oesophagus and tends to be better differentiated than adenocarcinoma. Verrucous carcinoma is a rare variant of well-differentiated SCC whereas spindle cell carcinoma is a variant of undifferentiated carcinoma. The latter has to be differentiated from sarcoma or carcino-sarcoma.

Most adenocarcinoma arises from Barrett's meta-plasia or glandular metaplasia in the oesophageal mucosa. These are mostly located in the distal third of the oesophagus or at the gastro-oesophageal junction (GOJ).

Dysplasia is a precancerous epithelial lesion which is histologically characterized by nuclear enlargement, hyperchromaticity and increased mitotic activity. Squamous cell dysplasia is found preceding a communal squamous cell carcinoma (SCC). Glandular dysplasia is associated with adenocarcinoma complicating Barrett's oesophagus. Dysplasia develops more frequently in metaplasia of the intestinal or the gastric than of the junctional type. Dysplasia is graded low, moderate or high grade with increasing relative risks for cancer. High grade dysplasia is considered as carcinoma in situ (Cis) but the natural history of this condition is still not well defined.

4. Anatomical location

Empirically, tumours of the oesophagus are allocated to four anatomical regions:

- Cervical oesophagus: extends from the lower border of the cricoid cartilage to the suprasternal notch (±18 cm from the upper incisor teeth). The post-cricoïd region (crico-pharyngeal muscle) is of particular importance since its involvement generally precludes surgical conservation of the larynx.
- Upper thoracic oesophagus: from the thoracic inlet to the tracheal bifurcation (±24 cm from the upper incisor teeth).
- Middle thoracic oesophagus: from the tracheal bifurcation to half-distance from the oesophago-gastric junction (±32 cm from the upper incisor teeth).
- Lower thoracic oesophagus: distal half of the distance between the tracheal bifurcation to the oesophago-gastric junction (±40 cm from the upper incisor teeth). This segment includes the abdominal oesophagus and measures approximately 8 cm in length.

Tumours of the gastro-oesophageal junction (GOJ) are currently classified as gastric cancer. However their natural behavior and therefore their therapeutic approach is similar to tumours of the oesophagus. Ideally tumours of the cardia should be defined as those of the initial 1 or 2 cm of the stomach (Hölscher et al., 1995a). There is however no strict consensus for this definition as many tumours have completely destroyed the Z-line (transition zone between normal squamous oesophageal epithelium and columnar gastric epithelium), thus making an exact measurement of the distance between the core of the tumour and the Z-line impossible. The most unequivocal classification system might consider as tumours of the cardia and GOJ, all adenocarcinomas having their core within 5 cm from the anatomical junction between oesophagus and stomach as seen on the surgical specimen (Steup et al., 1996). Tumours which are mainly located in the stomach are considered to be gastric cancer, even if they encroach into the oesophagus. Squamous cell carcinomas and Barrett's adenocarcinoma located mainly in the tubular oesophagus are considered to be oesophageal tumours and are hereby excluded from the group of GOJ tumours.

5. Tumour spread

Oesophageal carcinoma progresses by:

- Local spread in all directions. (Fig. 1). Intraluminal proliferation will cause symptoms of dysphagia which will usually lead to detection of the tumour. More 'ulcerative' tumour growth may result in few symptoms until the tumour has infiltrated mediastinal structures such as the left main bronchus or trachea, the recurrent nerves, aorta, pericardium or vertebras.
- Lymphatic spread: The oesophagus is marked by a rich network of submucosal lymphatics which allows easy tumour spread along the oesophagus to lymph nodes far from the primary tumour.

Regional lymph nodes for the oesophagus are, for the cervical oesophagus, the cervical nodes including the supraclavicular nodes, and, for the intrathoracic oesophagus, the mediastinal and perigastric nodes, excluding the celiac nodes.

Peri-oesophageal lymph node involvement is an early process. Overall 41% to 81% of patients (Zhang et al., 1994; Fok et al., 1994; Isono et al., 1991; Lerut et al., 1994; Akiyama et al., 1994; Baba et al., 1994) have metastatic lymph nodes at the time of the initial presentation. The chance for positive loco-regional nodes is close to 0% for intra-epithelial (T1a) tumours (Isono et al., 1991; Akiyama et al., 1994; Hölscher et al., 1995a), 21 to 56% for T1b tumours (Hölscher et al., 1995a; Isono et al., 1991; Akiyama et al., 1994; Baba et al., 1994; Hölscher et al., 1995a; Ide et al., 1994; Nishimaki et al., 1999), 58 to 78% for T2 (Hölscher et al., 1995a; Isono et al., 1991; Akiyama et al., 1994; Baba et al., 1994; Ide et al., 1994), 74 to 83% for T3 (Hölscher et al., 1995a; Isono et al., 1991; Lerut et al., 1994; Akiyama et al., 1994; Baba et al.,

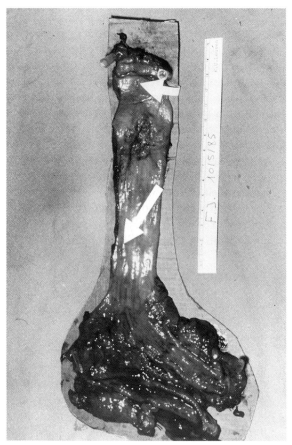

Fig. 1. Surgical specimen showing a SCC of the middle third of the oesophagus with two small satellite lesions (arrows) located in the upper and lower third of the oesophagus.

1994; Ide et al., 1994) and 83 to 100% for T4 tumours (Hölscher et al., 1995a; Isono et al., 1991; Baba et al., 1994; Ide et al., 1994). Oesophageal cancer also has a high propensity to invade distant lymph nodes without involving local nodes (skip metastasis); e.g. 24% of "early" submucosal tumours may have skip metastasis to distant cervical or abdominal nodes without local lymph node involvement (Nishimaki et al., 1999).

- Haematogenous spread is the mechanism of metastasis to distant organs, most frequently to liver, lung, bone and adrenals.

6. Clinical presentation

Early stage cancer is asymptomatic and is usually detected during endoscopies performed for other conditions of the GI tract or as part of surveillance programmes for Barrett's oesophagus. More advanced tumours become symptomatic either by obstructing the passage of bolus, or by direct in-

vasion of the organs surrounding the oesophagus. The most common symptom is progressive dysphagia, first to solids then to liquids. Swallowing may be painful (odynophagia) or lead to coughing in high-situated tumours or in the presence of fistula. Sialorrhea and regurgitation appear secondarily to oesophageal obstruction. Nocturnal regurgitation may then lead to inhalation pneumonia. Weight loss appears early, due to interference with normal food intake and later from tumour toxicity (nausea, horror carnis) thus leading to inanition and asthenia.

Invasion of mediastinal structures may present as tracheo-oesophageal fistulas (coughing related to swallowing, purulent broncho-pneumopathies, hemoptoe), recurrent nerve invasion (hoarseness), pericardial invasion (dysrythmias) or parietal pain (costo-vertebral invasion).

Clinical examination is negative in patients with early carcinoma of the oesophagus and the GO junction. A large number of patients, mostly with SCC, will present with signs of important alcohol and tobacco consumption. Halitosis may be noted in patients with obstructive tumours. Enlarged supraclavicular or cervical adenopathies and severe inanition are usually signs of advanced disease.

7. Diagnostic strategy and preoperative patient assessment

7.1. Diagnosis

As only early stage carcinoma has some chance of cure, a very low threshold should be adopted to perform fibreoptic upper GI endoscopy in all previously asymptomatic patients presenting with a positive anamnesis for dysphagia.

The vast majority of invasive oesophageal tumours are diagnosed by endoscopy (Fig. 2) or barium swallow. Endoscopy with biopsy is required in all patients for histological confirmation. Vital staining using Lugol or Toluidin blue may be helpful to guide biopsy in cases of early carcinoma thus increasing diagnostic accuracy. Barium swallow will usually show an irregularly lined oesophageal wall and is helpful mainly for topographic assessment of tumour extension and its relationship to the carina, as this may have therapeutic implications concerning the surgical access route.

When endoscopic biopsy identifies Barrett's oesophagus with high grade dysplasia, a second opinion by an expert pathologist is desirable because of important inter-observer variability in distinguishing

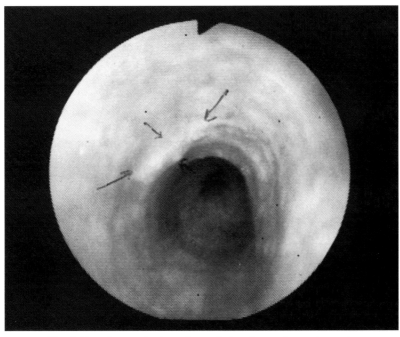

Fig. 2. Oesophagosopic view of an early invasive carcinoma (arrows).

intra-epithelial carcinoma and high grade dysplasia from moderate, low grade or no dysplasia. While the latter conditions require only surveillance, there is consensus that aggressive treatment should be instigated for high grade dysplasia since up to 50% of these surgical specimens will show foci of micro-invasive carcinoma at the time of operation.

All other diagnostic techniques are mainly for the purpose of staging loco-regional and distant tumour spread. Endo-oesophageal ultrasonography, thoracic and abdominal CT-scan, abdominal ultrasonography, MRI studies, cervical ultrasonography with fine needle aspiration biopsies of enlarged lymph nodes, bronchoscopy, ENT examination for proximal tumours, chest X-ray, radionuclide bone scan, invasive staging by laparoscopy or thoracoscopy or other, still investigational techniques such as 18-Fluoro-deoxy-glucose PET-scan (positron emission tomography) may serve this purpose.

7.2. Staging and classification

Adequate and extensive staging is required in every patient in order to be able to choose the most appropriate treatment modality and to give some indication of prognosis. The use of a uniform staging classification is further necessary to allow correct evaluation of the outcome of various treatment modalities and the subsequent comparison of results from different

Table 2

TNM stages for oesophageal cancer (UICC 1997)

Stage 0	Tis	N0	M0
Stage I	T1	N0	M0
Stage IIA	T2	N0	M0
	T3	N0	M0
Stage IIB	T1	N1	M0
	T2	N1	M0
Stage III	T3	N1	M0
	T4	any N	M0
Stage IVA	any T	any N	M1a
Stage IVB	any T	any N	M1b

centres. Consequently all tumours should currently be staged according to the 1997 edition (Table 2) of the International Union Against Cancer (UICC)'s TNM classification (Sobin and Wittekind, 1997), according to tumour depth (T), lymph node involvement (N) and existence of distant metastasis (M). This classification confronts preoperative staging by clinical and imaging assessment (cTNM) with final pathologic staging (pTNM) after resection. Any surgical specimen however will have to meet the minimal requirement of six mediastinal lymph nodes in order to allow pN assessment.

Several successive modifications of the TNM staging system from the 1970s through the 1990s have, however, made comparisons of outcome between different series in the literature extremely difficult.

7.2.1. T-staging

The depth of tumour penetration is evaluated as follows:

Tx primary tumour cannot be assessed
T0 no evidence of primary tumour
Tis Carcinoma in situ
T1 tumour invades lamina propria or submucosa
T2 tumour invades muscularis propria
T3 tumour invades adventitia (transmural tumour)
T4 tumour invades adjacent structures

From a surgical point of view, T-staging mainly aims at assessing tumour infiltration into mediastinal organs (T4) since this will preclude tumour resectability.

Thoracic CT scan: Classical signs of tumour invasion of the aorta, such as loss of the triangular fat plane between oesophagus, aorta and spine or a contact angle between tumour and aorta exceeding 90° over a height of two successive CT-images are considered to have an accuracy of approximately 80% for the assessment of aortic invasion. Suspicion of tracheo-bronchial invasion is based on displacement or distortion of the posterior wall of either trachea or bronchi (75–90% accuracy). Due to the absence of a natural fat plane between oesophagus and pericardium, CT-scan is less efficient for the detection of pericardial invasion except if a major pericardial effusion is present. Prospective comparative studies however, have seriously questioned the value of these radiological signs in preoperative staging since the T-factor was overestimated in many cases. MRI did not perform any better than CT-scan for the detection of T4 tumours since the accuracy of both CT-scan and MRI for the diagnosis of mediastinal invasion was less than 50%, which is no better than by chance (Lehr et al., 1988).

Endoscopic ultrasonography (EUS) is currently the most accurate technique in defining the T parameter: Reported accuracy rates for T staging by EUS ranges from 59 to 93% compared with 51 to 64% for CT-scan (Hölscher et al., 1994; Bardini et al., 1997; Murata et al., 1988; Hiele et al., 1997). For T1 and T2 tumours however, the sensitivity and specificity of EUS is less (70 to 82%) with an accuracy of only 74%. In the presence of a T1 tumour, only a 20 MHz probe can distinguish between T1a (intramucosal) and T1b (submucosal) infiltration. Since submucosal tumours present with lymph node involvement in 21 to 56% of cases (Hölscher et al., 1995a; Isono et al., 1991; Akiyama et al., 1994; Baba et al., 1994; Ide et al., 1994; Nishimaki et al., 1999), non-surgical therapies such as endoscopic mucosectomy or laser ablation should be contraindicated in T1b tumours.

The accuracy of EUS rises with the degree of tumour infiltration. For the diagnosis of T4 invasion it is 80 to 90%, provided the probe is able to pass the tumour. Indeed neoplastic strictures restrict the passage of the EUS-probe in 20 to 40% of mostly T3–4 tumours. Oesophageal dilatation is not recommended in this situation because of the high risk of perforation (Hiele et al., 1997).

A tracheo-bronchoscopy should be performed for all proximal and mid-oesophageal tumours in order to detect and histologically prove tumour invasion or tracheo-oesophageal fistulization. Although bronchoscopy has been reported (Hölscher et al., 1994) to have a low sensitivity (44%), it is the only method available to directly visualize any tumour infiltration and allow biopsies. A second primary tumour will further be found in the hypopharynx or tracheo-bronchial tree of 10 to 36% of patients with SCC (Hölscher et al., 1995b).

7.2.2. N staging

The presence of lymph node metastasis at the time of operation is known as one of the most important prognostic factors.

For oesophageal carcinoma regional lymph node involvement (N) is assessed as follows:

Nx regional lymph nodes cannot be assessed
N0 no regional lymph node metastasis
N1 regional lymph node metastasis

Tumours of the cardia or GOJ are currently classified as stomach carcinomas:

N0 no regional lymph node metastasis (in a regional lymphadenectomy specimen including at least 15 nodes)
N1 metastasis in one to six regional nodes
N2 metastasis in seven to 15 regional nodes
N3 metastasis in more than 15 regional nodes

Although EUS is superior to CT scan for the assessment of the N status, EUS is operator dependent and is limited by its inability to evaluate nodes distant from the oesophageal wall or behind air-filled structures (e.g. trachea). EUS evaluates lymph nodes not only by their size but also by shape and echogenicity patterns. Reported sensitivity, specificity and accuracy rates for correct assessment of mediastinal lymph node involvement by EUS are 64% to 88%, 47 to 93% and 64 to 88% respectively (Hölscher et al., 1994; Bardini et al., 1997; Murata et al., 1988;

Hiele et al., 1997; Luketich et al., 1997). For CT-scan these rates have been reported to be much lower (accuracy of 45 to 74%). Nevertheless, since most of these studies have been done in the 1980s and early 1990s, newer generations of CT scans may show improved performances and CT nodal assessment remains useful for purposes such as celiac node assessment in cases of non-passable tumour stenosis.

For the detection of cervical lymph node metastasis percutanous ultrasonography has a 74 to 79% sensitivity, a 91 to 94% specificity and an 88 to 89% accuracy (Natsugoe et al., 1999; Van Overhagen et al., 1993). Node contour and internal echo characteristics might be more valuable than formerly used criteria such as nodal size and roundness.

Staging thoracoscopy and laparoscopy has been shown to be superior to EUS, mainly due to better assessment of nodes with a diameter of less than one centimetre and its ability to stage obstructive tumours precluding the passage of the EUS-probe (Luketich et al., 1997). Since it is a costly and time consuming procedure with a specific morbidity and a potential risk for port-site metastasis, its use should be restricted to situations where a positive finding will have a direct therapeutic impact.

Although minimal invasive staging techniques might render more difficult oesophageal resection at a later stage, they should probably be used for a more accurate patient selection for multimodality treatment protocols (Krasna et al., 1996).

7.2.3. M-staging
The M factor assesses distant metastasis:

Mx distant metastasis cannot be assessed
M0 no distant metastasis
M1 distant metastasis

For tumours of the upper thoracic oesophagus:

M1a metastasis to cervical lymph nodes
M1b other distant metastasis

For tumours of the mid-thoracic oesophagus:

M1a not applicable
M1b non regional lymph node or other metastasis

For tumours of the distal oesophagus:

M1a metastasis to celiac lymph nodes
M1b other distant metastasis

For tumours of the GOJ:

M1 organ metastasis or non-regional lymph node metastasis (e.g. retro-pancreatic, mesenteric or para-aortic nodes).

The best strategy for the detection of distant metastasis (supraclavicular nodes and abdominal metastasis) might be the combination of CT-scan and EUS with reported sensitivity, specificity and accuracy rates of 83%, 81% and 82% respectively (Van Overhagen et al., 1993).

Staging laparoscopy has been shown to be useful to exclude otherwise undetectable peritoneal or small liver metastasis, mainly in case of locally advanced carcinoma of the GOJ. After extensive radiological staging, laparoscopy combined with laparoscopic ultrasonography may detect distant metastasis in 15 to 22% of patients with mainly GOJ tumours (Luketich et al., 1997; Romijn et al., 1998). Reported sensitivity, specificity and accuracy rates of staging laparoscopy with ultrasonography for carcinoma of the oesophagus and cardia were 81%, 100% and 95% respectively (Romijn et al., 1998).

Positron emission tomography scan (PET scan) using 18*F-deoxyglucose or other metabolites might soon become the most efficient tool for detecting distant metastasis using a single examination (Fig. 3). This is a field in fast evolution but early reports have shown that new metastases, which had not been detected by a complete conventional staging, may be found in up to 20% of patients, with sensitivity, specificity and accuracy rates of 88%, 93% and 91% respectively (Luketich et al., 1997). While this might be particularly useful for the differentiation of indeterminate long nodules and for tumour reevaluation after induction therapy protocols (Couper et al., 1998), PET-scan, although superior to CT for the detection of lymph node metastasis (Flanagan et al., 1997), at this time seems more efficient for the detection of distal metastasis than for N-staging.

7.2.4. Assessment of resectability
Oesophageal resection with either microscopically (R1) or macroscopically (R2) residual tumour leaves the patient with an operative risk but without any chance for five year survival whereas efficient medical techniques for palliation nowadays exist. Adequate preoperative staging should therefore aim at reliably assessing resectability. EUS has been reported to be superior to CT-scan in assessing resectability of both SCC and adenocarcinoma. Accurate prediction of non-resectability was possible in 91% of cases for EUS compared to 39% only for CT-scan (Hölscher et al., 1994; Tio and Tytgat, 1988).

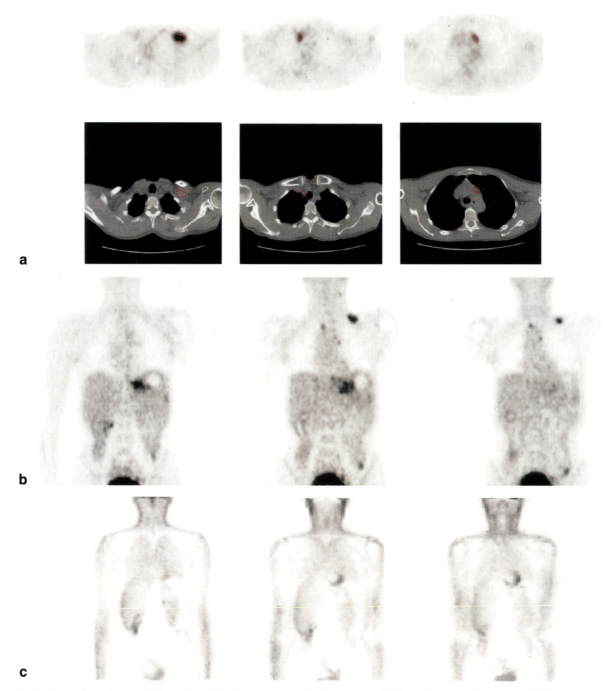

Fig. 3. Fluoro-deoxyglucose PET-scan of a GOJ adenocarcinoma. (a) Comparison of CT-scan (below) with transversal PET-scan images (above) precisely localize a left retro-clavicular, right para-tracheal and para-aortic lymph node metastasis, (b) frontal PET-scan views show the GOJ tumour as well as lesser gastric curve, right para-tracheal, aorto-pulmonary window, para-aortic, left jugular vein and left retro-clavicular lymph nodes. The latter were clinically undetectable. Para-tracheal nodes were histologically confirmed at mediastinoscopy, (c) after induction chemoradiotherapy a restaging PET scan showed almost no residual tumour activity.

7.2.5. Restaging after induction therapy

Chemotherapy and radiotherapy change the structure of the oesophageal wall by inducing edema and post-radiation fibrosis. Even the newest generations of CT-scans are unable to differentiate such therapy-induced changes from residual tumour (Jones et al., 1999). CT-scan and EUS may show a reduction of tumour volume and variations in number and size of lymph nodes but this does not correlate well with tumour response (Hölscher et al., 1994; Tio et al., 1991). The risks of both understaging (20%) and overstaging (36–44%) may lead to the withholding of potentially curative oesophagectomy in such patients (Jones et al., 1999; Van Raemdonck et al., 1997). Induction therapy should therefore be followed by surgical exploration in all medically fit patients without obvious organ metastasis or tumour progression on restaging since, even in patients with clinical T4 tumours, a rewarding 43% three-year survival may be achieved (Van Raemdonck et al., 1997). By assessing tumour metabolism rather than being a simple imaging technique (Fig. 3), PET-scan promises to improve the future assessment of tumour viability after induction therapy (Couper et al., 1998).

7.2.6. Problems of current clinical staging methods

Although CT-scan and EUS have improved the accuracy of clinical staging of oesophageal cancer over the last two decades, important problems remain to be solved.

– Classical staging techniques lead to overstaging in as many as 25 to 36% of patients (Lehr et al., 1988; Jones et al., 1999) with the potential risk of denying these patients their chance for possibly curative surgery or exposing them to the risk of tumour progression during what might be an unnecessary induction therapy. Histological proof, i.e. by EUS-guided fine needle aspiration, laparoscopy or thoracoscopy, is therefore required whenever imaging techniques suggest lymphatic or organ metastasis.

– Inadequate assessment of tumour depth remains a problem in some 20% of patients with superficial tumours. The inability to reliably assess lymph node involvement in T1b tumours still makes patient selection for non-radical treatment modalities such as endoscopic mucosectomy or photodynamic therapy very difficult.

– Current imaging techniques for lymph node assessment are unreliable for the estimation of the global number and mapping of positive nodes especially for nodes localized off the oesophageal wall. Since the total number of involved nodes or data such as the ratio involved/total nodes and the localization of positive nodes with respect to the tumour may have important implications on prognosis, these aspects need better preoperative

assessment. As long as accurate staging can only be obtained by radical resection, patient selection for multimodality treatments and the assessment of their outcome remains unreliable.

7.3. Medical assessment of operability

Assessment of medical operability should precede oncological staging since it is unnecessary to know that a tumour might be resectable if the patient is unable to undergo an operation. Patients with oesophageal cancer are frequently heavy drinkers and smokers. Liver cirrhosis, chronic obstructive or restrictive lung disease, coronary artery disease or other cardiomyopathies may frequently be discovered. A careful anamnesis should reliably evaluate general health status and detect exercise intolerance which is a strong predictor of pulmonary complications. The widely used classification of the American Society of Anesthesiologists is able to predict operative mortality as well as pulmonary complications. Age by itself is not a prohibitive factor as long as the functional status remains adequate (Smetana, 1999).

Cardiovascular and pulmonary function should be assessed as well as renal and hepatic function. Cardiovascular function is evaluated by ECG and, when necessary, cardiac ultrasonography, bicycle or other stress tests. Pulmonary function testing should include spirometry and carbon monoxide diffusion capacity. Although there is no real consensus which spirometric criteria contraindicate oesophageal resection, a forced expiratory volume in one second (FEV_1) and a forced vital capacity (FVC) of less than 70% of the predicted value and a ratio FEV_1/FVC below 0.65 suggest an increased risk for pulmonary complications (Smetana, 1999). Spirometry is useful to select those patients in whom aggressive preoperative treatment with bronchodilatators, corticosteroids and physical therapy may diminish the pulmonary risk. Deep-breathing exercises and incentive spirometry both reduce the relative risk of pulmonary complications by more than 50%, especially if these exercises are instructed preoperatively (Brooks–Brunn, 1995).

Portal hypertension is considered a contraindication for oesophageal resection in Child B and C patients (Belghiti et al., 1990). Nutritional status has to be assessed and the operative risk of patients with important weight loss may be reduced by a preoperative course of enteral or parenteral hypernutrition.

8. Prognosis

Tumour size is a prognostic factor as it is well correlated with lymph node involvement. Lymph node involvement is an important prognostic factor but due to the inability of current staging techniques to reliably assess lymph nodes preoperatively, this can only be done on specimens from radical surgery.

Reported 5-year survival rates of 42 to 72% (Hölscher et al., 1995a; Zhang et al., 1994; Fok et al., 1994; Akiyama et al., 1994; Baba et al., 1994; Ide et al., 1994; Lerut, 1998; Kato et al., 1991) for patients with negative nodes are much better than the 10 to 27% for those with positive nodes (Hölscher et al., 1995a; Steup et al., 1996; Baba et al., 1994; Lerut, 1998). Since cervical lymph nodes are involved in 26 to 37% (Isono et al., 1991; Lerut et al., 1994; Akiyama et al., 1994; Baba et al., 1994; Kato et al., 1991; Altorki and Skinner, 1997) of patients with resectable oesophageal cancer, adequate node assessment theoretically requires a radical resection with extensive abdominal, mediastinal and bilateral cervical lymph node dissection (three-field dissection). Those centers performing three-field dissections usually find some 10% higher rates of lymph node involvement for any T-stage than those centers performing only two-field dissections (Isono et al., 1991). In a group of 37 patients treated by resection with three-field dissection in our center, 16% of patients moved from M0 to M1b status (M+lymph according to the 1987 TNM-UICC classification) (Lerut, 1998).

For SCC, the tumour load, i. e. number of positive nodes, also seems to be an important prognostic factor since patients with only one positive lymph node survive longer than those with two or more involved nodes (Akiyama et al., 1994; Baba et al., 1994) respectively those with three or less positive nodes have a better prognosis than those with four or more involved nodes (Kawahara et al., 1998; Korst et al., 1998) For adenocarcinomas of the distal oesophagus and GOJ patients with four or less positive nodes also had a higher five-year survival after a radical resection than those with more than four involved nodes (Nigro et al., 1999). A ratio of involved to total removed nodes of less than 0.1 (Nigro et al., 1999) respectively 0.2 (Hölscher et al., 1995b) may also predict a better outcome.

Complete resection is another important prognostic factor since patients with locally advanced carcinoma (T3–T4) have a 20 to 31% chance for five year survival after complete (R0) resection compared to 0% after R1 or R2 resections (Hölscher et al., 1995a; Lerut et al., 1994; Ide et al., 1994; Nigro et al., 1999).

Histological tumour characteristics are only of marginal importance as prognosis is similar for SCC or adenocarcinoma of similar stages and location (Korst et al., 1998), except for early tumours where SCC might have a worse outcome than adenocarcinoma due to more frequently associated second primary tumours (Hölscher et al., 1995b). Genetic tumour characteristics however might gain importance in the near future as DNA aneuploidy, the presence of mutations of several tumour suppressing genes (p53, Rb, Cyclin D1) or over-expression of growth factors such as vascular endothelial growth factor (VEGF) have been shown to be associated with poor prognosis. Currently these findings, however, do not yet have any therapeutic implications.

9. Treatment of oesophageal cancer

9.1. Surgical treatment

9.1.1. Surgical techniques
The presence of lymph node involvement in most patients with resectable oesophageal cancer and the negative influence of lymphatic involvement on prognosis have lead to two attitudes towards resection techniques and the extent of associated lymphadenectomy. Those who believe that lymphatic involvement equals systemic disease claim that oesophageal resection is essentially palliative and consequently find it useless to seek for wide peritumoural resection and aggressive lymph node dissection. Most proponents of this attitude perform a transhiatal oesophagectomy (THE) as advocated by Orringer et al. (1993) with oesophageal stripping followed by retrosternal or usually posterior mediastinal gastric tube reconstruction with an oesophago-gastric anastomosis performed through a cervical incision. While this technique can be applied to most patients with carcinoma of the distal oesophagus it is contraindicated whenever tight adhesions or invasion of the tracheo-bronchial tree or the aorta are suspected as well as in most patients having had a previous oesophageal myotomy.

Others like Skinner and many Japanese surgeons believe that radical en bloc oesophagectomy with extensive lymphadenectomy can have a beneficial effect on cure rates even when there is lymph node involvement (Akiyama et al., 1994; Altorki and Skinner, 1997; Nigro et al., 1999; Lerut et al., 1992). Such radical resections are performed either through a left thoraco-abdominal incision (e.g. Sweet procedure) or separate right thoracic and abdominal incisions (Ivor–Lewis type of approach). Unlike surgery for gastric carcinoma, there are no standardized oesophageal resections and there is little consensus around the extension of lymphadenectomies to be performed with respect to tumour localization (Akiyama et al., 1994). While more or less extensive lymphadenectomies of the upper abdominal compartment and mediastinum (two-field lymphadenectomy) are recommended by many, additional cervical lymphadenectomies of the bilateral supraclavicular and cervical paratracheal regions are rarely performed outside Asia and some specialized Western centres. Nevertheless, the view that involvement of cervical lymph nodes remains regional disease with supra-carinal carcinomas, the improved staging and high five year survival rates after three-field lymphadenectomy which have been reported by several centres might support this approach.

Whatever is the attitude towards lymphadenectomy, the ability of oesophageal carcinoma to produce intra-mural skip lesions along the oesophagus, has lead many surgeons to perform systematically a sub-total oesophagectomy and to remove the lesser gastric curvature with all adjacent lymphatic tissues. Continuity is restored by most surgeons during the same procedure by creating a gastric tube and performing an intra-thoracic or cervical oesophago-gastric anastomosis either hand-sewn or using mechanical stapling devices. For patients with a history of previous partial gastrectomy (e.g. ulcer surgery) or when a total gastrectomy has to be performed (e.g. distal oesophageal tumours encroaching on the proximal stomach over a height of 5 cm or more) colon interposition or Roux-en-Y jejunal interposition are alternatives.

For tumours of the cervical oesophagus, the surgical strategy is determined by the length of tumour-free oesophagus underneath the crico-pharyngeal muscle which may in some cases require an additional laryngectomy. Oesophageal resections with laryngeal conservation are delicate procedures whose outcome may be hampered by difficult rehabilitation of swallowing and speech. Occasionally recurrent aspiration may require temporary or permanent tracheostomy.

For advanced carcinomas of the cervical oesophagus or hypopharyngeal tumours invading the larynx and oesophagus, a pharyngo-laryngectomy with total transhiatal oesophagectomy is standard treatment. A modified bilateral neck dissection is performed in

these cases and continuity is restored using the stomach when possible or the isoperistaltic colon when the stomach is too short or unusable.

Following a tendency of general enthusiasm for minimally invasive surgical techniques, the feasibility of oesophageal resections through video-assisted thoracoscopic surgery (VATS) and/or laparoscopy has been established. While preliminary results have not shown any improvement in postoperative morbidity and mortality rates, little is yet known about the oncological outcome. As a result, minimal invasive surgery for carcinoma of the oesophagus and GOJ presently remains strictly investigational.

9.1.2. Surgical results

Resectability. During the past decades the reported resectability rates for oesophageal cancer have progressively improved due to better preoperative staging and patient selection. From 1953 to 1978, only 39% of 83,783 reported patients were resectable (Earlam and Cunha–Melo, 1980), whereas 56% of 76,911 patients were so from 1980 to 1988 (Müller et al., 1990). According to more recent data the resectability rates have now reached 62 to 97% (Hölscher et al., 1995a; Lerut et al., 1994; Akiyama et al., 1994; Ide et al., 1994; Kato et al., 1991; Orringer et al., 1993).

Operative mortality and morbidity. While the hospital mortality rates of all series published between 1980 and 1988 (Müller et al., 1990) was 13.8%, today the post-operative mortality in expert centers is around 5%. Mortality will be higher in more extensive and palliative resections.

Reported complication rates range from 23 to 65% of all patients (Hölscher et al., 1995a; Steup et al., 1996; Zhang et al., 1994; Fok et al., 1994; Isono et al., 1991; Baba et al., 1994; Müller et al., 1990) and depend mainly on the criteria used to define a complication. Respiratory complications (pneumonia, atelectasis or respiratory insufficiency) occur in 24 to 37% of all patients (Steup et al., 1996; Isono et al., 1991; Akiyama et al., 1994; Altorki and Skinner, 1997; Müller et al., 1990). While trans-hiatal oesophagectomy has been introduced mainly to avoid respiratory complications, two prospective randomized studies (Goldminc et al., 1993; Chu et al., 1997) could not identify fewer cardiopulmonary complications after transhiatal compared with transthoracic oesophagectomy (Chu et al., 1997). Anastomotic leaks occur in 3 to 20% of cases (Hölscher et al., 1995a; Akiyama et al., 1994; Müller et al., 1990) independently if the anastomosis is performed in the neck or in the thorax. Surgical technique but also general factors related to the patient's nutritional status and vascular anastomotic supply influence the leakage rate. Anastomotic leaks are only rarely fatal if the anastomosis is in the neck. Recurrent nerve paralysis seems to occur more frequently after three-field than after two-field lymphadenectomy (14 versus 20%) (Isono et al., 1991).

Oncological results. The comparison of outcome from different surgical series is difficult because of heterogeneity in tumour types and localization, the variety of surgical techniques and repeated modifications of the tumour staging system. The cumulated five-year survival of all series before the nineties was 20% (Müller et al., 1990). More recent series reported overall five-year survival rates ranging from 26 to 45% (Hölscher et al., 1995a; Steup et al., 1996; Zhang et al., 1994; Akiyama et al., 1994; Baba et al., 1994; Ide et al., 1994; Lerut, 1998; Kato et al., 1991; Nigro et al., 1999; Orringer et al., 1993). Five-year survivals from our center are illustrated in Fig. 4. Barrett's carcinoma in many series has a better outcome due to the favorable influence of early carcinomas detected by endoscopic surveillance programs.

Reported 5-year survivals according to tumour stage are 60 to 90% for stage I disease (Baba et al., 1994; Ide et al., 1994; Kato et al., 1991; Orringer et al., 1993; Moghissi, 1992), 24 to 82% for stage IIa (Akiyama et al., 1994; Baba et al., 1994; Kato et al., 1991; Orringer et al., 1993), 38 to 71% for stage IIb (Akiyama et al., 1994; Kato et al., 1991; Orringer et al., 1993), 12 to 56% for stage III (Fok et al., 1994; Akiyama et al., 1994; Baba et al., 1994; Lerut, 1998; Orringer et al., 1993) and 0 to 31% for stage IV disease (Fok et al., 1994; Lerut et al., 1994; Akiyama et al., 1994; Baba et al., 1994; Kato et al., 1991; Orringer et al., 1993).

The impact of surgical radicality on long-term outcome seems important as it has been shown that radical R0 resections allow higher five-year survival rates than non-radical R0 resections (Hölscher et al., 1995a; Akiyama et al., 1994; Lerut, 1998; Altorki and Skinner, 1997; Lerut et al., 1992). Several Japanese authors have suggested that adding a bilateral cervical lymph node dissection to standard radical two-field dissection might improve the outcome. One randomized study (Kato et al., 1991) and a nationwide study in Japan (Isono et al., 1991) have shown that except for extremely early or very advanced carcinomas, the results of three-field lymph node dissection were better than those of two-field dissection. Akiyama found a better outcome after three-field dissection for patients with positive nodes as well as for those without nodal metastasis (Akiyama et al., 1994) and five year survival rates of 14 to 25% have been reached for those patients with positive celiac trunk or cervical nodes (Isono et al.,

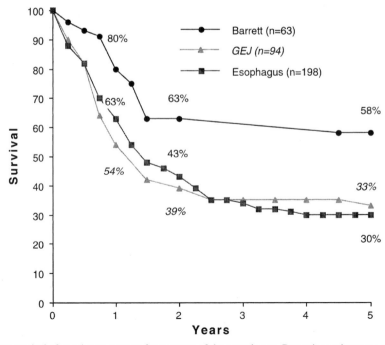

Fig. 4. Overall five year survival after primary surgery for tumours of the oesophagus, Barrett's carcinomas and tumours of the GOJ.

1991; Akiyama et al., 1994; Baba et al., 1994). There is however yet no evidence from large prospective randomized trials to prove that radical resection with three-field lymph node dissection definitely improves five-year survival.

9.2. Adjuvant and neoadjuvant therapies

Many therapeutic schemes using chemotherapy with or without radiotherapy have been tried, either alone or in conjunction with surgery, in order to improve the overall poor results of surgery for oesophageal carcinoma. Most chemotherapy regimens used combinations of cisplatin, 5-fluorouracil, vindesine or bleomycin while radiotherapy usually consisted of 20 to 60 Gray with various designs of dosage fractions and radiation fields. Although several phase II studies showed encouraging results with objective response rates of 50 to 60% and complete response rates of more than 20%, most prospective controlled trials were deceiving in terms of long-term survival.

Adjuvant therapies appear to be of limited use since a prospective randomized trial of postoperative chemotherapy with cisplatin-vindesine did not show any difference in survival (Ando et al., 1997) and two such studies (Tenière et al., 1991; Fok, 1993) did not show any benefit of giving post-operative radiotherapy either.

At least six phase III trials studying the use of preoperative chemotherapy did not show any improved survival compared with surgery alone (Lerut, 1998; Bhansali et al., 1996; Law et al., 1997). While surgical resectability was improved in the induction arm of two studies (Kelsen et al., 1998; Law et al., 1997), patient survival was not improved in any of these studies. A meta-analysis of 12 prospective randomized trials comparing Cisplatin-based adjuvant or neoadjuvant chemotherapy regimens with or without radiotherapy and/or surgery showed no significant survival benefits in the combined treatment arms (Bhansali et al., 1996).

The value of preoperative radiotherapy alone has been studied by a meta-analysis of five prospective randomized studies which had largely been updated for the occasion (Arnott et al., 1998). With a median follow-up of 9 years in 1147 patients, this meta-analysis suggested an overall reduction in the risk of death of 11% and a statistically almost significantly survival benefit of 3 and 4% at two and five years.

Combining the theoretical advantages of local irradiation with the radiosensitizing properties of chemotherapy together with its potential systemic effect on micrometastases, much has been expected of neoadjuvant chemoradiotherapy. Five prospective randomized trials however have not been able to show any survival benefit with preoperative chemoradiotherapy for squamous cell carcinoma (Nygaard et al., 1992; Apinop et al., 1994; Le Prise et al., 1994; Urba et al., 1997; Bosset et al., 1997) while the only trial to show a significant benefit for induction chemoradiotherapy in terms of improved median survival (16 versus 11 months) and three-year survival rates (32% versus 6%) had addressed oesophageal adenocarcinoma (Walsh et al., 1996). This trial however has been heavily criticized because of lacking precision in staging modalities, more advanced disease in the surgical group and the fact that survival in the surgical arm was much poorer than the reported results from the same centre with surgical treatment alone.

Although induction therapies were able to produce a complete pathologic response in 15 to 26% of the resected specimens in these trials, this did not improve the overall survival. Tumour progression under therapy in the approximately 20% of non-responders and a higher postoperative mortality in the induction arm might be responsible for this (Bosset et al., 1997).

Further efforts will have to refine the efficiency of induction protocols by developing new chemotherapy regimens (e.g. taxanes). Also, quality-of-life studies will need to identify that induction therapy is worthwhile in subgroups of patients which are most likely to respond to such therapies. Potentially unresectable T4 tumours may constitute such a subgroup of patients in which induction chemoradiotherapy allowed us to reach a 91% rate of R0 resections and a gratifying overall three-year survival of 32%, reaching even 53% after R0 resection (Lerut, 1998). Since more and more reports suggest that more extensive primary surgery might improve the results of standard resections from the past and as long as induction protocols do not yield better results than surgical resection alone, such induction therapy should not be administered in standard practice and outside carefully monitored study protocols.

9.3. Non-surgical 'curative' treatment

For early carcinomas of the oesophagus, several endoluminal treatment techniques have recently extended the therapeutic arsenal. Endoscopic mucosal resection may be used mainly for lesions with a limited surface extension while thermoablation techniques might also apply to more diffusely spreading lesions such as in degenerated Barrett's where several foci of early invasive carcinoma may be present. Endoluminal ablation techniques may use either laser thermocoagulation (Nd-Yag laser) or photodynamic energy enhancement. Oesophageal strictures may appear in one third of patients and results from follow-up are awaited. As discussed above, these techniques should only apply to lesions without extension into the submucosa because of expected failure due to lymph node metastasis in such T1b lesions (Hölscher et al., 1995b; Overholt et al., 1999). Until it is established that endoluminal therapies are as effective as surgery for early cancer, their use outside of study protocols, should be strictly restricted to inoperable patients.

For locally advanced carcinomas the exclusive use of radiotherapy or chemoradiotherapy without subsequent resection is currently under investigation. As the results of such treatment modalities will have to be compared to the results of radical surgery, the surgical techniques used in such studies should be very carefully defined.

9.4. Palliative treatments

Palliative resection or surgical bypass historically has been the best and most durable way to re-establish the ability to swallow in patients with unresectable stage IV disease. With a median life expectancy of approximately 6 months, only those patients with an uncomplicated and short postoperative hospital stay however may benefit from surgical palliation. The high in-hospital mortality rates (28 to 33%) of palliative surgery (Fok et al., 1994; Lerut et al., 1994; Sawant and Moghissi, 1994) encouraged the development of less morbid therapies. Many therapeutic options are nowadays available for patients with unresectable tumours and for those who are medically unfit for surgery: various regimens of chemotherapy or radiotherapy (either external irradiation or brachytherapy), a variety of oesophageal stents, laser therapy, photo dynamic therapy (PDT) or any combination of the above may be used.

Depending on the patient's general condition, the location and size of the tumour, the presence or absence of dysphagia or oesophago-airway fistula, the location and number of organ metastases as well as the symptoms they may produce, but also depending on the locally available technology and expertise, the choice of a palliative treatment can only be the best therapy for that particular patient

(Sawant and Moghissi, 1994). As a consequence of this, the comparison of the results of different palliative methods is very difficult and only a few prospective randomized studies have been reported. None of these treatments however is able to cure the patient and since the median life expectancy is short, maximum quality of life should be the most important objective to aim at. For stage IV patients with little or no symptoms, no treatment may therefore sometimes be the best treatment.

Chemotherapy (usually cisplatin-based) and/or external radiotherapy is frequently proposed to stage IV patients in good general condition. There is some evidence to suggest that chemoradiotherapy is superior to radiotherapy alone (Herskovic et al., 1992).

Symptomatic patients in poor general condition are usually candidates for endoscopic palliative procedures. Surgery may offer a better lasting relief of dysphagia than radiotherapy but is more invalidating during the first months after treatment. Surgery should therefore be reserved for patients with a reasonable life expectancy (Sawant and Moghissi, 1994; O'Rourke et al., 1992). There is some evidence that for advanced carcinomas, PDT using porfimer sodium (porphyrin compound) as a photosensitizing agent might be superior to Nd-Yag laser thermoablation. Although both techniques are efficient to relief dysphagia, PDT might produce less serious complications (e.g. perforations), more patients may complete therapy and a higher objective tumour response rate may be reached (Lightdale et al., 1995). Endobrachytherapy has further been shown to be as effective as laser therapy for the relief of dysphagia (Low and Pagliero, 1992).

10. Functional outcome and late sequels

Oesophagectomy is a major operation from which most patients will require several months to recover completely. Beside problems directly related to surgical complications (recurrent nerve palsy, infections) or to the toxicity of adjuvant therapies, bad appetite, feelings of early satiety due to reduced reservoir capacity of a tube gastroplasty and post-vagotomy diarrhea may lead in many patients to further weight loss during the first postoperative months. After this initial phase most patients however regain weight and finally up to 85% of those having been reconstructed by means of a tube gastroplasty brought up into the neck will show good to excellent functional results (De Leyn et al., 1992). Benign anastomotic strictures may develop in a number of patients and need to be differentiated from tumour recurrences. Usually they can be dealt with easily by one or several dilatations together with acid-suppressing medication.

Intolerance for dairy products and invalidating dumping syndrome however may remain resistant to therapy in some patients. Long-term survivors are mainly bothered by the consequences of acid and biliary reflux which at one year postoperative may lead to peptic stenosis and Barrett metaplasia of the oesophageal remnant in up to 50% of those with an intra-thoracic anastomosis. To reduce these problems is a further argument in favor of systematic reconstruction with gastro-oesophageal anastomosis in the neck.

11. Follow-up

Most centres perform routine postoperative programs with clinical, endoscopic and radiological assessment at regular time intervals after oesophageal resection since this is the only way to assess the results of treatment in a given centre. Control endoscopy with biopsies at regular time intervals will detect anastomotic recurrence. Mediastinal recurrences and lung metastasis are best detected by CT-scan. Liver metastasis are easily detected by ultrasonography and carcino-embryonary antigen is a useful tumour marker for recurrent adenocarcinoma.

It remains questionable however if such follow-up is of benefit to improve patient survival. Surgery will never be curative for recurrence and it remains unproved if palliative radiotherapy or chemotherapy prolong survival in non-symptomatic patients with recurrent oesophageal cancer. The potential psychological benefit for the patient to know that he is regularly taken care of in a follow-up program should however not be underestimated.

References and further reading

Akiyama H, Tsurumaru M, Udagawa H, Kajiyama Y. Radical lymph node dissection for cancer of the thoracic oesophagus. Ann Surg 1994; 220: 364–373.

Ando N, Iizuka T, Kakagawa T, Isono K, Watanabe H, Ide H, et al. A randomized trial of surgery with and without chemotherapy for localized squamous carcinoma of the thoracic oesophagus: The Japan Clinical Oncology Group Study. J Thorac Cardiovasc Surg 1997; 114: 205–209.

Altorki NK, Skinner DB. Occult cervical nodal metastasis in oesophageal cancer: Preliminary results of three-field lymphadenectomy. J Thorac Cardiovasc Surg 1997; 113: 540–544.

Apinop C, Puttisak P, Preecha N. A prospective study of com-

bined therapy in esophageal cancer. Hepatogastroenterology 1994; 41(4):391–393.

Arnott SJ, Duncan W, Gignoux M, Girling DJ, Hansen HS, Launois B, et al. Preoperative radiotherapy in oesophageal carcinoma: A meta-analysis using individual patient data (Oesophageal Cancer Collaborative Group). Int J Radiation Oncol Biol Phys 1998; 41: 579–583.

Baba M, Aikou T, Yoshinaka H, Natsugoe S, Fukumoto T, Shimazu H, et al. Long-term results of subtotal esophagectomy with three-field lymphadenectomy for carcinoma of the thoracic oesophagus. Ann Surg 1994; 219: 310–316.

Bardini R, Sovernigo G, Castoro C. Le bilan préthérapeutique dans le cancer du cardia. Ann Chir 1997; 134: 197–201.

Belghiti J, Cherqui D, Langonnet F, Fékété F. Esophagogastrectomy for carcinoma in cirrhotic patients. Hepatogastroenterology 1990; 37: 388–391.

Bhansali MS, Vaidya JS, Bhatt RG, Patil PK, Badwe RA, Desai PB. Chemotherapy for carcinoma of the oesophagus: A comparison of evidence from meta-analysis of randomized trials and of historical control studies. Ann Oncol 1996; 7: 355–359.

Bosset JF, Gignoux M, Triboulet JP, Tiret E, Mantion G, Elias D, et al. Chemoradiotherapy followed by surgery compared with surgery alone in squamous cell cancer of the oesophagus. N Engl J Med 1997; 337: 161–167.

Brooks-Brunn JA. Postoperative atelectasis and pneumonia. Heart Lung 1995; 24: 94–115.

Chu KM, Law SYK, Fok M, Wong J. A prospective randomized comparison of transhiatal and transthoracic resection for lower-third oesophageal carcinoma. Am J Surg 1997; 174: 320–324.

Couper GW, McAteer D, Wallis F, Norton M, Welch A, et al. Detection of response to chemotherapy using positron emission tomography in patients with oesophageal and gastric cancer. Br J Surg 1998; 85: 1403–1406.

De Leyn P, Coosemans W, Lerut T. Early and late functional results in patients with intrathoracic gastric replacement after oesophagectomy for carcinoma. Eur J Cardiothorac Surg 1992; 6: 79–85.

Desoubeaux N, Le Prieur A, Launoy G, Maurel J, Lefevre H, Guillois JM, Gignoux M. Recent time trends in cancer of the oesophagus and gastric cardia in the region of Calvados in France, 1978-1995: a population based study. Eur J Cancer Prev 1999; 8(6):479–486.

Earlam R, Cunha–Melo JR. Oesophageal squamous cell carcinoma: a critical review of surgery. Br J Surg 1980; 67: 381–390.

Flanagan FL, Dehdashti F, Siegel BA, Trask DD, Sundaresan SR, Patterson GA, et al. Staging of oesophageal carcinoma with 18-F-fluorodeoxyglucose Positron Emission Tomography. AJR 1997; 168: 417–424.

Fok M, Law SYK, Wong J. Operable oesophageal carcinoma: Current results from Hong Kong. World J Surg 1994; 18: 355–360.

Goldminc M, Maddern G, Le Prise E, Meunier B, Campion JP, Launois B. Oesophagectomy by a trans-hiatal approach or thoracotomy: a prospective randomized trial. Br J Surg 1993; 80(3): 367–370.

Herskovic A, Martz K, Al-Saraf M, et al. Combined chemotherapy and radiotherapy compared with radiotherapy alone in patients with cancer of the oesophagus. N Engl J Med 1992; 326: 1593–1598.

K. Moghissi, J.A.C. Thorpe and F. Ciulli (Eds.)
Moghissi's Essentials of Thoracic and Cardiac Surgery
© 2003 Elsevier Science B.V. All rights reserved

CHAPTER III.16

Management of inoperable oesophageal cancer

K. Moghissi

1. Introduction

At presentation, over 50% of patients with oeso-phageal cancer are deemed inoperable and of those undergoing resection, at most, only 15 to 20% will survive five years or more (Muller et al., 1990; Moghissi, 1992; Sharpe and Moghissi, 1996). Al-though the operative mortality and morbidity have reduced during the past two or three decades, the overall long-term survival rates have not significantly altered over this period.

One of the most challenging problems when faced with an unresectable cancer patient is the further management. For the majority with advanced and extensive disease, this management is the palliation of symptoms. The less invasive a method of pallia-tion, the more acceptable is such management. In a minority of cases, inoperability is due to the patients poor general condition. For these, survival benefit must be considered in addition to palliation.

Of the many symptoms in patients with oesopha-geal cancer, none is more distressing than dysphagia. Therefore, most palliative modalities aim to relieve dysphagia totally or substantially reduce its severity for as long as the patient lives. Additionally and ideally:
- The method should be repeatable if necessary,
- There should be no side effect or serious compli-cation attached to the method,
- The treatment should improve the quality of life,
- It should be acceptable to the patient allowing management outside of hospital institutions,
- The mortality of procedure should be accept-able to the patient. Many other attributes such as weight gain and performance status improvement are not realistically achievable for a sustained period in such inoperable patients.

There is no ideal palliative method available for all inoperable patients and in cancer located in vary-ing locations in the oesophagus. However, a number of available modalities can, alone or in conjunction with other methods, achieve an acceptable level of palliation. Prior to allocating a palliative method every patient who is a candidate for palliation of dysphagia should have been fully investigated and have had a diagnostic work up to indicate reason for inoperability. Selection of method should be based on the characteristics of the tumour, the location and the extent of the growth as well as the nature of the malignant stricture and endoluminal features of the lesion.

The above information can usually be obtained through chest radiography, barium contrast study and endoscopy. These should be carried out in all cases.

2. Methods

The following are treatment options:
2.1 Endoscopic dilatation with/without injection of toxic substances (e.g. alcohol)
2.2 External Beam Radiotherapy (EBR)
2.3 Brachytherapy
2.4 Chemotherapy
2.5 Tube and stent placement
2.6 Laser therapy
2.7 Bypass operations

It should be emphasised that the surgeon consid-ering treatment of oesophageal cancer should appre-ciate the range of indications and usefulness of each method in order to use them or advise their use as appropriate. It must also be noted that one or more of the above methods may have to be used in a patient in sequence or together to attain the best achievable result.

2.1. Endoscopic dilatation

To be effective, oesophageal dilatation has to be repeated at frequent intervals. When tumour mass is projecting into the lumen by a cauliflower type of tumour, endoscopic injection of alcohol into the tumour mass may be useful to cause necrosis of the growth thus decreasing the bulk and severity of obstruction. This method may still have a place in centres where more modern methods cannot be made available but generally more recent developments offer more effective methods of palliation. However it must be emphasized that dilatation is necessary in the initial step of many palliative treatments.

2.2. External Beam Radiotherapy (EBR)

Generalisation on the effectiveness of EBR in palliation of dysphagia is difficult since not much reliance can be placed on the published data because of variation in population characteristic, stage of disease or therapy regimens in different series. The prime indications of EBR are in localised tumour causing severe dysphagia. Palliation of dysphagia is irrespective of tumour type and is reported to be between 70 to 90% of cases and lasting for about six months. This may, however, be in selected patients who can tolerate high radiation dose (>4500 cGy). The suggested radiation dose is 5000 to 6000 cGY. Combined radiotherapy and chemotherapy appear not to be attended by a better outcome (Wara et al., 1976; Coia et al., 1993; Minsky, 1994; Minsky, 1996).

Mortality, morbidity and side effects of radiotherapy are understated and often completely missed in most reports concerned with EBR. Nonetheless, it is a fact that in advanced carcinoma complications such as radiation pneumonitis, bleeding and oesophago-airway fistula can occur in some patients following treatment. It is also worthwhile noting that dysphagia temporarily becomes more prominent during or soon after treatment. A variable percentage develop post radiotherapy stricture requiring dilatation. This incidence may be as high as 40%, when stricture is a mixture of malignant and benign and in the region of 10% when entirely benign. Such a stricture usually appears a few months after the complete eradication of intraluminal growth.

2.3. Brachytherapy

The aim of brachytherapy is to provide endoscopic radiotherapy to the entire intra-luminar component of the tumour, targeting the lesion while protecting the surrounding structures such as the heart, lungs and spinal cord. Only patients with important endoluminal tumour are selected for brachytherapy.

Pre-treatment evaluation of the extent of the growth in the oesophagus and dilatation of malignant stricture, if any, is necessary.

2.3.1. Equipment
- Endoscopic instruments: Either rigid or flexible fibreoptic instruments may be used both for evaluation and stricture dilatation using their appropriate bougie. Dilatation is necessary in order to endoscopically examine the lumen beyond the stricture.
- Brachytherapy equipment is comprised of:
  - An applicator which accommodates the insert tube that transfers the radiation source and is placed into the external tube (applicator),
  - A remote after-loading system.

2.3.2. The technique
Different techniques may be used to achieve the same objective. The one we have used (Renwick et al., 1992) is similar to that proposed by Giler and Pagliero (1985) and Pagliero and Rowland (1990) and consists of:
- Placement of the applicator under vision after oesophagoscopy and dilatation using a rigid oesophagoscope and with the patient under general anaesthetic.
- Control: Initially the applicator is fitted with a dummy source containing radio opaque beads located at 0.25 to 1 cm intervals. The beads represent the area covered by the radioactive source and should be shown radiologically to include the whole extent of the tumour as well as 2 to 3 cm at either end of the lesion.
- The optimal position of the applicator in the oesophagus as seen by the radio opaque beads within the dummy is checked by fluoroscopy or standard chest radiography.
- The applicator is fixed at the mouth end.
- General anaesthetic is then discontinued and with the applicator in place in the oesophagus, the patient is transferred to the radiotherapy remote control room where the treatment takes place. The dummy insert within the applicator is now replaced by the source carrier insert and the unit programmed and started.
- The prescribed dose can vary but in many centres it is 15 Gy in a single fraction 1 cm from the source axis. Some centres use a higher dose in divided

multiple fractions.
- After completion of treatment, the applicator is removed.
- The patient is discharged home a few hours later after a chest radiograph indicating no abnormal findings related to the procedure.
- We recommend the patient should take liquids and soft consistency food for a few days after the treatment prior to gradual progression to solid normal food.

Note that:
- The procedure can be undertaken under topical anaesthetic and sedation using flexible endoscope. The placement of the applicator is the undertaken using a guide wire.

2.3.3. Results
The improvement in swallowing (reduction in dysphagia grade) is achieved in about 80% of patients.

2.3.4. Complications
Consist of ulceration, fistulae and stricture which can occur in about one third of cases.

2.4. Chemotherapy

For over 15 years, chemotherapeutic agents have been under investigation and, as yet, no clear consensus has emerged on the optimal method of their application or the extent of their usefulness. Preoperative induction chemotherapy, either to improve survival in resected patients or to downgrade the tumour to achieve complete resection, has already been referred to in chapter III.15. The use of chemotherapeutic agents for palliation as a sole modality of treatment or adjunct to other methods is more controversial. In the 1980s a number of trials were carried out with inconsistent results and conclusions. There is, as yet, no clear evidence that chemotherapy in combination with other types of treatment can improve survival. Chemotherapy can temporarily relieve dysphagia but its complications and side effects are such as to often prohibit its employment.

2.5. Tubes and stents

Tubes and stents (Fig. 1) provide a passage for food through the oesophagus whose lumen is otherwise obstructed by tumour.

Intubation of the oesophagus for relief of dysphagia was first discussed in the mid-19th century but its use became practical in the 20th century. In the 1920s

Souttar (1924) introduced and used a tube made of metallic coil to establish patency in malignant obstruction of the oesophagus. In the 1950s Mousseau et al. (1956), and soon after Celestin (1959), introduced their oesophageal tubes. These tubes were to be inserted surgically by the so-called traction technique (Moghissi, 1960). Later tubes were designed to be inserted endoscopically. At the present time there are a number of tubes and stents available for use surgically or endoscopically (pulsion technique).

Most tubes are funnel-shaped whose expanded proximal end is designed to sit above the top of the obstruction and its distal end to be placed beyond the stricture. Stents are essentially tubes made of plastic or metallic coil with regular diameter throughout. New stents or tubes are regularly being designed and manufactured, each with some advantage and disadvantage compared with the existing ones. Selection should be on the basis of location and the length of the malignant stricture and expertise of the operator.

2.5.1. Placement of tubes and stents
There are basically two techniques for placement of tubes or stents. In both techniques, the location and extent of tumour within the lumen should be determined using contrast study and endoscopy.

Pulsion technique. The tube/stent is introduced orally and is pushed to sit within the whole length of the stenosed segment. The distal portion of the tube should sit below the lower end of stenosis in the normal oesophagus or in the stomach. The position of the tube is checked endoscopically and radiologically prior to patient discharge.

Traction technique. In this method, the tube is pulled from below (stomach) and placed in position.

The procedure is:
- Oesophagoscopy and dilatation (in very tight strictures). A bougie or a probe is introduced from the mouth to enter the stomach. The proximal end of this bougie is left outside of the mouth. This end is connected to the distal end of the oesophageal tube.
- Through a limited laparotomy, gastrotomy is performed and the distal end of the bougie is recovered from the stomach.
- The bougie is pulled out of the stomach through the gastrotomy via the abdomen and with it the lower end of the oesophageal tube, which passes through the oesophageal stricture. The placement can be assisted by the anaesthetist with a slight

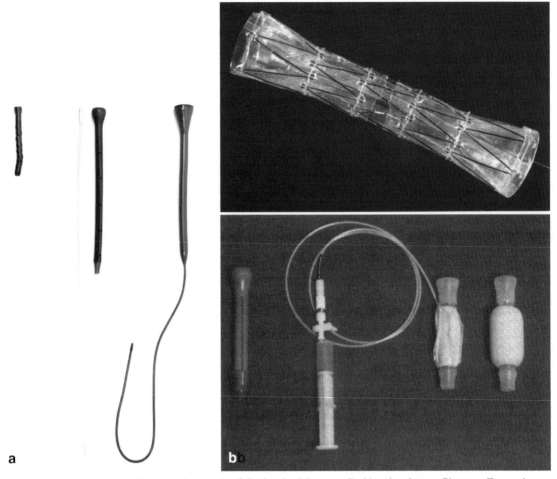

Fig. 1. Tubes and stents: (a) from left to right, Soutar tube, Celestin tube, Mousseau–Barbin tube; (b) top, Gianturco Z stent; bottom (left to right), Celestin tube, Wilson–Cook tube with inflatable balloon.

push from the mouth end of the tube by the endoscope. The procedure is easier when a rigid oesophagoscope is used to guide the passage through the pharynx.

• Once the tube is in position, its distal end in the stomach is cut and removed together with the attached bougie. As a rule many of the tubes such as Mousseau–Barbin or Celestin are placed by traction "rail road" technique. Stents and short tubes are placed using pulsion technique.

2.5.2. Indications for tube/stent
Tubes or stents may be used for:
(a) Inoperable and unresectable tumour causing severe dysphagia. The stricture may be extrinsic, endoluminal or both.
(b) Malignant strictures with oesophago-respiratory fistula.

2.5.3. Complications of tube/stent
– Perforation: this may occur at the time of placement or later by extrusion of the stent through the wall or by erosion of the oesophagus. When perforation occurs at the time of tube placement pneumomediastinum, pneumothorax and/or surgical subcutaneous emphysema appears. Perforation at a later stage results in mediastinitis, empyema and haemorrhagic complications.
– Blockage: either by large pieces of food or through tumour overgrowth above/below the tube or by tumour ingrowth through the coil of a stent.
– Haemorrhage: by ulceration and erosion of the wall and perforation of a large blood vessel. This can be fatal.
– Migration: some tubes when placed in the upper oesophagus can migrate upwards. Others will pass into the stomach causing obstruction of pylorus or creating a fistula.

Table 1
Oesophageal tubes/stents and their important features

Type of Prosthesis	Mode of placement	Important features	Advantages	Disadvantages	Remarks
Soutar	Pulsion	• Metallic coil	• Originally for intubation of cervical oesophagus	• Migration • Ingrowth of tumour	• Dilatation needed • Now not in use
Mousseau-Barbin	Traction	• Plastic tube with fine tail. • Funnel proximal end sits above the stricture	• Dilatation not needed • Blockage is rare • Ingrowth not possible • Suitable for extrinsic/intrinsic stricture	• Rigid and unyielding • Overgrowth ± • General anaesthetic required • Not suitable for cervical strictures	• Late complications: perforation, haemorrhage ± • Not much used now
Celestin	Pulsion/traction	• Plastic, flexible and yielding. • Small flange	• Suitable for short/long strictures • Perforation/haemorrhage is rare	• Migration ± up/down • Dilatation required • Not suitable for cervical strictures • Blockage by food ±	• Is still in use and is cheap compared with recently produced prosthesis • Probably best of all round prosthesis
Atkinson	Pulsion	• Plastic • Short tube with flange	• Easy to insert • Placement in cervical tumour ±	• Migration + • Overgrowth + • Dilatation required • Blockage ±	• Has been a favourite prosthesis for endoscopy • Inexpensive compared with other stents
Wilson-Cook	Pulsion	• Plastic • Short tube with/without balloon	• Easy to insert • Use in O–A fistula ± • Displacement rare	• Dilatation required • Placement in cervical tumours ± • Overgrowth ±	• In cases of fistulae, bronchoscopy aspiration required
Gianturco Z stent	Pulsion	• Zig-zag wiring with/without silicon covering • Self expanding • Has own placer/pusher	• Easy to insert • Use in cervical tumour ± • Use in O–A fistula ± • Minimal dilatation necessary	• Migration ± • Displacement ± • Blockage + • Tumour ingrowth + (in non silicon) Tumour overgrowth ±	• Expensive • Often more than one stent required • Removal problematic/not possible
Nitinol endostent (instent)	Pulsion	• Coil spring collar wire • Nickel titanium with pusher • Self retracting expanding	• Easy to insert	• Length shortens after insertion • Ingrowth/overgrowth ± • Migration ± • Dilatation required	• Use in O–A fistula ± • Is not possible to determine final length of stent once in place
Proctor-Living-stone	Traction/pulsion	• Plastic/latex • Expanded proximal end	• Easy to insert • May be used for O–A fistula • Migration rare	• Perforation ± • Haemorrhage ±	

Key to abbreviations: O–A = Oesophago–Airway, ± = Possible, + = Positive/Occurs, − = Negative/usually does not occur

Table 2

Comparison of Endoscopic YAG laser and Photodynamic Therapy (PDT) in unresectable/inoperable oesophageal cancer

	Yag Laser	PDT
Desobliteration	Immediate	2–3 days
Prior dilatation	Mandatory in most cases	Rarely required
Mode of application	Non-contact	Contact/Interstitial
Duration of effect	4–6 weeks	10–24 weeks
Complication	Perforation (3–10%)	Skin photosensitivity (3–10%)
Application in patients with stent/tube	Generally not possible	Always possible
Tumours in all locations of oesophagus	Difficult in cervical oesophageal tumours	No difficulty

2.5.4. Types of tube or stent

There are now a large number of tubes and stents for oesophageal intubation (Figs. 1a and 1b). Special circumstances such as cases with a high cervical malignant stricture or those with existence of oesophago-airway (O–A) fistulae demand both experience and specific types of prosthesis. In a great majority of cases, there is no advantage to use an expensive stent instead of a cheaper plastic tube and there is no published evidence suggesting superiority of results of one tube/stent against another.

In the most extensive published series of oesophageal intubation, comprising 2785 patients, Maharaj et al. (1988) used the Procter Livingstone tube showing results comparable with other published series. Since then other types of stent have become available which are more easily placed endoscopically and are self-expanding. It is the opinion of the author that for the majority of cases, the endoscopist/surgeon should use the tube or stent with which they have experience and expertise. In special cases, the use of a specific tube/stent may be advisable.

Table 1 shows some of the tubes/stents with their advantages and disadvantages. Not all are presently available in all countries but the table should serve as a guide.

2.6. Laser palliation of dysphagia

The general principle and techniques of endoscopic laser application are described in chapter IV.5. At this juncture, it should be emphasized that lasers are only useful in palliation of malignant dysphagia when the latter is due to endoluminal projection of exophytic tumour.

2.6.1. Types of laser

Two types of laser are commonly used: namely, Neodymium Yittrium Aluminium Garnet (YAG) laser, and Photodynamic Therapy (PDT).

YAG laser is used in its non-contact mode. Depending on the power setting and proximity of the delivery fibre to the target tissue, evaporation or a lesser degree of thermal injury and necrosis will ensue.

PDT for malignant obstructive oesophageal lesion consists of sensitization of malignant tissues followed by endoscopic illumination using appropriate laser light. The interaction between the chemical and the light produces necrosis of the tumour. Recanalization of the oesophagus and relief of dysphagia will follow.

The effect of YAG laser is almost immediate and lasts for four to six weeks. PDT effects appear after two or three days but generally last for ten to fourteen weeks. In both modalities, the application can be repeated for as long as there is endoscopic evidence of endoluminal and projecting tumour.

In suitable cases 90 to 100% recanalization has been reported in YAG laser. Similar results can be obtained with PDT (Table 2).

It must be emphasized that this high level of recanalization is possible only when the obstruction is entirely due to endoluminal projection and not to extrinsic pressure. In the experience of the authors, such an exclusively endoluminal malignant obstructive lesion in inoperable and unresectable oesophageal cancer is the exception rather than the rule; there is always additional mural and extrinsic compression by tumour and lymph nodes which accompany the intrinsic elements. However, return to quasi-normal swallowing is possible in a high percentage of cases since it does not require total patency of the oesophagus.

When YAG laser therapy is combined with photodynamic therapy both the effect and duration of relief is enhanced.

With regard to survival benefit, it is a general observation that desobliteration of the oesophagus has a survival benefit by reducing incidence of pulmonary complication which usually accompanies oesophageal obstruction. PDT appears to offer enhanced survival benefit.

2.6.2. Complications of laser therapy

The most important complication of endoscopic YAG laser therapy is oesophageal perforation. As can be expected, the incidence does vary according to the experience of the operator. It is also influenced by severity of the stricture and requirement for dilatation at the time of the laser therapy. The incidence of perforation in YAG laser therapy of oesophageal cancer is reported to be between 3 to 10%. PDT perforation is a rarity. In the author's series of 75 patients (115 treatments), no perforation has been observed (Moghissi et al., 2000).

Skin photosensitivity can complicate PDT but in experienced centres the incidence does not exceed 5% of cases. A higher incidence relates to patient non-compliance and/or lack of counselling

2.7. Bypass operation (oesophageal bypass surgery)

In certain circumstances and/or in selected patients there is a place for oesophageal bypass operation to palliate dysphagia. Whilst such procedures may be attended by a higher mortality than simpler methods of palliation when the malignant stricture is accompanied by an oesophago-airway fistula, they have the advantage of better swallowing and a more sustained level of relief of dysphagia.

There are a variety of operations in all of which the principle is to prepare a gastric, jejunum or a colonic tube to anastomose with the oesophagus above the obstruction.

2.7.1. Indications for bypass operations

- Patients with lower oesophageal tumour which, at exploration, are found to be unresectable. In many such cases, an end-to-side oesophago-gastric (fundus) anastomosis is possible. The oesophagus is severed above the tumour, the distal end is stapled or sewn over and the proximal end is anastomosed to a gastric tube made of the fundus (Fig. 2). When the exploration is carried out through left postero-lateral thoracotomy, the hiatus is enlarged and the fundus is pulled through the opening. The fundus is then anastomosed to the tumour-free lower oesophagus which has been prepared. Sometimes such an operation (oesophago-fundic-anastomosis) can be performed without dividing the oesophagus. In this case, a side anastomosis of oesophagus to stomach fundus is carried out.
- In tumours involving the stomach fundus, oe-

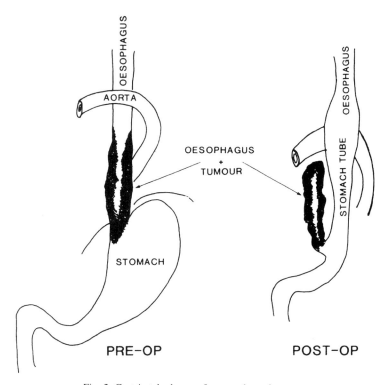

Fig. 2. Gastric tube bypass for oesophageal cancer.

of the oesophagus. Right and left recurrent laryngeal nerves run in the groove between the trachea and oesophagus and require identification in order to avoid injury.

2.2. Approach to the intrathoracic part of the oesophagus

For the purpose of the surgical approach the thoracic oesophagus may be divided into two parts:

2.2.1. The upper thoracic oesophagus

This is the part between the apex of the chest down to 3–4 cm below the arch of the aorta. This portion is more easily approached through a right posterolateral thoracotomy, with the patient placed in a left lateral position. The incision is made along the curvature of the ribs, some 4–5 cm below the angle of the scapula (Fig. 2a). The posterior part of the incision is made vertically between the spine and the vertebral border of the scapula.

The thoracic cavity is entered through the upper border of the 6th rib (periosteal stripping); i.e. the 5th intercostal space.

2.2.2. The lower thoracic oesophagus

This is the portion which is situated between the hiatus and up to 3 or 4 cm below the arch of the aorta. The best approach to this part is through a left posterolateral thoracotomy (Fig. 2b) with the patient placed in the right lateral position. The incision is

along the curvature of the ribs. The posterior end of the incision is made more vertically between the spine (vertebral column) and the vertebral border of the scapula. Allowance should be made with positioning and towelling of the patient for extension of the thoracotomy incision to the upper abdomen for a possible thoracolaparotomy. The selection of the intercostal space through which the pleural cavity is entered depends on several factors, such as:

- The location of the lesion in the oesophagus,
- The type of procedure which is planned to be undertaken, in particular whether there is going to be a resection of the oesophagus, and the level of the anastomosis with respect to the hiatus and the arch of the aorta. As a general rule the posterior end of the incision should be placed almost as high as the level of the intended anastomosis between the residual oesophagus (after oesophagectomy) and the proximal part of the substitute, such as the stomach, when the operation involves resection and reconstruction of the oesophagus.

Entry to the chest is usually made through the 6th intercostal space. In operations involving the oesophagus at or about the hiatus, entry into the pleural space is made through the 7th or 8th intercostal space. The inferior pulmonary ligament is incised and the lung retracted upwards and anteriorly.

It is important to note that in cancer surgery of the upper thoracic oesophagus provision should be made to access the cervical oesophagus on the right side of the neck. This provision should be made on the left side for those tumours approached by left thoracotomy or left thoracolaparotomy.

3. Mobilisation of the oesophagus

All surgery on the oesophagus involves mobilisation of a length of the oesophagus (with the lesion) and its separation from the neighbouring structures. In the neck, this is best achieved by encircling the oesophagus with plastic silicone tape or a fine silicone tube. This should be done without damage to either the membranous wall of the trachea or the muscularis of the oesophagus. To achieve this, the encircling is first made around the healthy part of the oesophagus. The mobilisation of the oesophagus is then facilitated by gently manoeuvring the encircling tape, which allows better visualisation of the neighbouring structures.

In the operation on the upper thoracic oesophagus, the azygos vein is divided between two ligatures.

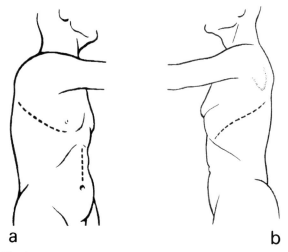

a   b

Fig. 2. (a) Right thoracotomy incision of approach to upper and mid-thoracic oesophagus. Note: (two-stage) Ivor Lewis-type of oesophagectomy. (b) Left thoracotomy for exposure of lower thoracic oesophagus.

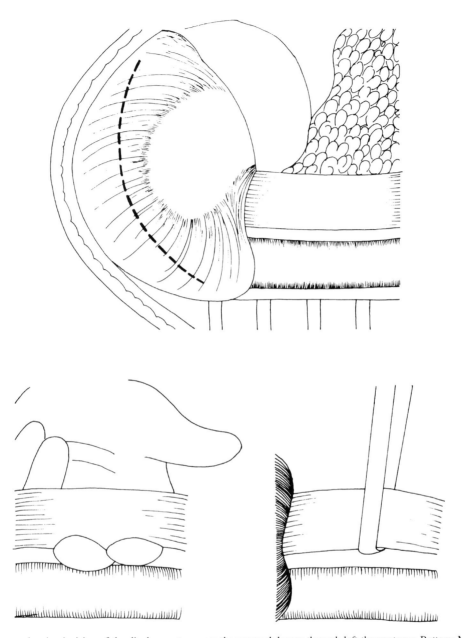

Fig. 3. Top: Diagram showing incision of the diaphragm to access the upper abdomen through left thoracotomy. Bottom: Mobilisation of the lower thoracic oesophagus.

The posterior half is then retracted back with or without its pleural covering. The mediastinal pleura is incised vertically over the oesophagus for the required distance. The oesophagus is encircled by a tape prior to mobilisation from the trachea and the aorta using sharp and blunt dissection, and aided by gentle traction on the tape. Care should be taken not to devascularize the oesophagus. For surgery of the lower thoracic oesophagus, mobilisation is best

carried out by passing an encircling tape around the oesophagus, allowing it to be lifted from its bed between the mediastinal pleurae (Figs. 3a and 3b).

The following is an easy method by which to encircle the oesophagus with a tape. A vertical incision is made over the mediastinal pleura of the lower oesophagus in the groove between the aorta and the oesophagus. Another incision is made in the pleural reflection over the triangular space (as seen at thoracotomy with the patient in a lateral position), situated between the pericardium anteriorly, the diaphragm inferiorly and the oesophagus posteriorly.

The fingers of the left hand are now introduced into the above-mentioned triangular space, so that their palmar surfaces pass around the oesophagus from anterior to right lateral and then to its posterior aspect, finding their way out through the incised mediastinal pleura between the oesophagus and the aorta. In this situation the dorsum of the fingers face the opposite pleura. One end of the tape is picked up between the fingers which are withdrawn with the tape between them, following their passage around the oesophagus. The two ends of the tape are now held by artery forceps. When the tape is gently pulled, it lifts the lower oesophagus allowing its easy mobilisation by sharp and blunt dissection.

The oesophageal vessels need division between ligatures. The use of an automatic 'ligating-dividing' instrument is of great help for dealing with the oesophageal arteries deriving directly from the aorta. In all operations, vascularisation of the oesophagus must be kept in mind. There is no hope for any suture line or anastomosis to survive without healthy vascularisation and good blood supply.

4. Technique of anastomosis

There are some unimportant controversies regarding the type of suture material and the most appropriate method of stitching in order to achieve a sound- and leak-proof oesophageal anastomosis. In the author's experience there are many methods of anastomosis which work well in experienced hands.

In all methods it is important:
- To avoid injury to the muscular wall of the oesophagus,
- To preserve (respect) the blood supply (arterial and also venous),
- To perform anastomosis in a disease-free part of the oesophagus.

The anastomosis may be carried out using hand-sewing technique or employing staplers.

The author's technique, which is shared by many, is to use two layers of interrupted stitches of non-absorbable (3.0) on atraumatic needles. In the first layer, the muscularis of the oesophagus is picked up and, as there is no serous membrane, the stitches are placed horizontally. In the second layer, the sutures pick up the complete thickness of the oesophagus, that is mucosa, submucosa and muscularis.

5. Oesophageal substitute (grafts)

At present there is no suitable manufactured oesophageal prosthesis which can replace and function in place of the resected oesophagus. Therefore, reconstruction of the alimentary tract following an oesophagectomy is limited to the use of an autotransplant of a tubular organ with its vascular pedicle. The stomach, jejunum or the colon satisfy the requirements and are used as an oesophageal substitute. When transplanted with their vascular pedicles, they can be anastomosed to the residual oesophagus (or the pharynx) and will assume the function of the oesophagus. Table 1 shows the advantages and disadvantages of oesophageal substitutes.

All transplants are positioned isoperistaltically. It is also important to ascertain that the transplanted substitute is not distorted in its passage from abdomen to/or through the chest to the neck. Insertion of a marker stitch on the anterior aspect of the substitute will assure identification of its correct position.

- The stomach has always been favoured for reconstruction of the alimentary tract. Its rich communicating blood vessels and the presence of a long vascular pedicle (the gastro-epiploic arcade) along its greater curvature make the stomach a strong candidate for oesophageal replacement. In addition, the stomach has two other attributes in its favour. Firstly, it can be transplanted to the neck when sufficiently mobilised and can be easily connected even to the pharynx. Secondly, when the stomach is used for reconstruction the operation usually involves one anastomosis only. There are, however, disadvantages associated with use of the stomach, the most cardinal of which are:
  - Loss of reservoir for food and the presence of a 'bag of fluid and gas' in the chest which is space-occupying,
  - Lack of effective peristaltic activities of the transplanted stomach can result in reflux of its content into the remnant oesophagus and pharynx.
- Jejunum: As a substitute, the jejunum has much to recommend it. It is already a tubular organ. Its vascularisation is rich and because of its peristalsis it can function in harmony with the oesophagus thus preventing reflux. However, it has two disadvantages. First, it cannot be transplanted directly with its mesenteric pedicle to distant sites such as the neck, or even the upper chest, with ease. Also, its use as a transplant involves several anastomoses.

Table 1

Advantages and disadvantages of various oesophageal substitutes

Type of substitute	Advantage	Disadvantage
Stomach	• Generous blood supply. • Can be transplanted to any level, including the pharynx. • Operation involves single anastomosis. • Low mortality even in the elderly.	• Reduction in stomach capacity at least initially. • Can be bulky and affects patients respiratory capacity as it is space-occupying. • Regurgitation of reflux may be a problem, particularly in low anastomosis. • Anastomotic stricture can occur.
Jejunum	• Good blood supply. • No regurgitation.	• Cannot be easily transplanted to any level especially in well-built individuals with fatty mesentery. • Multiple anastomoses required.
Colon	• Good blood supply. • Can be transplanted to any position including pharynx. • No regurgitation.	• Multiple anastomoses. • Late over-expansion of transplant

It is relevant to point out that an isolated loop of jejunum detached from its vascular pedicle may be used as a substitute in the neck when its artery and vein can be connected to neck vessels.

• The colon can be a suitable oesophageal substitute. Endowed with a loose mesentery and a vascular arcade which is connected to long vascular trunks, the colon can reach to any level. It also has a peristaltic activity which prevents reflux. However, like the jejunum, it has the disadvantage that its use necessitates many anastomoses.

6. Drainage of the chest following oesophageal surgery

Following all intra-thoracic oesophageal operations, the chest is drained using an underwater sealed drainage system. In cases of oesophagectomy, when there has been excision of the mediastinal pleura and communication between the two pleural cavities, a mediastinal drain is also required. This drain should preferably be a soft plastic or silastic tube and placed in the posterior mediastinum towards the opposite pleural space. The drainage of the abdominal cavity and the neck spaces may be necessary in some cases. It must be realised that after an oesophageal operation involving the neck, thorax and the abdomen, there is communication between all these spaces. Therefore, all drains in the neck spaces and the abdominal cavity in such cases will have to connect to an underwater sealed drainage system, otherwise air from these drains will find its way into the pleural cavities with resultant pneumothorax and collapse of the lung.

7. Resection and reconstruction of the oesophagus

There are now a number of well-established methods to resect the oesophagus and reconstruct the alimentary tract, each with its advocates. It is not within the scope of this book to describe in detail all techniques of oesophageal resection and reconstruction. Nevertheless, it is helpful to describe the basic principles of the more practised operations.

7.1. Oesophagectomy and oesophago-gastric anastomosis

7.1.1. Technique 1 — Oesophagectomy and low oesophago-gastric anastomosis
The operation is carried out through a left postero-lateral thoracotomy (Fig. 2b). The pleura is entered through the 7th or 8th interspace. Access to the abdomen is obtained through a peripheral and circumferential incision of the diaphragm avoiding the phrenic nerve (Fig. 3). This method was introduced by VC Thompson (1945) and has been extensively used by the author. The oesophagus bearing the lesion is mobilised and the hiatus cleared from fibro-fatty tissue. The blood vessels of the healthy oesophagus are carefully preserved. Alternative access is through left thoraco-laparotomy incision with/without division of the costal margin. The diaphragm is incised peripherally (Fig. 4).

In both approaches, the two edges of the diaphragmatic incision are retracted to allow inter-abdominal manipulations. Mobilisation of the stomach fundus and a variable portion of the body is carried out by

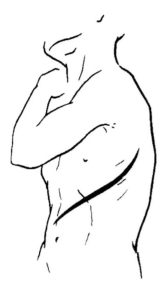

Fig. 4. Thoraco-laparotomy incision.

division between ligatures of gastrosplenic, gastro-colic and relevant gastrohepatic omenta. If necessary, the left gastric vessels may be ligated and divided but the gastro-epiploic arcade must be preserved.

Prior to delivery of the stomach to the chest, the hiatus is widened to allow this. The upper part of the stomach is now incised between two clamps (non-crushing on the stomach side). Alternatively, a TA 90 autosuture may be applied. The stomach incision is closed (the author uses two layers of absorbable 3.0 stitching) and oesophago-gastric (end-to-side) anastomosis is performed in two layers. The hiatus is now reconstructed and a few stitches are inserted to anchor the intra-thoracic stomach to the border of the now enlarged hiatus.

The diaphragmatic incision is then repaired in two layers using continuous non-absorbable material. For this, the author uses one layer of horizontal mattress sutures and then oversews this with another layer of continuous running sutures. The chest is then drained and closed.

7.1.2. Technique 2 — Oesophagectomy and high oesophago-gastric anastomosis in the chest

This technique is useful for oesophageal resection and its replacement by the stomach with high thoracic anastomosis (Fig. 5). The operation is based on the method described by Ivor Lewis (1946) who advocated it for resection of thoracic oesophageal cancer followed by oesophageal reconstruction using the stomach. The two stages of this operation are carried out as one procedure.

- Stage 1 — Abdominal stage
  The aim is to mobilise the stomach, completely ligating and dividing all blood vessels except for the right gastric and right gastro-epiploic arcade and its branches which enter the greater curvature of the stomach at right angles.

  With the patient lying on his back, an upper laparotomy is carried out and the stomach is fully mobilised. This involves ligation and division of the gastrosplenic, gastrocolic and gastrohepatic omenta with their contained blood vessels. The left gastric vessels are also divided between ligatures on the upper border of the pancreas, taking care not to damage the hepatic and splenic vessels. The right gastric artery is best preserved. The oesophageal hiatus of the diaphragm is then enlarged and the oesophagus is freed from all its attachments to the hiatus by sharp and blunt dissection. Two fingers of the right hand are inserted into the mediastinum through the hiatus posterior to the oesophagus, then anterior and finally, laterally, to assure freedom from adhesion. The abdomen is then closed.

- Stage 2 — Thoracic stage
  The patient is placed in left lateral position. The chest is opened by right posterolateral thoracotomy and the oesophagus is exposed through the 5th intercostal space. The oesophagus is mobilised from the hiatus to the level of the arch of the azygos vein; the latter is divided between two ligatures. Attention is paid to vascularisation of the oesophagus above the diseased area so that the anastomosis is within the healthy tissues. The stomach is now delivered into the chest through the hiatus and divided between two clamps, the distal clamp being a non-crushing one and the proximal a crushing one (alternatively TA 90 autosuture may be used). The line of the distal clamp (non-crushing) is closed with running through-and-through stitching reinforced by a second layer of seromuscular sutures using absorbable material. Note: when a stapler is used, a single layer of sero-muscular stitching will suffice.

  The anastomosis between the stomach and the oesophagus is made in a similar manner to that described for oesophago-gastric anastomosis in the left chest (see Technique 1 in section 7.1.1 above). The chest is then drained and closed.

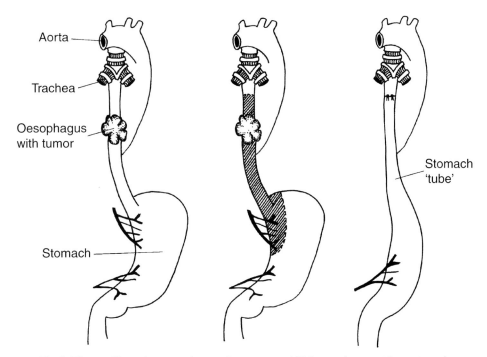

Fig. 5. Diagram illustrating stages in oesophagectomy and high oesophago-gastric anastomosis.

7.1.3. Three stage oesophagectomy (abdomino-thoraco-cervical approach)

This operation uses an abdominal midline incision to prepare gastric tube for oesophageal reconstruction, a right thoracotomy to excise the tumour and a cervical incision to access the oesophagus in the neck (Figs. 1a and 2a). The whole of the thoracic oesophagus (together with the tumour) is then excised and end-to-side oesophago-gastric anastomosis is carried out in the neck. The operation may be carried out by one team undertaking the procedure through three approaches. Alternatively, it can be carried out synchronously as a combined abdomino-thoraco-cervical oesophagectomy by two teams as was conceived by Milnes–Walker and Nanson (Nanson, 1988).

7.1.4. Trans-hiatal oesophagectomy (THO)

Although there is a tendency to suggest that trans-hiatal oesophagectomy is a relatively new procedure, in fact its principles date back to Grey–Turner (Turner, 1933). In recent years the operation has been popularised by Orringer (1984).

The approach is via a mid-line laparotomy and a cervical incision. The important steps of this operation are:

- Full mobilisation of the stomach (adding the Kocher manoeuvre to achieve extra mobility).

- Blunt dissection of the oesophagus in the posterior mediastinum through the abdominal wound after enlargement of the hiatus. It is important to note that:
  - THO is contra-indicated if there is evidence of fixation of tumour to adjacent mediastinal structures,
  - If the pleural spaces are accidentally opened they should be drained during the operation to prevent continuous accumulation of blood in the pleural spaces,
  - Extra care is required to avoid damage to the azygos vein and to the membranous posterior walls of the airway, namely the left main bronchus and lower part of the trachea in the region of the carina.
- The cervical incision is made along the anterior border of the sternomastoid muscle (the author prefers the right side approach),
  - The oesophagus is encircled and mobilisation proceeded from the neck and the abdomen until complete freedom of the thoracic oesophagus with its tumour from surrounding structures is achieved.
- The cervical oesophagus is stapled and divided (GIA surgical stapler). The proximal end is retracted gently upwards. The distal end is attached (sewn) to a wide tape.

- The cardiac end of the oesophagus is clamped. Below this clamp, the oesophago-gastric junction is double stapled and divided between the two rows of staples. The gastric end is then sewn over by a running stitch.
- The cardiac end of the oesophagus, assisted by the clamp, is pulled out towards the abdomen. This should allow complete withdrawal of thoracic oesophagus from the mediastinum with the tape attached to its cervical end out of the hiatus. The oesophagus (and the tumour) is now removed by cutting the tape. Note that one end of this tape is in the neck and the other in the abdomen.
- The abdominal end of the tape is then attached to the gastric tube.
- The gastric tube is next sewn to the tape and the stomach is carefully pushed to the mediastinum. A gentle pull on the tape from its cervical end places the stomach nicely in the mediastinum.
- Oesophago-gastric anastomosis is then carried out after trimming the oesophagus just above the stapled line.
- Drains are placed in the abdominal cavity, the mediastinum (through the hiatus) and neck space as well as the pleura (or pleurae) if required. All drains should be connected to an underwater system.

7.1.5. Synchronous combined pharyngo-laryngo-total oesophagectomy — pharyngo-gastric anastomosis

This is an operation for post-cricoid or upper cervical carcinoma. The operation is carried out by two teams; thoracic surgical (team 1) and otorhino-laryngologist (team 2).

- Team 1 starts with laparotomy and preparation of the stomach and then carries out transhiatal mobilisation of the oesophagus similar to the operation of trans-hiatal oesophagectomy (section 7.1.4 above).
- Team 2 starts simultaneously to mobilise the pharyngo-larynx and make an incision in the trachea below the larynx. The distal end of the trachea is then prepared for a permanent tracheostomy.
- Team 1 severs the oesophagus at the cardia and the whole of the oesophagus is pulled to the neck and can be extirpated together with the larynx, tumour and the laryngo-pharynx. The gastric tube is then fashioned and the stomach is next delivered to the neck. Pharyngo-gastric anastomosis is carried out and finally the permanent tracheostomy is fashioned. Drains are then placed as per trans-hiatal oesophagectomy and wounds repaired.

7.2. Replacement of the oesophagus by jejunum (jejunal interposition)

The approach to this operation can be made in three different ways:
(1) With the patient in the right lateral position, the chest is entered through the left posterolateral thoracotomy with access to the abdomen obtained through the diaphragm.
(2) With the patient in the oblique position a left thoracolaparotomy approach can be used, i.e. the incision of a low anterolateral thoracotomy is carried forward over the upper abdomen, the costal margin may be divided to obtain a very wide thoracolaparotomy exposure. It is however, preferable to make a separate abdominal incision which obviates the division of the costal margin.
(3) When the jejunal interposition is to be performed in the right chest, the operation may be carried out as a two-stage procedure with laparotomy and a separate right thoracotomy.

In the operation of jejunal interposition a suitable loop of jejunum is selected and divided at its two ends (with the mesentery and the contained blood vessels intact). The continuity of the bowel is then established by jejunojejunal anastomosis.

The portion of the diseased oesophagus is resected and the stomach end is closed. The isolated loop of the jejunum is now passed through the hiatus and anastomosed isoperistaltically to the oesophagus and the stomach. There is therefore, an oesophago-jejunal and a jejunogastric anastomosis. Attention should be paid to the vascular pedicle, its integrity and the way it passes through the hiatus, so that there is no distortion and twisting. This is even more crucial when jejunal loop is placed in the right chest through a separate thoracotomy (Fig. 6).

7.3. Oesophagectomy and reconstruction with the use of colonic transplant

The principle of this operation is the same as those for jejunal transplant (Fig. 3). The disease-bearing portion of the oesophagus is resected and the stomach end is closed. A suitable length of the selected colon is then isolated and divided at both its ends, carefully preserving the marginal arcade and its vascular trunk. The continuity of the bowel is established by colocolic anastomosis. The isolated loop is then anastomosed to the oesophageal remnant isoperistaltically. The distal end of the loop is anastomosed to the stomach end-to-side.

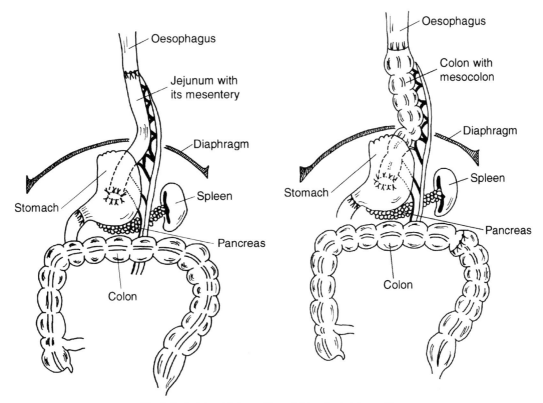

Fig. 6. Left: jejunal interposition, right: colonic interposition.

There are a variety of surgical approaches for oeso-phagocoloplasty depending on:

(a) The extent of the oesophageal excision: the max-imum being when the whole of the oesophagus is removed and the colon needs to be anastomosed to the pharynx,

(b) The type of disease: for a benign reflux stricture only a short segment is needed and the operation is best carried out through the left chest,

(c) Whether the transplanted bowel is placed in the posterior or the anterior mediastinum.

The usual approach for a short segment replace-ment is a left thoracotomy and access to the abdomen through the diaphragm.

A short segment of the colon, usually the splenic flexure with the ascending branch of left colic artery as the main arterial supply is selected. This seg-ment is isolated for transplant with its vascular pedicle (mesocolon) intact. Colon to colon anas-tomosis establishes the continuity of the large bowel. Isoperistaltic oesophago-colonic and colono-gastric anastomoses reconstruct the upper alimentary tract (Fig. 6).

References and further reading

Lewis I. The surgical treatment of carcinoma of the oesophagus. Br J Surg 1946; 34: 18–31.

Nanson EM. Synchronous combined abdomino thoraco-cervical esophagectomy: the team approach. In: Delarue NC, Wilkins EW, Wong J (eds.), International Trends in General Thoracic Surgery (Vol. 4). St. Louis: CV Mosby Company, 1988; pp. 215–219.

Orringer MB. Technical aids in performing transhiatal esophagec-tomy without thoracotomy. Ann Thorac Surg 1984; 38: 128–132.

Orringer MB, Marshall B, Iannettoni MD. Trans-hiatal eso-phagectomy for treatment of benign and malignant esophageal disease. World J Surg 2001; 25: 196–203.

Thompson VC. Carcinoma of the oesophagus. Resection and oesophago-gastrectomy. Br J Surg 1945; 32: 377–380.

Turner GG. Excision of the thoracic oesophagus for carcinoma with construction of an extrathoracic gullet. Lancet 1933; 9: 1315–1316.

CHAPTER III.18

Peri-operative management of patients undergoing oesophageal surgery

K. Moghissi

Under this heading is described:
(1) Pre-operative assessment and preparation
(2) Post-operative management
(3) Peri-operative nutritional management

1. Pre-operative assessment and preparation

1.1. Introduction

Distinction should be made between complex operations which involve oesophageal resection and reconstruction and simpler procedures without resection and reconstruction. Assessment and preparation of the patients for surgery in the latter group is no different from those undergoing pulmonary and general thoracic surgery described previously (see chapter I.17).

Patients undergoing resection of the oesophagus require establishment of the continuity of the upper alimentary tract using stomach jejunum or colon. This entails extensive surgical trauma in consequence of abdominal as well as thoracic surgical procedures. Many patients are dysphagic, some due to malignant obstructive lesions. Such patients are often malnourished and are prone to heightened post-operative complications. It follows that this subgroup needs special assessment and preparation relating to the complexity of the planned surgery. A rigorous assessment of cardiovascular, respiratory and other systems is required and attention should also focus on specific issues relating to the operation on the oesophagus and reconstruction of the upper digestive system.

1.2. Information and counselling

The majority of oesophageal resections are carried out in patients with obstructive diseases of the gullet with dysphagia. A high percentage of these patients are elderly and, for many with coexisting pathological conditions, eating is one of their few remaining pleasures. If they are constantly affected by dyspepsia, pain and/or dysphagia they will become depressed. Medical and nursing staff should explain the nature of the operation including post-operative requirements such as intravenous infusion, drainage tubes and nasogastric catheter. A patient in the twenty-first century should be well-informed regarding the risks and benefits of the proposed procedure. This information should be given in the course of an informal discussion with the hopeful prospect of re-establishment of oral food intake, which is the final objective of all oesophageal surgery.

1.3. Nutritional assessment and planning (see peri-operative nutritional management, section 3 further in this chapter)

1.4. Infection: prevention and prophylaxis

1.4.1. Hygiene of the mouth and oesophagus
Particular attention should be paid to oral and dental hygiene before surgery. Nursing staff should carry out repeated mouthwashes in patients with evidence of mouth or dental sepsis.

In patients with severe obstructive lesions the oesophagus may become very dilated and accommodate an enormous volume of foul-smelling liquid and food debris teeming with a multitude of pathogenic organisms. Regurgitation and subsequent inhalation of these organisms during the induction of anaesthesia can seriously affect the patient's recovery. In the course of surgery involving resection of the oesophagus, the oesophageal contents can soil and contaminate the pleural and mediastinal spaces. In patients with oesophageal obstruction, dietary intake should be restricted to liquid for a day or two before operation and oesophageal lavage should be carried out the day prior to surgery.

1.4.2. Prophylaxis and therapy of chest infection
Severely dysphagic patients are prone to chest infection on several accounts:
- Regurgitation and inhalation of oesophageal content in recumbent position, particularly at night,
- Lack of resistance to infection imposed by malnutrition and relative immunological incompetence,
- Existence of chronic bronchitis, emphysema and chronic obstructive pulmonary disease (COPD) in many patients prior to surgery.

Samples of sputum and regurgitant material (vomited by the patient) should be despatched to the laboratory for full microbiological studies including sensitivity to antibiotics. If there is overt chest infection, an appropriate antibiotic should be given for a few days prior to operation. Otherwise, a prophylactic regimen should be instituted

Prophylactic antibiotic use in surgery has been the subject of numerous publications some of which advise only a single dose at the start of the operation. However, many such studies have not specified the type of operation. In a study to assess the relevance of microbiological flora of the upper alimentary tract upon post-operative infection following major oesophageal surgery, Sharpe et al. (1992) showed that 67% of 140 patients with malignant oesophageal obstruction undergoing oesophagectomy had pathogenic organisms in the lumen of their oesophagus prior to surgery. Twenty-five patients (18%) developed post-operative infective complications. In 18 of these (66%), the infecting organisms were those which were recovered from the oesophageal lumen pre-operatively. In another prospective randomised study, the same group (Sharpe et al., 1992) showed that an effective antibiotic regimen for patients undergoing complex oesophageal surgery when the lumen of the oesophagus was opened, consisted of combined Cefuroxime 1.5 g and Metronidazole 1 g at induction of anaesthesia followed by four days of Cefuroxime 750 mg (twice daily) and Metronidazole

500 mg (four times daily). For oesophageal patients not undergoing resection, Cefuroxime alone at induction and for two post-operative days provided adequate prophylaxis.

1.5. Bowel preparation

In addition to the usual attention to bowel action and preparation before major surgery, special preparation of the colon is necessary for patients undergoing oesophago-coloplasty. The author's method of bowel preparation in these patients is as follows:
(a) If the patient is taking oral food, a low residue diet is given for three or four days prior to operation. In cases of severe dysphagia, total or supplementary parenteral or enteral nutrition is provided,
(b) Neomycin is given 1 g three times daily starting 72 hours before surgery.
(c) An enema is given 72 hours before operation followed by a twice daily bowel washout,
(d) A final washout is given the night before operation.

2. Post-operative management of patients undergoing oesophageal surgery

Post-operative management may be divided into the following categories:
(2.1) General management,
(2.2) Special management.

2.1. General post-operative management

Some aspects of general post-operative care and management are similar to the care of patients after pulmonary and general thoracic surgery (see chapter I.19) and need not be repeated. These concern:
- Transfer and return to the ward,
- Baseline observations and monitoring,
- Sedation, rest and sleep,
- General post-operative care and treatment.

2.2. Special post-operative management

The most crucial role of post-operative management after major oesophageal surgery is to re-establish the anatomical and functional state of the upper alimentary canal and prevent complications. The aim is for the patient to be able to eat normally and, to this end, special post-operative management may be discussed under:

(2.2.1) Alimentary tract management,
(2.2.2) Nutritional management (see section 3).

2.2.1. Alimentary tract management

- Oral hygiene is an important aspect of post-operative care in patients who have undergone oesophageal surgery. The mouth and throat are often contaminated by residual contents from the oesophagus. In addition, lack of oral food and liquid intake following surgery, together with dryness of the mouth and reduction of salivary secretions, produce an environment suited to growth of organisms.
- Nasogastric tube: In the early post-operative phase whilst intravenous feeding is in progress, the alimentary tract is 'at rest'. A nasogastric tube is, in most case, in situ. This should be disposed of as soon as possible. The tube is irritating, creates secretion and may be a factor in chest infection. When such a tube is in place, aspiration should be periodic, hourly at first then four to six hourly).The lumen should be open to air and not spigotted. This allows the exit of air with possible overflow of liquid. One method to prevent overflow is to connect the open end of the tube to a 20 to 50 ml syringe from which the plunger is removed and fixed in a vertical position to the patient's pillow allowing sufficient free length of the tube for the patient's movements. If the nasogastric tube is accidentally removed it should not be replaced unless there are good and pressing reasons to do so (e.g. distension and ileus).
- A patient undergoing major oesophageal reconstruction will be having total parenteral/enteral feeding during early postoperative days. This usually expands from 4 to 7 days during which time the regimen of nil by mouth is maintained. Prior to oral intake of fluid/nutrients, a contrast swallow is carried out to ascertain the integrity of repair or anastomosis.
- When oral feeding is resumed, the volume of food taken in each meal should be small. In some cases, the stomach may have been resected together with a portion of the oesophagus. In others, the oesophagus is reconstructed with the stomach tube and there is no reservoir to accommodate food and there is no sphincteric action of the lower oesophagus. It is therefore essential to provide small amounts of food at frequent intervals, otherwise reflux will become a serious problem.
- Whichever method has been used to replace the resected oesophagus, reconstruction of the alimentary tract necessitates anastomosis. It is important to prevent distension which can have several effects:
  - Imposing a strain on the suture lines,
  - Interfering with blood supply and venous return causing ischaemia, and hindering the anastamotic healing.
  - Causing distension of the bowels and interfering with fluid and nutrient absorption leading to disturbances of body fluid.

The abdomen should be examined daily by the resident doctor to assess distension and the presence of bowel sounds. If a nasogastric tube is in place, the volume and type of aspirate is checked. If there is evidence of distension but no aspirate can be recovered from the nasogastric tube, it is worthwhile withdrawing the tube for 2 or 3 cm and/or gently injecting 20 to 30 ml of warm saline and then aspirating. This often produces a remarkable result if the tube has been kinked or blocked.

- Prevention of regurgitation: When reconstruction of the alimentary tract involves use of the stomach as a substitute, there is no barrier to food regurgitation. The consequences of this are:
  - The sensation of gastric content in the throat and/or nausea and vomiting, particularly when the patient is in a reclining position,
  - A feeling of fullness after a meal with rejection of food and vomiting when the patient eats a greater volume than their reduced stomach can accommodate. Patients are advised to sleep in a propped-up position in bed. Medications such as Metoclopramide (Maxolon) are of benefit in reducing the sensation and also help emptying of the stomach,
  - Aspiration of the stomach contents into the airway with pulmonary infective complications.
- Irregular bowel action: After oesophagectomy the majority of patients develop constipation. Some, particularly after total gastrectomy, may have diarrhoea. During the post-operative phase, bowel action should be checked and its irregularities dealt with. Constipation can often be treated by dietary means but, if necessary, suppositories and small enemas may be given. Diarrhoea can sometimes be prevented by adhering to the principle of small and frequent meals. The addition of drugs such as codeine phosphate 30 mg two to three times daily will also be helpful. Prior to administrating drugs, the aetiology of the diarrhoea must be investigated and infective causes excluded.

3. Peri-operative nutritional management for patients undergoing major oesophageal surgery

3.1. Introduction

Peri-operative nutritional management is an important aspect of the care of patients undergoing major oesophageal surgery. Pre-operatively, many patients with malignant oesophageal obstruction are nutritionally deficient. Some patients receive adjuvant chemo/radiotherapy which upsets their normal food intake, at least temporarily, and consequently heightens their malnourishment. The operation itself introduces a catabolic state commensurate to the extent of the operation. For a few days post-operatively, the reconstructed upper alimentary canal cannot be used for delivery of nutrients. If there is a complication which affects the integrity of the new oesophagus, there will be additional anatomical problems with food delivery and burden of increased catabolic demand. It therefore follows that a proper nutritional programme must be undertaken for oesophagectomy patients. The specialist units which carry out oesophageal surgery should have a dedicated protocol for nutrition and a team experienced in assessing and planning the patients individual nutritional requirements and the route for delivery of nutrients.

3.2. Pre-operative nutritional assessment and planning

Pre-operative evaluation of nutritional status constitutes a mandatory part of the overall management of patients undergoing oesophageal surgery.

The objectives of nutritional assessment are:
- To identify and correct pre-operative deficiencies,
- To plan a comprehensive peri-operative nutritional scheme which includes the route of delivery of nutrient and appropriate regimen.

3.2.1. Nutritional markers

There exist a variety of clinical, anthropometrics and laboratory parameters by which nutritional status can be gauged. Many are used to elucidate nutritional deficiencies in metabolic disease or in a specific condition. Only a few are of practical relevance to oesophageal surgical patients.

Pre-operatively, the nutrition team should interview and assess the nutritional status of the patient in cooperation with the surgeon. Table 1 shows the common nutritional markers used to evaluate pre-operative nutritional status.

3.3. Peri-operative provision of artificial nutrition

Artificial feeding of oesophageal surgical patients, be it parenteral or enteral, is concerned with:
(3.3.1) Pre-operative to correct existing malnutrition,
(3.3.2) Post-operative to cover the normal or complicated post-operative period.

3.3.1. Pre-operative artificial nutrition
The requirement for this depends on:
- The severity of existing malnutrition,
- The level of nutrient intake expressed as the percentage of estimated energy and protein requirement,

Table 1

Assessment of nutritional status — Common indices of calorie/protein malnutrition

Ideal weight	Weight measurement in kg assessed by reference to standard tables and charts [a]
Weight loss	Expressed as a percentage using the formula: $\frac{\text{weight loss in kg}}{\text{usual weight}} \times 100$
Triceps skinfold	Measured then compared with standard charts for gender and size [a]
Mid-arm circumference	Measured then compared with standard charts for gender and size [a]
Body mass index	Calculated by weight / height^2
Serum Albumin	Measured and compared with normal range and average
Serum Protein	Measured and compared with normal range and average
Serum Transferrin	Measured and compared with normal range and average
Cell mediated immunity (skin test to antigen)	Candida skin test (usually −ve in malnutrition) *Note the limitation of significance of results* Tuberculin skin test (usually −ve) in malnutrition
Lymphocyte count	Measured and compared with the normal range (in malnutrition it is reduced)
Nitrogen balance	Directly measured from protein (nitrogen) intake and urinary output of nitrogen: $\frac{\text{Nitrogen intake}}{\text{Nitrogen output}}$ or $\frac{\text{Nitrogen intake}}{\text{Calculation of urinary nitrogen (urea)}}$ (−ve in malnourished)

[a] Reference to standard charts.

- The additional demand of adjuvant chemo/radiotherapy when, and if, applicable.

A number of studies have been carried out to quantitatively assess the level of pre-operative requirement in patients undergoing general and gastro-intestinal surgery. Most of these studies have determined the basic requirement to be:
- Energy = 30 to 35 kcal/kg body weight per day with 40 to 50% provided by carbohydrate,
- Nitrogen = 200–250 mg/ kg body weight per day.

Of all oesophageal conditions which concern the surgeon, two groups may require pre-operative nutritional support:
(a) Patients with malignant obstructive lesions and severe dysphagia,
(b) Patients with long standing benign oesophageal obstruction and dysphagia.

Malignant obstructive lesion. Some 65 to 70% of patients with cancer of the oesophagus are malnourished according to clinical anthropometric and laboratory criteria. In these patients there is a good correlation between severe (>10%) loss of body weight, decrease in mid-arm muscle circumference and negative nitrogen balance. For such depleted patients a period of seven to ten days pre-operative artificial feeding should be considered (Moghissi and Teasdale, 1980; Moghissi et al., 1992; McClave et al., 1999a,b).

Benign obstructive lesions. Severe malnutrition is uncommon amongst patients with benign lesions, even when dysphagia is severe. Occasionally some such patients present with a moderate degree of malnutrition. This sub-group requires pre-operative supplementary nutrition particularly if surgical therapy is going to involve resection of the oesophagus and reconstruction with the need for post-operative support.

Controversy regarding the method of pre-operative artificial nutrition, parenteral or enteral, continues. Our experience suggests that in patients with severe malnutrition (>10% of weight loss) suffering from critical-to-complete malignant dysphagia, pre-operative artificial nutrition is best carried out through the parenteral route. This is supported by a review/study of the literature and also by Gordon and Busby (1993) which tends to confirm this view.

It is important to note that great weight loss is rare in patients with benign dysphagia whose dysphagia is neither total nor insurmountable by dilatation.

Therefore, in an overall majority of benign obstructive lesions, oral or pre-operative enteral feeding can remedy any existing malnutrition.

3.3.2. Post-operative artificial nutrition

For the initial few days following major oesophageal surgery, an intravenous supply of fluid and nutrients for five to seven days is necessary. Thereafter the patient can be gradually introduced to enteral and then oral feeding supported by enteral nutrition followed by normal eating. It should be borne in mind that prior to oral intake, contrast swallow should be carried out to ensure the absence of anastomotic leak. Even when patients are taking food and liquid orally, intake will often still be insufficient to their requirements.

Fluid requirements: Calculation of fluid requirements should take account of:
- Basic requirement of fluid according to body weight or body surface,
- Volume of fluid loss in the drainage containers,
- Volume of aspirate from nasogastric tubes, etc.

Adjustment of the volume of fluid and the electrolyte content must be made according to the general clinical condition, urinary output and laboratory results.

The fundamental point is that many patients undergoing oesophageal resection and reconstruction are elderly with a degree of cardiac and renal dysfunction. The volume prescribed must take account of this and the patient must not be overloaded with fluid.

A number of patients with severe oesophageal obstruction due to cancer suffer from hypoproteinaemia, particularly hypoalbuminaemia which, because of dehydration, may not be demonstrable when they are first admitted to hospital. Additional fluid volume may cause oedema, including that of the lung.

Our experience suggests that a fluid volume of 35 to 40 ml/kg body weight covers the basic requirement of a patient in the immediate post-operative phase to which should be added the abnormal losses. Alteration should be made in special circumstances (e.g. complications). All fluid intake and output is recorded on a chart. It may at this juncture be pointed out that a fluid chart should allow for recording of the following details:
- Time, volume and type of fluid given by the nurse (in the case of i.v. fluid the commencing time should be recorded),
- Time, volume and type of fluid received or taken by the patient (in the case of i.v. fluid the time of completion should be recorded),

- Time and volume of urine output,
- Time, volume and type of aspirate from the naso-gastric tube.
- Volume and type of drainage from individual drains, calculated 12 to 24 hourly unless otherwise necessary (because of profuse drainage).

Nutritional requirement:

The ideal situation for a patient undergoing oesophageal resection is that they are well-hydrated and well-nourished (in positive or equilibrium nitrogen balance) at the time of undergoing surgical operation. Post-operatively, a patient will need to receive nutrients intravenously or artificially, either parenterally or enterally, until such time as food can be taken by mouth.

The energy and nitrogen requirements to cover the post-operative phase has been shown to be:

- Energy = 30 to 35 kcal/kg body weight per day with 40to 50% provided by carbohydrate,
- Nitrogen = 200 to 250 mg/kg body weight per day.

Our experience based on several studies concerning 300 oesophagectomies indicates that a basic energy intake of 40 to 45 kcal/kg bw per day and protein intake equivalent to 200 to 250 mg nitrogen/kg bw per day will satisfy the requirements and achieve positive or equilibrium nitrogen balance. When there are additional abnormal losses (either as drainage or large volume aspirate) their total volume should not only be counted as water loss but as protein-containing fluid and should be accounted for in the allowance. In the event of complication (such as fistulae) the volume of protein-rich fluid losses should also be added to the basic allowance. To the list of allowances should be added the energy and protein requirements which are necessary to cover such complications as infection with its associated hypercatabolism (see Table 2).

The route for delivery of nutrients in the post-operative period has also been the subject of much debate. Some surgeons rely entirely on an intravenous route to supply the immediate (5–7 days) post-operative period (Waitzberg et al., 1999). Others advocate enteral nutritional methods as soon as possible (often not specifying how long after operation). There is also no indication of the nutritional state of the patient prior to surgery. Recent studies (Pacellis et al., 2001; Heyland et al., 2001; Baigrie et al., 1997) suggest there is no difference between the morbidity and mortality rate between the two routes for delivery of post-operative nutrient. A problem with many of the studies concerned with nutrition for surgical patients is regarding a heterogeneous population undergoing many different types of surgery. The author's personal experience suggests that parenteral and enteral nutrition should be regarded as complimentary to each other.

Based on experience we have devised the following protocol for patients undergoing major surgical operation of resection and reconstruction:

- A central venous catheter is placed for intravenous nutrients either pre-operatively, for those requiring nutritional support prior to surgery, or at the time of operation,
- A fine tube jejunostomy feeding catheter is inserted at operation,
- During the first 5–7 post-operative days, total and partial parenteral nutrition is given, the latter together with jejunostomy feeding. Intravenous nutrients are reduced from day three to four and jejunostomy feeding is increased so that by day six to seven, enteral nutrition is fully established and intravenous feeding discontinued. Thereafter, oral feeding is resumed with gradual increase in the volume and consistency as shown in Table 3.

Particular attention must be paid to the nutritional value of food intake when oral feeding is resumed as, at this time, there is a tendency to lose ground. Arrangements should be made with the nutritional team to provide a high calorie and protein content for these patients. Also, based on post-operative nutritional studies, the author believes that in many cases there is a need for nutritional support by supplementary feeding using manufactured nutrient solutions, even when the patient's alimentary tract is fully operational.

3.4. Route of delivery of nutrient

Selection of the method and route of delivery of nutrient in the pre-operative period requires careful planning. Consideration should be given to:

- The type of surgical procedure which is planned

Table 2

Recommended daily nutritional requirements for the first 7–10 post-operative days

Basic	{	Basic calories: 40–45 kcal/kg body weight
		Basic protein: equivalent of 0.2–0.25 g nitrogen/kg body weight
	+	Losses through drainage and aspirate
	+	Losses through complication
	+	Additions because of hypercatabolism

Table 3

Suggested post-operative nutritional schedule for patients undergoing major oesophageal resection and reconstruction

I.V. and enteral nutrition:

TPN + fluid via jejunostomy	For 2–3 days
Partial i.v. nutrition + enteral nutrition	From 3rd to 6th post-op day
Then the introduction of oral fluid + enteral nutrition	From 6th to 7th post-op day

Oral and enteral nutrition:

Grade I diet: Liquid diet + enteral nutritional support	2 days
Grade II diet: Purée liquidised food + enteral nutritional support	1 to 2 days
Grade III diet: Semi-solid food + oral nutritional support	1 to 2 days
Grade IV diet: Solid diet + oral nutritional support (usually required)	Thereafter

- The patients' requirement
- The estimated post-operative period when the alimentary tract will not be functional
- Experience of the nutritional and surgical team.

The route of pre-operative delivery should take account of the whole peri-operative period and not pre-operative alone.

3.4.1. Parenteral nutrition

This is delivered by intravenous (i.v.) route which, in turn, requires circulatory access. A well-placed i.v. catheter is an essential requirement for i.v. feeding. Peripheral veins are not suitable for the infusion of hypertonic nutritional solutions as they require frequent repositioning. Therefore, central venous catheterisation should be carried out which means using the superior vena cava which is commonly cannulated for i.v. feeding via jugular or subclavian veins. Several methods are used to place the catheter. Figure 1 shows the points of insertion for central venous catheterisation. Two points are used in common practice:

- Percutaneous insertion of the catheter usually through a subclavian vein,
- Cut-down technique for insertion of a catheter into the external (or internal) jugular vein, both of which have been well documented in the literature.

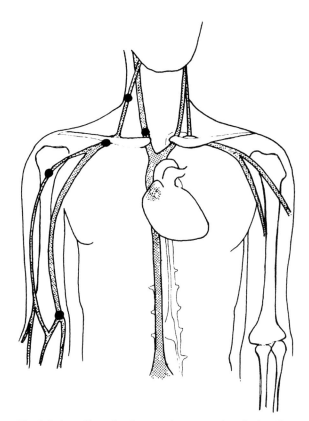

Fig. 1. Points of insertion for central venous catheterisation (from above downwards): external jugular vein, internal jugular vein, subclavian vein (direct insertion), cephalic vein, basilic vein.

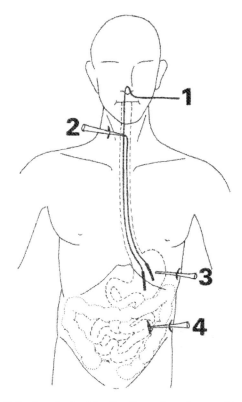

Fig. 2. Routes of enteral feeding (from above downwards): nasogastric tube, oesophagostomy, gastrostomy, jejunostomy.

Whether a cut-down or a percutaneous technique is used for establishing the intravenous infusion, the procedure is considered as a surgical operation and strict antiseptic techniques must therefore be observed.

In all cases, the position of the catheter in the central vein should be checked radiologically, before starting the infusion. Nutrient solutions are particularly favourable for the culture of micro-organisms and the catheter itself is an easy port of entry for the introduction and spread of organisms within the body. Catheter insertion and all manipulation (e.g. change of infusion) should be meticulous with regard to sterile techniques.

Subcutaneous tunnelling of the catheter. For some time, subcutaneous tunnelling of a length of i.v. ca-theter, just distal to its point of entry into the vein, has been advocated (Scribner et al., 1970; Moghissi, 1979). The aims of this method are to:
- Separate the point of entry into the vein from the point of entry into the skin, thereby preventing movement of the catheter in and out of the vein
- Prevent contamination.

3.4.2. Enteral feeding
There are many ways of providing nutrients via the alimentary tract. Figure 2 shows the different routes for enteral feeding.
- *Nasogastric tube feeding:* is probably the commonest method of enteral feeding in hospitals. The standard nasogastric tubes (Ryle's tubes) used for decompression of the gastro-intestinal tract, are wide bored and generally unsuitable for

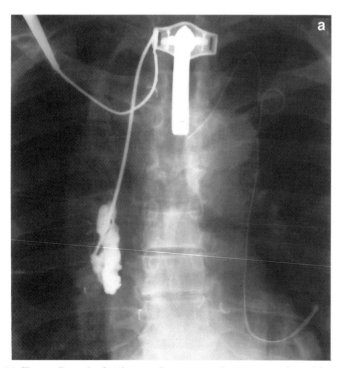
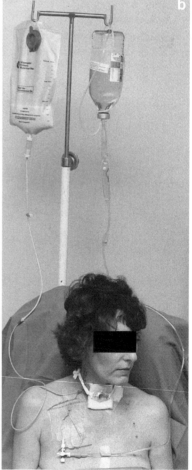

Fig. 3. (a) Chest radiograph of a pharyngo-laryngo-oesophagectomy patient with tracheostomy. The central intravenous line is shown in the left subclavian-innominate vein and contrast medium filled cervical fine tube gastrostomy in place. (b) Fine tube cervical gastrostomy in a patient with pharyngo-laryngectomy and total oesophagectomy. Note cervical gastrostomy (right neck) as well as intravenous fluid into right subclavian/superior vena cava line.

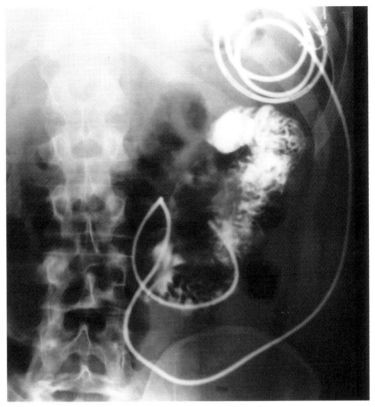

Fig. 4. Fine tube jejunostomy placed at the time of oesophagectomy.

enteral feeding purposes. Instead, fine bore tubes are designed with a diameter of 1 to 2 mm which can be used satisfactorily.

- *Gastrostomy:* is a most convenient and useful method provided that competence of the oe-sophago-gastric sphincteric action can be assured. It may be carried out by standard technique or minimal access (laparoscopic technique) or per-cutaneously employing a fine tube. In patients with gastric tube cervical anastomosis or those with post-cricoid carcinoma undergoing total oe-sophagectomy and pharyngo-laryngectomy, a fine tube cervical gastrostomy can be fashioned to serve for the intake of nutrients or to prevent over-distension (Fig. 3).

- *Jejunostomy (Fig. 4):* This is carried out using a variation of the standard Wangensteen's method (Moghissi and Boore, 1983; Moghissi et al., 1985) and employs a fine catheter. A limited upper mid-line laparotomy is carried out and a loop of jejunum, 10 to 12 cm distal to its commencement, is chosen and exteriorized. A small (narrow ring) purse string suture is applied in the seromuscular coat of the antimesenteric border of the bowel

using a catgut suture. A stab incision is made at the centre of the purse string. The incision should only be large enough to admit a fine feeding tube of 1 or 2 mm in diameter. With the wire still *in situ* the tube is inserted for a distance of 10 to 15 cm in the jejunum, towards the ileum. The wire is withdrawn and the purse string suture is tied around the tube. A second purse string suture is applied around the first one and, in turn, tied with the aim of invaginating or tunnelling the tube. The end of the tube is now brought out of the abdomen through a separate stab skin incision. The jejunum around the fine tube is then transfixed to the peritoneum and abdominal wall, using the needle ends of the purse string catgut sutures.

Both in gastrostomy and jejunostomy, when arti-ficial feeding is to be discontinued, the tube is with-drawn and a small dressing is applied over the ab-dominal wound. This wound will heal in a few days.

It is important to emphasize that in many cases of major oesophageal surgery both parenteral and en-teral nutrition delivery routes should be established. The two routes of delivery are used sequentially in the early post-operative phase. In some cases such as the patient illustrated in Fig. 3a, parenteral and enteral nutrition were used sequentially. Also, cervical fine tube gastrostomy was established. In this case the gastrostomy was used both for aspiration (in early post-operative phase) and for enteral feeding in later post-operative stage.

References and further reading

Abbot WE, Levets S, Krieger H. Metabolic changes in surgical patients in relation to water, electrolytes, nitrogen and calorie intake. Metabolism 1959; 8: 847–861.

Baigrie RJ, Devitt PG, Watkin DS. Enteral versus parenteral nutrition after oesophagogastric surgery: a prospective randomised comparison. Aust NZ J Surg 1997; 67: 736.

Belsey RHR. Hiatus hernia. Modern trends in Gastroenterology. London: Butterworth, 1952.

Bhasin DK, Sharma BC, Gupta MM, Sinah SK, Sing K. Endoscopic dilatation for treatment of anastomotic leaks following transhiatal esphagectomy. Endoscopy 2000; 32: 469–471.

Boyle MJ, Franceschati D, Livingstone AS. Transhiatal versus transthoracic esophagectomy; complications and survival rates. Ann Surg 1999; 65: 1137–1141.

Carr CS, Ling DKE, Boulos P, Singer M. Randomised trial of safety and efficacy of immediate post-operative enteral feeding in patients undergoing gastro-intestinal resection. BMJ 1996; 312: 869–870.

Casson AG, Porter GA. Evolution and critical appraisal of anastomotic technique following resection for esophageal adenocarcinoma, abstract, 2002. Presented at 12th World Congress, World Society of Cardiothoracic Surgeons, Lucerne.

Gordon P, Busby MD. Overview of randomised clinical trials of total parenteral nutrition for malnourished surgical patients. World J Surg 1993; 17: 173–177.

Heyland DK, Montalvo M, MacDonald S, Keefe L, Su XY, Drover JW. Total parenteral nutrition in the surgical patient: a meta analysis. Can J Surg 2001; 44: 86–87.

Johnston IDA, Tweedle DEF, Spivy J. Intravenous feeding after surgical operation. In: Wilkinson, AW (ed.), Parenteral Nutrition. Edinburgh: Churchill Livingstone, 1972; p. 189.

MacFie J. Enteral versus parenteral nutrition. Br J Surg 2000; 87: 1121–1122.

Mann J, Truswell S. Essentials of human nutrition. New York: Oxford U Press, 1998.

McClave SA, Sexton LK, Spain DA, et al. Enteral tube feeding in the intensive care unit: factors impending adequate delivery. Crit Care Med 1999a; 27: 1252–1256.

McClave SA, Snider HL, Spain DA. Pre-operative issues in clinical nutrition. Chest 1999b; 115: 645–705.

Miller JO, Jain MK, de Gara EJ, Morgan D, Urschel JD. Effect of surgical experience on results of oesophagectomy for oesophageal carcinoma. J Surg Oncol 1997; 65: 20–21.

Moghissi K, Hornshaw J, Teasdale PR, Dawes EA. Parenteral nutrition in carcinoma of the oesophagus treated by surgery: nitrogen balance and clinical studies. Br J Surg 1977; 64: 125–128.

Moghissi K. A technique of superior vena caval catheterisation for prolonged intravenous feeding. J R Coll Surg Edin 1979; 24: 178–179.

Moghissi K, Teasdale PR. Parenteral feeding in patients with carcinoma of the oesophagus treated by surgery: energy and nitrogen requirements. J Parenteral Ent Nutr 1980; 4: 371–375.

Moghissi K, Teasdale P, Dench M. Comparison between pre-operative nasogastric feeding and parenteral feeding in patients with cancer of the oesophagus undergoing surgery. J Parenteral Ent Nutr 1982; 6: 335.

Moghissi K, Boore J. Parenteral and enteral nutrition for nurses. London: William Heinemann Medical Books, 1983.

Moghissi K, Dietel M, Taylor GA. Esophageal problems: use of nutritional support. In: Dietel M. (ed.), Nutrition in clinical surgery. Baltimore: Williams Wilkins, 1985; pp. 303–319.

Pacellis F, Bossola M, Papa V, Malerba M, Modesti C, Sgadari A, Bellantone R, Doglietto GB. Enteral versus parenteral nutrition after major abdominal surgery: an even match. Arch Surg 2001; 136: 933–936.

Scribner BH, Cole JJ, Christopher TJ, et al. Long-term parenteral nutrition. The concept of an artificial gut. JAMA 1970; 212: 457–463.

Sharpe DAC, Renwick P, Matthews KHR, Moghissi K. Antibiotic prophylaxis in oesophageal surgery. Eur J Cardiothorac Surg 1992; 6: 561–564.

Swanson SJ, Sugarbaker DJ. The three hole esophagectomy: the Brigham and Women's Hospital approach (modified McKeown technique). Chest Surg Clin N Am 2000; 10: 531–552.

Waitzberg DL, Plopper C, Terra RM. Post-operative total parenteral nutrition. World J Surg 1999; 23: 560–564.

Williams SR. Basic nutrition and diet therapy (11th ed.). Mosby Inc., 2001.

K. Moghissi, J.A.C. Thorpe and F. Ciulli (Eds.)
Moghissi's Essentials of Thoracic and Cardiac Surgery
© 2003 Elsevier Science B.V. All rights reserved

CHAPTER III.19

Complications of oesophageal surgery

K. Moghissi

1. Introduction

One of the objectives of post-operative management is to prevent complications which could jeopardise recovery from surgical operation or, at least, delay them. Most complications set in gradually, beginning with some aberrations in the post-operative course. Undetected or unsuccessfully checked these aberrations become complications.

2. Haemorrhage

As with other types of surgery, post-operative haemorrhage following major oesophageal operations may be reactionary or secondary. The characteristics of the two types of bleeding have been described previously (section 2 in chapter I.20). In major oesophageal surgery involving thoraco-laparotomy haemorrhage may be:

• Externally visible and apparent in drainage container or through the wound,
• Concealed within the chest or abdomen,
• Concealed within the alimentary canal manifesting as haematemesis or malaena.

In the presence of symptoms and signs of bleeding the aetiology and site of bleeding must be investigated urgently using imaging techniques and endoscopic examinations. Serious reactionary haemorrhage often requires re-opening of the wound and arrest of bleeding.

Secondary haemorrhage after oesophagectomy and reconstruction is usually due to:

– Infection causing ulceration and bleeding from the suture line,
– Anastomotic ulcer,
– Fistula between the neo-oesophagus at the site of the anastomosis and a blood vessel such as the pul-

monary artery or the aorta. Such a fistula can cause severe haemorrhage with fatal consequences.

– Occasionally there is haemorrhage from a coincidental duodenal ulcer away from the site of the anastomosis.

3. Cardiovascular complications

3.1. Cardiac

Some oesophageal patients are weak, elderly and have cardiac diseases. Ischaemic heart disease and atrial fibrillation may be pre-existing but because of the distress imposed by malignant or benign oesophageal obstruction, the patient may still be selected for operative treatment. Serious cardiac complications in these cases can be halted by proper monitoring peri-operatively and through appropriate and prompt action. Patients with manifest cardiac complications should be referred to a cardiologist.

3.2. Vascular

Thrombo-embolic complications (see section 4.2 in chapter I.20).

4. Respiratory system complications

These are the commonest cause of morbidity and mortality following major oesophageal surgery involving resection and reconstruction.

Immediately after operation there may be difficulty of spontaneous breathing in which case patient ventilation is supported by endotracheal intubation and assisted ventilation. Some surgeons advocate routine post-operative assisted ventilation for 24 hours but others, including the author, do not.

4.1. Sputum retention

- Early after operation: upper airway obstruction due to excessive secretion and/or inhalation of oesophagogastric content may cause ventilatory difficulty leading to hypoxia. Bronchoscopic suction is usually required to clear the airway.
- A few days after operation: retention of sputum and collection of excessive mucopurulent secretions in the respiratory tract, particularly in heavy smokers, bronchitics and the emphysematous will cause respiratory insufficiency. Post-operative physiotherapy with administration of mucolytic agents should prevent this complication. Repeated bronchoscopy and occasionally temporary tracheostomy (mini tracheostomy) for suction of tenacious secretions may be inevitable.

4.1.1. Pulmonary infective complications

Pneumonitis, pneumonic consolidation and lung abscess, though infrequent, are major causes of post-operative mortality and morbidity following major oesophageal operations. Pulmonary infection usually occurs a week or so after operation. It is multifactorial in origin and is partly due to poor post-operative management. Amongst the factors involved are lack of mouth hygiene and infection of intravenous lines by contamination. Besides preventative measures, appropriate antibiotics based on microbiological studies are prescribed and active chest physiotherapy should be pursued.

4.2. Pleural infection (see also section 8 in chapter I.20)

In the absence of oesophageal leak and fistula an empyema is a rare event. Nevertheless, empyema and extension of a subphrenic collection in the pleural space should be borne in mind in cases of post-operative clinical and laboratory manifestations of infection. Purulent collections should be evacuated by aspiration or drainage and the causative agents need to be identified and dealt with appropriately.

4.2.1. Chylothorax

This complication most often arises from injury to the thoracic duct. It usually subsides by conservative measures such as aspiration or drainage and expansion of the lung. Sometimes it requires operative treatment (see chapter I.24).

5. Alimentary tract complications

5.1. Distension

Early after operation, distension of the bowels and ileus are the major concern. Alimentary canal decompression is undertaken. Proper monitoring of fluid balance and biochemical profile should be carried out.

5.2. Reflux oesophagatis and ulceration

Reflux oesophagitis and ulceration in the remnant stomach can be treated by appropriate H_2 receptor antagonist drugs or proton pump inhibitors. Sometimes granulation tissue and ulcer occur at the site of the anastomosis causing bleeding. Anastomotic bleeding may be treated conservatively with drugs and endoscopic cauterisation or NdYAG laser fulguration. When conservative policy fails the difficult decision of surgical operation has to be made. The problem is to locate the site of the ulceration and bleeding.

5.3. Leaks and fistulae

Of all post-operative complications, the breakdown of anastomosis and fistula formation are the most taxing, both to the patient and the surgeon. Prevention must be the keyword in the management of leaks. The cause of many fistulae can be traced to the operating theatre and to technical problems during the surgical procedure. Devascularisation, crushing of tissue and anastomosis in infected surroundings and between pathological tissues are important causative factors. Some fistulae occur because of infection and abscess formation near the suture line and/or at the site of the anastomosis, others are due to tumour residue necrosis (i.e. incomplete resection).

Apart from technical problems, the causes of leaks and fistulae may be grouped under:
- Infection,
- Malnutrition,
- Lack of pulmonary expansion.

The incidence of fistulae is negligible when patients are operated on by an experienced team and are cared for in units where oesophageal surgery is commonplace. By being aware of the complications and their seriousness one can prevent them or apply early therapeutic measures.

The clinical presentation of fistulae differ according to the site of the fistulous opening. The possibilities are:

- Oesophago-mediastinal,
- Oesophago-pleural,
- Oesophago-airway,
- Oesophago-vascular.

It is noteworthy that leaks may be clinically silent but radiologically apparent by contrast study. Such occult leaks pose a difficult management problem when in the chest, since exploration is a major procedure. Occult leak in the neck should be explored (Casson and Porter, 2002). Except for total breakdown of the anastomosis, an exceptional occurrence, fistulous complications manifest 7–10 days after operation. Slight-to-moderate fever may herald more serious manifestations. Chest radiograph and its comparison with previous radiographs will show some pleural reaction or frank hydro(pyo)thorax. The diagnosis can be confirmed by further radiological investigation using appropriate contrast medium; the use of video-radiography is advantageous to identify the leak in difficult cases.

Oesophago-airway fistulae will present with symptoms predominantly referred to the respiratory system. Oesophagovascular fistulae are very rare and are difficult to diagnose until fatal or near-fatal haemorrhage occurs. It should be noted that:

- Fistula can occur occasionally in patients who had non-resectional oesophageal operation, e.g. repair of hiatal hernia, either by surgical accident or spontaneously (e.g. post operative vomiting),
- After an operation involving resection and reconstruction contrast swallow radiography should be carried out before the start of oral intake, to ensure that the anastomosis is not leaking,
- A surgical team undertaking oesophageal resection must be familiar with diagnosis and treatment of leak,
- Treatment of leak and fistula should commence upon suspicion of its existence.

For therapeutic purposes the size, proximal site and track and distal site of the fistulae must be precisely located. Appropriate contrast medium swallows and meticulous radiological investigations are essential. Endoscopy, carried out by the surgeon is mandatory.

There are principally three methods of treatment:

(a) Conservative method which is based on:
- Drainage of the distal site of the fistulous opening and the space or cavity (e.g. neck, chest or abdomen) to which it flows,

- Provision of high calorie and high protein nutrition parenterally or enterally (jejunal),
- Control of infection by an appropriate antibiotic and disinfection of the space if applicable,
- Oesophagoscopic inspection of the proximal site of the fistula and application of an irritant (20% sodium hydroxide solution) to the site, when the fistula is found at endoscopy to be small (<5 mm), surrounded by granulating tissue.

(b) Radical surgical method which consists of:
- Surgical exploration and exposure of the fistula,
- Interruption of the fistulous communication with excision of the track followed by re-anastomosis,
- Provision of proper drainage,
- High calorie and nitrogen content nutrition either parenterally or by enteral routes,
- Control of infection by antibiotics.

(c) In a very sick patient, the conservative method (as above) is added to by oesophageal derivation. That is, isolation of the fistula-bearing part of the oesophagus, by proximal oesophagostomy (in the neck) and prevention of reflux.

In all cases the progress is monitored by contrast study and biochemical and clinical parameters.

6. Malnutrition

Post-operative malnutrition should be considered as a complication of major oesophageal surgery. The causes may be multiple:

- Lack of supply or intake which occurs during the changeover regimen from parenteral/enteral to oral feeding. This is one of the major causes and is due to the fact that patients are simply not in a position to receive all their requirements during the changeover period. The changeover must be a gradual and slow process from one to the other. In practice, oral feeding is supplemented by enteral/or intermittent parenteral feeding before being considered as the sole route of nutritional intake.
- It must be realised that:
  – After oesophageal resection and reconstruction the patient cannot accommodate a large volume of food intake. Small meals should be given at frequent intervals,
  – Lack of appetite and disinterest in eating may develop due to nausea, reflux and/or absence of the stomach following operation which cre-

ates a feeling of fullness. Appropriate drugs, attention to diet and the mode of alimentation, together with an appetite stimulant are helpful. Post-operative nutritional study and rehabilitation should prevent such malnutrition.

When there are clinical indications that malnutrition is present, the patient must be nutritionally assessed and treated using supportive enteral or, if necessary, parenteral feeding.

7. Infective complications

These complications may be:
- Chest infection (pleuro-pulmonary),
- Urinary infection,
- Abdominal and subphrenic infection (abscesses),
- General infection (septicaemia),
- Wound sepsis.

Every precaution must be exercised to prevent post-operative infection, or to recognise it early in order to abort it before its full development. The general principles of management are:
- Identification of the site of infection,
- Identification of the pathogenic organisms and their sensitivities to antibiotics — for this, a sample of purulent material and/or blood are dispatched for microbiological studies,
- Drainage of the purulent collection from the neck, pleural and/or subphrenic spaces,
- Correction of anaemia and nutritional deficiencies,
- Administration of antibiotics according to a planned scheme.

The likelihood of infection being derived and propagated via the intravenous infusion (contamination), particularly during intravenous feeding, must not be forgotten.

8. Wound complications

Patients undergoing major oesophageal surgery may have any of a number of thoracic or abdominal incisions. Any of these wounds can present with a degree of non-healing dehiscence or various degrees of sepsis which are likely to be multiple and extensive.

A complete 'burst chest' with disruption of all layers of the wound is rare.

Dehiscence of the wound affecting the skin and superficial layer of muscles is occasionally encountered. When clean and uncomplicated by purulent discharge this is repaired by simple closure. At-

tention is paid to muscular dehiscence which can be hidden under the intact skin and subcutaneous tissues. In this case, the overlying skin should be incised in order to obtain access to the whole length of the disrupted muscle. Necrotic or fibrotic devitalized muscles, as well as skin edges, are excised. Suturing is carried out in layers or by a series of interrupted through-and-through (deep tension) sutures, without a drain; the sutures are tied firmly to approximate but not too tightly to crush.

The repair of an infected wound (septic wound) which is discharging or contains purulent collection is more complicated and the wound needs to be examined carefully. An abscess appearing under the skin may sometimes track down to the pleural space and even to a leak at the site of anastomosis.

A sinogram outlining the track is helpful in finding the location of a deeply situated discharging sinus.

Operations in which the costal margin has been severed and then repaired may have a dehiscence or septic area of cartilaginous costal margin. Here, the stitches and necrotic cartilage have to be explored and excised before the wound is repaired otherwise healing cannot be expected.

As a rule, a patient with a septic wound does not require antibiotics. Patients whose wounds are deeply infected, particularly from an empyema, benefit from systemic antibiotic in addition to drainage, which is the mainstay of treatment.

9. Bed sores

Of all thoracic surgical patients, those undergoing oesophageal surgery are more prone to the development of bed sores. Malnutrition with loss of weight, lack of mobility and circulatory inadequacy are contributory factors. The care of the skin by nurses and inspection by the surgical team must be included in the planned management of these patients.

References and further reading

Abbot WE, Levets S, Krieger H. Metabolic changes in surgical patients in relation to water, electrolytes, nitrogen and calorie intake. Metabolism 1959; 8: 847–861.

Baigrie RJ, Devitt PG, Watkin DS. Enteral versus parenteral nutrition after oesophagogastric surgery: a prospective randomised comparison. Aust NZ J Surg 1997; 67: 736.

Belsey RHR. Hiatus hernia. Modern trends in gastroenterology. London: Butterworth, 1952.

Bhasin DK, Sharma BC, Gupta MM, Sinah SK, Sing K. Endoscopic dilatation for treatment of anastomotic leaks following transhiatal esphagectomy. Endoscopy 2000; 32: 469–471.

Boyle MJ, Franceschati D, Livingstone AS. Transhiatal versus transthoracic esophagectomy; complications and survival rates. Ann Surg 1999; 65: 1137–1141.

Casson AG, Porter GA. Evolution and critical appraisal of anastomotic technique following resection for esophageal adenocarcinoma, abstract, 2002. Presented at 12th World Congress, World Society of Cardiothoracic Surgeons, Lucerne.

Gordon P, Busby MD. Overview of randomised clinical trials of total parenteral nutrition for malnourished surgical patients. World J Surg 1993; 17: 173–177.

Heyland DK, Montalvo M, MacDonald S, Keefe L, Su XY, Drover JW. Total parenteral nutrition in the surgical patient: a meta analysis. Can J Surg 2001; 44: 86–87.

Johnston IDA, Tweedle DEF, Spivy J. Intravenous feeding after surgical operation. In: Wilkinson AW (ed.), Parenteral Nutrition. Edinburgh: Churchill Livingstone, 1972; p. 189.

MacFie J. Enteral versus parenteral nutrition. Br J Surg 2000; 87: 1121–1122.

Mann J, Truswell S. Essentials of human nutrition. New York: Oxford University Press, 1998.

Miller JO, Jain MK, de Gara EJ, Morgan D, Urschel JD. Effect of surgical experience on results of oesophagectomy for oesophageal carcinoma. J Surg Oncol 1997; 65: 20–21.

Moghissi K, Hornshaw J, Teasdale PR, Dawes EA. Parenteral nutrition in carcinoma of the oesophagus treated by surgery: nitrogen balance and clinical studies. Br J Surg 1977; 64: 125–128.

Moghissi K. A technique of superior vena caval catheterisation for prolonged intravenous feeding. J R Coll Surg Edin 1979; 24: 178–179.

Moghissi K, Teasdale PR. Parenteral feeding in patients with carcinoma of the oesophagus treated by surgery: energy and nitrogen requirements. J Parenteral Ent Nutr 1980; 4: 371–375.

Moghissi K, Teasdale P, Dench M. Comparison between pre-operative nasogastric feeding and parenteral feeding in patients with cancer of the oesophagus undergoing surgery. J Parenteral Ent Nutr 1982; 6: 335.

Moghissi K, Boore J. Parenteral and enteral nutrition for nurses. London: William Heinemann Medical Books, 1983.

Moghissi K, Dietel M, Taylor GA. Esophageal problems: use of nutritional support. In: Dietel M. (ed.), Nutrition in clinical surgery. Baltimore: Williams Wilkins, 1985; 303–319.

Pacellis F, Bossola M, Papa V, Malerba M, Modesti C, Sgadari A, Bellantone R, Doglietto GB. Enteral versus parenteral nutrition after major abdominal surgery: an even match. Arch Surg 2001; 136: 933–936.

Sharpe DAC, Renwick P, Matthews KHR, Moghissi K. Antibiotic prophylaxis in oesophageal surgery. Eur J Cardiothorac Surg 1992; 6: 561–564.

Swanson SJ, Sugarbaker DJ. The three hole esophagectomy; The Brigham and Women's Hospital approach (modified McKeown technique). Chest Surg Clin N Am 2000; 10: 531–552.

Waitzberg DL, Plopper C, Terra RM. Post-operative total parenteral nutrition. World J Surg 1999; 23: 560–564.

K. Moghissi, J.A.C. Thorpe and F. Ciulli (Eds.)
Moghissi's Essentials of Thoracic and Cardiac Surgery
© 2003 Elsevier Science B.V. All rights reserved

CHAPTER IV.1

Video assisted thoracic surgery (VATS)

W.S. Walker

1. Introduction

Video assisted thoracic surgery, often referred to by either the acronym VATS or as videothoracoscopic surgery, allows the thoracic surgeon to perform complex intra-thoracic operations through small incisions with consequently reduced pain, trauma, hospitalisation and recovery time. The impact of this new technique on current thoracic surgical practice may be judged from the extent to which it has largely replaced conventional open surgery in many areas, particularly the more straightforward pulmonary procedures.

As with laparoscopic surgery in the abdomen, VATS became possible with the advent in 1990/1991 of surgical video cameras based on small reliable charge-coupled device video chips. These could be attached to the end of 5 or 10 mm surgical telescopes providing a real time video display of the operative field on a monitor. This image, coupled with new endoscopic instruments, made it possible for the surgeon to undertake bimanual intra-thoracic operative procedures as distinct from the inspection, biopsy or relatively simple therapeutic interventions allowed by conventional thoracoscopy (Loddenkemper, 1998).

Although there are differences between the surgical approaches advocated by various VATS authors, in most instances, the surgeon operates using the video screen image. It is indeed the coordination of hand-eye movement according to the image presented on the video monitor which distinguishes VATS procedures from other approaches undertaken via a limited thoracotomy. These may be described as reduced access but they are not the truly minimal access endoscopic procedures which characterise videothoracoscopic operations.

In this chapter, we will consider those factors contributing to the efficient conduct of VATS procedures, briefly review current VATS practice, identify potential future developments and highlight those features which contribute to good clinical practice.

2. Basic operative considerations

2.1. Surgical philosophy

VATS provides an alternative approach strategy and operative technique for undertaking established thoracic surgical operations. The operative technique is usually entirely analogous to a standard open procedure thereby allowing the VATS procedure to share the previously developed knowledge based on optimal conduct of a procedure. It is crucial that VATS procedures are undertaken within this framework from both an intellectual perspective and also the current climate of audit, governance and litigation so that the standard considerations of safety, technical efficiency and reliability that are relevant to an open operation are applied equally to a VATS procedure.

2.2. Access

Access to the chest is gained via a "port". This may be a physical entity in the form of a metal or plastic tube or a simple open incision of about two cm. In general, a simple incision has the advantage of allowing a greater degree of freedom of movement for an instrument in the port site whereas a physical port may offer more protection to the tissues, facilitate passage of instruments in muscular or fat individuals and, if metallic, provide a ground to prevent diathermy induced inadvertent charging of instruments. Intercostal nerve damage is reduced by avoiding leverage at the port site, use of narrow rib inter-spaces and forced reinsertion of instruments. More complex operations benefit from the creation of a 4 to 5 cm intercostal incision sometimes referred to as a "utility" or "access" incision usually placed ante-riorly or laterally in the 4th or 5th interspace. This facilitates the insertion of larger endoscopic staplers and other instruments including conventional clamps and the removal of complete operative specimens.

Port placement varies somewhat with different procedures and between authors but the fundamen-tal principle is that of triangulation (Landreneau et al., 1992, 1993), i.e. operating with the optic and in-struments entering the chest through ports located at the corners of a notional triangle and orientated to-wards the operating point which forms the apex of a pyramid (Fig. 1). This practice ensures that the sur-geon operates in the direction of vision and reduces the risk of crossing instruments with resulting mutual interference ("fencing", Fig. 2a). It is also possible to alternate the instrument and optic between the various ports, allowing different views and angles of attack. It is generally recommended to place the optic centrally as illustrated in Fig. 1 but this position provides less depth information than a slightly side on view which can be helpful in detailed dissection (Fig. 2b).

In laparoscopic surgery, operating space is gener-ated by expanding the abdomen with CO_2; in VATS it is gained by collapsing the lung. This means that safe VATS surgery requires a well-collapsed lung in order to provide operating space, visualization and access. Most VATS surgeons prefer the use of a dou-ble lumen endobronchial tube for this purpose but other options exist. Insufflation with CO_2 (Wolfer et al., 1994) at a flow rate below 2 l/min and an in-trapleural pressure of less than 10 mmHg is one al-ternate technique and may be particularly useful for gaining limited space quickly, e.g. in sympathectomy. This technique can be potentially hazardous as it may mimic a tension pneumothorax; it is also somewhat awkward as gas-tight port tubes are necessary. High frequency jet ventilation provides a further alternative strategy and provides a mid-volume slightly vibrating lung. Both of these techniques avoid the potential dif-ficulties of double lumen intubation but neither afford an equivalent degree of pulmonary collapse and lung volume control. Intrapleural suction should be car-ried out either below a fluid level or (assuming the CO_2 technique is not used) with one port open and unobstructed so as not to reduce intrapleural pressure and hence cause re-expansion of the collapsed lung.

2.3. Instruments

Although various specialised dissection instruments both endoscopic and more conventional, including

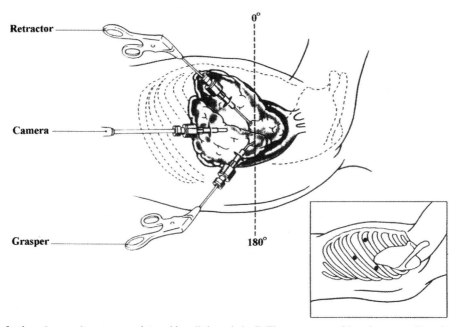

Fig. 1. The use of a three (or more) port approach to achieve "triangulation". The ports are positioned so as to allow the operator to place the operative area at the apex of a notional pyramid defined by the optic and operating instruments the relative positions of which can be rotated as required.

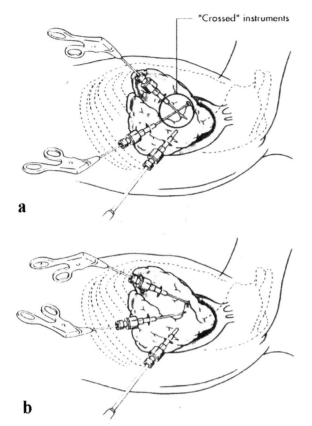

"Crossed" instruments

a

b

Fig. 2. (a) Fencing occurs when the operating instruments and/or optic cross and mutually interfere with each other. (b) Position of optic for side-on view.

Table 1

Endoscopic stapler sizes and useage

Cartridge colour	Stapler leg length [a]	Typical thoracic tissue
Grey	2 mm	Small pulmonary arteries
White	2.5 mm	Large pulmonary arteries; pulmonary veins; azygos vein
Blue	3.5 mm	Peripheral lung parenchyma; segmental bronchi; oesophageal wall
Green	4.8 mm	Main bronchus and lobar bronchi; central pulmonary parenchyma; stomach

[a] Autosuture sizes — Ethicon sizes are comparable but differ fractionally.

those with relocated hinges and altered blade geometry, are available, few of these are strictly necessary as open instruments can often be utilised. Endoscopic dissectors and scissors are, however, essential for detailed dissection and endoscopic tissue graspers and suckers can be of value but many other endoscopic instruments originate in laparoscopic surgery and are inappropriate for thoracoscopic use. Disposable instruments are relatively inexpensive and significantly lighter than reusable ones, quite apart from the fact that adequate cleaning can be a major issue with reusable endoscopic instruments. In the author's opinion, disposable endoscissors are far superior to reusable ones which are very difficult to maintain in a sharp condition. We have found that long fine vascular clamps make useful general purpose instruments for dissection, passing slings and controlling vascular structures while a sponge holding forceps (Rampley type) serves well as a relatively atraumatic lung retractor or as a swab holder when cleaning the operative field.

Endoscopic linear staplers are essential for prac-

tical modern videothoracoscopic lung surgery. These fire either four or six parallel rows of staggered staples and cut between the middle rows leaving haemo- and aerostatic sealed ends. These are available in 30, 35, 45 and 60 mm length cartridges and in different staple leg lengths according to the tissue to be divided and should be selected accordingly (Table 1).

The hilar structures radiate in a centrifugal manner whereas instruments tend to approach the hilum in a centripetal manner. Thus the instrument and the structure to be dissected or divided tend to be in direct opposition instead of at mutual right angles which would be the normal orientation at an open procedure. This situation can be managed by selecting the best site for instrument insertion and by manipulating the structure with a sling in order to bring it into as near to right angles as possible to the stapler.

3. Safety issues

3.1. Contraindications and conversion

Contraindications to a VATS procedure are largely a matter of common sense. The surgeon must have access, good vision, and an achievable technical objective. If these conditions cannot be met, the procedure either cannot begin or should be abandoned and converted to an open procedure. Conversion to open thoracotomy may be required for a variety of reasons (Table 2). In general these may be considered under three headings: visualization difficulties, intraoperative complications and situations where a VATS procedure is considered inappropriate. In any instance where safety or oncological principles are at risk, conversion to an open procedure is mandatory. Conversion is usually a measured and controlled pro-

Table 2

Possible reasons for conversion to open thoracotomy

Condition	Effect	Options prior to conversion
Visualization problems:		
Failure to achieve single lung ventilation	No operative vision	Attempt to reposition tube
Pleura obliterated by adhesions	No operative vision	Attempt division
Obesity	Chest wall may be thicker than length of port tube	Consider use of laparoscopic tube
Anticoagulation	Bleeding from videoscope port and dissection area obscuring view	Try to control with suction or swabs
Intraoperative Complications:		
Lesion cannot be found	Operation cannot proceed	Try further deflation of lung and direct finger palpation
Dissection area stuck (most likely with inflammatory conditions)	Risk of inadvertent vessel injury	Nil – conversion mandatory
Brisk bleeding	Operative safety risk	Nil – conversion mandatory
Equipment failure	Operative safety risk	Nil – conversion mandatory
VATS procedure inappropriate:		
Lesion unexpectedly large or advanced	Compromises safety and oncological principles	Nil – conversion mandatory
Procedure required exceeds competency of operator	Compromises safety and may compromise oncological principles	Nil – conversion mandatory

cess but occasionally an intraoperative problem may require urgent thoracotomy. An open thoracotomy tray must, therefore, be immediately available and the patient should be draped and positioned so that rapid conversion is always feasible. Conversion is often thought of as demonstrating the potential inadequacy of a VATS approach with the implication that it is inherently less safe; it should rather be considered to indicate correct and safe decision making. Ultimately the patient has progressed to the surgical strategy which would otherwise have been selected, i.e. open thoracotomy, but at least has had the chance to benefit from minimal access techniques. The safety record of VATS procedures has been reviewed in several series of mixed procedures (Table 3) with low average mortality (0.26%) and intraoperative complication (4.77%) rates. Conversion rates vary somewhat with procedure complexity but rarely exceed 15%. (Inderbitzi and Grillet, 1996; Krasna et al., 1996; Yim and Liu, 1996; Jancovici R et al., 1996).

3.2. Bleeding

Serious bleeding during major VATS procedures is uncommon. Possible causes include staple misfires which are very rare (Craig and Walker, 1995) and inadvertent injury to vessels. In the author's opinion, major vascular structures (pulmonary veins and main or stem pulmonary arteries) should be gently clamped proximally with a vascular clamp prior to division with an endostapler. Equally, the surgeon must be able to visualise the entire length of the stapler or scissor jaws before using these devices and must be aware of the position of instrument tips. Minor bleeding is not haemodynamically important but may still constitute a safety issue if it causes the operative field to be obscured.

3.3. Training

Many complications and pitfalls can be avoided by adequate training. Specific training in video surgery

Table 3

Reported operative complication rates in VATS procedures

Author	Patients	Type	Mortality	Complication	Conversion
Inderbitzi, 1996	5280	Meta-analysis (145 papers)	0.3%	3.61%	1.04%
Krasna, 1996	321	Single series	nil	3.1%	8.1%
Yim, 1996	1337	Twin institution	0.07%	4.3%	Not stated
Jancovici, 1996	937	Four institution	0.5%	10.9%	12.4%
Average adjusted for patient numbers:			0.26%	4.77%	–

is required to master orientation, proprioception, operative techniques and correct use of instruments and is recommended by both the UK and US cardiothoracic societies. VATS procedures benefit from the magnification and illumination provided by the videothoracoscope. Indeed, visualization of some parts of the chest, especially the apex, is undoubtedly superior using videothoracoscopic approaches. Magnification is, however, inherently associated with a reduced operating field and therefore the surgeon must be aware of this and develop a proprioceptive sense for instrument location much as tends to be required when operating with magnifying loupes. There are skills which are specific to the VATS approach notably hand/eye co-ordination based on a video image and the ability to reconstruct a three--dimensional concept of operative anatomy from a two-dimensional monitor representation. Not all individuals possess these abilities despite being excellent open surgeons so that awareness of personal limitations is an important safety element.

4. Oncological issues

The use of VATS techniques in the definitive management of malignancy remains a cause of concern to many thoracic surgeons (Mack et al., 1997). The most controversial aspects relate to the adequacy of a formal resection for malignancy as compared to an open procedure and to the risk of wound implantation with tumour cells. The results of major resection are reviewed in detail below under Major Pulmonary Resection. There can be no doubt that, even with biopsy material, care must be taken to prevent the risk of wound implantation. Specimens should be placed into polythene bags before extraction through ports, and biopsies should be taken via a port tube thereby ensuring that the wound is shielded.

The available data does not, in fact, suggest that VATS poses any greater risk of wound implantation than open thoracotomy but scrutiny and awareness are certainly higher for this new form of surgery. The question of port site seedlings was addressed by Downey on behalf of the VATS Study Group (Downey et al., 1996) and by Collard in a more detailed review (Collard and Reymond, 1996). Taken together with more recent case reports, fewer than 30 cases have been published and over half of these occurred in patients operated on for conditions at known increased risk of wound implantation, i.e. intrathoracic metastatic disease or mesothelioma. Lewis calculated the risk of port site implantation

in VATS overall to be in the order of 0.08% (Lewis et al., 1997).

A more important issue may be the need to ensure that the attraction of a VATS approach is not allowed to influence the choice of operative procedure. A peripheral pulmonary carcinoma, for example, is best treated by lobectomy on the basis of current available data (Ginsberg and Rubinstein, 1991; Warren et al., 1994; Landreneau et al., 1997) and if a surgeon is not competent to perform a VATS lobectomy, it would be incorrect to undertake a wedge resection simply in order to achieve a VATS operation. Similar arguments apply to oesophageal carcinoma other than in-situ disease and to advanced intrathoracic carcinoma where extensive mediastinal clearance may be considered to be in the patient's best interest.

5. Applications and results of video assisted thoracic surgery

5.1. Pleural disease

VATS provides the surgeon with a comprehensive view of the pleural space and affords the opportunity to biopsy pleural lesions and also concurrent pulmonary or other abnormalities. It is important to remember, however, that thoracoscopy has been used for many years in the diagnosis of pleural disease and, in the author's opinion, remains a more efficient method of obtaining a simple pleural biopsy in that only one rather than three port sites are required and no imaging equipment is necessary. The use of VATS techniques in early phase empyemas, i.e. before the lung has become encased by a mature cortex, has been demonstrated by various authors in both adults (Mackinlay et al., 1996; Lawrence et al., 1997) and children (Gandhi and Stringel, 1997). These series show that adhesions can be broken down, pus evacuated and light pulmonary cortex can be shaved off. Results are good with an end result which is probably best thought of as intermediate between simple tube drainage and a formal decortication but without the major trauma of the latter. In the later stages, however, thoracotomy remains the treatment of choice (Cassina et al., 1999)

5.2. Pulmonary

5.2.1. Pneumothorax
VATS is applicable to both primary and secondary pneumothorax. Various techniques are available for dealing with primary pneumothorax. The most com-

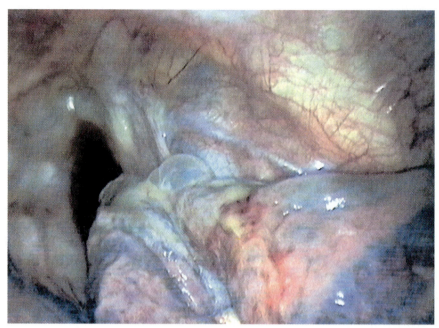

Fig. 3. Typical apical bullous complex. Note the adhesions to the apex of the pleural cavity. These must be divided with care as to avoid bleeding and cautery should be used sparingly so as to avoid injury to the brachial plexus.

mon surgical options are to control the leaking bullous complex with a Roeder knot endoscopic loop tie or with an endoscopic stapler (Fig. 3) and then to perform a pleural abrasion or pleurectomy procedure. Insufflation with kaolin is commonly practised in European centres for primary pneumothorax but is viewed with more caution in the UK due to reluctance to leave foreign material in the pleural cavity in young patients.

The results of VATS for primary pneumothorax surgery have been presented in several series (Naunheim et al., 1995; Mouroux et al., 1996; Bertrand et al., 1996). These report low perioperative complication rates (6 to 11%) and recurrence rates of 0 to 3% at between 17 months and 2 years mean follow up. These data are clearly early in the potential natural history of primary pneumothorax follow up and longer review will be necessary to confirm continuing low recurrence rates. Preliminary results would appear to suggest, however, that they are similar to those obtained with open surgery and according to one limited retrospective analysis, a VATS approach may also offer cost savings (Schramel et al., 1996).

Secondary pneumothorax represents a more difficult patient group with advanced age and often associated chronic obstructive airways disease. The method of treatment is similar but the air leak is usually due to a leak in an obvious bullous complex. Having controlled the primary leak, the options for

achieving pulmonary adhesion are similar but may also include insufflation of kaolin (talc) as a possible alternative. As with open surgery, the risks are greater but given the reduced trauma of the VATS approach, recourse to a surgical option is often more feasible than with an open thoracotomy.

Giant bullae are rare but relatively straightforward to excise using a VATS approach. The procedure is usually facilitated by first puncturing the bulla as this generates space within the pleural cavity and allows the operator to identify the base of the bulla more easily. Excision of the bulla(e) is then usually undertaken using an endoscopic stapler (Menconi et al., 1998; De Giacomo et al., 1999). Alternatively, the bulla can be secured using a Roeder or other slip knot or shrunk with a laser.

5.2.2. Lung volume reduction
Reduction pneumoplasty or lung volume reduction (LVR, Fig. 4) seeks to improve pulmonary function in emphysematous patients by removing particularly badly diseased portions of lung. In theory, removal of these portions allows the remaining lung to ventilate more effectively whilst the improvement in chest wall dynamics enhances breathing and lowers the perception of dyspnoea. Although of considerable recent interest this is not a new concept having originally been described some 30 years ago (Brantigan and Mueller, 1957; Brantigan et al., 1961). At that

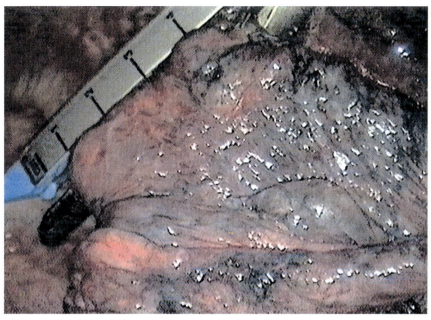

Fig. 4. Use of 60 mm endoscopic stapler in VATS lung volume reduction.

time, air leakage and mortality prevented it being successful but the development of surgical instrumentation and intensive care have made it a feasible proposition.

Interest was rekindled by reports describing successful open bilateral reduction using staplers (Cooper et al., 1995, 1996) and the subsequent literature on this subject is prolific attesting to the interest and controversy it has aroused. It should be noted, however, that prior to this time VATS laser LVR had already been described (Wakayabashi and Brenner et al., 1991) and subsequent publications confirmed the feasibility of VATS LVR using laser or endostaplers in either staged sequential or bilateral operations (Stammberger et al., 1997; De Giacoma et al., 1999) although the stapled approach would appear to offer superior results (McKenna et al., 1996). Unilateral VATS LVR is not as effective as a bilateral LVR (McKenna et al., 1996; Kotloff et al., 1997) which also has very similar operative mortality (3%) and morbidity. Whatever the mechanisms underlying this procedure, it would appear to work — albeit for an uncertain number of years. Although the absolute gains in lung function are modest, being usually of the order of a 0.4 to 0.6 l improvement in FEV1, this can equate to a major percentage gain of 16 to 31% for unilateral and 25 to 57% for bilateral procedures and often produces a gratifying subjective improvement in dyspnoea.

There are obvious theoretical advantages to operating on debilitated respiratory cripples using a VATS approach as opposed to an open median sternotomy. This appears to be confirmed in the literature (Kotloff et al., 1996; Wisser et al., 1997) where VATS bilateral LVR is reported as being associated with equal or reduced perioperative mortality, a lower incidence of respiratory failure and more rapid improvement in respiratory function when compared with open bilateral surgery. Interestingly, at least one US study (Lapp et al., 1998) identifies the VATS LVR approach as being cheaper than open surgery due to shorter in patient stay and reduced morbidity.

Currently, there are several major randomized studies in progress which are intended to address the question of the comparative value of LVR as compared with rehabilitation. These include the US National Emphysema Treatment trial (NETT), the Swedish National trial, the Canadian Lung Volume Reduction Surgery trial and the UK Papworth-based study. These will require several years before producing definitive results but will be useful indicators of the scientific value of this procedure. Interestingly, recruitment to several of these trials has been hampered by patient reluctance to remain within the rehabilitation arm.

5.2.3. Wedge excision

Wedge excision is undertaken for two primary indications: interstitial biopsy and excision of a solitary intrapulmonary nodule. The technique in either instance is straightforward, involving three port sites and the application of typically three or four endoscopic stapler firings in order to excise a wedge of lung tissue.

Interstitial lung biopsy performed as a VATS procedure allows the surgeon to select the area to be biopsied rather than be restricted to the area immediately subjacent to a small thoracotomy as was the case with open approaches. The portion excised should be towards an edge or corner of a lobe and representative of the observable disease process while avoiding areas of end stage damage. Care is necessary in cases with very fibrotic lung as the stapler knife may not then cut effectively. Generally, a hospital stay of two to four days is required and morbidity and inpatient stay are reduced compared with open surgery while diagnostic accuracy is similar at over 96% (Kadokura et al., 1995; Mouroux et al., 1997). Perhaps most eloquently, there has been an increase in the referral rate for lung biopsy since the advent of VATS reflecting physician satisfaction with the outcomes achieved.

VATS wedge excision of pulmonary nodule is applicable to the excision of small indeterminate isolated lesions (Mack, 1999) and to definitive management of early (T1) peripheral carcinomas in debilitated patients. The primary problem is not the technique but rather localisation of the lesion itself. Localisation strategies proposed include preoperative radiological localisation using either a hook wire or dye marker and intraoperative localisation using digital palpation. It is very difficult to locate lesions below 1 cm in diameter at surgery unless these are obviously placed close to the surface of the lung. Failure to do so is an absolute indication for conversion to an open thoracotomy. Attempts at improving intraoperative localisation with ultrasonography or mechanical fingers have not proved particularly useful to date. As with lung biopsy, wedge excision of an intrapulmonary nodule requires that the lesion is located near to the edge or surface of a lobe. Lesions located towards the central portion of a lobe are not suitable as the thickness of the lung becomes excessive for the stapler and the risk of damage to major vascular structures increases. If there is doubt as to whether the nodule has been excised the specimen should be sent for frozen section analysis to confirm or refute the presence of the lesion. With appropriate selection this has proved to be a safe and reliable approach with a conversion rate below 1% (Mack et al., 1993) reduced pain and earlier discharge (Santambrogio et al., 1995).

Wedge excision as definitive treatment of a peripheral carcinoma carries the same caveats regarding risk of local recurrence (Ginsberg and Rubeinstein, 1991; Landreneau et al., 1997) whether performed as an open or videothoracoscopic procedure. As noted above, therefore, the desire to undertake a VATS procedure should not dictate the operation to be performed. If a lobectomy is necessary this may require conversion to open thoracotomy unless the surgeon is adept at VATS lobectomy.

5.3. Bronchogenic carcinoma

5.3.1. Diagnosis and staging
Video assessment allows the surgeon to establish a histological diagnosis by wedge resection of small peripheral lesions as previously discussed or by direct core biopsy of larger or more central lesions (photo needle bx). It can also contribute to mediastinal assessment where it does not replace mediastinoscopy but can usefully supplement nodal staging by providing access to the lower mediastinal stations and subaortic window (Champion and McKernan, 1996; Rendina et al., 1994).

5.3.2. Defining operability
Regrettably, open and shut thoracotomy for disease deemed to be inoperable at the time of thoracotomy continues to be commonplace. In the UK, for example, national statistics indicate (annual return for 1997–1998) that this rate currently exceeds 10% (61). This unfortunate situation can largely be avoided by routine use of VATS assessment of all malignant cases (Loscertales et al., 1997) and exclude local inoperability prior to opening the chest. It can also help define the required level of resection (lobectomy vs. pneumonectomy) required which may aid decision making in compromised patients who might withstand lobectomy but not a pneumonectomy (Waller et al., 1997). These issues can be usefully considered during a diagnostic and staging evaluation but even if the staging and diagnosis are considered certain without recourse to VATS assessment, it is a simple matter to undertake a VATS inspection immediately prior to a planned open thoracotomy and hence exclude easily identified causes of irresectability. In the author's opinion, this form of pre-resectional VATS assessment should now be mandatory before proceeding to a formal thoracotomy.

5.3.3. Major pulmonary resection

Few centres have significant expertise with major pulmonary resection using VATS techniques with VATS lobectomy in the UK, for example, accounting for less than 2% of all lobectomy procedures (Society of Cardiothoracic Surgeons returns). There are two fundamental reasons for this: concern regarding the oncological safety of this approach and the steep learning curve required to master the technical aspects of a difficult, challenging and potentially hazardous procedure. Currently, three different techniques are used to achieve a VATS lobectomy. These have been reviewed in detail elsewhere (Walker, 1999) but in brief, the different techniques may be summarised as: endoscopic hilar dissection, minithoracotomy and en bloc hilar stapling. The endoscopic hilar dissection technique (McKenna, 1994; Kirby et al., 1995; Roviaro et al., 1995) utilises endoscopic surgical techniques to mobilise and individually divide the hilar structures in a manner exactly analogous to a standard open lobectomy. Typically three ports are used together with an enlarged 4 to 5 cm port placed on the lateral or anterior chest wall to facilitate passage of large instruments and the extraction of the operative specimen (Fig. 5). The ribs are not spread and the surgeon operates entirely according to the view presented on a video monitor. In the mini-thoracotomy approach (Giudicelli et al., 1994; Yim and Liu, 1997) the hilar structures are also individually divided but the surgeon operates under direct vision by peering through a small thoracotomy with the video camera serving only as a supplementary aid to vision and as an internal light source. The

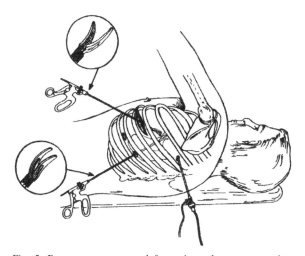

Fig. 5. Port arrangement used for major pulmonary resection. The enlarged anterior port (sometimes referred to as an 'access' or 'utility' incision) is used for specimen extraction.

mini thoracotomy has limited skin length of about 8 cm but the intercostal incision is approximately 15 cm and is opened using a special rib spreader. This is not, therefore, strictly speaking an endoscopic procedure and involves an incision which is ultimately little different from a small open thoracotomy thereby obviating much of the point behind a VATS approach. The third method (Lewis, 1998), which is sometimes referred to as a simultaneously stapled lobectomy, utilises video imaging and endoscopic techniques but is quite different in that the hilar structures are not separately dissected and divided but are rather stapled en masse with the lobe being cut away from the staple line. Critics of this approach express concern regarding the ability to adequately stage and clear nodal tissue at the hilar level.

It may be that confusion arising from the diversity of approaches has further impeded the uptake of VATS lobectomy but in experienced hands all three are associated with excellent results (Yim et al., 1998; Roviaro et al., 1998; Walker, 1998) All appear safe as confirmed by a survey (Mackinlay, 1997) of 1530 VATS lobectomy cases, demonstrating an average conversion rate of 11% (range 1% to 30%). Fifty one (3.3%) intraoperative accidents occurred due either to surgical manoeuvres or to instrument failure but only 17 (1.1%) of these required immediate conversion and none were fatal. The great majority of conversions therefore were not related to potentially dangerous events but rather to technical or oncological circumstances which indicated that elective conversion to an open approach would be the better option. This same series demonstrated only two instances of cancer implants in port wounds (incidence 0.13%) both of which occurred before routine use of plastic bags for specimen delivery. Operative mortality and complication rates are lower than those generally reported with open thoracotomy and, perhaps most encouragingly, the mid-term survival data suggests results which are at least as good as with open resection.

We and others (Walker et al, 1996; Ohbuchi et al., 1998; Demmy and Curtis, 1999) have noted decreased pain scores and opiate usage, reduced high dependence scores, more rapid mobilisation, earlier discharge and reduced cytokine activation (Fig. 6).

6. Oesophageal disease

6.1. Benign oesophageal disease

Oesophageal cysts and leimyomas are uncommon but have been successfully excised via endoscopic

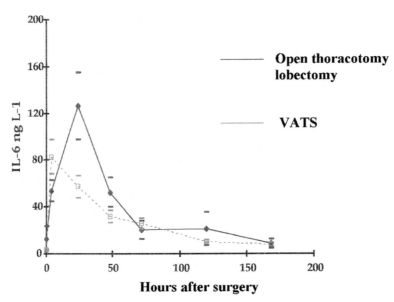

Fig. 6. Cytokine (IL6) levels following VATS and open thoracotomy lobectomy. The values obtained in the VATS vases were consistently and significantly lower than in the open cases (data in press — European J Clinical Research).

procedures (Merry et al., 1999; Bardini and Aso-lati, 1997; Roviaro et al., 1998). The management of the most significant condition, gastro-oesophageal reflux, has been radically changed by the advent of minimal access fundoplication which has been shown to be effective with low morbidity but this is, however, far more commonly performed through an abdominal approach using complete (Nissen) or incomplete (Toupet) wraps (Kassis and Luketitch, 1999; Richardson and Bowen, 1998). A modified Belsey IV procedure has been described as a VATS approach with promising initial results (Nguyen et al., 1998) but it seems doubtful whether this technique will rival the laparoscopic operations. Myotomy for achalasia can be equally well performed by both laparoscopic and VATS approaches (Shoenut et al., 1997; Stewart et al., 1999). There are, unfortunately, no randomized data available in the literature to determine which approach is better. The results of thoracoscopic myotomy are equivalent to those of balloon dilatation (Shoenut et al., 1997) and most authors consider a laparoscopic approach to be superior on the basis of more rapid mobilization and lower conversion rates (Raiser et al., 1996; Stewart et al., 1999). One rationalization is to reserve the thoracoscopic approach for those patients with a short oesophagus or gross obesity (Roberts and Cuschieri, 1995). We have found the VATS approach to offer excellent visualization and to be associated with rapid mobilisation and early return of peristaltic function with, usually, a three day in-patient stay.

As described initially by Cuschieri, the procedure is facilitated by inserting an endoscope before positioning the patient. This allows relaxation of the lower oesophageal sphincter to be confirmed following the myotomy and makes it easier to check for mucosal breaches by using the insufflation function whilst the chest is filled with water.

6.2. Oesphageal carcinoma

VATS has been advocated as a useful advanced lymph node staging technique in oesophageal carcinoma which complements laparoscopic assessment. Both are about 94% accurate in determining lymph node status (Krasna, 1997) and should, theoretically, be a procedure which would benefit greatly from a VATS approach. Oesophageal resection by VATS should logically be advantageous as the surgical injury in open resection is substantial and the patients are often debilitated. Various descriptions have been offered but while combined laparoscopic and VATS procedures are possible (Lloyd et al., 1994; Nguyen et al., 1999) these are often impractical and interest has largely focused on utilising VATS to mobilise the thoracic oesophagus in conjunction with open abdominal mobilisation of the stomach and an open cervical anastomosis (Cuschieri, 1993; Collard, 1996). The operative view of the oesophagus through a right chest approach is excellent with only the azygos vein requiring division but early hopes of reduced pulmonary complications and in-patient stay have not been rewarded. Later reports have, therefore, largely confirmed that while VATS oesophagectomy is feasible it does not appear to confer any advantages (Collard, 1996; Robertson et al., 1996; Peracchia et al., 1997). Peracchia and colleagues, for example (1997), reviewed 107 thoracoscopic oesophagectomies collected from the literature. Conversion was required in 12 (11.2%) with no intraoperative deaths. However, the procedures tended to be lengthy and ultimate morbidity and inpatient stay were little better than with open resection. In particular, the incidence of chest complications and ventilation in this review was not improved. The current evidence does not, therefore, support the use of VATS oesophageal mobilisation. It is also evident that the uptake of oesophageal mobilisation has been modest indicating general dissatisfaction with the procedure. One variation that may prove useful, at least as a niche procedure, is videoscopic mediastinal oesophageal dissection as described by Buess for benign and in situ or early (T1) stage oesophageal cancer (Manncke et al., 1994). This procedure requires a special dissection instrument inserted via a cervical incision and gastric mobilization via a laparotomy.

7. Mediastinal conditions

Thymic resection has been described either entirely as a VATS procedure or utilising VATS as an adjunct to transcervical mobilisation (Mantegazza et al., 1998; Mack and Scruggs, 1998). These strategies have been successfully used for thymic hyperplasia and for small thymomas. Concern has been expressed regarding the completeness of resection achieved particularly in the context of malignancy (Kohmann, 1997). The available data does not support these concerns but follow up is short and time will resolve this issue. An alternate consideration is whether a VATS approach is actually less traumatic than either trans-cervical or trans-sternal approaches both of which are well-tolerated with low residual pain whereas any intercostal approach including VATS will have an associated risk of neuropraxia. The cosmetic advantage of a VATS approach in young females with myasthenia may, however, be more compelling.

Simple mediastinal cysts are relatively easy to either excise or deroof using VATS techniques and their successful management has been described in numerous case reports. Teratodermoid lesions are usually associated with dense surrounding inflammatory tissue which makes a videothoracoscopic approach both excessively difficult and dangerous.

Mediastinal tumours can be either biopsied or excised depending upon size, location and the underlying diagnosis (Demmy et al., 1998).

8. Miscellaneous

8.1. Sympathectomy

Sympathetic chain interruption or segmental excision of levels T2–T4 can be performed either supine or prone. The supine approach is often undertaken with the patient in a semi-erect position and allows rapid bilateral cautery interruption of the chain. It has been used extensively with a thoracoscopic technique by Drott and Claes (1996) and is the usual approach for most surgeons carrying out VATS procedures when either two or three ports are created on each side. In view of cosmetic considerations, a 5 mm videoscope is preferable and it is helpful to place the incisions in the infra-mammary crease. Recently, the use of a 2 mm endoscope has been described (Pillay et al., 1997). The prone approach has been advocated by Cuschieri (1994) and offers the advantage that the lung drops away from the posterior chest which may facilitate segmental excision as he recommends. Either approach works well and there is little evidence to suggest that trunk interruption is any less effective than segment excision. Thoracic sympathectomy is very effective for palmar hyperhidrosis. It offers much less certain benefit for axillary hyperhidrosis (Zacherl et al., 1998) and the value of this procedure in many other claimed indications including Raynaud's syndrome, angina, flushing and chronic pain are anecdotal. Preoperative counselling is a particularly important aspect of this procedure, however, so that the risks of compensatory hyperhidrosis, wound pain and Horner's syndrome are well understood. Compensatory hyperhidrosis may occur in 30 to 40% of cases and can be reduced by selective division of the rami rather the chain itself (Gossot et al., 1997) using a technique originally described by Wittmoser (Schurr and Buess, 1993). This approach is also associated, however, with higher relapse rates (Gossot et al., 1997).

8.2. Splanchnicectomy

Intractable abdominal pain from malignant disease or chronic pancreatitis has been improved in several limited series by division of the splanchnic nerves

— splanchnicectomy — with satisfactory result even with division of the left side only (Noppen et al., 1998; Le Pimpec et al., 1998). The long term value and general applicability of this procedure to visceral abdominal pain is still under investigation.

8.3. Trauma

The use of VATS techniques requires a patient able to withstand at least partial one-lung ventilation. Most major trauma patients do not come into this category but there are some with sufficiently stable cardiorespiratory status to benefit from VATS assessment and treatment. The chief applications of VATS or thoracoscopy in trauma thus far described are: evaluation of suspected ruptured diaphragm, management of chest tube induced bleeding, evacuation of haemothorax, assessment of penetrating thoracic wounds and intrathoracic foreign bodies and evacuation of empyema. The use of VATS in haemothorax extends from the acute event where it may be used to identify the cause of bleeding and to apply clips to bleeding vessels in acute cases. Intrathoracic clots can be evacuated in the early post injury phase so reducing the chance of cortex formation. The results of thoracoscopy both conventional and by VATS have been reviewed by Villavicencio (1999) and colleagues who collected over 500 patients from the literature. They noted that thoracoscopic evaluation was generally highly efficient as a diagnostic tool with a low missed injury rate of only 0.8% and it proved over 80% effective as a therapeutic approach in the limited range of applications for which it was used, mainly chest tube bleeding, evacuation of retained hemothoraces, and evacuation of empyemas. Both conventional and video thoracoscopes appear equally effective (Karmy-Jones et al., 1998). Recently, the application of this technique to acute gunshot wounds of the chest has been described (Brusov et al., 1998) and routine use of VATS pericardial window and inspection in suspected cardiac trauma cases has been recommended by Morales and colleagues (1997). They reported a series of 108 patients with penetrating wounds near the heart but no obvious signs of cardiac injury. Diagnostic thoracoscopic pericardial window was undertaken to rule out cardiac injury. In 33 patients (30.6%), the procedure identified hemopericardium. Sensitivity for the procedure was 100%, specificity 96%, and accuracy 97%. There were no deaths and no complications due to the procedure.

8.4. Diaphragm

Apart from identifying diaphragmatic injury as noted above, various case reports describe VATS repair of various diaphragmatic herniae (Hussong et al., 1997; Silen et al., 1995) and even repair of a ruptured diaphragm (Kurata et al., 1996). This approach is, however, probably only applicable to relatively small defects.

8.5. Spinal surgery

Conventional anterior thoracic spinal surgery has required an open thoracotomy approach. This can be obviated in some instances by the use of a VATS approach which enables the thoracic and spinal surgeons to co-operate while retaining the minimal access approach. VATS techniques have been described in excision of thoracic discs, spinal correction surgery in children and (Kokoska et al., 1998; Rosenthal and Dickman, 1998) including the thoracolumbar junction (Huang et al., 1997). This same philosophy can be extended to neurogenic tumours with an intra medullary component where a laminectomy and direct mobilisation of the intraspinal portion by the spinal surgeon can be followed by a VATS approach and excision of the tumour by the thoracic surgeon.

8.6. Pericardium

Patients requiring pericardial drainage are usually either cases with malignant effusions or chronic benign effusion. Malignant effusions are, in the author's opinion, probably best dealt with via a subxyphoid approach as this is a less invasive procedure which offers good short term palliation for minimal pain. Chronic pericardial effusion and those cases of malignant effusion associated with an undiagnosed pulmonary or pleural origin may benefit from a VATS approach. This allows the surgeon to sample any intrapleural disease and to perform a pericardial window (Fig. 7) for drainage long term (Nataf et al., 1998).

8.7. Thoracic duct

Injury to the thoracic duct is rare and usually related to oesophagectomy although spontaneous leakage is described, notably with lymphoma (Hillerdal, 1997). Various case reports testify to the value of a VATS approach to occluding the thoracic duct usually by

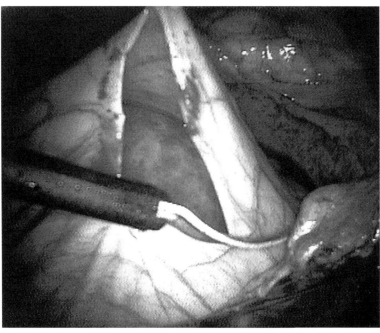

Fig. 7. Operative image of VATS left pericardial window.

the application of clips across the duct close to the right diaphragm (Lapp et al., 1998).

9. Future perspectives

Video-assisted surgery has already replaced open approaches to many lesser thoracic operations and in some centres, has proved a safe technique for complex major procedures. Further development will depend on improvements in instrument design and imaging technology and on better training with coordinated strategies for developing videoscopic skills. Instrument advances should include: staplers that have smaller ends and angulate easily, videoscopes that are less than 5 mm while preserving full view and illumination and effective 3-D systems. It is to be hoped, also, that improved operative techniques and lung sealants may allow the patient to reap the full benefits of the VATS approach in terms of reduced hospital stay and early return to normal activity. Ultimately, however, randomized prospective trials will be necessary to test the true benefits of VATS procedures. Scientific proof rather than clinical belief will be required within contemporary financially restricted healthcare systems if both purchasers and managers are to accept greater investment in minimal access techniques.

References and further reading

Bardini R, Asolati M. Thoracoscopic resection of benign tumours of the esophagus. Int Surg 1997; 82: 5–6.

Bertrand PC, Regnard JF, Spaggiari L et al. Immediate and long term results after surgical treatment of primary spontaneous pneumothorax by VATS. Ann Thorac Surg 1996; 61: 1641–1645.

Brantigan OC, Mueller E. Surgical treatment of pulmonary emphysema. Am Surg 1957; 23: 789–804.

Brantigan OC, Kress MB, Mueller EA. The surgical approach to pulmonary emphysema. Dis Chest 1961; 39: 485–501.

Brenner M, Kayaleh RA, Milne EN et al. Thoracoscopic ablation of pulmonary bullae; radiographic selection and treatment response. J Thorac Cardiovasc Surg 1994; 107: 883–890.

Brusov PG. Kuritsyn AN, Urazovsky NY, Tariverdiev ML. Operative videothoracoscopy in the surgical treatment of penetrating firearms wounds of the chest. Military Medicine 1998; 163: 603–607.

Cassina PC, Hauser M, Hillejan L, Greschuchna D, Stamatis G. Video-assisted thoracoscopy in the treatment of pleural empyema: stage-based management and outcome. J Thorac Cardiovasc Surg 1999; 117(2): 234–238.

Champion JK, McKernan JB. Comparison of minimally invasive thoracoscopy versus open thoracotomy for staging lung cancer. Int Surg 1996; 81: 235–236.

Collard JM, Reymond MA. Video-assisted thoracic surgery (VATS) for cancer. Int Surg 1996; 81: 343–346.

Collard JM, Lengele B, Otte JB, Kestens PJ. En bloc and standard esophagectomies by thoracoscopy. Ann Thorac Surg 1993; 56: 675–679.

Collard JM. As originally published in 1993: En bloc and standard esophagectomies by thoracoscopy. Updated in 1996. Ann Thorac Surg 1996; 61: 769–770.

Cooper JD, Trulock EP, Triantafillou AN et al. Bilateral pneumectomy (volume reduction) for chronic obstructive pulmonary disease. J Thorac Cardiovasc Surg 1995; 109: 106–119.

Cooper JD, Patterson GA, Sundaresan RS et al. Results of 150 consecutive bilateral lung volume reduction procedures in patients with severe emphysema J Thorac Cardiovasc Surg 1996; 112: 1319–1330.

Craig SR, Walker WS. Potential complications of vascular stapling in thoracoscopic surgery. Ann Thorac Surg 1995; 59: 736–738.

Cuschieri A. Endoscopic subtotal oesophagectomy for cancer using the right thoracoscopic approach. Surg Oncol 1993; 2 (Suppl. 1): 3–11.

Cuschieri A, Shimi SM, Crosthwaite G, Joypaul V. Bilateral endoscopic splanchnicectomy through a posterior thoracoscopic approach. J R Coll Surgeons of Edin 1994; 39: 44–47.

De Giacomo T, Venuta F, Rendina EA, et al. Video-assisted thoracoscopic treatment of giant bullae associated with emphysema. Eur J Cardiothoracic Surg 1999; 15: 753–756.

Demmy TL, Krasna MJ, Detterbeck FC et al. Multicenter VATS experience with mediastinal tumors. Ann Thorac Surg 1998; 66: 187–192.

Demmy TL, Curtis JJ. Minimally invasive lobectomy directed toward frail and high-risk patients: a case-control study. Ann Thorac Surg 1999; 68: 194–200.

Downey RJ, McCormack P, LoCicero III J. Dissemination of malignancies following video-assisted thoracic surgery: a report of 21 cases. J Thorac Cardiovasc Surg 1996; 111: 954–960.

Drott C, Claes G. Hyperhidrosis treated by thoracoscopic sympathicotomy. Cardiovasc Surg 1996; 4: 788–790.

Gandhi RR, Stringel G. Video-assisted thoracoscopic surgery in the management of pediatric empyema J Laparoendoscop Surg 1997; 1: 251–253.

Ginsberg R, Rubinstein L. A randomised trial of lobectomy versus limited resection in patients with T1N0 non small cell lung cancer. Lung Cancer 1991; 7 (Suppl.): 83.

Giudicelli R, Thomas P, Lonjon T et al. Video-assisted minthoracotomy versus muscle sparing thoracotomy for performing lobectomy. Ann Thorac Surg 1994; 58: 712–718.

Gossot D, Toledo L, Fritsch S, Celerier M. Thoracoscopic sympathectomy for upper limb hyperhidrosis: looking for the right operation. Ann Thorac Surg 1997; 64: 975–978.

Hazelrigg S, Boley T, Henkle J et al. Thoracoscopic laser bullectomy: a prospective study with three-month results. J Thorac and Cardiovasc Surg 1996; 112: 319–321.

Hill RC, Jones DR, Vance RA et al. Selective lung ventilation during thoracoscopy: effects of insufflation on hemodynamics. Ann Thorac Surg 1996; 61: 945–948.

Hillerdal G. Chylothorax and pseudochylothorax. Eur Respir J 1997; 10: 1157–1162.

Huang TJ, Hsu RW, Liu HP et al. Video-assisted thoracoscopic treatment of spinal lesions in the thoracolumbar junction. Surg Endoscopy 1997; 11: 1189–1193.

Hussong RL Jr., Landreneau RJ, Cole FH Jr. Diagnosis and repair of a Morgagni hernia with video-assisted thoracic surgery. Ann Thorac Surg 1997; 63: 1474–1475.

Inderbitzi RGC, Grillet M-P. Risk and hazards of video-thoracoscopic surgery: a collective review. Eur J Cardiothorac Surg 1996; 10: 483–489.

Jancovici R, Lang-Lazdunski L, Pons F et al. Complications of

video-assisted thoracic surgery: a five year experience. Ann Thorac Surg 1996; 61: 533–537.

Jones DR, Graeber GM, Tanguilig GS et al. Effects of insufflation on haemodynamics during thoracoscopic procedures. Ann Thorac Surg 1993; 55: 1379–1382.

Kadokura M, Colby TV, Myers JL et al Pathological comparison of video-assisted thoracic surgical lung biopsy with traditional open lung biopsy. J Thorac Cardiovasc Surg 1995; 109: 494–498.

Karmy-Jones R, Vallieres E, Kralovich K et al. A comparison of rigid -v- video thoracoscopy in the management of chest trauma. Injury 1998; 29: 655–659.

Kaseda S, Aoki T, Hangai N. Video-assisted thoracic surgery (VATS) lobectomy: the Japanese experience. Seminars in Thoracic and Cardiovascular Surgery 1998; 10: 300–304.

Kassis ES, Luketitch JD. Minimally invasive surgical treatment of gastroesophageal reflux disease. Chapter 13 in: WS Walker (Ed.), Video-assisted Thoracic Surgery. Oxford: Isis Medical Media, 1999; pp. 173–187.

Kirby TJ, Mack MJ, Landreneau RJ et al. Lobectomy — video-assisted thoracic surgery versus muscle sparing thoracotomy. A randomized trial. J Thorac Cardiovasc Surg 1995; 109: 997–1002.

Klena JW, Cameron BH, Langer JC, Winthrop AL, Perez CR. Timing of video-assisted thoracoscopic debridement for pediatric empyema. J Am Coll Surg 1998; 187: 404–408.

Ko CY, Waters PF. Lung volume reduction surgery: a cost and outcomes comparison of sternotomy versus thoracoscopy. American Surgeon 1998; 64(10): 1010–1013.

Kohman LJ. Controversies in the management of malignant thymoma. Chest 1997; 112: 296S–300S.

Kokoska ER, Gabriel KR, Silen ML. Minimally invasive anterior spinal exposure and release in children with scoliosis. J Soc Laparoendoscopic Surgeons 1998; 2: 255–258.

Kotloff RM, Tino G, Bavaria JE et al. Bilateral lung volume reduction surgery for advanced emphysema. A comparison of median sternotomy and thoracoscopic approaches. Chest 1996; 110: 1399–1406.

Kotloff R, Tino G, Hansen-Flaschen J et al. Short-term functional outcomes following unilateral vs bilateral lung volume reduction surgery (LVRS). Am J Resp Crit Care Med 1997; 155(part 2 Supp): A602.

Krasna MJ, Deshmukh S, McLaughlin JS. Complications of thoracoscopy. Ann Thor Surg 1996; 61: 1066–1069.

Krasna MJ. The role of thoracoscopic lymph node staging in esophageal cancer. Int Surg 1997; 82: 7–11.

Kurata K, Kubota K, Oosawa H, Eda N, Ishihara T. Thoracoscopic repair of traumatic diaphragmatic rupture. A case report. Surg Endoscopy 1996; 10: 850–851.

Landreneau RJ, Mack MJ, Hazelrigg SR et al. Video-assisted thoracic surgery: basic technical concepts and intercostal approach strategies. Ann Thorac Surg 1992; 54: 800–807.

Landreneau RJ, Mack MJ, Keenan RJ, Hazelrigg SR, Dowling RD, Ferson PF. Strategic planning for video-assisted thoracic surgery. Ann Thorac Surg. 1993; 56: 615–619.

Landreneau RJ, Sugarbaker DJ, Mack MJ, et al. Wedge resection versus lobectomy for stage I (T1 N0 M0) non-small-cell lung cancer. J Thorac Cardiovasc Surg 1997; 113: 691–698.

Lapp GC, Brown DH, Gullane PJ, McKneally M. Thoracoscopic management of chylous fistulae. Am J Otolaryngology 1998; 19: 257–262.

Lawrence DR, Ohri SK, Moxon RE, Townsend ER, Fountain

SW. Thoracoscopic debridement of empyema thoracis. Ann Thorac Surg 1997; 64: 1448–1450.

Le Pimpec Barthes F, Chapuis O, Riquet M, et al. Thoracoscopic splanchnicectomy for control of intractable pain in pancreatic cancer. Ann Thorac Surg 1998; 65: 810–813.; 113: 528–531.

Lewis RJ, Caccavale RJ, Sisler GE et al. Does VATS favor seeding of carcinoma of the lung more than a conventional operation? International Surgery 1997; 82: 127–130.

Lewis RJ, Caccavale RJ, Sisler GE, Bocage J-P, Mackenzie JW. 100 video-assisted thoracic surgical non-rib spread simultaneous lobectomies. Ann Thorac Surg 1997; 63: 1415–1421.

Lewis RJ, Caccavale RJ. Video-assisted thoracic surgical non-rib spreading simultaneously stapled lobectomy (VATS(n)SSL). Sem Thorac Cardiovasc Surg 1998; 10: 332–339.

Lloyd DM, Vipond M, Robertson GS, Hanning C, Veitch PS. Thoracoscopic oesophago-gastrectomy — a new technique for intra-thoracic stapling. Endosc Surg Allied Tech 1994; 2: 26–31.

Loddenkemper R. Thoracoscopy — state of the art. Eur Respir J 1998; 11: 213–221.

Loscertales J, Jimenez-Merchan R, Arenas-Linares C, Giron-Arjona JC, Congredado-Loscertales M. The use of video assisted thoracic surgery in lung cancer. Evaluation of resectability in 296 patients and 71 pulmonary exeresis with radical lymphadenectomy. Eur J Cardiothorac Surg 1997; 12: 892–897.

Mack MJ, Hazelrigg SR, Landreneau RJ, Acuff TE. Thoracoscopy for the diagnosis of the indeterminate solitary pulmonary nodule. Ann Thorac Surg. 1993; 56: 825–830.

Mack MJ, Scruggs GR, Kelly KM, Shennib H, Landreneau RJ. Video-assisted thoracic surgery: Has technology found its place? Ann Thorac Surg 1997; 64: 211–215.

Mack MJ, Scruggs G. Video-assisted thoracic surgery thymectomy for myasthenia gravis. Chest Surg Clin North Am 1998; 8: 809–825.

Mack MJ. Thoracoscopic management of the solitary pulmonary nodule. In: W S Walker (ed.), Video-assisted Thoracic Surgery. Oxford, Isis Medical Media, 1999.

Mackinlay TA, Lyons GA, Chimondeguy DJ et al. VATS debridement versus thoracotomy in the treatment of loculated postpneumonia empyema. Ann Thorac Surg 1996; 61: 1626–1630.

Mackinlay TA (abstract). VATS lobectomy: an international survey Presented at the IVth International Symposium on Thoracoscopy and Video Assisted Thoracic Surgery, Sao-Paulo, May, 1997.

Manncke K, Raestrup H, Walter D et al. Technique of endoscopic mediastinal dissection of the oesophagus. Endos Surg and Allied Technologies 1994; 2: 10–15.

Mantegazza R, Confalonieri P, Antozzi C, et al. Video-assisted thoracoscopic extended thymectomy (VATET) in myasthenia gravis. Two-year follow-up in 101 patients and comparison with the trans-sternal approach. Ann NY Acad Sci 1998; 841: 749–752.

McKenna RJ. Lobectomy by video assisted thoracic surgery with mediastinal node sampling. J Thorac Cardiovasc Surg 1994; 107: 879–882.

McKenna RJ, Brenner M, Gelb A et al. A randomized prospective trial of stapled lung reduction versus laser bullectomy for diffuse emphysema. J Thorac Cardiovasc Surg 1996; 111: 317–322.

McKenna RJ, Brenner M, Fischel RJ, Gelb AF. Should lung volume reduction for emphysema be unilateral or bilateral? J Thorac Cardiovasc Surg 1996; 112: 1331–1340.

McKenna RJ Jr, Fischel RJ, Wolf R, Wurnig P. Video-assisted thoracic surgery (VATS) lobectomy for bronchogenic carcinoma. Sem Thorac Cardiovasc Surg 1998; 10: 321–325.

Menconi GF, Melfi FM, Mussi A, Palla A, Ambrogi MC, Angeletti CA. Treatment by VATS of giant bullous emphysema: results. Eur J Cardiothoracic Surg 1998; 13: 66–70.

Merry C, Spurbeck W, Lobe TE. Resection of foregut-derived duplications by minimal-access surgery. Paediat Surg Int 1999; 15: 224–226.

Morales CH, Salinas CM, Henao CA, Patino PA, Munoz CM. Thoracoscopic pericardial window and penetrating cardiac trauma. J Trauma-Injury Infection Crit Care 1997; 42: 273–275.

Mouroux J, Elkaim D, Padovani B et al Video-assisted thoracoscopic treatment of spontaneous pneumothorax: technique and results of 100 cases. J Thorac Cardiovasc Surg 1996; 112: 385–391.

Mouroux J, Clay-Meinesz C, Padovani B et al. Efficacy and safety of video thoracoscopic lung biopsy in the diagnosis of interstitial lung disease. Eur J Cardiothorac Surg 1997; 11: 22–26.

Nataf P, Cacoub P, Regan M, et al. Video-thoracoscopic pericardial window in the diagnosis and treatment of pericardial effusions. Am J Cardiol 1998; 82: 124–126.

Naunheim KS, Mack MJ, Hazelrigg SR et al. Safety and efficacy of video assisted thoracic surgical techniques for the treatment of spontaneous pneumothorax. J Thorac Cardiovasc Surg 1995; 109; 1198–1203.

Naunheim KS, Ferguson MK. The current status of lung volume reduction operations for Emphysema. Ann Thorac Surg 1996; 62: 601–612.

Nguyen NT, Schauer PR, Hutson W, et al. Preliminary results of thoracoscopic Belsey Mark IV antireflux procedure. Surg Lap, Endos and Percutaneous Techniques 1998; 8: 185–188.

Nguyen NT, Schauer PR, Luketich JD. Combined laparoscopic and thoracoscopic approach to esophagectomy. J Am Coll Surg 1999; 188(3): 328–332.

Noppen M, Meysman M, D'Haese J, Vincken W. Thoracoscopic splanchnicolysis for the relief of chronic pancreatitis pain: experience of a group of pneumologists. Chest 1998; 113: 528–531.

Ohbuchi T, Morikawa T, Takeuchi E, Kato H. Lobectomy: video-assisted thoracic surgery versus posterolateral thoracotomy. Jap J Thorac Cardiovasc Surg 1998; 46: 519–522.

Peracchia A, Rosati R, Fumagalli U, Bona S, Chella B. Thoracoscopic dissection of the esophagus for cancer. Int Surg 1997; 82: 1–4.

Peracchia A, Rosati R, Fumagalli U, Bona S, Chella B. Thoracoscopic esophagectomy: are there benefits? Sem Surg Oncol 1997; 13: 259–262.

Pillay PK, Kumar K, Tang KK. Video-endoscopic and mini-endoscopic sympathectomy for hyperhidrosis. Stereotactic and Functional Neurosurgery 1997; 69(1–4 Part 2): 274–277.

Raiser F, Perdikis G, Hinder RA, et al. Heller myotomy via minimal-access surgery. An evaluation of antireflux procedures. Arch Surg 1996; 131: 593–597.

Ravini M, Ferraro G, Barbieri B et al. Changing strategies of lung biopsies in diffuse lung diseases; the impact of video-assisted thoracoscopy. Eur Resp J 1998; 11: 99–103.

Rendina EA, Venuta F, De Giacomo T, et al. Comparative merits

may also be an important source of pain. Analgesia is therefore very important and has been partly based on an epidural or peridural thoracic catheter. Further analgesic combinations are made, e.g. with acetaminophen, or non-steriodal analgesics if there are no contraindications. Because of the narrow therapeutic margin of parenteral opioids between analgesic and respiratory depressive effect they have to be given with caution. Small repeated doses of 2 to 4 mg intravenous morphine has been used by other groups, although most patients require only oral analgesics as early as two days after the procedure.

Gastrointestinal complications represented a significant fraction of the mortality of one center even in patients without history of peptic ulcer disease or constipation. Not only a routine gastrointestinal prophylaxis (antacids, H2 blockers, proton-pump inhibitors), but also prevention of constipation seems of highly important.

Prophylactic antibiotic therapy may be considered. Regular postoperative bacterial sampling of valid sputum for culture and eventual antibiogram may aid in discussions about antibiotic change in case of chest radiography infiltrates and clinical suspicion of pneumonia in order to prescribe a clearly directed treatment. A rather generous antibiotic treatment in those frail patients seemed adequate to us: infiltrates, fever, leukocytosis and high or ascending C-reactive protein values may be the base for such a treatment. Whereas some groups give an oral antibiotic for bronchitis prophylaxis in every patient, we do not perform any antibiotic bronchitis prophylaxis. Intravenous steroids are necessary when patients have had preoperative oral steroid medication and can normally be changed within 24 hours to oral dosage again. In case of complications adequate supportive steroid medication is important.

Postoperative episodes of pulmonary embolism have been observed. Due to the important reduction of the pulmonary vascular bed by their disease, COPD certainly poses an important additional risk to that of pulmonary embolism in general. Besides heparin and early mobilization, we use anti-thrombotic stockings. As pulmonary embolism after hospital discharge was also observed in some LVRS patients, oral anticoagulation may be considered and weighed against its risks.

Physiotherapy is very helpful to mobilize secretions, to re-expand collapsed pulmonary parenchyma, and to mobilize the patient early in order to maintain the patient's general force and prevent thrombo-embolic disease. Incentive spirometers, breathing exercises, and early and rather "aggressive" mobilization are important mainstays of therapy. With a good interdisciplinary approach of management as is also mandatory for lung transplant patients, 30 days and in-hospital mortality is below 5%.

1.5. Predictors of outcome

Pre-operative predictors of peri-operative morbidity and mortality have been analyzed in 47 consecutive patients undergoing bilateral LVRS, via median sternotomy, by Szekely et al. (1997). A six-minute walking distance of 200 m or less and hypercarbia with a resting room $PaCO_2$ of 45 mmHg or more were associated with prolonged hospital stay and increased mortality. In these patients, more than one third died after the operation, compared to a zero mortality for the rest of the study population.

Neither lung function parameters nor arterial blood gas and single breath diffusing capacity predicted outcome. In contrast, heterogeneous pattern of the upper lobe, as assessed by chest computed tomography and lung perfusion scan, was associated with superior outcome compared to predominantly lower lobe disease or diffuse emphysema. The authors conclude that after patients have been selected on the basis of morphological evidence of heterogeneity, no functional parameter allowed further refinement of selection criteria.

Overall improvement was significant only for stapler procedures, and improved outcome was correlated with greater smoking history and younger age. Interestingly, preoperative FEV_1 and gas exchange variables did not predict outcome in these patients. Increased thoracic gas volume as assessed by CT scan grading was the primary predictor of response in patients treated by laser ablation. The authors conclude that younger patients with evidence of advanced emphysematous lung disease and hyperinflation will improve most after LVRS.

Ferguson et al. (1998) performed exercise testing in 27 patients before and after LVRS. None of the preoperative lung function parameters correlated with changes in exercise performance after LVRS, and only a weak correlation was observed between preoperative dead space/tidal volume ration and improvement in maximal oxygen uptake.

1.5.1. Radiological assessment of emphysema morphology as a predictor of outcome
Emphysema morphology, i.e. the heterogeneity of emphysema, has so far been the most reliable pre-

dictor for postoperative outcome in the population of operated LVRS patients. Patients with heterogeneous disease profited more than patients with completely homogeneous emphysema morphology, although also for the latter group a sustained benefit for at least two years could be demonstrated. Besides clinical and physiological features, appropriate patient selection includes morphological aspects of emphysema.

Many centers select patients for LVRS only if marked differences in the severity of emphysema are present in chest computer tomography (CT) and lung perfusion scan. Several groups have developed and applied sophisticated methods to classify and grade emphysema as assessed by CT scan of the chest; however, to our knowledge most of them have not been validated.

Based on a validated, simple, computed tomography based radiological emphysema classification (Table 2) we were able to demonstrate that also patients with intermediately heterogeneous or even homogeneous emphysema experienced a clinically relevant improvement not only at three months after the intervention but at least two years after LVRS.

Table 2

Validated emphysema classification

The following definitions were applied:

1. *Homogeneous:*	No regional or only very minor differences in the severity of emphysema (i.e., decreased density, loss of vascular lung structure) are appreciable.
2. *Intermediately heterogeneous:*	A distinct regional difference in the severity of emphysema may be present maximally in the area of one or more than one but not in adjacent lung segments of either lung.
3. *Markedly heterogeneous:*	A distinct regional difference in the severity of emphysema is present in at least two adjacent lung segments of either lung.

The following features were assessed in addition for *intermediately* **or** *markedly* **heterogeneous cases:**

Predominant upper lobe type:	Emphysema is preferentially located in the upper lobe with or without involvement of the apical segments of the lower lobes.
Predominant lower lobe type:	Emphysema is preferentially located in the lower lobe and may or may not involve the lingula or the middle lobe, respectively.
Bullae:	One or few single bullae are additionally present with a diameter of less than 7 cm.
Asymmetry:	Concerning the two lungs.

At 24 months postoperatively, FEV_1 and dyspnoea readings continued to be significantly better than preoperatively in all three morphologic groups. Survival was highest in markedly heterogeneous emphysema.

Only limited published data is available on the effect of LVRS on lung function in patients with homogeneous or intermediately heterogeneous as compared to markedly heterogeneous emphysema morphology. Patients with a homogeneous type of emphysema have been excluded *a priori* from LVRS in a high proportion of centers, as documented in a recent European survey. (Hamacher et al., 2000). Homogeneous emphysema morphology accounted for about two thirds of their rejections from surgery in one center reporting on 300 cases. This was between two and three times more frequently the reason for rejection than medical contraindication to operation. The rationale not to operate on patients with homogeneous emphysema is based on pathophysiological considerations and the observation, that the degree of heterogeneity is a predictor of short-term functional improvement

Our recent study (Hamacher et al., 1999) showed functional and subjective benefit of statistical and clinical significance in homogeneous and intermediately heterogeneous emphysema, and not only in the group with marked heterogeneity (Table 3). Whereas clinical outcome in terms of MRC dyspnoea score was not different between all three groups during the studied follow-up period, functional outcome at 24 months and survival turned out to be predicted as well by morphology. Gradual decline of FEV_1 was observed in all three groups and averaged 63–194 ml per year or 1.9–5.7% of predicted FEV_1 per year.

?#1

Overall mortality differed between the three morphology groups and was least in the markedly heterogeneous morphology group. Whether less lung functional status preoperatively or less profit by LVRS have been related to different survival remains open. The findings add survival to the outcome variables. Also, the question on whether survival is influenced by LRVS in general cannot yet be definitely answered. One study of patients not operated due to missing insurance coverage versus operated patients suggests that a survival advantage exists after LVRS. The importance of survival differences is however relative in the light of any treatment that is primarily intended to be palliative.

In conclusion, two years after LVRS, FEV_1 and dyspnoea score continued to be significantly better than preoperatively in all three morphologic groups, whereas short-term as well as two years functional

Table 3

Clinical and functional outcome according to chest computed tomography morphology of emphysema [a]

	Homogeneous (n = 12; 7 female; age: 66±2 years)			Intermediately Heterogeneous (n = 7; 4 female; age: 66±2 years)			Markedly heterogeneous (n = 18; 2 female; age: 66±2 years) [c]		
	Preop.	3 Months	24 Months	Preop.	3 Months	24 Months	Preop.	3 Months	24 Months
VC (l)	2.57±0.18	2.99±0.20 [e]	2.72±0.21	2.53±0.32	3.03±0.43	2.76±0.30	3.38±0.23 [c]	4.27±0.27 [e]	3.90±0.26 [b]
(% pred.)	79±4	93±3 [e]	85±5	80±6	94±6	89±4	85±5	106±4 [e]	98±4 [b]
FEV$_1$ (l)	0.68±0.04	0.93±0.05 [e]	0.77±0.06	0.70±0.08	1.07±0.15 [b]	0.96±0.15	0.92±0.07 [c]	1.62±0.17 [e,f]	1.25±0.14 [b,c]
(% pred.)	26±1	38±2 [e]	32±2 [b]	29±2	44±4 [e]	41±5 [b]	31±2	52±4 [e,c]	41±4 [b]
FEV$_1$ decline # (ml/year)			81±18			63±31			194±30 [c,d]
(% pred./year)			3.2±0.8			1.9±1.0			5.7±0.9 [d]
TLC (l)	7.67±0.34	7.18±0.35 [b]	7.34±0.40 [b]	7.38±0.54	6.66±0.57	6.90±0.59	8.55±0.31	7.97±0.29 [e]	8.22±0.32
(% pred.)	136±4	130±3	129±3 [b]	134±5	121±6 [b]	125±5	130±5	120±4 [b]	125±5
RV (l)	5.09±0.24	4.15±0.23 [b]	4.54±0.30 [b]	4.88±0.29	3.59±0.40 [b]	3.98±0.46	5.19±0.28	3.70±0.24 [e]	4.20±0.29 [e]
(% pred.)	234±8	193±9 [b]	203±11 [b]	229±14	167±15 [b]	181±15	217±14	153±12 [e]	172±14 [e]
RV/TLC	0.67±0.01	0.58±0.02 [e]	0.62±0.02 [b]	0.67±0.03	0.54±0.04 [b]	0.58±0.04	0.61±0.02	0.47±0.03 [e,f]	0.51±0.03 [e,c]
6-min Walking distance (m)	274±26	370±26	317±36	314±35	354±33	330±65	252±21	365±18 [b]	352±25 [b]
Dyspnoea (MRC score)	3.5±0.2	1.6±0.4 [e]	2.0±0.3 [e]	3.7±0.2	1.4±0.5 [e]	2.0±0.6 [b]	3.4±0.2	1.5±0.2 [e]	1.9±0.2 [e]

[a] Mean values ± standard error. # Decline of FEV$_1$ calculated from the difference between the values at 3 months and at 24 months postoperatively

[b] $p \leq 0.05$ versus corresponding preoperative value

[c] $p \leq 0.05$ versus homogeneous

[d] $p \leq 0.05$ versus intermediately heterogeneous

[e] $p \leq 0.01$ versus corresponding preoperative value

[f] $p \leq 0.01$ versus homogeneous.

profit was greatest in markedly heterogeneous emphysema patients. A unified emphysema nomenclature and classification in regard to LVRS would make results between groups comparable and probably patient selection more appropriate.

1.6. Results

1.6.1. Lung function

The improvement in FEV_1 has drawn most attention from the reports on reduction surgery. Most series on short-term results after staple lung volume reduction as shown in Table 4 show important and significant improvements of FEV_1 and reduction of hyperinflation three to six months after LVRS. In a recent meta-analysis of more than 900 patients, the overall interquartile range of FEV_1 rose by 0.23 to 0.36 l from 24 to 28% of predicted preoperatively, to 35 to 40% of predicted at 3 to 6 months (Young et al., 1999).

Brenner et al. (1999) analyzed short-term and long-term rate of change in pulmonary function after unilateral or bilateral LVRS either by stapling, NdYAG contact mode laser procedures, or a combination of both. Bilateral stapling revealed the highest improvement in FEV_1, and even unilateral stapling was superior to unilateral combined procedures. Laser ablation led only to slight improvements. On the other hand, the long-term rate of decline in FEV_1 after surgery was highest in bilateral stapler operations, and a general correlation between the magnitude of initial improvement in FEV_1 and rate of decline was found. The authors conclude that the higher rates of long-term deterioration after initial higher improvement raise questions regarding optimal long-term procedures.

Functional results for two years and more are still sparse. The authors' own data indicate that in all three morphology groups the functional benefit at two years is still above baseline. In the large cohort of Cooper et al. 40 patients with three year follow-up were recently published showing still highly significant increase in FEV_1 from 0.76 l (26% predicted) at baseline to 0.95 l (35% predicted) (Cooper et al., 1999). These effects were also observed between baseline and three year's residual volume measurements (298% vs. 215% of predicted) and total lung capacity (14% vs. 126% of predicted).

Thus far, no published data allow conclusions on the contribution of LVRS on the "naturally" occurring decline in FEV_1. In very advanced emphysema, FEV_1 decline may be biased by the "survivor ef-

Table 4

Published data on outcome

Reference	% Increase in FEV_1	n patients	Unilateral/bilateral	Operative technique used
Cooper et al., 1996	51%	150	Bilateral	Median sternotomy
McKenna et al., 1996	Unilateral 29%; Bilateral 57%	166	79 Bilateral; 87 Unilateral	VATS
Roué et al., 1996	About 51%	13	Bilateral ($n = 2$); Unilateral ($n = 9$)	Thoracotomy ($n = 10$); median sternotomy ($n = 1$)
Argenziano et al., 1996	61%	85	Bilateral	Clamshell/thoracotomy
Miller et al., 1996	97%	53	Bilateral	Median sternotomy
Yusen et al., 1996	64%	84	Bilateral	Median sternotomy
Wisser et al., 1996	About 54%	60	Bilateral	Median sternotomy ($n = 15$); VATS ($n = 27$); thoracotomy $\pm$ VATS ($n = 18$)
Daniel et al., 1996	49%	17/26	Bilateral	Median sternotomy
Kotloff et al., 1998	34%	174	Bilateral	Median sternotomy ($n = 86$); VATS ($n = 88$)
Demertzis et al., 1998	About 50%	25	Bilateral ($n = 23$); Unilateral ($n = 2$)	Median sternotomy ($n = 23$); 2 anterolateral thoracotomies
Norman et al., 1998	26%[a]	14	Bilateral	Median sternotomy
Stammberger et al., 1998	About 50%	85	Bilateral	VATS
De Perrot et al., 1998	53%	18	Bilateral	Ant. muscle-sparing thoracot.
Mineo et al., 1998	50%	14	Unilateral (for asymmetric emphysema)	VATS
Stamatis et al., 1999	Unilateral 25%; Bilateral 75%	95	Unilateral ($n = 24$); Bilateral ($n = 70$)	Median sternotomy ($n = 38$); Bilateral thoracotomies ($n = 26$); Unilateral thoracotomies ($n = 20$); VATS ($n = 10$)

[a] Pre-bronchodilator data recorded.

[b] n.i.: not indicated.

fect": if patients with lower FEV_1 survive, they seem to fare better in terms of FEV_1 decline since they cannot lose as much FEV_1 as patients with higher FEV_1. This effect might account for falsely observed or interpreted differences between groups and underlines the difficulty of interpreting low FEV_1.

1.6.2. Gas exchange

In the initial paper of LVRS by Joel Cooper (Cooper et al., 1995), a significant improvement in arterial oxygen content has been noted with no significant change in carbon dioxide.

The evolution and role of resting arterial blood gases (ABG) over a longer period after LVRS have not yet been well defined. Gas exchange at rest has only been elucidated for a perioperative period up to three to six months postoperatively in LVRS patients but studies focusing on that subject for a longer period of time have not yet been published.

The main findings of a recent study of our group were a slight temporary allover improvement of alveolar ventilation up to one year and increased mean PaO_2 at three and six months after LVRS, effects that were most pronounced three months postoperatively. Weak relations of $PaCO_2$ changes with lung volumes such as VC and FEV_1 underlined the obvious role of lung mechanics for alveolar ventilation. Mean PaO_2 was also temporarily improved at three and six months after LVRS. Importantly, the fraction of patients with resting PaO_2 of ≤ 55 mmHg fulfilling criteria for long term oxygen treatment (LTOT) was unchanged six months after LVRS compared to pre-operatively. The individual's gas exchange parameter AaDO2, and therefore, PaO_2 were not predictable by any of the assessed ventilatory or other biometric parameters.

In conclusion, LVRS only temporarily improved alveolar ventilation in a majority of our patients, i.e. for 12 months, and PaO_2 was temporarily improved up to six months postoperatively, whereas overall gas exchange remained unchanged. As on an individual basis LVRS improved or worsened gas exchange and alveolar ventilation, no clear benefit of LVRS on gas exchange has been observed. This study underlines that not only the main short-term but also the sustained beneficial effects of LVRS are, contrary to blood gas parameters, based on lung mechanics. This should be taken into consideration when giving patients advice before LVRS, especially in case of the hope to be able to abandon long-term oxygen therapy after LVRS.

1.6.3. Exercise capacity

Benditt and coworkers investigated the physiologic mechanisms of improved exercise capacity after LVRS by progressive cardiopulmonary exercise testing on 21 consecutive patients (Benditt et al., 1997). Significant improvements were seen in maximal work, maximal oxygen consumption, and maximal ventilation, whereas the dead space to tidal volume ratio at peak exercise decreased as a result of an increase in tidal volume.

Interestingly, the increase in maximal ventilation during exercise was the result of increased tidal volumes only since breathing frequencies at peak exercise were not higher after the operation. Based on the analysis of breathing patterns and gas exchange, the gain in exercise capacity is mediated primarily by improved respiratory mechanics.

Ferguson et al. (1998) investigated exercise performance in 27 patients who underwent bilateral staple LVRS by median sternotomy. The combination of increased tidal volume and reduced dead space ventilation resulted in significant increase in alveolar ventilation and decrease in $PaCO_2$.

1.6.4. Dyspnoea

Breathlessness is subjective and may improve by a great variety of mechanisms. Whereas all historical surgical approaches to emphysema failed to improve objective measurements of outcome, most patients reported relief of dyspnoea. For the patient, relief of dyspnoea is obviously more important than changes in any lung function parameters. In published studies on LVRS, dyspnoea declined, as assessed by the modified Medical Research Council Dyspnoea Score, between 1.0 and 2.4 points, which is in good agreement with data of our group of nearly two points improvement Other tools like the Borg scale, Chronic Respiratory Questionnaire and Mahler baseline/transitional dyspnoea index corroborate this finding. Long-term improvement of dyspnoea has been reported by several groups, and our recent data underline a clear benefit in most of the patients for at least two years (Hamacher et al., 1999).

Interestingly, most studies on outcome after LVRS did not reveal good correlations between any parameter of lung function or exercise capacity and subjective improvement of dyspnoea. Data from our group demonstrated similar improvements in the Medical Research Council Dyspnoea Score regardless whether the individual improved in term of obstruction, hyperinflation, or both. Measurements of breathing and performance during exercise, especially assessment of dynamic hyperinflation, seem to be closer to the sensation of dyspnoea than parameters of lung function. Martinez et al. demonstrated less dynamic hyperinflation during exercise after LVRS, as assessed by end-expired lung volume (Martinez et al., 1997). Probably, these parameters are a better explanation for subjective improvement after LVRS than parameters of lung function.

1.6.5. Quality of life

The effect of LVRS on long-term health related quality of life is not well known. Whereas two studies reported on combined preoperative rehabilitation and LVRS and used the same instruments as in the present study, a few publications covered aspects of quality of life in LVRS with short-term follow-up to six months.

In our patient population, we prospectively assessed a cohort of 32 LVRS patients followed up for two years by the SF-36 questionnaire. (Ware et al., 1993). We observed a severe impact on health-related quality of life before the intervention. Parallel to the known important and sustained improvements in dyspnoea, exercise tolerance, and lung function, the intervention exerted very meaningful and sustained clinical improvements on health-related quality of life. Six of eight domains of the SF-36 showed a sustained improvement over two years, which was also the case with the prevalence of anxiety in a disease characterized by relentless progression and, therefore, expected decline of quality of life.

The best predictor for short-term outcome after LVRS in terms of the assessed gain in daily exercise performance, as assessed with "physical functioning" of the QOL questionnaire was preoperative CT morphology, which demonstrated that patients with marked emphysema heterogeneity had the most probable benefit in terms of their exercise tolerance. This finding corroborated the prospectively studied results which showed in general most lung functional profit in patients with markedly heterogeneous emphysema, but an important, albeit smaller profit in patients with homogeneous morphology as well, as discussed before.

Severe preoperative dyspnoea is a leading symptom of the studied patients, a central content of health-related quality of life, related to exercise capacity, and one main target of LVRS. Dyspnoea as well as several parameters from lung function and walking tests also significantly and persistently improved after LVRS. Surprisingly, RV/TLC ratio and FEV_1 paralleled the improvements as well as the moderate decline in the two years following LVRS in several dimensions of health-related quality of life, including central aspects of mood. These findings underline the surprisingly strong interaction between emotional perception and lung functional parameters of COPD patients before and after LVRS.

In conclusion, the impressively high impact of severe COPD with emphysema on patients' general and health related quality of life has been shown to be significantly and persistently improved after LVRS in the physical and mental dimensions that patients consider important.

1.6.6. Lung elasticity and resistance

Otto Brantigan believed that improvements in lung elastic recoil were responsible for the reduction of airway obstruction following lung volume reduction. A study performed by Sciurba and coworkers (1996) demonstrated a statistically highly significant improvement in the coefficient of retraction in a cohort of 20 patients. This improvement in elastic recoil is accompanied by a decrease in chest wall elastic recoil and these changes may be responsible for improvements in lung function and airway conductance.

1.6.7. Breathing pattern and ventilatory muscle recruitment

Hamacher et al. (1999) evaluated the changes in breathing pattern before and after bilateral thoracoscopic LVRS in nineteen patients. The contribution of abdominal volume changes to tidal volume increased from a mean of 43% to 58%, and the fraction of inspiratory time with abdominal paradoxical motion decreased from 12% to 5%. The postoperative reduction of the phase shift between rib cage and abdominal motion and greater contribution of abdominal volume changes to tidal volumes are consistent with a greater force-generating capacity of the diaphragm. Benditt et al. (1997) studied breathing and ventilatory muscle recruitment pattern in eight patients before and three months after bilateral LVRS at rest and during exercise. The observed rightward shift in the slope of end-expiratory esophageal versus gastric pressure indicates increased use of the diaphragm after surgery. The authors conclude that the improved efficiency of breathing due to changes in breathing and ventilatory muscle recruitment is likely to be an important contributor to the observed increased work capacity after LVRS.

1.6.8. Ventilatory drive

Martinez et al. (1997) analyzed eight patients before and three to five months after bilateral LVRS and compared this cohort to 13 healthy control subjects. The elevated baseline central ventilatory drive, as assessed by mouth occlusion technique, was lowered to normal values after the operation, and the response to increased CO_2 levels was significantly decreased. These changes in ventilatory drive may at least partially be responsible for relief of dyspnoea following LVRS. More recently, Lahrmann et al. (1999) investigated the neural drive to the diaphragm in 14 patients before and after LVRS. This central drive, as assessed by root mean square analysis of the esophageal electromyogram, was decreased one month after the operation, with a further significant decrease six months and one year after LVRS. The capacity of the respiratory pump to generate inspiratory pressure is increased, thereby, less central ventilatory drive is necessary for generation of sufficient inspiratory pressures. The authors conclude that reduction of dyspnoea following LVRS may be attributed to a reduction in central ventilatory drive.

1.6.9. Chest wall and diaphragm movement

Lando and coworkers (1999) analyzed thoracic movement, as expressed by the ratio of mid-sagittal lung area at full inspiration to that at full expiration (I/E ratio) on fast magnetic resonance imaging. Before the operation, the diaphragm was flattened at end-inspiration, and only a small excursion of the diaphragm was noted during breathing. Besides significant improvements in lung function, arterial oxygen content and six-minute walking distance, a significant increase in the I/E ratio six months after bilateral staple LVRS was corroborated by improved diaphragmatic excursion. Analyzing plain chest roentgenograms of 25 patients before and three to six months after bilateral LVRS, Lando et al. investigated on changes in diaphragm length (Lando et al., 1999). Restoration of the diaphragm curvature with a significant increase in the length of the most vertically orientated portion of the diaphragm muscle were observed. This increase in diaphragm length correlated directly with postoperative reductions in static lung volumes and with increased trans-diaphragmatic pressure and maximal voluntary ventilation.

1.6.10. Reconfiguration of bony thorax

Lando and coworkers analyzed changes in anteroposterior and transverse thoracic diameters as assessed by plain chest roentgenograms (25 patients) and chest CT scans (14 patients) following bilateral LVRS via median sternotomy (Llando et al., 1999). Three months after surgery, transverse diameters were only slightly reduced, whereas the anteroposterior diameters in the middle and lower region of the rib cage were significantly decreased. These reductions correlated with the reduction in total lung capacity and residual volume, suggesting that a reduction in overall lung volume by surgery caused the reduction in chest diameters.

1.6.11. Survival following LVRS

It is known that FEV_1 is the best single predictor of life-expectancy in patients with severe COPD. Therefore, it might be speculated that LVRS has a beneficial effect on long-term survival after operation by improving lung function.

Brenner and coworkers analyzed a cohort of 256 patients who underwent bilateral staple LVRS (Brenner et al., 1999). Within a median follow-up of 623 days, one-year survival was 83% (missing patients assumed to be dead) and two-year survival 76%, respectively. Further analysis revealed improved survival in younger patients, patients with higher baseline FEV_1 and PaO_2, and higher short-term improvement in FEV_1. A substantial mortality, especially in patients with a high-risk profile, is noted.

In a recent study, Serna and colleagues compared survival after unilateral versus bilateral volume reduction by video-assisted thoracoscopy (Serna et al., 1999). A total of 260 patients were included in the analysis with an average follow-up of about 29 months. Overall survival two years after bilateral procedures was 86%, and significantly lower with 73% in patients who underwent unilateral LVRS. Whereas most of the published studies suggest a positive effect of LVRS on survival, the question whether LVRS is superior to optimized medical treatment alone in terms of survival can only be answered by randomized trials, since patient characteristics in studies elucidating survival in medically treated COPD patients are not comparable.

1.6.12. Alpha-1-Antytrypsin deficiency subgroup analysis

In this hereditary disorder, decreased serum levels of α_1-protease inhibitor, a glycoprotein synthesized in the liver, lead to an imbalance between protease and antiprotease activity. Destruction of the connective tissue framework of the lung by neutrophil elastase and other proteolytic enzymes predisposes to the development of emphysema. Whereas patients with heterogeneous subtypes usually do not suffer from emphysematous disease, smokers and even non-smokers with the homozygous phenotype PiZZ rapidly decline in lung function due to severe destruction of mainly the lower lobes.

In comparing the results of 12 consecutive patients with homozygous PiZZ Antitrypsin deficiency with 18 patients suffering from smoker's emphysema, three months after the procedure, results were the same in both groups. However, as early as six months after LVRS, patients with Antitrypsin deficiency deteriorated in lung function, and one year after the operation, only the six-minute walking distance was slightly improved. Patients with smoker's emphysema had a significant benefit still at two year's follow-up. These results are in good agreement with a smaller series presented by Gelb et al. (1999). Four patients had only modest improvement of FEV$_1$ within a mean follow-up of 27 months, but vital capacity increased from 68 to 88% of predicted.

On the other hand, patients with Antitrypsin deficiency have an accelerated course of the underlying disease with a rapid loss of lung function, therefore, the decline after operation may reflect mainly the natural course of the underlying disease being an important predictor not for short-term, but for long-term outcome after LVRS.

1.7. Economic aspects

In the United States of America, nearly 13 million people suffer from COPD, and about 1.65 million are thought to have emphysema predominantly. Therefore, LVRS may have a significant impact on overall health care costs. Benditt and colleagues (1997) analyzed the economic aspects of LVRS and calculated the median total charge for the procedure to be nearly $27,000. The author concludes that if only 10% of the 1.65 million people suffering from emphysema would undergo LVRS, this would sum up to more than $4.6 billion. On the other hand, LVRS may reduce hospital stay, medications and need for oxygen therapy due to exacerbation of COPD.

Overall costs excluding physicians' fees for 52 consecutive patients undergoing LVRS by median sternotomy were calculated with a median of nearly $20,000, ranging from about $12,000 to $122,000. Costs were related significantly to duration of ICU stay and length of hospitalization, therefore, identification of factors leading to prolonged hospital stay may help to reduce overall costs of LVRS.

A study by Ko et al. (1998) compared median sternotomy and video-assisted thoracoscopy in terms of surgical and patient outcome as well as the associated costs. A total of 42 patients with severe emphysema underwent LVRS (19 via sternotomy and 23 via thoracoscopy). Both groups were comparable preoperatively. Postoperatively, the sternotomy patients had more days on the ventilator, more days on the intensive care unit, higher incidence of prolonged air leak, and longer hospital stay. Neither surgical approach conferred any long-term medical advantage; however, the average total hospital costs and charges were reduced in the VATS group ($27,178 versus sternotomy, $37,299). This study concluded that the overall charges and costs of the VATS approach is less than that of sternotomy.

1.8. LVRS and lung transplantation

The waiting period for lung transplant candidates with end-stage pulmonary emphysema continues to increase, therefore, alternative treatment options to reduce morbidity and mortality are needed. Lung volume reduction surgery has been advocated as an alternative to lung transplantation in patients with severe emphysema. In a study conducted by Gaissert et al. (1996), functional improvement by either unilateral or bilateral lung transplantation was much better compared to LVRS, however, LVRS may have a sufficient impact on symptoms and daily activities in these patients, avoiding transplantation-specific complications and need for immunosuppresion. Patients undergoing thoracoscopic LVRS did not need prolonged mechanical ventilation after the operation, in-hospital morbidity was less, and they were discharged significantly earlier. Prior LVRS does not preclude further successful lung transplantation therefore, this procedure is worth a try in most of the patients with end-stage pulmonary emphysema.

On the other hand, lung volume reduction may be used as an adjunct to lung transplantation to further improve functional outcome. Anderson et al. (1997) performed unilateral LVRS in the native lung in three patients 36 to 55 months after unilateral lung transplantation for severe emphysema. They conclude that LVRS of the native lung is a beneficial intervention in cases where hyperinflation of the native lung led to significant functional impairment with compression of the transplanted lung.

References and further reading

Anderson MB, Kriett JM, Kapelanski DP, Perricone A, Smith CM, Jamieson SW. Volume reduction surgery in the native lung after single lung transplantation for emphysema. J Heart Lung Transplant 1997; 16(7): 752–757.

Argenziano M, Moazami N, Thomashow B, Jellen PA, Gorenstein LA, Rose EA et al. Extended indications for lung volume reduction surgery in advanced emphysema. Ann Thorac Surg 1996; 62: 1588–1597.

Argenziano M, Thomashow B, Jellen PA, Rose EA, Steinglass KM, Ginsburg ME et al. Functional comparison of unilateral versus bilateral lung volume reduction surgery. Ann Thorac Surg 1997; 64: 321–327.

Benditt JO, Wood DE, McCool FD, Lewis S, Albert RK. Changes in breathing and ventilatory muscle recruitment patterns induced by lung volume reduction surgery. Am J Respir Crit Care Med 1997; 155(1): 279–284.

Brantigan OC, Mueller EA, Kress MB. A surgical approach to pulmonary emphysema. Am Surgeon 1957; 23: 789–804.

Brenner M, McKenna RJJ, Chen JC, Osann K, Powell L, Gelb AF et al. Survival following bilateral staple lung volume reduction surgery for emphysema. Chest 1999; 115(2): 390–396.

Carter MG, Gaensler EA, Kyllonen A. Pneumoperitoneum in the treatment of pulmonary emphysema. N Engl J Med 1950; 243, 15: 549–558.

Clagett OT. Surgical treatment of emphysematous blebs and bullae. Dis Chest 1949; 15: 669–683.

Cooper JD. Technique to reduce air leaks after resection of emphysematous lung. Ann Thorac Surg 1994; 57: 1038–1039.

Cooper JD, Trulock EP, Triantafillou AN, Patterson GA, Pohl MS, Deloney PA et al. Bilateral pneumectomy (volume reduction) for chronic obstructive pulmonary disease. J Thorac Cardiovasc Surg 1995; 109(1): 106–119.

Cooper JD, Lefrak SS. Lung-reduction surgery: 5 years on. Lancet 1999; 353(Suppl 1): SI26–SI27.

Criner GJ, Cordova FC, Furukawa S, Kuzma AM, Travaline JM, Leyenson V et al. Prospective randomized trial comparing bilateral lung volume reduction surgery to pulmonary rehabilitation in severe chronic obstructive pulmonary disease. Am J Respir Crit Care Med 1999; 160(6): 2018–2027.

Criner G, Cordova FC, Leyenson V, Roy B, Travaline J, Sudarshan S et al. Effect of lung volume reduction surgery on diaphragm strength. Am J Respir Crit Care Med 1998; 157: 1578–1585.

Ferguson GT, Fernandez E, Zamora MR, Pomerantz M, Buchholz J, Make BJ. Improved exercise performance following lung volume reduction surgery for emphysema. Am J Respir Crit Care Med 1998; 157: 1195–1203.

Gaissert HA, Trulock EP, Cooper JD, Sundaresan RS, Patterson GA. Comparison of early functional results after volume reduction or lung transplantation for chronic obstructive pulmonary disease. J Thorac Cardiovasc Surg 1996; 111(2): 296–305.

Gelb A F, McKena R J, Brenner M, Fischel R, Zamel N. Lung function after bilateral lower lobe lung volume reduction surgery for alpha 1-antitrypsin emphysema. Eur Resp J 1999; 14: 928–933.

Hamacher J, Bloch KE, Stammberger U, Schmid RA, Laube I, Russi EW et al. Two years outcome of lung volume reduc-

tion surgery in different morphologic emphysema types. Ann Thorac Surg 1999; 68: 1792–1798.

Hamacher J, Russi EW, Weder W. Lung volume reduction surgery: A survey on the European experience. Chest 2000; 117(6): 1560–1567.

Hazelrigg SR, Boley TM, Henkle JQ, Lawyer C, Johnstone D, Naunheim KS et al. Thoracoscopic laser bullectomy: a prospective study with three-month results. J Thorac Cardiovasc Surg 1996; 112(2): 319–327.

Ingenito EP, Evans RB, Loring SH, Kaczka DW, Rodenhouse JD, Body SC et al. Relation between preoperative inspiratory lung resistance and the outcome of lung-volume-reduction surgery for emphysema. N Engl J Med 1998; 338(17): 1181–1185.

Ko CY, Waters PF. Lung volume reduction surgery: a cost and outcomes comparison of sternotomy versus thoracoscopy. Am Surg 1998; 64(10): 1010–1013.

Kotloff RM, Tino G, Bavaria JE, Palevsky HI, Hansen-Flaschen J, Wahl PM et al. Bilateral lung volume reduction surgery for advanced emphysema — a comparison of median sternotomy and thoracoscopic approaches. Chest 1996; 110: 1399–1406.

Lando Y, Boiselle PM, Shade D, Furukawa S, Kuzma AM, Travaline JM et al. Effect of lung volume reduction surgery on diaphragm length in severe chronic obstructive pulmonary disease. Am J Respir Crit Care Med 1999; 159(3): 796–805.

Lando Y, Boiselle P, Shade D, Travaline JM, Furukawa S, Criner GJ. Effect of lung volume reduction surgery on bony thorax configuration in severe COPD. Chest 1999; 116(1): 30–39.

Lahrmann H, Wild, Wanke T, Tschernko E, Wisser W, Klepetko W et al. Neural drive to the diaphragm after lung volume reduction surgery. Chest 1999: 116: 1593–1600.

Little AG, Swain JA, Nino JJ, Prabhu RD, Schlachter MD, Barcia TC. Reduction pneumoplasty for emphysema — early results. Ann Surg 1995; 222(3): 365–374.

Maki DD, Miller WTJ, Aronchick JM, Gefter WB, Miller WTS, Kotloff RM et al. Advanced emphysema: preoperative chest radiographic findings as predictors of outcome following lung volume reduction surgery. Radiology 1999; 212(1): 49–55.

Martinez FJ, Montes de Oca M, Whyte RI, Stetz J, Gay SE, Celli BR. Lung-volume reduction improves dyspnoea, dynamic hyperinflation, and respiratory muscle function. Am J Respir Crit Care Med 1997; 155: 1984–1990.

McKenna RJ Jr., Brenner M, Fischel RJ, Gelb AF. Should volume reduction for emphysema be unilateral or bilateral? J Thorac Cardiovasc Surg 1996; 112: 1331–1339.

Naunheim KS, Ferguson MK. The current status of lung volume reduction operations for emphysema. Ann Thorac Surg 1996; 62(2): 601–612.

Naunheim KS, Kaiser LR, Bavaria JE, Hazelrigg SR, Magee MJ, Landreneau RJ et al. Long-term survival after thoracoscopic lung volume reduction: a multi-institutional review. Ann Thorac Surg 1999; 68(6): 2026–2031.

Petermann J. Zur Freudschen Operation bei Lungenemphysem. Dtsch Med Wochenschr 1925; 51: 221.

Reich L. Der Einfluss des Pneumoperitoneums auf das Lungenemphysem. Wien Arch f Innere Med 1924; 8: 245–260.

Roberts JR, Bavaria JE, Wahl P, Wurster A, Friedberg JS, Kaiser LR. Comparison of open and thoracoscopic bilateral volume reduction surgery: complications analysis. Ann Thorac Surg 1998; 66(5): 1759–1765.

Sciurba FC, Rogers RM, Keenan RJ, Slivka WA, Gorcsan J, Ferson PF et al. Improvement in pulmonary function and elastic recoil after lung-reduction surgery for diffuse emphysema. N Engl J Med 1996; 334(17): 1095–1099.

Serna DL, Brenner M, Osann KE, McKenna RJJ, Chen JC, Fischel RJ et al. Survival after unilateral versus bilateral lung volume reduction surgery for emphysema. J Thorac Cardiovasc Surg 1999; 118: 1101–1109.

Szekely LA, Oelberg DA, Wright C, Johnson DC, Wain J, Trot-man-Dickenson B et al. Preoperative predictors of operative morbidity and mortality in COPD patients undergoing bilateral lung volume reduction surgery. Chest 1997; 111(3): 550–558.

Wakabayashi A, Brenner M, Kayaleh RA, Berns MW, Barker SJ, Rice SJ et al. Thoracoscopic carbon dioxide laser treatment of bullous emphysema. Lancet 1991; 337: 881–883.

Ware JE Jr., Snow KK, Kosinski M, Gandek B. SF-36 Health Survey. Manual and interpretation guide (1st ed.). Boston: The Health Institute, New England Medical Center, 1993.

Young J, Fry-Smith A, Hyde C. Lung volume reduction surgery (LVRS) for chronic obstructive pulmonary disease (COPD) with underlying severe emphysema. Thorax 1999; 54: 779–789.

K. Moghissi, J.A.C. Thorpe and F. Ciulli (Eds.)
Moghissi's Essentials of Thoracic and Cardiac Surgery

CHAPTER IV.3

Interventional bronchoscopy

K. Moghissi

1. Introduction

The principle of interventional bronchoscopy consists of the use of the bronchoscope as a means of access to the tracheo-bronchial lumen in order to carry out therapeutic procedures. The rigid bronchoscope alone or in conjunction with the flexible fibre optic bronchoscope (FFB) remains the instrument of choice in the majority of therapeutic bronchoscopies. Nevertheless, since the widespread use of the flexible fibre optic instrument for diagnostic bronchoscopy many physicians exclusively employ FFB for therapeutic endoscopy.

The technique of bronchoscopy, its main features and the advantages and disadvantages of both the rigid and fibre optic instruments have been referred to in Table 3 in chapter I.2.

2. Bronchoscopic intervention

The main bronchoscopic treatment methods are:
(1) Therapeutic bronchial lavage and debridement,
(2) Cryotherapy,
(3) Brachytherapy,
(4) Laser Therapy (see Lasers in Cardiothoracic Surgery – chapter IV.5),
(5) Placement of stent (see Tracheo-bronchial stenting – chapter II.2).

2.1. Therapeutic bronchial lavage and debridement

2.1.1. The aims are:
- To clear the tracheo-bronchial tree of debris and infected secretion or blood clot which embarrasses the respiration in a patient who cannot expectorate adequately to clear the airway,
- To carry out bronchial lavage using warm normal saline alone or with appropriate antiseptic agents and/or medication,
- Post-operative removal of retained sputum,
- To obviate continuous antibiotic therapy in severe bronchiectatic patients especially when there is evidence of intermittent haemoptysis and atelectasis and when secretions are infected by a mixture of microbial and fungal organisms.

2.1.2. Method
- Bronchoscopy is carried out using the rigid instrument under general anaesthesia with intermittent positive pressure ventilation through the bronchoscope (see section 2.3.4 in chapter I.2),
- The bronchoscope tip is placed in the lower trachea and a sample taken of tracheobronchial secretions — if necessary this sampling can be from different main or lobar bronchi individually,
- Suction and clearing of tracheobronchial secretions is carried out,
- The lavage proper consists of placing the tip of the instrument into the right and then the left main bronchus, for no more than 1 cm into the lumen, thus allowing ventilation of the opposite side through the side holes of the instrument. Using a 50 ml syringe warm, sterile saline solution is injected into the lumen of the bronchoscope. For each side a volume of 200 to 500 ml of saline is introduced 50 ml at a time, followed by suction with a catheter introduced into the bronchoscope and connected to suction apparatus. During the injection of fluid and its suction, the anaesthetist interrupts ventilation. In practice, 50 to 100 ml of fluid is introduced and sucked out, during which time positive pressure ventilation is interrupted momentarily.

The scheme is:

A	No ventilation →	(a) 50–100 ml of fluid in
↓		(b) Suction of fluid
B	No injection and no suction →	(c) Ventilation

This is repeated until 250 to 500 ml of saline has been used for each side.

It is important to measure the volume of fluid which is aspirated to ascertain that it approximately equals the input volume. During the procedure the patient is monitored as per bronchoscopy under general anaesthetic (section 2.3.4 in chapter I.2).

It is to be noted that bronchoscopic toilet in a general intensive care unit should be a routine practice. It is usually performed by a physician/anaesthetist using the flexible bronchoscope. However, the author believes that for thoracic surgical patients in the postoperative phase, the use of the rigid bronchoscope is safer and more appropriate and should be performed by the surgical team. In such cases, the procedure may be carried out under local (topical) anaesthesia.

2.2. Cryotherapy

2.2.1. Principle
Cryotherapy is based on the principle that a gas will cool on sudden expansion when passing from high to lower pressure (Joule-Thomson effect). Advantage is taken of this principle to form ice crystals in the cells and in extra-cellular interstitial fluid which in turn provokes tissue necrosis. The cryoprobe used for bronchoscopic cryotherapy is an insulated cannula which is fuelled by liquid nitrogen or nitrous oxide which cools the probe tip down to $-80°C$.

The aim of cryotherapy is the production of cold injuries in obstructing intraluminal tumour tissue followed by necrosis and desobliteration of the bronchus.

2.2.2. Method
- Rigid bronchoscopy under general anaesthesia is the preferred method. The obstructive malignant lesion should have been biopsied and assessed by previous bronchoscopy.
- The cryoprobe is introduced and applied to the tumour.
- There are a selection of probes 2 to 5 mm diameter in straight, right-angled and flexible forms which are used according to the size of the tumour. The time of crystal formation is between 15 to 20 seconds.
- Re-bronchoscopy is usually needed four to five

days later for debridement and removal of necrotic and part necrotic tissue.

2.2.3. Results and complications
The effect of cryotherapy is apparent within 3 or 4 days and tumours larger than 1 or 2 cm need re-treatment within 3 to 4 weeks. Very good desobliteration resulting in expansion of collapsed lung/lobe can be achieved. There is a theoretical advantage of combining cryotherapy with radiotherapy due to hyperaemia which follows the freeze. Bleeding, pneumothorax and respiratory failure have been reported as complications of bronchoscopic cryotherapy.

2.3. Brachytherapy

This is the provision of a radiotherapy source close to the tumour within the bronchial tree. The technique employs high dose radiation (HDR) by means of a computer guided after-loading device. The source for HDR brachytherapy is commonly Iridium 192. Some use local anaesthetic and flexible fibre optic bronchoscopy (FFB) to insert the guide-wire and flexible 2 mm diameter catheter. Others prefer general anaesthetic and endotracheal intubation or rigid bronchoscope in order to introduce a larger 4 mm diameter catheter. In either method, the position of the catheter close to the tumour is verified using the FFB, following which, the instrument and/or the endotracheal tube is removed and the after-loading catheter secured against displacement at the nose or mouth. X-ray confirms the position of the tube. Co-operation between the surgeon (or the physician), physicist and radiotherapist is essential to achieve the optimal radiation dose for a given tumour.

Brachytherapy may be used for palliation or, in some circumstances, combined with external beam radiotherapy for curative intent. It can also be used with other endobronchial methods of palliation such as laser therapy.

2.3.1. Results
Brachytherapy can achieve good palliation in patients with malignant endoluminal obstruction and lung collapse.

2.3.2. Complications
- Fatal haemorrhage is reported to be between 3 to 50%. However, it is important to note that fatal haemorrhage can occur in advanced lung cancer cases even without specific treatment.
- Fistulae between airways and mediastinal spaces

and mediastinal viscera can follow brachytherapy but these are rare.

- Radiation bronchitis is a more common complication which, when accompanied by necrosis and scarring can result in stenotic lesions. The incidence can reach 30% with some patients requiring regular dilatation.

3. General remarks on interventional bronchoscopic methods for lung cancer treatment

There are currently important bronchoscopic treatments available for treating malignant endoluminal tumours. These consist of laser therapy using NdYAG laser and photodynamic therapy (PDT), brachytherapy, cryotherapy and placement of stent. These methods may be used individually or in combination. The selection of methods is partially dependent on pathology, topography and extent of the lesion in the airway and the aims of treatment. All the different methods aim to overcome obstruction of the airway. Some can arrest haemorrhage and thus treat haemoptysis.

At the time of writing, no published data based on trials are available to suggest which of the methods is the most appropriate for symptom palliation or which affords better survival benefit. A trial which was initiated by the Medical Research Council in Britain was aborted without reaching its level of recruitment numbers (Moghissi et al., 1999). However, whilst symptom relief is achieved by all, experience, backed by published literature, indicates that therapeutic methods vary in rapidity of effect and duration of relief as well as their ability to palliate specific symptoms.

In principle, laser therapy, brachytherapy and cryotherapy are best suited to cases in which the airway obstruction is essentially due to endoluminal projection of the tumour. Stent is a more appropriate option for cases in which there is an extrinsic compressive lesion. Because of their biological action on cancer tissue brachytherapy and PDT, in addition to achieving desobliteration of the lumen, influence tumour growth and inhibit its expansion. These treatment modalities may be used in inoperable cancer patients with early stage cancer who are unsuitable for major resectional surgery. Combination therapies used sequentially, concomitantly or as staged procedures can be advantageous in carefully selected patients. This particularly applies to the use of NdYAG laser to debulk large tumours followed by PDT or brachytherapy. Alternatively, stent can be used after laser debulking in order to overcome extrinsic obstruction.

References and further reading

Macha HN. The German experience. The therapeutic approach of endobronchial HDR — Brachytherapy. In: Hetzel MR (ed.), Minimally Invasive Techniques in Thoracic Medicine and Surgery. London: Chapman & Hall, 1995; pp. 216–231.

Mehta MP, Petereit DG, Chosy L, et al. Sequential comparison of low dose rate and hyperfractionated high dose rate endobronchial radiation for malignant airway occlusion. Int J Radiat Oncol Phys Biol 1992; 23: 133–139.

Mehta MP, Macha HN. Brachytherapy — The American experience. Brachytherapy — The German experience. In: Hetzel MR (ed.), Minimally Invasive Techniques in Thoracic Medicine and Surgery. London: Chapman & Hall, 1995; pp. 205–246.

Moghissi K, Bond MG, Sambrook RJ, et al. on behalf of Medical Research Council Lung Cancer working party. Treatment of endotracheal or endobronchial obstruction by non-small cell lung cancer: lack of patients in an MRC randomized trial leaves key questions unanswered. Clin Oncol 1999; 11: 179–183.

Paradelo JC, Waxman MJ, Thorne BJ, et al. Endobronchial irradiation with 192 Ir in the treatment of malignant endobronchial obstruction. Chest 1992; 102: 1072–1074.

Speiser BL, Spratlin GL. Radiation bronchitis and stenosis secondary to high dose rate endobronchial irradiation. Int J Radiol Oncol Biol Phys 1993; 25: 589–597.

biopsies in very vascular tumours, or in patients with superior vana caval obstructive syndrome.

2.1.6. Pulmonary embolism

This is rarely the cause of massive haemoptysis. However, treatment by heparinisation or fibrinolytic agents in such cases can produce large haemoptysis.

2.1.7. Post pulmonary resectional haemoptysis

This requires specific mention since its discovery and prompt diagnosis will usually have favourable outcome.

Small repeated haemoptysis may occur from a few weeks to a few months after pulmonary resection. In benign cases haemoptysis is usually due to infection and granulation tissue formation at the bronchial stump. In malignant conditions, recurrence and broncho vascular fistula may be the cause.

Haemoptysis is the mode of presentation of empyema and broncho pleural fistula but the blood is usually mixed with pleural fluid and/or pus. In early broncho-pleural fistula after pneumonectomy a large volume of heavily bloodstained fluid is expectorated which can spill over into the healthy lung, causing considerable respiratory distress.

2.2. Cardiovascular system conditions

Congenital heart condition and/or cardiac valvular disease may cause haemoptysis. Cases of acute and massive haemorrhage have been reported in patients with Fallot's tetralogy, artero-venous fistulae or pulmonary vascular abnormalities, such as aberrant bronchial arteries may be the cause of a major bleed.

3. Diagnosis of haemoptysis

Most cases of haemoptysis are the result of broncho-pulmonary disease and require ordered and comprehensive investigation. In this regard clinical history, imaging and endoscopy are particularly important. Cardiovascular and blood dyscrasia need thorough investigation when respiratory system examination yields a negative result.

4. Management

This should be considered under:
(1) First aid and initial management

(2) Localisation of bleeding and investigation of the cause
(3) Arrest of haemorrhage and treatment

4.1. First aid and initial treatment

This is particularly relevant to sudden and massive haemoptysis in which appropriate emergency procedures could make a substantial difference in outcome.

The immediate aim is initially to clear the airway, thus preventing asphyxiation and allowing unobstructed ventilation. Then to support the cardiovascular system in order to maintain haemodynamic stability. The following scheme is recommended:

- The mouth and airway should be cleared by suction,
- If the site of bleeding (i.e. right or left lung) is known, the patient should be made to lie on the affected side with the head lower than the level of the chest thus preventing the blood spilling to the good side and providing a clear airway to the healthy lung,
- Suction bronchoscopy should be carried out through a rigid bronchoscope. The rigid instrument allows suction and clearing of the airway as well as oxygenation with positive pressure through the venturi port of the bronchoscope. It also permits efficient lavage of the bronchial tree,
- Bronchial lavage with cold (4°C) saline solution. This not only clears the blood but also reduces bleeding by bronchial artery vaso constriction,
- A wide-bore intravenous catheter should be placed into the internal jugular vein for rapid transfusion, if required, and also for central venous pressure recording,
- An arterial cannula is inserted for sampling blood gas analysis and monitoring arterial pressure,
- Sedation and antitussive drugs will be needed when ventilation is satisfactory. Morphine, in appropriate dosage, is an effective drug to sedate and prevent excessive coughing which aggravates bleeding.

Once emergency measures have been successful in achieving their objective and the immediate life-threatening situation is under control the second phase of management is put into operation. This consists of:
- Monitoring respiratory and haemodynamic parameters,
- Despatch of a sample of blood mixed with bronchial secretion aspirate for microbiological study.

A broad spectrum antibiotic is given parenterally after sampling has been undertaken.

It is important to note that a less dramatic haemoptysis, though not life threatening, will nevertheless require vigilance and active investigation and treatment. Also, sometimes small bleeding is a prelude to massive haemoptysis.

4.2. Location of bleeding and arrest of haemorrhage

Chest radiography and bronchoscopy will, in most cases, indicate the source within the bronchial tree. In acute haemoptysis, there is no time for undertaking a detailed investigation to implement aetiologically based treatment; the arrest of haemorrhage takes priority. In less dramatic cases, repeat bronchoscopy using the fibreoptic bronchoscope is carried out and imaging other than a plain chest X-ray is arranged both to localise the site of bleeding and to determine the aetiology when bleeding is from the respiratory system. More generalised investigation will be needed when bleeding cannot be attributed to respiratory system pathology.

4.3. Arrest of haemorrhage and treatment

In acute situations and, occasionally in some chronic cases, it is necessary to arrest the haemorrhage before undertaking more definitive treatment procedures or therapeutic measures.

Some or all of the following methods may be used to arrest bleeding:
- Bronchoscopy and lavage using cold normal saline solution (1–4°C)
- Laser photo-radiation (NdYAG laser) in doses of 15 to 20 W × 2 to 3 second pulse is very useful in bleeding from granulation tissue and some tumours. The aim is charring and coagulation rather than evaporation. Care should be taken not to use too high a power which can perforate a bronchus or blood vessel.
- Use of vaso-constricting agent applied to the area of bleeding is particularly useful in haemorrhage following bronchial biopsy,
- Tamponade:
  (a) using balloon through the bronchoscope
  (b) packing the bronchial lumen of the bleeding area with gauze soaked in vaso-constrictive drugs such as adrenaline or clotting agent. This is carried out through a rigid bronchoscope
- Isolation of the main bronchus using double lu-men endobronchial tube. In this method, one of the main bronchi which leads to the site of bleeding is blocked and one lung ventilation carried out
- Emergency thoracotomy and resection of broncho pulmonary pathology: an emergency operation is warranted when the bleeding cannot be controlled by other means and when the pathology is identified and judged to be correctable by surgery. Prior to surgical operation, however, it is necessary to exclude such conditions as bleeding diathesis. It is also important to examine serial chest radiographs, if available, taken prior to the haemoptysis. Pre-operative bronchoscopic examination is mandatory to locate the side and site of the bleeding.

The surgeon who proposes to undertake an emergency operation for acute and life-threatening haemoptysis needs to know:
- The pathological cause of bleeding,
- The location of the lesion which is causing the bleeding.

The undisputed indication for surgery is important haemoptysis resulting from traumatic injuries of broncho-vascular pulmonary structures.

During a 25-year period this author has had nine occasions in which it was necessary to carry out an emergency pulmonary resection for acute haemoptysis, excluding traumatic injuries. These included two neoplasms, one lung abscess, two cases of bronchiectasis, two cases of tuberculous cavity and two cases of aspergilloma.

5. Intervention on bronchial arteries

Many cases of haemoptysis originate from bronchial arteries. This forms the basic rationale for intervention on bronchial arteries.

5.1. Bronchial artery embolisation

The procedure is advocated for cases in which haemoptysis relates to bronchial arterial abnormalities. Prior to operation, selective bronchial artery angiography should be carried out. The immediate result of embolization in acute and large volume bleeding is good-to-excellent and the haemoptysis ceases in 80 to 90% of cases.

5.2. Bronchial artery ligation

In some rare cases, haemoptysis is attributed to dilated and tortuous bronchial vessels. In these cases the vessels may be approached and ligated either through standard thoracotomy, or via VATS.

References and further reading

Chang AB, Ditchfield M, Robinson PJ, Robertson CF. Major haemoptysis in a child with cystic fibrosis from multiple aberrant bronchial arteries treated with traneximic acid. Pediatr Pulmonol 1996; 6: 416–420.

Haponik EF, Fein A, Chin R. Managing life-threatening haemoptysis: has anything really changed? Chest 2000; 118: 1431–1435.

Jean-Baptist E. Clinical assessment and management of massive haemoptysis. Crit Care Med 2000; 28: 1642–1647.

Jougon J, Ballester M, Delcambre F, et al. Massive haemoptysis: what place for medical and surgical treatment. Eur J Cardiothorac Surg 2002; 22: 345–351.

Kato A, Kudo S, Matsumoto K, Fukahori T, Shimizu T, Uchino B. Bronchial artery embolization for haemoptysis due to benign diseases: immediate and long term results. Cardiovasc Interven Radiol 2000; 23: 351–357.

Lee TW, Wan S, Choy DK, Chan M, Arifi A, Yim AP. Management of massive haemoptysis: a single institution experience. Ann Thorac Cardiovasc Surg 2000; 6: 232–235.

Mal H, Rullon I, Mellot F et al. Immediate and long-term results of bronchial artery embolization for life-threatening haemoptysis. Chest 1999; 115: 996–1001.

Sidman JD, Wheeler WB, Cabalka AK, Soumekh B, Brown CA. Management of acute pulmonary haemorrhage in children. Laryngoscope 2001; 111: 33–35.

K. Moghissi, J.A.C. Thorpe and F. Ciulli (Eds.)
Moghissi's Essentials of Thoracic and Cardiac Surgery

CHAPTER IV.5

Laser in cardiothoracic surgery

K. Moghissi, K. Dixon and M.R. Stringer

1. Introduction

The word 'laser' is an acronym of Light Amplification by the Stimulated Emission of Radiation. Following absorption of light (photon) energy by an atom or molecule, an excited state is created that is either related to a change in electron orbit, or describes a specific type of molecular vibration. This unstable excited state can return spontaneously to the lower (equilibrium) energy level, with the emission of a photon, or can be induced to make the same transition by another incident photon. Importantly, the resultant stimulated photon has the same wavelength and is emitted in the same direction as that which induced its release.

The rate of stimulated emission is dependent upon the number of excited states created; in order for an amplification process to proceed it is therefore necessary that the number of excited states within the laser medium be increased at the expense of the equilibrium state. Such a population inversion can only be achieved by a method of pumping which involves the delivery of sufficient energy to the medium. The method of pumping (as well as the wavelength of laser output) depends upon the laser medium.

It is the first few photons to be emitted (spontaneously) that initiate the process of light amplification but if no control were placed upon the direction of propagation, the resultant light would be emitted in all directions. The direction of beam propagation can be imposed by placing the laser medium within an optical resonant cavity, formed by two mirrors, facing each other along a central axis (Fig. 1).

Reflection at the mirrors turns the photons back into the cavity so that they can enhance the chain reaction of stimulated emission. In this way, the beam grows in intensity with each traverse of the medium. In order to allow the emission of the laser beam, one of the mirrors (the output coupler) is partially reflecting.

Lasers are named according to the specific laser medium which can take many forms:

- Solid-state lasers: consist of ions contained within a host medium of solid crystal or glass which is optically pumped using either an intense source of light such as xenon flash tube or by using another laser. The most common medical lasers of this type are:
  - Ruby laser (694.3 nm): a medium of aluminium oxide (Al_2O_3) doped with chromium (Cr^{3+}) ions.

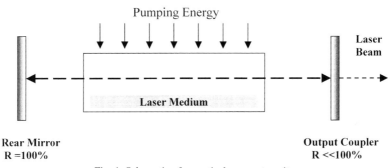

Fig. 1. Schematic of an optical resonant cavity.

– Nd : YAG (1064 nm), Er : YAG (2.94 μm), Ho : YAG (2.1 μm) lasers: a medium of Yttrium Aluminium Garnet doped with Neodynmium (Nd^{3+}), Erbium (Er^{3+}) of Holmium (Ho^{3+}) ions.

- Gas lasers: consist of an atomic or molecular species in the gaseous, vapour or plasma state. Lasing action can be stimulated by passing an electric current through the laser medium. Examples of these are:
  – Argon ion laser (principal emission lines at 488 and 514 nm)
  – Carbon dioxide (CO_2) laser (10.6 μm)
  – Copper vapour laser (511 and 578 nm)
  – Excimer lasers (e.g. ArF 193 nm, KrF 248 nm, and XeCl 308 nm)
- Dye lasers: comprise organic dyes in solution or suspension which are optically pumped by flash tube or by another laser. Each dye may be tuned over a limited wavelength range (~30 nm) and a wide range of dyes is available allowing, with the appropriate choice of pumping source, laser emission from ultra-violet through to infrared wavelengths.
- Diode lasers: employing suitably doped semiconducting materials are pumped by the passage of an electric current.

2. Characteristics of laser light

Three fundamental properties characterise laser emission:

- Coherence: it has already been stated that a stimulated photon is emitted with the same wavelength and in the same direction as the photon that induced the emission. Coherence is the term used to describe the relationship between the two waveforms and it may be discussed in terms of both time (temporal coherence) and space (spatial coherence).
- Monochromaticity: this is a consequence of temporal coherence and implies a single output wavelength.
- Collimation: this is a consequence of spatial coherence and represents the directionality of the beam as defined by the angular beam divergence.

The combination of very low divergence and narrow bandwidth results in an output that has a very high spectral intensity. Even low-power devices exhibit a spectral intensity of much greater magnitude than can be obtained from a non-laser light source. One of the principle benefits of laser light in medical applications is the ability to focus the beam to a spot of small diameter. This is useful in allowing efficient light delivery via a narrow optical fibre.

3. Laser–tissue interaction

The effect of laser light upon tissue depends upon a number of factors, principally the output characteristics of the laser (wavelength, average power, pulse energy and duration and spot-size) and the optical properties of the tissue. The latter determines the depth to which laser light affects the tissue. Briefly, incident laser light can be reflected, scattered or absorbed. Reflection is a type of scattering that occurs at the tissue surface; irradiation of a reflective tissue surface results in a loss that demands the input of a higher laser power to achieve the desired effect. Scattering below the surface has the effect of diffusing the incident beam so that biological effects may be induced at sites other than the target resulting in collateral damage.

4. The biological effects of lasers

Many lasers affect tissue through thermal effect. The laser energy is absorbed by the tissue and is converted into heat. Other lasers affect tissue by photochemical effects in combination with a photosensitising chemical which interferes with cell and tissue metabolism — a technique known as photodynamic therapy. It is therefore convenient, if somewhat simplistic, to classify medical lasers into:

4.1 Thermal lasers.

4.2 Metabolic (non-thermal)/dye lasers and diodes.

4.1. The visible and tangible evidence of the effects of thermal lasers are:

- Coagulation: this results from denaturisation of tissue protein causing destruction and necrosis.
- Haemostasis: arrest of haemorrhage caused by laser is partially due to fibrin formation and also from vaso constriction.
- Vaporisation: high power laser energy produces total burn and evaporation of water thus creating a crater in the target tissue, the border of which is formed by charred and totally and partially necrosed tissue. When vaporisation occurs over a narrow area the effect is similar to surgical incision.

4.2. Metabolic/dye lasers and diodes

The effects of these lasers are:

- Interference with tissue/cell metabolism by a number of mechanisms which affect cell respiration and produce cytotoxic agents.
- Ischemia and necrosis due to the release of vaso-active substances affecting small vessels.

The wavelength produced by a dye laser is dependent on the dye used. In photodynamic therapy a photochemical needs to be incorporated into the target tissue prior to exposure of that tissue to the laser light. It is the interaction between the wavelength of light which matches the absorption band of the chemical, usually in the presence of oxygen, that is responsible for the photochemical effects.

5. Laser equipment for clinical application

This is comprised of three essential components:

(1) Laser generator: this generates laser light of a specific wavelength.
(2) Delivery system: to transmit the emitted laser light to the patient.
(3) Applicators: these are the devices which carry the delivered laser light to a specific site in the body. Applicators are part of the delivery system manipulated by the clinician.

5.1. Types of lasers in cardiothoracic surgery

Amongst a variety of available lasers, currently the most commonly used lasers in thoracic and cardiac surgery are:

5.1.1 CO$_2$ lasers.
5.1.2 NdYAG and HoYAG lasers.
5.1.3 Dye and diode lasers employed in photodynamic therapy.

5.1.1. Carbon Dioxide (CO$_2$) Lasers

This laser emits light at a wavelength of 10.6 micrometers (10600 nm) in the infrared range of the electromagnetic spectrum. Its properties are:

- Strongly absorbed by water.
- Great cutting power.
- Weak haemostatic activity.

The great disadvantage of this laser is that it cannot be delivered through optical fibres thus restricting its endoscopic application. At the present time, the application of the CO$_2$ laser in thoracic surgery is limited to its application to the upper airway, principally larynx and trachea.

5.1.2. NdYAG laser

This is the most extensively used laser in thoracic surgery. Its prominent properties are:

- Emits light at a wavelength of 1064 nm.
- Will transmit through water.
- Good haemostatic effect.
- Can be delivered through optical fibres.
- Can be used in either contact or non-contact mode.

NdYAG, being a colourless light, is usually coupled with a Helium–Neon red light laser acting as an aiming beam. In thoracic surgery NdYAG laser is used endoscopically, broncho-oesophagoscopically, thoracoscopically and intra operatively.

5.1.3. Diode laser (805 nm)

The introduction of the high-power gallium–arsenide (GaAs) diode array allows the possibility of a much more compact and easily applied laser system, the output of which induces a comparable clinical effect to the NdYAG source.

6. Lasers in bronchopulmonology

6.1. NdYAG laser

6.1.1. Tracheo-bronchoscopic laser therapy

Tracheo-bronchoscopic laser therapy using NdYAG laser was begun in the 1970s (Nath et al., 1973; Toty et al., 1979), and since then, the method has received universal acceptance for the treatment of endoluminally projecting lesions in the tracheo-bronchial tree.

Its main indications are:

- Inoperable lung cancer with tumour component obstructing trachea, main or lobar bronchi.
- Benign tracheo-bronchial tumours.
- Tracheal/main bronchial inflammatory strictures.
- Haemorrhage due to granulation tissue/tumour in the bronchi.

Bronchoscopic NdYAG laser can be carried out with use of the flexible fibreoptic instrument under local anaesthesia as was originally practiced by Nath et al. (1973). However, the safest and most reliable method, which is also the least distressing for the patient, is to carry out tracheo-bronchoscopic YAG laser therapy under general anaesthesia with the use of the rigid bronchoscope (Toty et al., 1979, 1981; Hetzel et al., 1985; Moghissi et al., 1986).

The task is greatly facilitated if a specially designed instrument is used. Alternatively, the rigid instrument may be used through which ventilation is maintained. The fibreoptic instrument is introduced through the rigid bronchoscope to localise the target and to provide a means by which the laser fibre is passed through its biopsy channel.

The procedure is undertaken as follows:
- Carry out bronchoscopy under general anaesthesia and maintain ventilation through the bronchoscope (see bronchoscopy, Fig. 4 in chapter I.2).
  - (a) Either introduce the laser delivery fibre through the dedicated channel (if the bronchoscope is designed for laser therapy).
  - (b) Alternatively, place the flexible fibreoptic instrument into the rigid scope before introducing the laser fibre into the biopsy channel of the fibreoptic instrument. The tip of the delivery fibre must be seen to be at least 1.5 cm through the end of the flexible fibreoptic bronchoscope otherwise the high temperature at the laser fibre tip will damage the fibreoptic bronchoscope.

    In either case, the laser radiation is of non-contact mode.
- The tip of the fibre is directed towards the target and the Helium–Neon (He–Ne) aiming beam focused on the area, but not touching it. The He–Ne beam will be seen as a red circle.
- Note that the smaller the diameter of the circle, the more focused is the beam at the target. Therefore, less power (in Watts) will be needed to achieve evaporation. A power of 20 to 40 W for 2 to 4 seconds is used. This is repeated several times until the lesion is evaporated.
- If charring rather than evaporation is required, the same power may be used but the tip of the laser fibre kept further away from the target.
- The author prefers using higher power energy of 40 W focusing closely on the target for evaporation of bulky tumours within the trachea/main bronchi and a lower power for charring of flatter lesions within lobar and segmental orifices.
- Following completion of therapy, pieces of tumour and debris should be removed with biopsy forceps through the rigid bronchoscope and thorough cleansing and lavage of the bronchial tree carried out. This is important because, distal to the point of obstruction, there is often collection of pus and infected material. It is also logical in such cases to obtain a sample of secretions for microbiological studies.

Results: The mortality of bronchoscopic Yag laser therapy is reported to be between 1–3% (Personne et al., 1986). In the author's series of just over 700 patients, no procedure-related mortality was observed.

Complications: There are a variety of reported complications associated with tracheo-bronchial laser therapy:

Major fatal haemorrhage approximately	1%
Minor haemorrhage	4–6%
Pneumothorax/fistula	<1%
Fire	<1%
Others (infection)	1–2%

- Symptomatic and functional results are generally good to excellent.
- Survival depends almost entirely on the nature (pathology) of the lesion.
- In the case of cancer, the overall stage of tumour, extent and localisation of metastases will govern the outcome.

6.1.2. Thoracoscopic uses of YAG laser

Video assisted thoracoscopic surgery (VATS) method can be used to deliver YAG laser to the pleural cavity.
The indications are:
- Control of superficial air leak (alveolar leaks) in pneumothorax.
- Deflation and shrinkage of blebs, emphysematous bullae and small, peripheral pulmonary air cysts.
- To create pleurodesis by parietal pleural abrasion (Torre, et al., 1989; Sharpe et al., 1994).
- Dissection of adhesions.

At present, only a limited number of patients have received the benefit of thoracoscopic laser therapy.

6.1.3. Intra-operative use of YAG laser

A pilot study carried out by Moghissi et al. (1988) showed the potential of NdYAG laser in pulmonary surgery. Low power laser energy promotes clotting and seals air leaks. High power radiation will evaporate tissue and incise the lung with little bleeding or air leak (Fig. 2). Later, both experimental and clinical work showed that YAG laser may be used to locally excise coin lesions.

In practice, NdYAG laser can be used intra-operatively for:
- Local excision of nodular lesions (Moghissi, 1989).
- In conjunction with conventional pulmonary surgery (Moghissi, 1990).
- In pulmonary metastasectomy (Moghissi, 1990, Branscheid, 1992).

When its use is envisaged for local excision of pulmonary nodular lesions, the patient should be investigated for malignancy since the majority of such nodules are malignant.

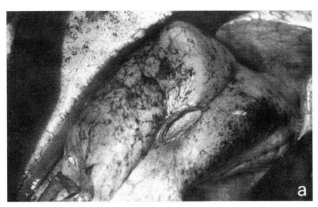 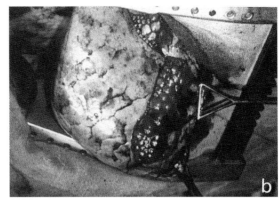

Fig. 2. (a) Intra-operative view of the inflated lung. In the centre, an incision has been made using high power non-contact YAG Laser. Note that the incision has not caused bleeding or air leak. (b) Same view of the lung in which a superficial incision has been made using cutting and coagulating (blend) electro-diathermy. In contrast to (a) there is both bleeding and airleak from the surface.

Limited, muscle-sparing thoracotomy with an appropriately placed incision usually suffices to expose the tumour. Despite negative CT evidence for lymphadenopathy intra-operative exploration should be made for lymphadenectomy of enlarged/pathological lymph nodes. Local excision is carried out by using high power 70 to 90 W of energy. A circular incision is made some 2 cm away from the visible border of the tumour. The incision is deepened and the tumour removed. Only small sub-segmental arteries and sub-segmental bronchi require stitching or clipping.

Apart from excision of nodular primary lesions, the method is highly suitable for metastasectomies.

NdYAG in conjunction with pulmonary surgery is employed for separation of segments to prevent excessive air leak, for haemostasis and for reducing lymphatic leaks following excision of lymph nodes.

6.2. Photodynamic therapy (PDT)

The basis of PDT is photosensitisation of tissue by a chemical with a defined absorption band for a specific wavelength of laser light. When such sensitised tissue is exposed to the appropriate laser light, injury and necrosis will occur due to interaction between the photochemical and light. In this process, the presence of oxygen is crucial and the formation of singlet oxygen appears to be the basis of cytotoxicity and the resultant necrosis. Several photosensitizers have been used experimentally and clinically such as Photofrin and mTHPC (mesotetra hydroxy phenol phthalocyanine) 5-ALA (Amino Levulinic Acid) each requiring a specific laser light wavelength for their activation. ALA is a naturally occurring pre-

cursor in the process of Heme (hemoglobin) biosynthesis pathway. It is converted to the endogenous photosensitizer protoporphyrin IX. This can be activated by red, green and blue light.

The commonest photosensitiser in use for endoscopic PDT is Photofrin requiring a matching 630 nm laser light (red). A variety of laser light sources have also emerged, the latest being Diode lasers combining efficiency with manageability and mobility of the equipment.

In 1975, Dougherty and colleagues showed that by administering haematoporphyrin derivatives (HPD) systemically as a photosensitiser in mice with transplanted mammary tumours, eradication of the tumour was achieved with little damage to the surrounding tissue. This was also shown to be the case in a variety of other tumours (Dougherty et al., 1978). The first PDT treatment in human lung cancer was carried out by Hayata and colleagues in 1982.

At the same time Balchum et al. (1984) and Cortese et al. (1982, 1986) demonstrated the feasibility and potential benefits of endobronchial PDT in cases of bronchial carcinoma. Since then, a number of authors have shown total response and long survival of patients with early stage carcinoma treated by endoscopic PDT. Others have also demonstrated benefits in terms of palliation of symptoms as well as survival benefits in those patients with inoperable tumours when treated by endoscopic interstitial PDT (Balchum, et al., 1984; McCaughan et al., 1997; Moghissi et al., 1999).

6.2.1. Bronchoscopic PDT for lung cancer
The steps of the procedure are (Fig. 3):
• Full clinical, radiological and endoscopic investi-

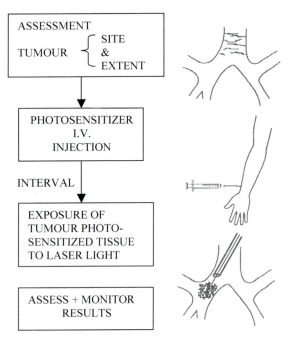

Fig. 3. Protocol for bronchoscopic photodynamic therapy for lung cancer.

gation: bronchoscopy should include biopsy sampling and determination of location and extent of tumour in the airway.

- Intravenous injection of the photosensitiser: currently the most commonly used photosensitizer is Photofrin administered 2 mg/kg BW).
- Bronchoscopic illumination carried out 24 to 72 hours later: this may be performed using the flexible instrument and under topical anaesthetic. However, the author's preference is to carry out the procedure under general anaesthetic using both rigid and flexible bronchoscopes. The rigid bronchoscope is inserted first into the trachea for the maintenance of ventilation. The flexible fibreoptic bronchoscope (FFB) is then placed into the rigid bronchoscope and advanced towards the tumour. The light delivery fibre is passed through its biopsy channel. This fibre has an end cylindrical diffuser for interstitial therapy which may be placed in the substance of the tumour for treatment (Fig. 4). When surface application is required for PDT of a superficial tumour a laser fibre with an end diffuser (microlens) is placed over the cancer so that the light hits the target area.

It is important to emphasize that it would be unwise to use FFB under topical anaesthesia for obstructive main stem lesions since it would be difficult to deal with any ventilatory or haemorrhagic complications during the procedure. Furthermore the suction channel of FFB does not permit proper clearing of thick secretion and debris (Moghissi et al., 1991).

The light and light dose. Wavelength of light used with Photofrin is a red light at 630 nm.

Many investigators, including the authors, use a dose of 200 Joules per cm of tumour tissue (400 mW output/cm of the diffuser for 500 seconds).

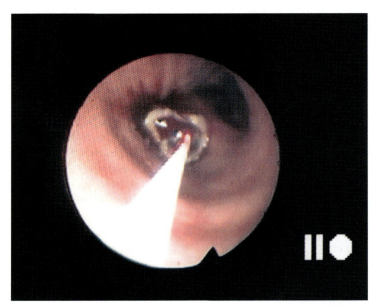

Fig. 4. Shows cylindrical diffuser in obstructed bronchus for interstitial therapy.

Experience is needed to optimise time and energy to achieve necrosis of the tumour in its entirety.

Post-operative management. Patients with bulky tumour occupying main bronchi require a repeat bronchoscopy 4 to 6 days later in order to rid the bronchus of necrotic debris and to carry out further illumination of residual tumour, if required. Clearly, this debridement in larger obstructive tumours cannot be carried out satisfactorily via FFB with its narrow aspiratory channel and the minute cup biopsy forceps. Rigid open-ended bronchoscope with its larger biopsy device is the instrument of choice.

Patients are monitored at 2 to 3 monthly intervals and additional PDT, Nd YAG laser or other treatment given as appropriate.

Indications. Bronchoscopic PDT has been employed for malignant tracheo-bronchial lesions irrespective of the histological type of the tumour. In early superficial cancer, long survival/cure can be achieved (Hayata et al., 1984; Cortese et al., 1986; Kato et al., 1996). In inoperable, unresectable cases palliation can be achieved; additionally there is survival benefit in those with better performance status (Moghissi et al., 1999). Pre-requisites for endoscopic PDT are: visible presence of endoluminal tumour and confirmation of malignancy by histological examination. Illumination for early lesions is by the superficial application of light via the optical fibre with end (micro-lens) diffuser and for bulky extensive tumours is by insertion of the cylindrical diffuser into the bulk of the tumour (interstitial therapy). There is generally no procedure-related mortality (Moghissi et al., 1999).

Complications. The following complications have been reported:

- Photosensitivity skin reaction: The incidence is dependent on patients' compliance in avoiding sunlight and upon rigour of counselling. Although this has the potential to be an important drawback, its incidence can be reduced (<4%) by thorough counselling and education of the patient (Moghissi et al., 1999, 2001).
- Haemorrhage has been reported when treatment was undertaken in patients with bulky inoperable tumours (Balchum et al., 1984), though recent reports of a large series has not shown such complication (McCaughan et al., 1988; Moghissi et al., 1999).

- Post treatment dyspnoea and breathlessness. This is a rare event but can occur in patients with severe obstructive lesion due to a bulky endoluminal tumour. After treatment, debris and secretions maybe retained in the bronchus, thus obliterating the lumen. In such patients, repeat bronchoscopy for debridement 3 to 5 days later should be routine. Further re-bronchoscopy/aspiration should be carried out as appropriate.
- Infective complication due to retention of secretion. This can be prevented by carrying out thorough aspiration and cleansing of the bronchial tree at the conclusion of bronchoscopic PDT. Active physiotherapy and prophylactic antibiotic should be given in those with severe bronchial obstruction and distal infection.

7. Laser therapy of the oesophagus

At the present time, laser radiation for treatment of oesophageal pathology is delivered endoscopically, which means that only endoluminal lesions may be accessed. For this reason, the major part of experience in laser therapy is in its endoscopic application.

Two types of lasers are currently used in the oesophagus. These are NdYAG (YAG) laser and dye lasers used in photodynamic therapy (PDT).

7.1. Endoscopic YAG laser

The thermal effect of YAG laser evaporates, coagulates and generally necroses the target lesion (Fig. 5). Although in its original developmental phase YAG laser was applied to a number of different lesions, present day indications are generally in malignant tumours though some benign tumours respond well.

7.1.1. Technique

General or local/topical anaesthetic may be used. We prefer to perform endoscopic laser therapy under general anaesthesia imposing neither time restriction nor presenting discomfort to the patient or operator. The flexible fibreoptic instrument is employed with the delivery fibre inserted through its biopsy channel. This instrument is suitable for treatment of all lesions located in the oesophagus except those at the pharyngo-oesophageal junction and proximal cervical oesophagus.

Some of the important practical points relating to treatment of obstructive tumours are:

- Most cases require dilatation prior to laser therapy.

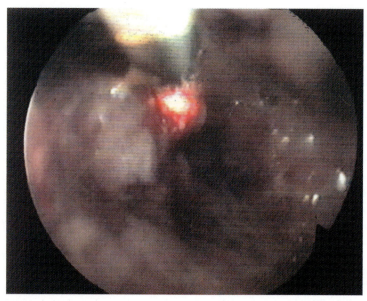

Fig. 5. NdYAG laser treatment of oesophageal cancer. The red circle is the aiming beam. At the centre is the laser destroying the tumour. The right hand side of the tumour is blackened following treatment.

- One should allow at least 1 to 1.5 cm of the delivery fibre to extrude from the exit point of the biopsy channel of the oesophagoscope in order to prevent thermal damage to the instrument.
- Ideally, treatment should start at the most distal point (retrograde treatment). However, in many cases the proximal part of the tumour may have to be dealt with first.
- Start by short bursts of 20 W × 2 to 3 seconds, raising the power if required.
- It is mandatory to clearly visualise the lumen and the projecting tumour.
- Direct the aiming beam (Helium–Neon) to the portion of tumour or lesion which is projecting into the lumen and not at the oesophageal wall.
- At intervals between pulses, wash and aspirate.
- Smoke: if a rigid open-ended instrument is used, for instance in the pharynx/cervical oesophagus, the delivery fibre is introduced via an appropriate metallic applicator. There is usually some smoke which needs disposal (we use a metallic suction tube in conjunction with the rigid instrument to aspirate oesophageal secretions, liquid and fumes).
- When a fibreoptic endoscope is used, washing and aspiration will clear the view.
- In laser therapy of lesions of the pharyngo-oesophageal junction under general anaesthesia, a metallic endotracheal tube is used in preference to plastic to avoid accidental fire.

7.1.2. Indications
- Malignant and benign tumours:
  – In advanced malignant cases the aim is palliation (relief of dysphagia).
  – In early stage cancer patients who are operable but otherwise unsuitable for resection or who reject surgical operation, the aim is curative intent.
- Projecting granulation into the lumen, e.g. at the site of oesophago-gastric anastomosis.
- Bleeding of oesophageal ulcer.

The power setting for haemostasis should be below 20 W but attention should be paid to the relationship between the power setting and the distance between the delivery fibre end and the target, referred to previously (see section 6.1.1 in this chapter).

7.1.3. Results
- In dysphagic patients with malignant obstruction, laser therapy is intended to dispose of the obstructive lesion, which, in turn, provides relief of dysphagia. The treatment may need to be repeated at 4 to 8 week intervals. It can be repeatedly effective providing that the dysphagia is due to intraluminal tumour growth and not through extrinsic compression by glands or oesophageal wall involvement. There appears to be a relationship between the length of the tumour and the dysphagia free interval (Lightdale et al., 1987; Spinelli et al., 1995).

- Effect on survival is difficult to assess since there may be benefits which indirectly effect survival due to better swallowing and nutrition and the prevention of respiratory complications caused by obstructed oesophagus and decrease of tumour mass. There is no evidence that YAG laser therapy is attended by survival benefit in advanced stage tumours by slowing its growth rate.
- The important point to note is that nearly 80% of patients can swallow until death and, in many, failure relates to the extrinsic obstructive nature of the tumour.

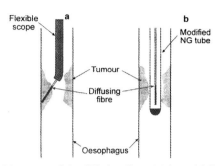

Fig. 6. Placement of the diffusing fibre: (a) interstitially in the tumour, (b) intraluminally within the oesophagus.

7.2. Photodynamic therapy (PDT)

The principle of PDT has been previously described in this chapter. In practice, the application of PDT in the endoscopic treatment for oesophageal lesions is carried out as follows (Moghissi et al., 1995, 2000).

7.2.1. Technique
- The patient is given an injection of a photosensitizer. The author uses Photofrin 2 mg/kg of body weight. This is licensed and is currently the most commonly used photosensitiser.
- Illumination takes place 24 to 72 hours after administration of the drug.
- The patient should have had full assessment of the lesion, by means of clinical examination, imaging and endoscopic investigation to provide information on:
  - Diagnosis.
  - The severity of dysphagia.
  - Extent of endoluminal involvement of the oesophagus by the lesion, i.e. the length and the dimension of its projection into the lumen.
  - In the case of cancer, staging and operability.
  - General condition of the patient.
- It is important to know the length and the extent of endoluminal projection of the lesion, since these determine the type of diffuser to be employed and whether the illumination is going to be interstitial, where the diffuser is inserted into the tumour mass, or intraluminal (surface applications), where the tumour mass circumferentially involves the lumen.
- The delivery system is an optical fibre with end cylindrical diffuser. The length of the diffuser should match the length of the lesion. At the present time, diffuser lengths are from 0.5 to 3 cm. It follows that, in the presence of a 5 cm lesion, two sequential placements of the diffuser

would be required to illuminate the lesion in its entirety.
- 200 J/cm is the usual illumination dose to be given; that is 400 milliWatts per 1 cm length of diffuser for 500 seconds.
- There are two types of illumination (Fig. 6):
  (a) Interstitial illumination when the tumour consists of a large mass. In this case the diffuser is inserted into the tumour mass. It is important to select an appropriate size of diffuser to match the length of tumour.
  (b) Surface application when the tumour is not bulky but superficial. Here too the size of the lesion determines the length of the diffuser to be used.

7.3. Indications

- PDT has a place in both early and advanced oesophageal cancer. In early cancer, complete response with long survival amounting to cure can be expected. However, as yet, there is no published data involving a large series of patients with early stage cancer treated by PDT. This is due to the fact that early stage cancers are generally submitted to surgical resection except for those cases not suitable for operation or who refuse surgery.
- The role of PDT in advanced cancer is essentially one of palliation of dysphagia (Table 1). However, there appears to be survival benefit for those patients with a good general condition (Moghissi et al., 2000).

There are two subsets of patients with advanced oesophageal cancer in whom PDT has an important place. Firstly, patients who have been stented but who subsequently develop recurrence of dysphagia due to an overgrowth of tumour above, below or within the prosthesis. No other modality improvement in left ventricular function or in exercise capacity.

– Some studies have shown an increase in left ventricular ejection fraction.

– The mechanisms by which the anginal pain is relieved following TMLR are not clearly understood.

– Despite the advantages that CO_2 laser has compared with HoYAG laser, the latter permits light delivery through optical fibres which is both attractive and more practical. HoYAG laser thus allows TMLR via minimal access approach or can be used as PMLR.

– It is important to appreciate that PMLR may be carried out by a non-surgical team. However, at the time of writing, it is best practiced by cardiac surgical teams or, alternatively, to have such a team ready at hand for when required.

References and further reading

Balchum OJ, Doiron DR. Photoradiation therapy of obstructing endobronchial lung cancer. Lasers Med Surg 1982; 357: 53–55.

Balchum OJ, Doiron DR, Hutch GC. Photoradiation therapy of endobronchial lung cancer employing the photodynamic action of haematoporphyrin derivative. Lasers Surg Med 1984; 4: 13–30.

Barr H, Shepherd NA, Dix A et al. Eradication of high grade dysplasia in columnar lined (Barrett's) oesophagus by photodynamic therapy with endogenously generated photoporphyrin IX. Lancet 1996; 348: 584–585.

Branscheid D, Krysa S, Wollkopf G et al. Does NdYag laser extend the indications for resection of pulmonary metastases? Eur J Cardiothorac Surg 1992; 6: 590–597.

Clarke SC, Schofield PM. Laser revascularisation. Brit Med Bull 2001; 59: 249–259.

Cortese DA, Kinsey JG. Endoscopic management of lung cancer with haematoporphyrin derivative photo therapy. Mayo Clinic Proc 1982; 57: 543–547.

Cortese DA. Bronchoscopic photodynamic therapy of early lung cancer. Chest 1986; 90: 629–631.

Dougherty TJ, Grindey GB, Fiel R, Boyle DG. Photoradiation therapy cure of animal tumours with haematoporphyrin and light. J Nat Cancer Inst 1975; 55: 115–121.

Dougherty TJ, Kaufman JE, Goldfarb A et al. Photoradiation therapy for the treatment of malignant tumours. Cancer Res 1978; 38: 2628–2630.

Ferguson MK, Naunheim KS. Resection for Barrett's mucosa with high grade dysplasia; Implications for prophylactic photodynamic therapy. J Thorac Cardiovasc Surg 1997; 114(5): 824–829.

Hayata Y, Kato H, Konaka C et al. Bronchoscopic photoradiation for tumour localisation in lung cancer. Chest 1982; 82: 10–13.

Hayata Y, Kato H, Konaka C et al. Photoradiation therapy with haematoporphyrin derivative in early and stage I lung cancer. Chest 1984; 86: 169–177.

Hertzel MR, Nixon C, Edmonstone WM et al. Laser therapy in 100 tracheobronchial tumours. Thorax 1985; 40: 341–345.

Hovarth KA, Cohn LH, Cooley DA, Crew JR, Frazier OH et al. Transmyocardial Laser Revascularization. Result of a multicentre trail with transmyocardial revascularization used as sole therapy for end-stage coronary artery disease. J Thorac Cardiovasc Surg 1997; 113: 645–652.

Horvath KA, Aranki SF, Cohn LH et al. Sustained angina relief 5 years after Trans Myocardial Laser Revascularisation with a CO_2 laser. Circulation 2001; 12: 181–184.

Kato H, Okunaka T, Shimatani H. Photodynamic therapy for early stage bronchogenic carcinoma. J Clin Laser Med Surg 1996; 14: 235–238.

Lightdale CJ, Zimbalist E, Winawer SJ. Outpatient management of oesophageal cancer with endoscopic NdYAG laser. Am J Gastroenterol 1987; 82: 46–50.

McCaughan JS Jr, Hanley PC, Bethel BH, Walker J. Photodynamic therapy of endobronchial malignancies. Cancer 1988; Vol 62: 691–701.

McCaughan J, Williams TE. Photodynamic therapy for endobronchial malignant disease. A prospective fourteen year study. J Thorac Cardiovasc Surg 1997; 114: 940–947.

Mirhoseini M. Laser applications in thoracic and cardiovascular surgery. Med Instr 1983; 17: 401–403.

Mirhoseini M, Shelgikar S, Cayton MM. New concepts in revascularization of the myocardium. Ann Thorac Surg 1988; 45: 415–420.

Mirhoseini M, Shelgikar S, Cayton MM. Transmyocardial lasers revascularization: A review. J Clin Laser Med Surg 1993; 11: 15–19.

Moghissi K, Jessop K, Dench M. A new bronchoscopy set for laser therapy. Thorax 1986; 41: 485–486.

Moghissi K, Dench M, Goebells P. Experience in noncontact NdYag laser in pulmonary surgery: A pilot study. Eur J Cardiothorac Surg 1988; 2: 87–94.

Moghissi K. Local excision of pulmonary nodular (coin) lesion with noncontact Yttrium Aluminium Garnet laser. J Thorac Cardiovasc Surg 1989; 97: 147–151.

Moghissi K. Experience in limited lung resection with the use of laser. Lung 1990; supp: 1103–1109.

Moghissi K, Parsons RJ, Dixon K. Photodynamic therapy for bronchial carcinoma with the use of rigid bronchoscope. Lasers Med Sci. 1991; 7: 381–385.

Moghissi K, Papiri N. A clinico-pathological study of the origin of adeno-carcinoma of the mid thoracic oesophagus and results of surgical resection. Chirurgie 1992; 118: 298–303.

Moghissi K. Surgical resection for stage 1 cancer of the oesophagus and cardia. Br J Surg 1992; 79: 935–937.

Moghissi K, Sharpe DAC, Pender D. Adeno-carcinoma, carcinoma and Barrett's oesophagus: a clinico-pathological study. Eur J Cardiothorac Surg 1993; 7: 126–132.

Moghissi K, Dixon K, Hudson E, Stringer MR. Photodynamic therapy for oesophageal cancer. Laser Med Sci 1995; 10: 671.

Moghissi K, Dixon K, Stringer M, Freeman T, Thorpe A, Brown S. The place of bronchoscopic photodynamic therapy in advanced unresectable lung cancer: experience of 100 cases. Eur J Cardiothorac Surg 1999; 15: 1–6.

Moghissi K, Dixon K, Thorpe JA, Stringer MR , Moore PJ. The role of photodynamic therapy (PDT) in inoperable oesophageal cancer. Eur J Cardiothorac Surg 2000; 17: 95–100.

Moghissi K. PDT in Bronchopulmonary cancer. In: Clinical Photodynamic Update. Eurocommunica Publications, 2001: pp. 18–21.

Nath G, Gorish W , Kiefhaber P. First laser endoscopy via fibre optic transmission system. Endoscopy 1973: 5: 208–213.

Overholt BF, Panjehpour M. Photodynamic Therapy for Barrett's oesophagus: follow up in 100 patients. Gasterointest Endosc 1999; 49: 1–7.

Personne C, Colchen A, Leroy M, Vourc'h G, Toty L. Indication and technique for endoscopic laser resection in bronchology. A critical analysis based on 2284 resections. J Thorac Cardiovasc Surg 1986; 91: 710–715.

Regula J, MacRobert AJ, Gorchein A, et al. Photosensitisation and photodynamic therapy of oesophageal, duodenal and colorectal tumours using 5 aminolevulinic acid induced protoporphyrin IX: A pilot study. Gut 1995; 36: 67–75.

Sachinopoulou A, Beek R, Tukkie DW, Meijer PF, et al. Transmyocardial revascularization. Lasers Med Sci 1995; 10: 83–89.

Schneider J, Diegeler A, Krakor R, Walther T, Kluge R, Mohr FW. Transmyocardial laser revascularisation with Holmium:YAG laser: loss of symptomatic improvement after 2 years. Eur J Cardiothorac 2001; 19: 164–169.

Sen PK, Udwadia TE, Kinare SG, Parulkar GB. Transmyocardial revascularization. A new approach to myocardial revascularization. J Thorac Cardiovasc Surg 1965; 50: 181–189.

Sharpe DAC, Dixon C, Moghissi K. Thoracoscopic use of laser in intractable pneumothorax. Eur J CardioThorac Surg 1994; 8: 34–36.

Spinelli P, Mancini A, Dalfonte M. Endoscopic treatment of gastrointestinal tumours. Indications and results of laser photocoagulation and photodynamic therapy. Sem Surg Oncol 1995; 11: 307–318.

Summers JH, Henry AC 3rd, Roberts WC. Cardiac observations late after operative Transmyocardial Laser Revascularisation. Am J Cardiol 1999; 84: 489–490.

Torre M, Belloni P. NdYag laser through thoracoscopy. A new curative therapy in spontaneous pneumothorax. Ann Thorac Surg 1989; 47: 887–889.

Toty L, Personne CL, Herzog P. Utilisation d'un faiseau laser (Yag) a conducteur souple pour le traitement endoscopique de certaines lesions tracheobronchiques. Rev Fr Mal Respir 1979; 7: 475–482.

Toty L, Personne C, Colchin A, Vourc'h G. Bronchoscopic management of tracheal lesions using the NdYag laser. Thorax 1981; 36: 175–178.

Wiseth R, Forfang K, Ilebekk A, et al. Myocardial laser revascularisation in the year 2000 as seen by a Norwegian specialist panel. The process of evaluation and implementing new methods in clinical practice. Scand Cardiovasc J 2001; 35: 14–18.

Topics in Cardiac Surgery

K. Moghissi, J.A.C. Thorpe and F. Ciulli (Eds.)
Moghissi's Essentials of Thoracic and Cardiac Surgery

CHAPTER V.1

Interventional cardiology

P. Wilde and P. Boreham

1. Introduction

Structural modification of the heart to treat disease was for many years the exclusive province of the cardiac surgeon. With the dramatic advances in cardiac surgery in the second half of the twentieth century, there has been a parallel development of minimally invasive techniques of treating certain cardiac conditions.

The report of the first human coronary angioplasty performed by Andreas Gruentzig (Gruentzig, 1978) in 1977 heralded a major change in the approach to revascularisation in coronary heart disease. The approach suggested by Gruentzig (Gruentzig et al., 1979) was initially considered radical, dangerous and unlikely to succeed but the treatment of coronary artery disease over the next two decades changed so radically that coronary angioplasty is now performed more frequently than coronary artery bypass surgery in many developed countries. The balloon dilatation of the mitral valve in rheumatic heart disease is the most established interventional form of treatment for heart valve disease in adults. In paediatric cardiology there is a wider range of interventional procedures from valvular and stricture dilatation to occlusion of fistulae and septal defects.

These procedures have brought a great change in emphasis in the management of adult heart disease. We have now entered an era of the combined approach to treatment. Surgeons and interventionists must work together to discuss treatments and patient management to achieve optimal patient care at the most reasonable cost.

2. Percutaneous Transluminal Coronary Angioplasty (PTCA)

2.1. Pathophysiology

The basic principle of coronary angioplasty is the disruption of plaque and displacement of the material into the wall of the artery, usually with an accompanying disruption of some layers of the vessel wall. The process is aided by the enlargement and remodelling of the native artery which occurs naturally as the plaque forms, giving room for the displacement process to occur. In most cases the disruption of a plaque exposes the contents of the plaque to the bloodstream, releasing many highly active substances that tend to promote clotting with inflammatory and smooth muscle cell proliferation. It is thought that the release of these activating factors and the local production of thrombus have an effect on acute complications and possibly on the later development of restenosis at the site of intervention.

Once the vessel is opened and the plaque is displaced sufficiently to provide an adequate blood flow, the cellular response to the local trauma must be sufficiently modified to prevent early thrombosis until the lumen has re-endothelialised. This is usually achieved by anticoagulation and anti-platelet therapy. The cellular proliferation process following the local trauma is the basis of the restenosis that remains a problem in some cases. In cases where a metallic stent is deployed, there can be even more intense reactions, causing early thrombosis and late intimal hyperplasia and restenosis. Much research in coronary angioplasty is concerned with the control or modification of these cellular reactions.

2.2. Indications and patient selection

2.2.1. Clinical indications

The main clinical indications for coronary angioplasty are very similar to those for coronary artery bypass grafting. Stable angina and unstable angina are the commonest indications. All patients offered coronary angioplasty should normally be potential surgical candidates. There are however some exceptions to this, some patients being too ill or frail (poor left ventricle, renal failure or other co-existing disease) to be candidates for cardiac surgery, but they may still benefit from revascularisation.

More recently it has proved possible to treat some patients with coronary angioplasty for whom coronary surgery would be dangerous or inappropriate. Patients with acute myocardial infarct of less than four hours duration may be suitable for 'primary coronary angioplasty' or 'rescue coronary angioplasty' (coronary angioplasty following failed thrombolysis) whilst others with a recent infarct and continuing angina may be treated by coronary angioplasty. In symptomatic patients with previous CABG, graft or native vessel angioplasty is sometimes more appropriate than repeat surgery (see Fig. 1).

2.2.2. Lesion indications

Certain lesions are less suitable than others for coronary angioplasty and make surgery a better option. Lesions in the left mainstem are usually contraindicated for coronary angioplasty because complication occurring here can be catastrophic, although some have been successfully treated by coronary angioplasty. Bifurcation lesions, distal lesions and lesions in very tortuous vessels can all be difficult to treat.

Chronic occlusions may be difficult or impossible to cross with the guide wire and certainly have a much lower success rate than patent vessels. The site, length and duration of the occlusion are often crucial in making the decision between referring for coronary angioplasty or coronary artery bypass grafting. The overall success rate of coronary angioplasty in occlusions is in the region of 40–80%. There are various strategies for improving the success rate of the initial procedure; these include stiffer, hydrophilic coated, vibrating or olive tipped guide wires. Other techniques such as the use of excimer lasers or high-speed rotational burrs (Rotablator) require the occlusion to be crossed first with a guide wire. In general, the technology of catheters, wires, balloons and stents is improving rapidly which allows increasingly complex lesions to be treated (see Fig. 2).

2.3. Technique

Successful coronary angioplasty is dependent on the combination of appropriate skill and experience with the best available technology. It is essential that the technique is undertaken by a physician with the appropriate level of skill and training. Training requirements are usually stated by national societies of cardiology.

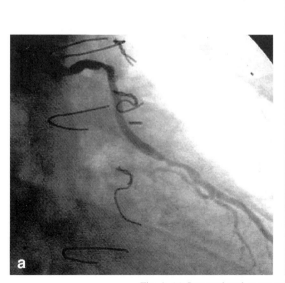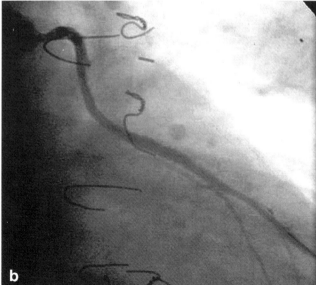

Fig. 1. (a) Stenosed saphenous vein graft. (b) Dilated and stented vein graft.

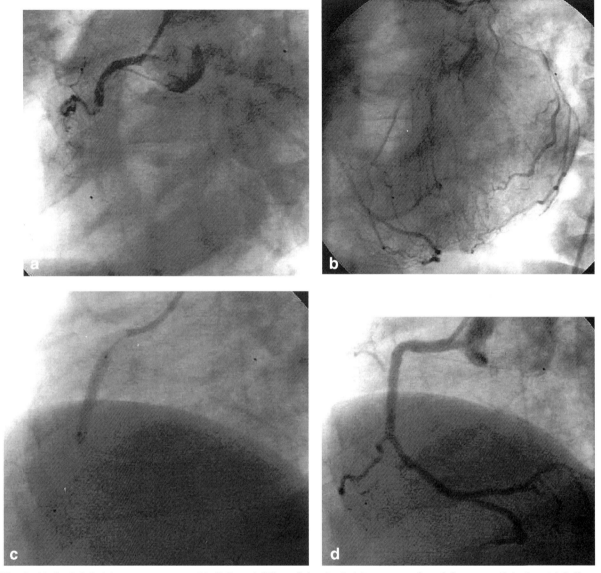

Fig. 2. (a) Occluded right coronary artery. (b) Collateral filling of the distal right coronary from left coronary injection. (c) Balloon expanding the stent. (d) Reopened right coronary artery.

The basic requirements are:
- A catheter laboratory with high resolution imaging (preferably digital, with reference image and quantitative angiography capability).
- A well-trained team capable of monitoring patient condition and treating any complications, including major cardiovascular events.
- A full range of angioplasty hardware, including guide catheters, guide wires, balloons and stents.
- Appropriate adjunctive technologies, including pharmacological agents.
- Access to a cardiac surgical team, either in the same building or at least within close reach in the event of a major emergency.

The first step in coronary angioplasty is the acquisition of high quality images of the lesion(s). The imaging needs to be of a sufficiently high quality to judge not only the severity of the lesion and the distal arteries affected but the morphology of the lesion itself. The plaque must be very clearly visualised in order to identify its size, shape and site and its relationship with the main vessel and important branches. Calcification in or near the lesion needs identification. Important technical factors to

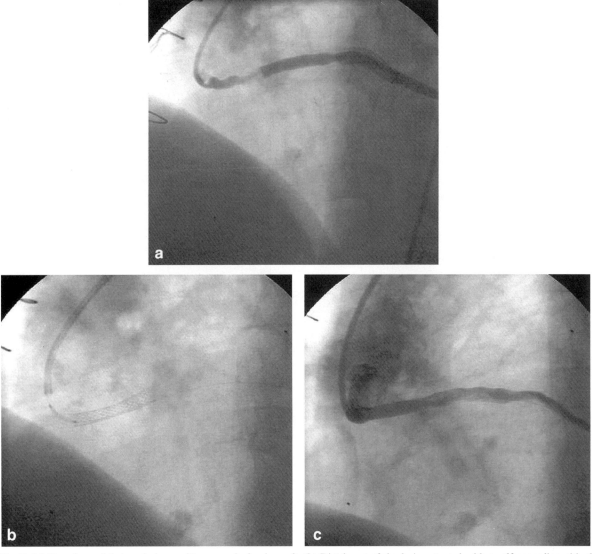

Fig. 3. (a) Complex ostial stenosis in an obtuse marginal vein graft. (b) Distal part of the lesion stented with a self-expanding nitinol stent and a second stent prepared for implantation at the ostium. (c) Final result showing full re-opening of the vein graft.

be assessed are the curvature tortuosity and size of the artery, and the anatomy and orientation of the proximal vessel, the ostium and the aortic root.

The next step will be the selection of an appropriate guide catheter and approach (see Fig. 3). The procedure is performed under local anaesthesia and most procedures are performed from the femoral artery by direct puncture. The brachial (cut down) and radial routes can also be used and the latter is gaining in acceptance. The guiding catheter is normally 6 French in size but occasionally a larger catheter is required. The tip of the guide catheter must engage atraumatically in the ostium and must

afford sufficient backup to support the advancing devices in the coronary artery. Appropriate selection of imaging views together with correct guide catheter deployment is one of the most important determinants of a successful outcome.

The patient is normally heparinised and will have been pre-treated with aspirin and with additional ticlopidine or clopidogrel. Intracoronary nitrate therapy is often helpful to maximally dilate the artery. At this stage the 0.014" steerable guide wire can be advanced and manipulated through the lesion. The uninflated low profile balloon is then advanced along the wire to the lesion and through it. The lower the balloon profile, the easier it is to cross very severe stenoses. In the case of complete occlusions, it may be possible to cross with a simple wire technique but frequently other more complex techniques with stronger wire and more support may be needed.

The balloon itself is described as non-compliant or semi-compliant. This means that it inflates to a predetermined size at a nominal pressure and beyond this it only increases in diameter very slightly as the pressure increases. Most balloons reach nominal size at 6 atmospheres but many can be inflated to much higher pressures. Short balloon dilatations can produce symptomatic ischaemia but it is surprising that in the majority of cases there is little discomfort. Balloon size must be chosen carefully to avoid either inadequate dilatation or an inappropriate dissection. Angiographic control of the result of dilatation will determine the need for stenting. It is nowadays common to deploy a stent if the result is judged as 'sub-optimal'. This is a somewhat subjective decision and there is still much debate about the precise indications for stenting. Unexpanded stents are now increasingly low in profile and there is a trend towards 'direct' or 'de novo' stenting without preliminary dilatation using a small balloon.

Once the dilation is complete, with or without a stent, it is important to confirm a good result. There must be no impairment of flow, there must be no threatening occlusive lesion and the patient must not exhibit signs or symptoms of continuing ischaemia. At this stage the wire can be removed and after final angiography, the catheter can also be removed. Anticoagulation must be allowed to wear off and catheter withdrawal must be delayed for 4–6 hours unless the vessel puncture is closed with a closure device. In the case of the radial approach, direct pressure to the artery can be applied immediately. Most patients will be fully mobile within 12 hours of the procedure and are often discharged within 24 hours.

2.4. Adjunctive devices and techniques

The rotablator is a device with a high-speed rotational burr which travels over a central guide wire. It has been shown to be particularly useful in ostial stenoses, calcified, long and small vessels and also in bifurcating lesions to debulk the stenoses. There have been some reports of distal embolisation by the micro-emboli produced by the system which can cause the 'no reflow' phenomenon.

Directional coronary atherectomy (DCA) devices have a balloon along one edge of the catheter and a cutting device on the other edge. The balloon inflates, pressing the cutting surface against the arterial wall and associated atheroma. A cutter removes a region of tissue and collects it in a compartment in the catheter. The device can be useful if there is a large eccentric plaque but it requires large diameter delivery catheters. It has been associated with distal embolisation and has a significant restenosis rate when used without stenting.

Intracoronary ultrasound (IVUS) techniques are now well developed and allow high-quality imaging of both the lumen of the coronary artery and the normal and pathological structures of the vessel wall. The device is a low-profile ultrasonic transducer that uses the same guide wire as the balloon catheter. IVUS has been used extensively to assess coronary arteries before and after the angioplasty process and stent deployment. Many institutions have IVUS equipment available for use during difficult procedures or in uncertain situations. The additional time and expense in using the equipment makes it unsuitable for routine application in most centres.

Areas of future development are also focused on the problem of diffuse severe total coronary artery disease that is not suitable for coronary artery bypass grafting or coronary angioplasty. To this end there has been work performed in transmyocardial laser channel formation from both the epicardial surface inwards and the endocardial surface outwards. There is also significant research on gene therapy that would encourage collateral or new vessel growth. These are in early stages of evaluation.

2.5. Adjunctive drug therapy

In the early years of development of coronary angioplasty, medical therapy supporting the procedure consisted of anticoagulation with heparin and warfarin as well as conventional anti-anginal agents. Despite such treatments, a significant proportion of patients continued to have thrombotic complications. Heparinisation continues to be a mainstay of the procedure but oral anticoagulants have been shown to have no useful advantages. Recent attention has focused on the importance of platelets in the formation and propagation of thrombus during coronary angioplasty.

Various exogenous factors, such as thromboxane (TxA2), adenosine diphosphate (ADP), adrenaline, collagen and thrombin, stimulate 'inactive' platelets resulting in activation of certain surface receptors. The approach of maintaining the 'inactive' state has been shown to confer significant benefit on patients with coronary artery disease. Aspirin is an irreversible cyclo-oxygenase inhibitor that inhibits the production of thromboxane by platelets and endothelium and was the first drug proven to reduce ischaemic episodes. Aspirin is now universally used before and during most angioplasty procedures. More recently ADP receptor antagonists have been developed (e.g. Clopidogrel and Ticlopidine, members of the thienopyridine family). These are irreversible ADP receptor antagonists and block this avenue of platelet activation. They have an effect in addition to aspirin and they have been shown to reduce the incidence of early occlusion of stents.

A second technique involving the neutralising of 'activated' platelets has been shown to be very effective in coronary angioplasty. Platelet aggregation is dependent on the GPIIb/IIIa receptor, which is found exclusively on platelets and megakaryocytes and mediates the final common pathway in this process. Once the GPIIb/IIIa receptor is active it can then bind to one end of fibrinogen molecules which attaches with the other end to other active platelets. Certain agents can stop thrombus formation in an unstable situation and may even disperse recently formed thrombus. The impressive results of large clinical trials involving the use of GPIIb/IIIa inhibitors has bolstered enthusiasm for the use of these as the primary adjunctive therapy to coronary angioplasty, particularly in complex cases and unstable syndromes.

2.6. Complications (see Table 1 and Fig. 4)

The three main procedure-related complications are thrombosis, dissection and spasm. Aspects of prevention or resolution of thrombosis have already been covered. Flow-limiting dissections have been recognised as a major factor in sudden occlusion of vessels undergoing angioplasty. Improved image quality has helped in earlier detection of dissections.

This coupled with improved devices (in particular, stents) has led to the introduction of routine coronary artery stenting. Not only do stents provide an important treatment for obvious dissections but the use of stents for 'suboptimal' results and even in elective stent implantation has resulted in the reduction of flow-limiting dissections. Early identification of problems and prompt stent deployment has been crucial in this change. Vessel spasm is a less common complication but this can usually be identified relatively easily and it is usually amenable to intracoronary drug therapy.

Increased risk of acute complications of all types is seen in diabetic patients, patients with unstable angina or recent myocardial infarction and those procedures with signs of dissection or filling defect post procedure. Stent implantation in small vessels (less than 3 mm in diameter), saphenous vein grafts and ostial lesions are also associated with increased early occlusion rates. Procedure-related complications are commonly measured by major adverse cardiac events which include death, myocardial infarction and emergency revascularisation.

The main late complication is restenosis, which typically occurs in the first few months following angioplasty. This remains one of the main limitations of coronary angioplasty and is the focus of continuing research attempts to find a solution. Stenting has reduced restenosis rates but other research areas are in the field of local therapy either by radiation (brachytherapy) or local drug delivery. Late complications are generally measured by reintervention rates, either by surgery or angioplasty. Symptomatic assessments and quality of life indicators are also useful.

2.7. Meta-analysis of randomised trials of coronary artery bypass grafting and coronary angioplasty vs. medical treatment

Coronary artery bypass grafting improves survival of symptomatic patients with severe, multi-vessel

Table 1

PTCA complications with or without stent and with or without GPIIb/IIIa receptor blocker abciximab

Complication	Coronary angioplasty	Coronary angioplasty + stent	Coronary angioplasty + IIb/IIIa*	Coronary angioplasty + stent + IIb/IIIa*
Abrupt closure	4–8%	1–3.4%	~0.5%*	~0%*
Death or Acute MI or urgent revascularisation	6–8%	6–7%; 10.8%*	6.9%*	5.3%*
Late revascularisation rate	~20%	~12%; 10.6%*	15.4%*	8.7%*

Figures without * are derived from several major trials, including BENESTENT (1994) and the STRESS Trial (1994).
Figures with * come from the EPISTENT Investigators (1998).

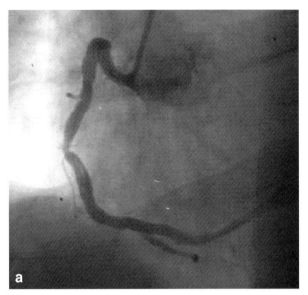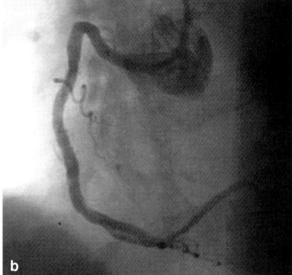

Fig. 4. (a) Mid right coronary artery lesion. (b) Implanted stent.

coronary artery disease or left mainstem disease (Yusuf et al., 1994). An improvement in survival has not been observed in surgically treated patients with single-vessel disease and chronic stable angina.

Coronary angioplasty has been shown to be superior to medical therapy in patients with single-vessel disease with severe symptoms, improving exercise performance and quality of life, but an improvement in survival is not established (Parisi et al., 1992). This also has been highlighted by a trial of angioplasty versus medical treatment (RITA, 1993; RITA-2, 1997).

The treatment of multi-vessel coronary artery disease with coronary angioplasty is current practice in cases which are unsuitable for coronary artery bypass grafting. In some combinations of lesions, particularly where the left anterior descending artery is free of stenosis, multi-vessel PTCA may be the most appropriate treatment. In patients with single vessel disease and mild or no symptoms, medical therapy may offer relatively better, or at least equivalent benefit, particularly with new pharmacological therapies and aggressive risk-factor reduction.

Future cardiac events can be prevented with aggressive risk-factor reduction and coronary artery bypass grafting but this has not yet been proved with coronary angioplasty. Progression of coronary artery disease and identification of future culprit lesions are at best difficult to predict based solely on angiography, and diagnostic and treatment options should be considered carefully for each patient.

2.8. Meta-analysis of coronary artery bypass grafting vs. coronary angioplasty

The acute results of PTCA are so good and the complication rate so low, that use of this technique has been justified to address even more complex stenoses in patients with multi-vessel disease. As a consequence, a difficult question arises: when is coronary artery bypass grafting (CABG) suitable and when should PTCA be preferred?

The outcome following PTCA and CABG in patients with multi-vessel disease has been compared in several randomised trials such as the *Argentine Randomised Trial of Percutaneous Transluminal Coronary Angioplasty versus Coronary Artery Bypass Surgery in Multivessel Disease* (ERACI) (Rodriguez et al., 1993), the *German Angioplasty Bypass Surgery Investigation* (GABI) (Hamm et al., 1994), the *Coronary Angioplasty versus Bypass Revascularization Investigation* (CABRI, 1995), and the *Emory Angioplasty versus Surgery Trial* (EAST) (King et al., 1994) trials.

In essence, comparison of PTCA and CABG in all these trials indicates no difference in mortality and incidence of myocardial infarction. All of these studies showed that the number of patients requiring re-interventions was markedly increased in the PTCA group (37%, 44%, 33%, and 49%, respectively, compared to 3%, 4%, 3%, and 1.1% in the CABG group).

The *Bypass Angioplasty Revascularisation Investigation* (BARI, 1996) study involved a larger num-

Table 2

BCIS audit returns 1997 (only from units with complete data)

	All elective coronary angioplasty	Unstable angina	Chronic total occlusion	PTCA of restenosis	Primary PTCA for myocardial infarction
Number of patients	1505	1284	235	204	63
Procedural success	92%	83%	80%	92%	79%
Post coronary angioplasty myocardial infarction	0.8%	1.2%	0.9%	1.5%	0%
Post coronary angioplasty coronary artery bypass grafting	0.9%	0.9%	0%	1%	0%
Post coronary angioplasty Mortality	0.13%	1.1%	0%	0%	9.5%

Courtesy of the British Cardiovascular Interventional Society.

ber of patients and a 5-year follow-up period. This study confirms the previously obtained results. The event rates for CABG and PTCA were 1.3% v. 1.1% for mortality, 4.6% v. 2.1% ($P < 0.01$) for Q-wave myocardial infarction, and 0.8% v. 0.2% for stroke, respectively. The 5-year survival rate was also found to be similar: 89.3% in patients assigned to CABG and 86.3% in those assigned to PTCA ($P < 0.19$).

The *Stent or Surgery Trial* (SoS, 2002) compared stent-assisted percutaneous coronary intervention (PCI) with CABG in patients with multivessel disease. Mortality rates were similar in both groups and the repeat revascularisation rates were 21% in the PCI group and 6% in the CABG group, indicating an improvement on earlier PCI vs. CABG studies. It should also be remembered that the morbidity for PTCA is low, possibly lower than CABG, and the costs are also less. This means that referral for repeat PTCA may not be resisted by patient and physician as much as referral for repeat CABG.

2.9. Registry data for coronary angioplasty

Although registry data is not as scientifically objective as that from prospective randomised trials, it has the advantage of demonstrating results in a large number of procedures and also reflects current practice. The British Cardiovascular Interventional Society (BCIS) collates the majority of results of coronary angioplasty procedures performed in the UK. The disadvantage of such registries is that the data are usually not complete, but Table 2 shows data only from a subgroup of centres returning complete or near-complete data.

3. Balloon dilatation of valve stenosis

In theory all valve stenoses are potentially suitable for valve dilatation, but in practice it is only mitral

stenosis that is regularly treated by this method. The most successful technique was first described in 1984 (Inoue et al., 1984). Occasional cases of severe aortic stenosis are treated in adult patients but the long term results are poor and this treatment is generally reserved for severely ill patients where palliation is needed.

3.1. Mitral valve commissurotomy

Experience has shown that in general the most suitable valves for this treatment are those affected by a relatively pure form of rheumatic mitral stenosis. Careful assessment of the valve morphology by echocardiography is required to determine the severity of stenosis and the involvement of the leaflets, the commisures and the sub-valvular apparatus. Significant fibrosis or calcification of the valve, its commisures or the sub-valvular apparatus is a relative contraindication to the procedure. If there is no more than very mild regurgitation and the valve morphology is suitable, then balloon dilatation is the treatment of choice.

Once the patient is selected for the procedure, a further examination by trans-oesophageal echocardiography is indicated. This is done to examine the valve in more detail, exclude undetected regurgitation, measure the valve annulus, and most importantly, exclude thrombus in the left atrium and appendage.

At the beginning of the procedure a preliminary diagnostic left heart catheter is generally performed. The commonest technique uses the Inoue latex balloon which requires a venous approach and a puncture of the inter-atrial septum using a long trans-septal needle from the femoral vein. This is usually done with ultrasound or angiographic guidance because the left atrium will generally be large and the atrial anatomy will be distorted. Once a long sheath is advanced to the left atrium, it is

Table 3

(a) Early results of PMC				(b) Long-term results of PMC					
Study	No. of patients	Valve area (cm^2)		Study	No. of patients	Followup (months)	Survival (%)	Freedom from operation	NYHA Class I–II and freedom from operation
		before PMC	after PMC						
Iung et al. 1996	216	1.0 ± 0.3	2.0 ± 0.7	Cohen et al. 1993	136	60	76	51	–
Vahanian 1996	1088	1.0 ± 0.2	1.9 ± 0.3	Palacios et al. 1995	327	48	90	79	66
				Iung et al. 1999	600	60	94	74	66
				Pan et al. 1993	350	60	94	91	85

possible to compare left atrial and left ventricular pressures simultaneously using the pre existing left heart catheter. After confirming the haemodynamics, the balloon is manipulated through the stenotic mitral orifice and the distal portion of the balloon is inflated. It is then pulled back firmly into the orifice and fully expanded to a predetermined size. The 'waist' of the balloon is usually 28 or 30 mm in diameter. The procedure takes only a few seconds and the balloon is deflated in the left atrium. Cardiac output will be transiently interrupted while the mitral flow is obstructed. A single inflation may be all that is required but some operators advocate a progressive series of inflations with increasing balloon size and ultrasound guidance. The haemodynamic measurements and a second left ventriculogram will reveal any increase in mitral regurgitation.

The procedure is performed with systemic heparinisation (given after the trans-septal puncture is successfully achieved) and protamine is needed after the procedure to facilitate sheath removal and haemostasis. The patient will be left with a small atrial septal puncture but this rarely causes a problem and may close in time.

3.2. Results of balloon mitral valve commissurotomy

The technique is now well established and there are many published results. Early results of percutaneous mitral valvotomy (PMC) show an improvement in valve area similar to that which can achieved by surgical valvotomy (see Table 3a).

Long-term results are also good with a high proportion of patients showing good quality long-term survival without the need for mitral valve surgery (see Table 3b).

The decision to perform mitral valve balloon commissurotomy must ultimately depend on a number of factors including clinical and anatomical variables as well as operator expertise. This approach must

be considered as complementary with surgery. In some cases redilatation following previous surgical or balloon commissurotomy can be performed but the results in this group are less clear and are probably poorer than for the initial valvotomy.

References and further reading

BARI Investigators. Comparison of coronary bypass surgery with angioplasty in patients with multivessel disease, the Bypass Angioplasty Revascularization Investigation (BARI) Investigators. N Engl J Med 1996; 335: 217–225.

BENESTENT Study Group. A comparison of balloon-expandable stent implantation with balloon angioplasty in patients with coronary artery disease. N Engl J Med 1994; 331: 489–495.

The British Cardiovascular Interventional Society (BCIS) registry data at *www.bcis.org.uk*

CABRI Trial Participants. First-year results of CABRI (Coronary Angioplasty versus Bypass Revascularisation Investigation). Lancet 1995; 346(8984): 1179–1184.

Cohen JM, Glower DD, Harrison JK, Bashore TM, White WD, Smith LR, Rankin JS, Sabiston DC Jr. Comparison of balloon valvuloplasty with operative treatment for mitral stenosis. Ann Thorac Surg 1993; 56(6): 1254–1262.

EPISTENT Investigators. Randomised placebo-controlled and balloon-angioplasty-controlled trial to assess safety of coronary stenting with use of platelet glycoprotein-IIb/IIIa blockade, the EPISTENT Investigators, Evaluation of Platelet IIb/IIIa Inhibitor for Stenting. Lancet 1998: 352(9122): 87–92.

Gruentzig AR. Transluminal dilatation of coronary artery stenosis (letter). Lancet 1978; 1: 263.

Gruentzig AR, et al. Nonoperative dilatation of coronary artery stenosis: percutaneous transluminal coronary angioplasty. N Engl J Med 1979; 301: 61–67.

Hamm CW, et al. A randomized study of coronary angioplasty compared with bypass surgery in patients with symptomatic multivessel coronary disease, German Angioplasty Bypass Surgery Investigation (GABI). N Engl J Med 1994; 331: 1037–1043.

Inoue K, et al. Clinical application of transvenous mitral commissurotomy by a new balloon catheter. J Thorac Cardiovasc Surg 1984; 87: 394–402.

Iung B, Cormier B, Ducimetiere P, Porte JM, Nallet O, Michel PL, Acar J, Vahanian A. Immediate results of percutaneous mitral commissurotomy. Circulation 1996; 94(9): 2124–2130.

Iung B, Garbarz E, Michaud P, Helou S, Farah B, Berdah P, Michel PL, Cormier B, Vahanian A. Late results of percutaneous mitral commissurotomy. Analysis of late clinical deterioration: frequency, anatomic findings, and predictive factors. Circulation 1999; 99(25): 3272–3278.

Jones RH, et al. Long-term survival benefits of coronary artery bypass grafting and percutaneous transluminal angioplasty in patients with coronary artery disease. J Thorac Cardiovasc Surg 1996; 111: 1013–1025.

King SB 3rd, et al. A randomized trial comparing coronary angioplasty with coronary bypass surgery, Emory Angioplasty vs Surgery Trial (EAST). N Engl J Med 1994; 331: 1044–1050.

Palacios IF, Tuzcu ME, Weyman AE, et al. Clinical follow-up of patients undergoing percutaneous mitral balloon valvotomy. Circulation 1995; 91: 671–676.

Pan M, Medina A, Suarez de Lezo J, Hernandez E, Romero M, Pavlovic D, Melian F, Franco M, Cabrera JA, Romo E, et al. Factors determining late success after mitral balloon valvulotomy. Am J Cardiol 1993; 71(13): 1181–1185.

Parisi AF, et al. A comparison of angioplasty with medical therapy in the treatment of single-vessel coronary artery disease, Veteran Affairs ACME Investigators. NEJM 1992; 326: 10–16.

RITA Trial Participants. Coronary angioplasty versus coronary artery bypass surgery: Randomised Interventional Treatment of Angina (RITA) trial. Lancet 1993; 341(8845): 573–580.

RITA-2 Trial Participants. Coronary angioplasty versus medical therapy for angina: the second Randomised Intervention Treatment of Angina (RITA-2) trial. Lancet 1997; 350(9076): 461–468.

Rodriguez A, et al. Argentine randomized trial of percutaneous transluminal coronary angioplasty versus coronary artery bypass surgery in multivessel disease (ERACI): in-hospital results and 1-year follow-up, ERACI Group. J Am Coll Cardiol 1993; 22: 1060–1067.

SoS Investigators. Coronary artery bypass surgery versus percutaneous coronary intervention with stent implantation in patients with multivessel coronary artery disease (the Stent or Surgery trial). Lancet 2002; 360(9338): 965–970.

The STRESS Trial. A randomized comparison of coronary-stent placement and balloon angioplasty in the treatment of coronary artery disease, Stent Restenosis Study Investigators. N Engl J Med 1994; 331: 496–501.

Vahanian A. Percutaneous mitral commissurotomy. Eur Heart J 1996; 17: 1465–1469.

Yusuf S, et al. Effect of coronary artery bypass graft surgery on survival: overview of 10-year results from randomised trials by the Coronary Artery Bypass Graft Surgery Trialists Collaboration. Lancet 1994; 344: 563–570.

K. Moghissi, J.A.C. Thorpe and F. Ciulli (Eds.)
Moghissi's Essentials of Thoracic and Cardiac Surgery
© 2003 Elsevier Science B.V. All rights reserved

CHAPTER V.2

Imaging in cardiovascular disease

I.U. Haq and N.M. Wheeldon

Despite advances in diagnostic imaging techniques and an increasing number of novel investigations to aid diagnosis and management, the chest X-ray remains the most common initial imaging investigation in the vast majority of patients with heart disease. It is important to use a systematic approach when interpreting the chest X-ray to avoid missing relevant findings. The cardiac position, site and configuration should be noted. Structures in the mediastinum which may be visualised include the trachea, aorta, pulmonary arteries, superior vena cava and azygous vein. If enlarged, other structures such as the thyroid, thymus and lymph nodes can be seen. The lung fields should be checked to assess the vascular pattern and masses, the lung contours for signs of blurring or loss of definition, and the cardiac borders, mediastinal margins and diaphragms. Finally, the bases should be examined, in female patients the breast shadows should be examined, and the soft tissues should be checked for masses.

1. Chest radiography

Refer to Figs. 1a and 1b.

1.1. Heart size

The transverse cardiac diameter, that is, the horizontal distance between the extreme right and left borders, is normally less than 15 cm. Serial X-rays can quantify changes in heart size. The cardiothoracic ratio is the ratio of the transverse cardiac diameter and transverse chest diameter measured from the inside rib margin at the widest level of the chest. This is generally less than 50%.

An enlarged heart is due to an increase in chamber size or pericardial effusion. The heart may appear enlarged when epicardial fat shadows are present, particularly in obese patients. Chest X-rays are normally taken in the PA projection. An AP projection is sometimes necessary when the patient cannot mobilise from bed; this can produce a magnification artefact.

1.2. Chamber size

1.2.1. Left atrium
- The left atrium is situated posteriorly, resulting in the right heart appearing denser than the left.

An increase in left atrial size may result in the following:
- the right heart border having a double shadow as the left atrium produces a second convex shadow that does not extend down as far as the diaphragm.
- the left atrial appendage producing a convex bulge on the left heart border just below the hilum.
- the left main bronchus being elevated and the angle between the right and the left main bronchi increased.

1.3. Other chambers

Enlargement of the right ventricle produces anti-clockwise rotation of the heart about its vertical axis so that the apex is lifted above the diaphragm. With left ventricular enlargement, clockwise rotation of the heart means that the left ventricular contour elongates and the cardiac apex is displaced downwards and outwards. Assessment of right atrial size is very unreliable. It may produce a larger than normal extension of the heart shadow to the right of the midline and a horizontal upper right heart border.

aortic knuckle (the lower of the two bulges is due to post-stenotic dilation of the proximal descending aorta), and inferior rib notching due to pressure erosions of the walls of the intercostal grooves produced by the enlarged tortuous collateral arteries. It usually affects the third to eighth ribs, and is usually bilateral and symmetrical.

1.8. Ischaemic heart disease

A chest X-ray should be taken in all patients admitted with suspected myocardial infarction. It is useful for:
(a) Identification of evidence of acute heart failure: e.g. the presence of pulmonary oedema.
(b) Detecting complications: e.g. signs of pulmonary venous hypertension secondary to acute mitral regurgitation or VSD, a localised bulge to the left ventricular border in left ventricular aneurysm, sometimes with calcification, and pericardial and pleural effusions in Dressler's syndrome.
(c) Excluding non-cardiac causes of chest pain.

1.9. Valvular heart disease

1.9.1. Mitral stenosis
The heart size is usually normal. There may be calcification of the mitral valve and left atrial enlargement. Elevation of pulmonary venous pressure may lead to signs of pulmonary venous distension and pulmonary oedema. In long-standing severe disease, there is pulmonary arterial hypertension producing enlargement of the main and proximal pulmonary arteries. This may lead to right heart failure with dilatation of the right sided chambers.

1.9.2. Mitral regurgitation
The heart is enlarged and there may be marked aneurysmal dilatation of the left atrium and ventricle in severe chronic regurgitation. In chronic regurgitation features of pulmonary hypertension and oedema are less common than in mitral stenosis. In acute regurgitation, pulmonary oedema is present without an increase in heart size.

1.9.3. Aortic stenosis
There may be aortic valve calcification and a displaced cardiac apex due to left ventricular hypertrophy. The ascending aorta may be prominent due to post-stenotic dilatation.

1.9.4. Aortic regurgitation
The heart is enlarged due to left ventricular dilatation and the ascending aorta is prominent. There may be mild left atrial enlargement and calcification of the aortic valve. Signs of pulmonary venous hypertension occur late in the course of the disease.

1.9.5. Prosthetic valves
All valves apart from homografts are radio-opaque and can be seen on the chest X-ray. It may be possible to detect abnormalities, e.g. strut fractures and bioprosthetic calcification.

2. Cardiovascular MRI and CT

Computed tomography (CT) and magnetic resonance imaging (MRI) are newer cardiac imaging techniques which are increasingly in use. They can be used as an adjunct to other investigations in ischaemic heart disease, in the evaluation of cardiac dimensions and function, pericardial disease, congenital heart disease, paracardiac and cardiac masses and for aortic imaging.

2.1. Ischaemic heart disease

Magnetic resonance angiography of the coronary arteries has recently reached clinical practice. At present it can consistently image only the proximal coronary arteries. It can be used to evaluate the patency of bypass grafts. Both CT and MRI can demonstrate regional wall thinning and complications of infarction such as left ventricular aneurysm and mural thrombus. Left ventricular segmental dysfunction such as reduced wall thickening and wall motion can be assessed with gated images. Electron beam CT may be used to detect coronary artery calcification suggesting the presence of coronary artery disease.

2.2. Assessment of cardiac function

Measurement of ventricular volumes with these techniques are very accurate and correlate well with post-mortem findings. Derived volumes are more accurate than standard 2-D echocardiography as they are based on three dimensions and therefore do not rely on geometrical assumptions to derive three-dimensional volumes from one or two planes. Wall thickness and myocardial mass can be accurately estimated. Indices such as stroke volume can be calculated from the ventricular volumes.

2.3. Valvular heart disease

Although echo is the investigation of choice for valvular heart disease, with advancing MRI technology, blood velocities through stenotic valves can be measured and thereby pressure gradients can be deduced. If there is a single regurgitant valve, ventricular volumetry can be performed: the difference in right ventricle and left ventricle stroke volumes is equal to the regurgitant volume through the valve. The degree of aortic regurgitation can be assessed by the volume of retrograde flow in the ascending aorta during diastole.

2.4. Pericardial disease

MRI or CT may be of help in locating local disease as a cause of pericardial effusion, even though echo is the imaging modality of choice. Solid pericardial disease is difficult to evaluate with echo but can be visualised with CT or MRI. Pericardial thickness greater than 3 mm can help differentiate constrictive pericardial disease from restrictive cardiomyopathy.

2.5. Congenital heart disease

MRI may occasionally provide additional information to echocardiography in children. It is often more useful in adults in whom echocardiography is limited. It can accurately define anatomy and quantify flow though shunts and surgical bypass conduits.

2.6. Aortic imaging

CT and MRI are excellent at imaging thoracic aortic pathology. MRI is particularly suitable in dissection, aortitis and coarctation and is ideal in surveillance because of its reproducibility and the absence of ionising radiation. MRI is a particularly accurate imaging method for aortic dissection and can be used in an emergency or in chronic dissection to monitor aortic dilatation and to plan surgery. CT with intravenous contrast is also commonly used to diagnose aortic dissection. CT and MRI can be used as screening tools in mediastinal trauma. MRI is ideal for imaging the anatomy of coarctation.

3. Myocardial perfusion scintigraphy

Isotope-labelled perfusion tracers with scintigraphic imaging to demonstrate areas of reduced myocardial perfusion is a sensitive and reliable method of demonstrating myocardial ischaemia, which can guide prognosis and treatment in patients with exertional chest pain. The sensitivity and specificity is higher than is achieved with exercise stress testing. In the diagnosis of coronary artery disease with tomographic imaging, sensitivity is 93% and specificity 88%. However, it is not a standard screening test in patients with exertional chest pain for reasons of cost and radiation exposure. As a second-line investigation, it is helpful when additional or alternative information to that provided by a standard exercise test is required.

Cardiovascular stress can be provided either by exercising the patient on a treadmill or may be achieved pharmacologically with an inotrope (e.g. dobutamine), or a vasodilator (e.g. dipyridamole or adenosine). The isotope should ideally distribute in the myocardium in linear proportion to bloodflow over the range of values experienced in health and disease. There should be efficient myocardial extraction from the blood on first passage through the heart, stable retention within the myocardium during data acquisition, rapid elimination allowing repeat studies under different conditions, ready availability, competitive pricing, and good imaging characteristics. No current tracer possesses all of these properties and compromises have to be made.

Thallium 201 and ^{99M}Tc-MIBI are common tracers, although ^{99M}Tc-tetrofosmin is gaining in use. It is lipophilic and rapidly cleared from the blood after intravenous injection, uptake in the myocardium is rapid, and there is little redistribution. It is regionally distributed within the myocardium in proportion to bloodflow at the time of injection.

The isotope is injected at peak exercise and images are taken with a γ camera after 30–45 minutes. These images are compared with rest images taken some days later after a second injection of isotope. Interpretation can be enhanced by the use of single-photon emission CT. Areas of myocardial ischaemia are identified by reduced uptake of isotope in stress images but not rest images. Reduced uptake in the same anatomical distribution on both stress and rest images indicates areas of myocardial infarction.

Myocardial perfusion scintigraphy is useful for assessing prognosis in patients with exertional chest pain. A normal scan indicates an excellent prognosis with a 10-year cardiac mortality of less than 1%. The extent and severity of perfusion defects and the presence of multi-territory abnormalities all assist the estimation of prognosis. The test is often used to prioritise patients for coronary angiography. Conversely, the functional significance of coronary artery stenoses identified angiographically can be determined.

4. Coronary angiography

Refer to Figs. 4a, 4b, and 4c.

Coronary angiography remains the 'gold standard' for diagnosis, estimating prognosis and plan-

ning treatment strategies in patients with exertional chest pain. The cardiac surgeon should be completely *au fait* with interpreting coronary angiograms since they indicate the severity and extent of coronary artery stenoses and, if the best treatment for the patient is coronary artery bypass grafting, the images allow the surgeon to determine which vessels need grafting.

The technique involves the insertion of specially shaped cardiac catheters into the coronary vessels. Then 5–10 ml of contrast medium is injected to

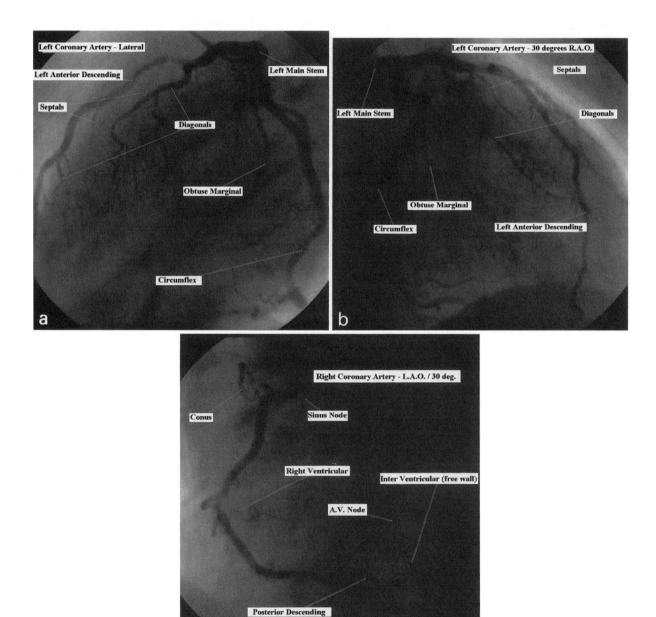

Fig. 4. (a) Left coronary artery system: lateral projection. (b) Left coronary system: 30° right anterior oblique projection. (c) Right coronary artery: 30° left anterior oblique projection.

outline the arterial tree for imaging. Views of the same coronary artery are taken from different angles using repeated injections of dye. Dye may also be injected into the left ventricle to assess left ventricular function. The procedure is performed under local anaesthetic, most commonly via the femoral artery approach.

4.1. Indications

Angiography is useful in patients in whom non-invasive testing (e.g. exercise tests, myocardial scintigraphy) is equivocal, or in those who have a history highly suggestive of coronary artery disease, when non-invasive tests are negative. This is because of false positives and negatives with non-invasive tests; the rate of these is largely dependent on the pre-test probability of coronary artery disease. Angiography in the patient with multiple admissions for 'chest pain — ? cause' when other avenues have been exhausted will help confirm or refute the presence of coronary artery disease and can be a cost-effective means of management.

4.2. Prognosis

Angiography will enable the severity, extent and location of coronary stenoses to be determined and the impact of the disease on left ventricular function. In conjunction with non-invasive testing, this information yields prognostic information, and helps determine the optimal treatment plan for the individual patient.

4.3. Possible revascularisation

The results of coronary angiography are important in the planning of treatment strategies in patients with coronary artery disease. The decision to proceed with the test depends on the estimated risk of future cardiac events. In addition to the history, factors to take into account are the severity of angina, unstable angina, early post-infarction angina, the presence of ischaemia-related heart failure and general coronary risk factors such as age, sex, smoking status, hypertension, hyperlipidaemia, diabetes and disease in vascular beds other than the heart.

Surgical revascularisation has been shown to improve symptoms and to enhance survival in patients with stenosis of the left main coronary artery and in those with proximal three-vessel coronary artery disease with impairment of left ventricular function.

4.4. Percutaneous transluminal coronary angioplasty (PTCA)

The technique of PTCA is initially similar to coronary angiography. Once the guiding catheter is seated in the coronary artery ostium, a guide wire is passed down the artery and a balloon is directed down the wire to the target lesion. Dilatation of the balloon enlarges the arterial lumen by stretching the vessel wall and by forcing the atherosclerotic plaque into the medial layer. Patients are pre-treated with aspirin and intravenous boluses of heparin. The acute occlusion rate is about 5% per lesion attempted and the restenosis rate is around 30%. The complication rate has fallen since the advent of stents.

The feasibility and success of PTCA depends on both angiographic variables and the clinical setting. Angiographic predictors of restenosis include lesions on sharp bends in vessels, ostial lesions at major bifurcations, proximal or mid-vessel lesions in vein grafts, restenosis after PTCA and chronic total occlusions. Tortuous vessels proximal to the target lesion may be difficult to reach with the balloon. Calcification may lead to failure of dilatation. Lesions in the left main stem or in a last remaining vessel supplying the whole of the left ventricle have greater procedural mortality.

Clinical variables associated with a higher complication rate include advancing age, past myocardial infarction or heart failure and patients with unstable angina.

4.5. Stents

Stents are fenestrated tubes or cages that can be expanded by a balloon to provide a scaffold within coronary arteries. The introduction of stents has led to a decrease in the incidence of abrupt vessel closure. However, stents are not free of complications. Subacute occlusion may occur up to ten days after stent implantation. The incidence is reduced with antiplatelet therapy, e.g. the combination of aspirin and ticlopidine, or aspirin and clopidogrel. Restenosis is more common when long stents are used. Very occasionally, the stent may dislodge from the balloon during the procedure and embolise into the systemic circulation.

5. Echocardiography and Doppler ultrasound

Echocardiography is an invaluable investigation in many clinical situations and may preclude the need for more invasive tests. The transducer contains a piezo-electric crystal which acts as the source for ultrasound. A small amount of the sound energy is reflected at interfaces between tissues of different acoustic impedance. The transducer also acts as the receiver of this reflected ultrasound. Sound travels through soft tissue and blood at a constant speed. It is therefore possible to determine the depth of a structure by the time delay between emission of the ultrasonic signal and the return of its echo to the transducer. This delay determines the position of a spot on the display screen and the magnitude of the signal determines the brightness of the spot.

5.1. 2-D echocardiography

By placing the transducer in between rib spaces at different sites on the chest wall, the heart can be imaged in cross-section in different planes. The most common views are:

- Parasternal long-axis, in which the right and left ventricles, mitral and aortic valves and the proximal ascending aorta are seen through the long axis of the heart (Fig. 5a).
- Parasternal short-axis, obtained by rotating the probe through 90°. Tilting the transducer allows imaging of the aortic valve, mitral valve and the cavity of the left ventricle (Fig. 5b).
- With the transducer at the apex, all four cardiac chambers can be viewed in section, as well as the atrial and ventricular septa and the pulmonary

veins. Rotation of the probe through 90° produces images in the 'apical long axis' and 'apical two-chamber' planes.

- Less common is subcostal imaging which allows good views of the atrial septum and caval veins, and the descending aorta and pulmonary trunk.

5.2. M-mode echocardiography

On an M-mode trace, echoes returning across a chosen scan line are displayed in a recurring pattern with the ECG. By concentrating on directing a single beam of ultrasound in a single direction, temporal and spatial resolutions are enhanced. More precise measurements can often be made compared to 2-D images. However, only a small part of the heart can be imaged at any one time, making it difficult to elucidate relationships between cardiac structures, or to draw conclusions when the heart is affected patchily. In practice, M-mode and 2-D echocardiography are complementary.

5.3. Doppler techniques

The Doppler principle allows the velocity of flow within the heart to be estimated accurately. The shift in frequency of a waveform (i.e. the transmitted ultrasound) is proportional to the velocity of the source (e.g. the reflecting surfaces of moving blood cells) relative to the observer (e.g. the ultrasound transducer). The echo machine displays calculated velocities of flow rather than the shift in frequency.

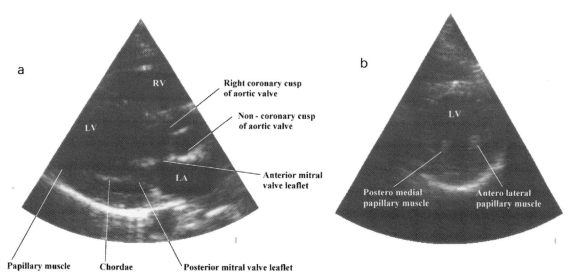

Fig. 5. (a) Parasternal long axis view of the heart. (b) Parasternal short axis view of the heart at left ventricular level. The posteromedial and anterolateral papillary muscles can both be seen.

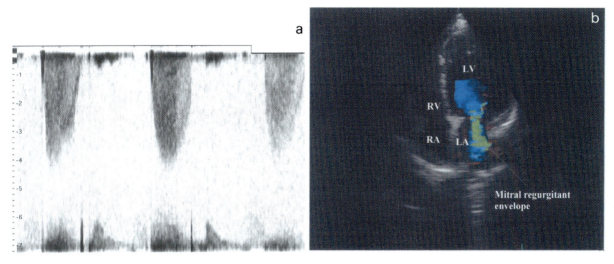

Fig. 6. (a) Continuous wave recording from the apex in a patient with aortic stenosis, showing velocity on the vertical axis and time on the horizontal axis. The high velocity signal of 4.2 ms^{-1} is from blood passing through the stenotic valve, giving an estimated pressure difference across the valve of 70 mmHg. (b) Mitral regurgitation colour flow map. There is significant regurgitation as shown by a region of flow recruitment in the left ventricle, a wide neck at the level of the valve and a large intra-atrial portion. This is a slightly oblique apical four chamber view. The apical approach is used to look at the apex and free wall and at the right ventricle which tends to be sliced obliquely in other views.

With pulsed Doppler, the velocity of bloodflow is assessed at one site, selected by positioning the sample volume at the desired depth along the cursor line superimposed on a two-dimensional display of the heart. Flow towards the transducer is displayed above the baseline and flow away from it is displayed below. Pulsed Doppler is useful for measuring normal and low velocities (1–3 ms^{-1}).

Continuous wave Doppler uses a transducer that emits a constant stream of ultrasound in a single direction. It simultaneously receives the returning echoes continuously. It can record very high velocities of flow. The drop in pressure across an obstruction such as a stenotic valve is proportional to the increase in velocity of blood as it flows across it. Thus gradients across stenosed valves can be estimated (Fig. 6a).

5.3.1. Colour flow mapping

In colour flow mapping, the cross-sectional image is divided into numerous sample volumes, arranged at uniform intervals along each scan line. At each site, pulsed Doppler is used to estimate the mean velocity of all the blood cells moving within it. This is assigned a colour which is displayed in the corresponding pixel on the echocardiographic image. Flow towards the transducer is displayed in red and flow away is displayed in blue. Turbulence results in a mosaic of different colours. The technique allows identification of abnormal patterns of flow which may then be interrogated with pulsed and continuous wave Doppler (Fig. 6b).

5.3.2. Indications

Transthoracic echocardiography can be used in a variety of clinical settings.

- *Congenital heart disease:* In patients with congenital heart disease, echocardiography has supplanted cardiac catheterisation in many situations.
- *Ischaemic heart disease:* In patients with ischaemic heart disease, echocardiography is useful in assessing contractile function. Affected myocardium may show abnormalities of wall motion. These changes often occur early on in patients in the process of myocardial infarction. Stress echocardiography to assess regional changes in left ventricular function can be used to detect areas of viable myocardium. It adds substantially to the sensitivity and specificity of exercise testing. Echocardiography may also be useful in assessing the complications of myocardial infarction. For example, it can distinguish between cardiogenic shock caused by severe left ventricular damage, right ventricular infarction and cardiac rupture with tamponade. It is useful, in patients who develop a new pansystolic murmur after infarction, to distinguish between acute mitral regurgitation and ventricular septal rupture.

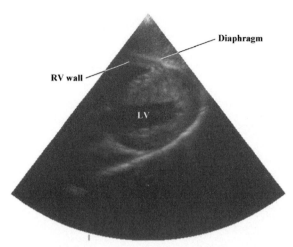

Fig. 7. Subcostal view of the left ventricle in a patient with hypertrophic cardiomyopathy. Note the significant hypertrophy of both the septum and posterior wall and small left ventricular cavity size.

- *Heart failure:* Echocardiography should be carried out in all patients with a new diagnosis of heart failure. It helps distinguish between 'systolic heart failure' due to impaired left ventricular contractile function and 'diastolic heart failure' as a result of poor compliance of an ageing and inelastic ventricle or of a hypertrophied ventricle in a patient with hypertension. Diagnosis of the aetiology of heart failure is often possible, such as severe aortic stenosis, other valvular heart disease, or left ventricular aneurysm. By assessing global left ventricular function, echo is also useful in determining prognosis.
- *Hypertrophic cardiomyopathy:* The thickness of the myocardium can be measured in different parts of the heart. Classical features are systolic anterior motion of the mitral apparatus and dynamic obstruction of the left ventricular outflow tract shown by Doppler techniques (Fig. 7).
- *Pericardial disease:* Echocardiography is a sensitive means of detecting pericardial effusion. In patients with tamponade, there is right ventricular and atrial diastolic collapse and exaggerated falls in the velocity of flow across the mitral and tricuspid valves on inspiration.
- *Valvular heart disease:* Echo is useful for diagnosing and quantifying valve stenosis and regurgitation. This is best carried out by a combination of 2-D and M-mode studies, colour flow mapping and spectral Doppler. The consequences of valvular pathology on ventricular dimensions and function may also be assessed. Echo is also useful in diagnosing mitral valve prolapse, studying

prosthetic valves and in demonstrating vegetations in patients with infective endocarditis. Complications of infective endocarditis can also be shown, such as fistulas and abscesses, although transoesophageal echo is more sensitive (Fig. 8).
- *Intracardiac masses:* Thrombus in the heart can be demonstrated and echo is therefore useful in patients with unexplained sources of embolism (Fig. 9). Myxoma is readily demonstrated on 2-D echo.

5.4. Transoesophageal echocardiography

Transoesophageal echocardiography (TOE) accounts for about 5% of all echo studies. The patient is fasted, false teeth and other foreign bodies are removed from the mouth, and the pharynx is sprayed with a topical anaesthetic. The patient may be given sedation. The probe is then passed into the oesophagus which lies directly behind the left atrium providing an optimal site for ultrasonic examination of the heart and thoracic aorta. The principal complications are failed oesophageal intubation, excessive sedation, arrhythmias, oesophageal mucosal tears, vomiting, aspiration and, very occasionally, oesophageal rupture. Complications are uncommon, and the procedure can often be performed safely as an out-patient. The latest multiplane probes incorporate a single transducer that can be rotated electronically through 180° and thus produce images of heart through multiple cross-sections.

5.4.1. Indications and clinical applications of transoesophageal echocardiography
TOE can be used when transthoracic studies are inadequate or impractical such as intraoperative studies, patients with chest deformities or pulmonary disease, or patients on mechanical ventilation. Other indications include the following:

Valve disease. TOE is used to assess the suitability for balloon valvuloplasty in patients with mitral stenosis. It can assess the extent of commisural fusion and cusp thickening, calcification, mobility and involvement of subvalvular structures. In patients with mitral regurgitation being considered for surgical treatment, TOE can be used to assess the suitability of the valve for repair (as opposed to replacement). In patients with prosthetic valves, there is often a lot of acoustic shadowing behind the valve making imaging difficult with transthoracic studies. TOE is more sensitive in mitral prosthetic valve

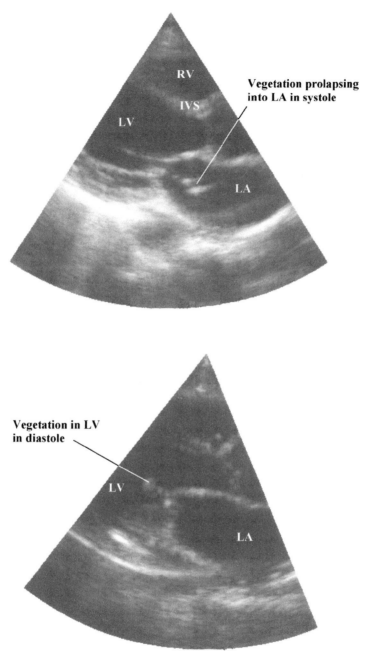

Fig. 8. Classic appearance of a vegetation attached to the anterior mitral valve leaflet. The echogenic mass is seen in the left ventricle in diastole and prolapses into the left atrium in systole.

dysfunction although aortic prosthetic valves can be difficult to evaluate from the oesophagus. It is also used to diagnose paraprosthetic and transvalvular regurgitation, prosthetic valve dehiscence, thrombi and vegetations adherent to prosthetic valves, and degeneration of the leaflets of tissue valves.

Infective endocarditis. TOE can detect vegetations less than 1 mm wide and is thus more sensitive than transthoracic echo. It is also more accurate in the detection of endocarditis-related complications, e.g. abscess formation, valve perforation and flail leaflets.

Suspected cardiac source of embolism. TOE is indicated in patients who have sustained a recent cere-

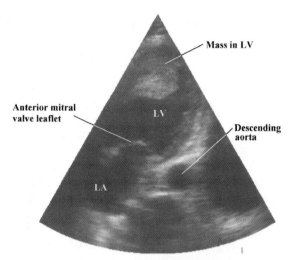

Fig. 9. Thrombus at the left ventricular apex. The patient had sustained a myocardial infarction with consequent apical akinesis. The mass is more echodense than the surrounding myocardium and there is a division between it and the myocardium — classic features of thrombus.

brovascular accident or peripheral embolism if there is clinical evidence of valve disease or atrial fibril-lation. It may also be useful if an abnormality on transthoracic imaging requires further information. In patients undergoing elective cardioversion of atrial fibrillation, TOE can be used to assess the presence of thrombus in the left atrium and atrial appendage. A more pragmatic approach, however, is to anticoagulate patients for 4 weeks prior to cardioversion.

Aortic disease. TOE can be performed in acute dissection to confirm the diagnosis and to define the extent of the dissection and plan the surgical approach. This should only be undertaken in cardiac centres. Patients with a low likelihood of aortic dissection, or suspected dissection involving the descending aorta only, may be investigated by TOE, MRI or contrast CT.

Other indications. TOE is increasingly being used in patients with complex congenital heart disease. It may also be used to monitor left ventricular function during non-cardiac surgery, and immediately post-operatively to confirm a satisfactory result after valve repair or replacement.

CHAPTER V.3

A. Anaesthetic management for cardiac surgery

C. Paoloni and S. Ghosh

1. Introduction

With the evolution of a wide range of cardiac procedures to rectify disease states ranging from congenital anomalies to ischaemic heart disease and valvular lesions, anaesthesia for cardiac surgery has developed into a speciality in its own right. This section provides a broad summary of the anaesthetic principles applicable to the peri-operative care of cardiac surgical patients.

Anaesthesia for patients with cardiac pathology is inherently hazardous (Radr et al., 1999) because of the haemodynamic consequences associated both with the administration of anaesthetic agents and the transition from spontaneous respiration to the application of intermittent positive pressure ventilation (IPPV). There are several mechanisms by which anaesthesia (Guarracino et al., 1998) can lead to cardiac dysfunction in previously asymptomatic patients or acute deterioration in those with pre-existing symptoms.

Anaesthetic agents may cause:
- depression of myocardial contractility, either as a direct effect or through sympathetic blockade (Engoren et al., 1998)
- vasodilatation, usually as a result of depression of central vasomotor centres, or as a direct effect on smooth muscle
- bradycardia, usually via a vagally mediated effect
- tachycardia, through vagal blockade, direct or indirect sympathomimetic actions, or as a reflex response to vasodilatation (Engoren et al., 1998; Guarracino et al., 1998)
- arrhythmias, through sensitisation of the myocardium to circulating catecholamines or as a direct effect
- intra-myocardial redistribution of coronary blood flow, usually causing a diversion or 'steal' from the subendocardium

The application of IPPV is necessary for the safe maintenance of adequate ventilation with the chest open, but has cardiovascular effects which include (Branson et al., 1999; Michalopoulos et al., 1998):
- alteration of venous return to the heart, as a result of increased mean intra-thoracic pressure
- alteration of pulmonary artery pressure, through transmission of positive alveolar pressure to pulmonary vessels

The choice of individual anaesthetic agents has not been conclusively demonstrated to affect outcome after cardiac surgery. The key principles of anaesthetic management are that the potential for decline in cardiovascular status is anticipated and that the chosen technique aims to minimise the haemodynamic disturbance. Avoidance of those factors likely to result in decompensation, utilisation of intrinsic compensatory mechanisms, an understanding of the pathophysiology of the cardiac lesion and recognition of the patient's cardiac reserve are essential for optimal anaesthetic management.

2. Pre-operative anaesthetic assessment and preparation

Refer to Guarracino et al. (1998) and Michalopoulos et al. (1998).

The pre-operative anaesthetic assessment should focus on:
- the underlying cardiac pathology
- the degree of limitation of cardiac function
- concomitant pathology, especially cerebrovascular disease, renal dysfunction, pulmonary disease and diabetes
- current drug therapy
- laboratory investigations

Particular emphasis should be placed on identification of patients who may be further optimised from a medical standpoint. Whilst little improvement in cardiac function may be gained without surgery, some patients may benefit from aggressive medical treatment, e.g. to correct cardiac failure and reduce pulmonary oedema pre-operatively, amelioration of coincidental pulmonary disease, stabilisation of diabetes, blood transfusion for anaemia or correction of electrolyte imbalances (Zaidi et al., 1999).

2.1. Drug therapy

Drugs most commonly prescribed for cardiac surgical patients include diuretics, anti-arrhythmics, vasodilators, anti-coagulants, lipid lowering agents, hypoglycaemic agents, bronchodilators and, less commonly, steroids.

Pre-operative cessation of drug therapy that has maintained the patient in an optimal state until the time of surgery is not recommended. The adverse effects of sudden discontinuation of Beta-blockers or calcium channel antagonists are well recognised and it is common practise to continue all cardiovascular drugs up to the day of surgery. One notable exception is the group of Angiotensin Converting Enzyme (ACE) inhibitors; patients on ACE inhibitors tend to have persistently low systemic vascular resistances in the post-cardiopulmonary bypass (CPB) period and some require vasopressors, e.g. noradrenaline, to maintain an adequate blood pressure.

It is thus becoming widely accepted that ACE inhibitors should be discontinued a few days pre-operatively (Zaidi et al., 1999).

Aspirin should have been discontinued 7 to 12 days pre-operatively. Patients on warfarin should ideally have omitted 2 or 3 doses to allow the prothrombin time to fall to less than 1.5 times the control value. Heparin is usually allowed to continue until the time of surgery.

Most hypoglycaemic agents can safely be continued until the night before surgery. With sugars being monitored regularly, longer-lasting agents, e.g. metformin, are best discontinued at least 24 hours pre-operatively.

Patients on steroids, e.g. for lung disease or connective tissue disorders, require additional steroids in the peri-operative period to avoid the development of hypoadrenalism in response to the stress imposed by surgery.

3. Premedication

The aim of premedication (Engoren et al., 1998; Guarracino et al., 1998) is to produce sedation and anxiolysis such that the tachycardic and hypertensive responses to stress are obtunded. This is generally achieved using benzodiazepines (e.g. lorazepam, diazepam or temazepam), opiates (e.g. Morphine or fentanyl), or a combination of benzodiazepine and opiate. Anticholinergic agents are widely used for their anti-sialogue effect. Hyoscine or glycopyrrolate are more suitable than atropine because of their lesser effect on heart rate.

4. Monitoring for anaesthesia

The minimal standards of monitoring required for cardiac surgery include ECG, pulse oximetry, capnography, invasive arterial and central venous pressure measurement, core temperature and urine output. The timing of placement of invasive monitoring in relation to induction of anaesthesia varies according to the preferences of individual anaesthetists. Some institutions routinely utilise pulmonary artery flotation (PA) catheters intra-operatively. More recently trans-oesophageal echocardiography (TOE) has begun to gain acceptance, not only as a means of assessing valvular function prior to and following valve repair, but as a means of monitoring left heart filling and ventricular performance. Use of PA catheters and/or TOE is certainly beneficial in selected cases but is of questionable value as a routine practice.

Monitoring of the electrical activity of the brain to detect cerebral hypoperfusion during CPB is of limited value in predicting post-operative neurological outcome. The use of near-infra-red spectroscopy to non-invasively monitor cerebral surface oxygen saturation using probes placed on the scalp and trans-cranial Doppler to measure middle cerebral arterial blood velocity are both under evaluation during cardiac surgery.

5. Choice of anaesthetic and conduct of anaesthesia and CPB

A wide variety of agents for the induction and maintenance of anaesthesia (Engoren et al., 1998) and for muscle relaxation have been employed for cardiac surgery. The haemodynamic effects of individual agents are well-documented; but studies of the influence of anaesthetic technique on morbidity and mortality after either coronary or valvular surgery have demonstrated that choice of individual agents is of relatively little importance in determining outcome. In the absence of contrary evidence, it would appear that rational combination of any of the available agents, bearing in mind the pathophysiology of the underlying disease and the need for maintenance of haemodynamic stability, is the key to cardiac anaesthesia.

Induction of anaesthesia for cardiac surgery is most commonly done by a combination of benzodiazepine (e.g. midazolam or diazepam) and moderate-to high-dose opiate (e.g. fentanyl or sufentanil), followed by an infusion of an intravenous agent (e.g. Propofol), to maintain anaesthesia using a total intravenous anaesthetic technique (TIVA). Alternatively anaesthesia may be maintained using an inhalational agent such as Isoflurane. If an inhalational agent is chosen, then this can be administered via the oxygenator gas flow during CPB whilst the lungs are not ventilated.

Nitrous oxide is generally avoided for cardiac procedures because of its myocardial depressant effects when administered with moderate doses of opiates and because of its propensity to diffuse into and cause expansion of gaseous microemboli.

The induction of anaesthesia by bolus injection of conventional anaesthetic induction agents (e.g. etomidate, thiopentone, propofol) is less widely practised for cardiac surgery than for other types of surgery. This is because of the adverse haemodynamic consequences likely to be encountered in this group of patients who poorly tolerate the sudden vasodilatation and myocardial depression associated with these agents.

Muscle relaxation for intubation, facilitation of Intermittent-Positive Pressure Ventilation (IPPV) and prevention of diaphragmatic movement is achieved using non-depolarising agents that competitively antagonise the effects of acetylcholine at the neuromuscular junction. The most commonly used muscle relaxant for cardiac surgery is Pancuronium which has a relatively long duration of action, produces minimal vasodilatation and, when administered with moderate doses of opiate, maintains a stable heart rate or slight tachycardia; the overall effect being minimal change in mean arterial pressure.

Hypertensive responses to skin incision, sternotomy and aortic manipulation should be anticipated and controlled by administration of additional opiate or use of an infusion of a titratable, short-acting hypotensive agent, e.g. sodium nitroprusside or glyceryl trinitrate. Undesirable tachycardia is best treated using the short-acting beta-blocker Esmolol.

- Arterial blood gases are measured after commencement of IPPV and a baseline activated clotting time (ACT) determined before anticoagulation with heparin. Blood gases and ACT are repeated at set points: post-heparinization, 10 minutes after initiation of CPB, at 30-minute intervals during CPB, immediately prior to separation from CPB and after return to physiological circulation.

- Following surgical exposure of the heart and prior to aortic cannulation, Heparin 3 mg/kg is given and the ACT is checked to ensure a rise to greater than 380 seconds. Following arterial and venous cannulation, CPB is commenced. On establishment of full flow through the CPB circuit, ventilation is discontinued and the lungs allowed to deflate.

- Optimal perfusion pressures and flow rates during CPB for preservation of organ function have yet to be conclusively established. Perfusion at moderate flow rates (flow index 1.8 to 2.2 l/min/m^2) and low pressures (40 to 50 mmHg) is satisfactory.

- Haemodilution to a Haematocrit of 22 to 25% as a result of blood being diluted with the CPB priming fluid and, in some centres deliberate venesection, may enhance blood flow through small capillaries by reducing blood viscosity.
 Moderate hypothermia with core cooling to 28–30°C enhances organ, particularly cerebral, preservation, though there is currently a trend to maintain normothermia during CPB for uncomplicated coronary surgery and, in some cases, even for valve surgery.

- Cerebral blood flow during CPB is determined by perfusion flow rate, arterial pCO$_2$ and perfusion pressure. Management of arterial blood gases during CPB may follow the alpha-stat or pH-stat principles. Moderate hypercapnia (pCO$_2$ of 5.5 to 6.5 kPa at temperature corrected to 37°C) ensures cerebral vasodilatation and enhanced cerebral blood flow and may reduce the incidence of neurological injury.
 Other measures that can be taken to minimise cerebral injury during CPB include rigorous monitoring and control of blood glucose and sodium. The administration of the barbiturate Thiopentone (30 to 40 mg/kg) reduces cerebral oxygen requirement and is of benefit if given prior to circulatory arrest.
 Perfusion pressure during CPB is controlled by

the use of vasopressors such as phenylephrine or metaraminol, or vasodilators such as phentolamine or diazoxide, as required.

- On completion of surgery on the heart itself the following parameters should be met before weaning from CPB:
  – core temperature 37°C
  – base deficit <5 mmol/l
  – serum potassium 4.5 to 5.5 mmol/l
  – haematocrit >24%
  – stable rhythm/moderate tachycardia (80 to 90 beats/min)
  – perfusion pressure >45 mmHg
  – mechanical ventilation of lungs re-established
- On transition from CPB to physiological circulation, protamine 3 mg/kg is given to reverse heparinization and the ACT is checked to ensure a return to baseline values. Additional protamine is given in small doses if required. Adverse effects of protamine include a reduction in systemic vascular resistance and increase in pulmonary vascular resistance and this may produce a marked fall in blood pressure.

The haematocrit is restored to normal values by the administration of residual blood from the CPB circuit, autologous blood if this has been venesected prior to CPB and the use of Bank blood if required. If diuresis has been poor during CPB this can be induced using frusemide or mannitol to reduce the amount of retained water from the CPB prime and cardioplegic solution.

- Anaesthesia is generally maintained until transfer of the ventilated patient to the Intensive Care Unit.

6. Post-operative sedation, analgesia and weaning from ventilation

6.1. Sedation and ventilation

Sedation and ventilation (Branson et al., 1999; Price et al., 1999) are generally continued until satisfactory core and peripheral body temperatures are attained and the patient is haemodynamically stable. A wide variety of regimens are in use for sedation and analgesia. Choice should be based on the relative haemodynamic effects of individual agents and whether early or delayed extubation are desired. Combinations of opiates (e.g. morphine or fentanyl) and benzodiazepines (e.g. midazolam or diazemuls) given intermittently or by continuous intravenous infusion, or infusion of an anaesthetic agent (e.g. propofol) are suitable. Bolus injection of Haloperi-

dol is useful in treating the small number of patients who display evidence of 'post-pump' psychosis on recovery from sedation.

6.1.1. Analgesic requirements

Analgesic requirements are generally not high after sternotomy (O'Connor, 1999) and intravenous infusion of opiate continuously or by a patient-controlled system on emergence from sedation is usually only required for the first 24 hours post-operatively. Thereafter analgesia using paracetamol, codeine and non-steroidal inflammatory drugs suffices.

6.2. Extubation

In some centres ventilation is routinely continued for a set period of time. For uncomplicated cases there is little evidence to suggest that delaying extubation is beneficial. In general, once the following parameters have been attained, sedation can be discontinued and the patient safely extubated:

- minimal bleeding
- acid-base status, electrolytes and haematocrit are within physiological limits
- blood gases are satisfactory at an inspired oxygen concentration <50%
- core temperature >35°C and core–peripheral temperature gradient <6°C
- analgesia has been given, rate and depth of spontaneous respiration are clinically satisfactory, patient is able to respond to command and is not distressed
- no coincidental disease requiring an extended period of weaning from ventilation, e.g. chronic respiratory insufficiency, and there is no evidence of lobar collapse, undrained pneumothorax or haemothorax
- blood pressure and cardiac rhythm are acceptable and stable

Extubation after uneventful cardiac surgery can usually be achieved by transition from mechanical ventilation to a short period of spontaneous respiration with the endotracheal tube in place and connected to a low-resistance circuit with a controlled oxygen flow, e.g. T-piece.

Patients often require a high inspired oxygen concentration after CPB because of shunting through the pulmonary circulation that develops most significantly as a result of:

- reperfusion injury sustained by the lungs following re-establishment of physiological circulation after a period of isolation during CPB

- the use of vasodilators, e.g. glyceryl trinitrate, sodium nitroprusside to control blood pressure, and anaesthetic agents

If mechanical ventilatory support is required to aid weaning from IPPV until adequate spontaneous respiration is established, then the following modes of ventilation are commonly available (Branson et al., 1999; Michalopoulos et al., 1998; Price et al., 1999):

6.2.1. Synchronised Intermittent Mandatory Ventilation (SIMV)

This mode allows the patient to breathe spontaneously between the pre-set mandatory tidal volumes delivered by the ventilator. Breaths are timed to coincide with the patient's own inspiratory effort and can be used with or without CPAP or PEEP.

In the weaning process the frequency of mandatory breaths is gradually reduced so that spontaneous ventilation takes over.

- Abolition of all respiratory efforts and heavy sedation can be avoided
- Reduction in mean intrathoracic pressure results in less cardiovascular depression
- Reduced risk of barotrauma

6.2.2. Pressure support ventilation (PSV)

Spontaneous breaths are augmented by a pre-set constant positive pressure of between 5 and 20 cm H_2O, the delivery of which is triggered by the patient's inspiratory effort and applied either for a fraction of the inspiratory time or until the inspiratory flow falls below a set level.

- Respiratory rate, inspiratory time and inspiratory flow rate are determined by the patient
- Tidal volume is determined by the level of pressure support, lung mechanics and patient effort
- Reduces the work of breathing
- Can be used with SIMV

6.2.3. Mandatory minute volume (MMV)

This is a modification which ensures a pre-set minute volume is received by the patient irrespective of minute-to-minute variations in the level of spontaneous ventilation.

6.2.4. Bimodal positive airway pressure ventilation (BIPAP)

Spontaneous breaths are augmented by pre-set positive pressures for inspiratory (IPAP) and expiratory (EPAP) phases separately. This provides pressure support for the inspiratory phase of a breath and PEEP in expiration in a cyclical pattern.

- Inspiratory positive airway pressure (IPAP) is initially set at 10–15 cm H_2O (=PS)
- Expiratory positive airway pressure (EPAP) is initially set at 5 cm H_2O (=PEEP)
  Adjustments are made in 2 cm H_2O increments

Choice of mode of delivery (change from IPAP to EPAP) is determined by the clinical indications:

- Spontaneous: set IPAP and EPAP as above, patient triggers
- Spontaneous/timed: set as above and set breaths per minute (BPM) at 2–5 below spontaneous rate
- Timed: set as above and set BPM slightly greater than spontaneous rate

6.2.5. Positive end expiratory pressure (PEEP)

This should be considered if oxygenation of arterial blood (>90% Hb saturation) proves difficult to achieve despite inspired oxygen concentration greater than 50%.

A pressure of between 5–10 cm H_2O is pre-set for the end expiratory phase of the respiratory cycle.

- Expands under-ventilated lung units
- Increases functional residual capacity (FRC)
- Decreases venous admixture if shunting is due to alveolar collapse
- May benefit patients with cardiac failure with low cardiac output as the reduction in pre and afterload can decrease wall tension and increase the balance of myocardial oxygen supply and demand

Potential problems:

- Increased risk of barotrauma.
- Increased intrathoracic pressure reduces venous return and increases pulmonary vascular resistance which reduces cardiac output.
- PEEP >10 cm H_2O is associated with increased pulmonary vascular resistance, which may result in increased right ventricular afterload with right ventricular dilatation. Deviation of the inter ventricular septum into the left ventricle may impair left ventricular filling and cardiac output.

6.2.6. Continuous positive airway pressure (CPAP) (Fig. 1)

This is applied using a flow generator and CPAP valve attached to a T-piece circuit on the endotracheal tube. This method is useful in weaning patients who have required PEEP while being ventilated. CPAP may also be applied by means of a tight-fitting face mask with appropriate CPAP valve (2.5–10 cm H_2O).

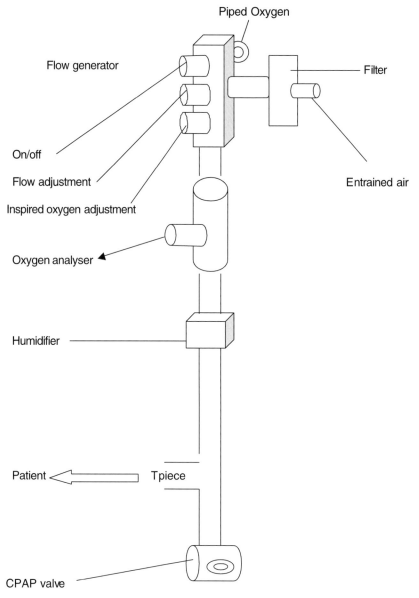

Fig. 1. Continuous positive airway pressure (CPAP) Circuit.

- Improves oxygenation and lung mechanics by recruitment collapsed alveoli and improved distribution of inspired gas.
- Decreases airway resistance during inspiration.
- Respiratory rate falls, tidal volume and vital capacity increases.

- Mean intrathoracic pressure is lower with CPAP than IPPV plus PEEP and so haemodynamic depression is minimised.

B. Anaesthetic management of thoracic procedures

1. Introduction

Thoracic surgery poses particular challenges to the anaesthetist because of the need to safely establish and maintain ventilation in patients with compromised lung function and to provide one-lung anaesthesia in patients with limited respiratory reserve (Coucher et al., 1997; Kavanagh and Sandler, 1996; Zollinger et al., 1998). Thoracic operations range from diagnostic procedures such as bronchoscopy, thoracoscopy, and mediastinoscopy, to therapeutic resection of intrathoracic tissue by minimally invasive techniques or by thoracotomy. This section concentrates on the indications for, and techniques of, one-lung ventilation and also highlights the importance of the provision of good quality post-operative pain relief in reducing post-operative respiratory complications (Grant, 1999; Slinger, 1999).

2. One-lung ventilation

The indications for one-lung ventilation can be broadly summarised as:
- prevention of soiling of one lung by spillage of material from the other
- control of the distribution of ventilation
- facilitation of surgical access for operations on the lung or other intra-thoracic structures

One-lung ventilation is currently most commonly achieved by placement of a double lumen endobronchial tube. Inflation of both the tracheal and endobronchial cuffs effectively separates the lungs. Clamping off the gas supply to one lumen and opening it to atmosphere diverts ventilation to the opposite lung and causes the isolated lung to collapse. Double lumen tubes can be difficult to correctly position, particularly on the right side. The shorter right main bronchus with its earlier origin of the upper lobe bronchus than on the left requires careful positioning of the endobronchial limb to ensure that the cuff does not occlude the orifice of the upper lobe bronchus. Right-sided tubes have a slot on the endobronchial limb or cuff to specifically provide ventilation for the upper lobe bronchus. Correct positioning of the tube is ideally checked by fibre optic bronchoscopy (Simon et al., 1992).
- A less commonly used technique for lung or lobar isolation is the use of a bronchial blocker; in the absence of commercially produced devices, many centres use fogarty catheters positioned bronchoscopically through a single lumen endotracheal tube to occlude the desired lobar or main bronchus. This technique is particularly useful in paediatric practice as smaller sized double lumen tubes are not readily available.
- An alternative technique for maintaining ventilation of both lungs whilst facilitating surgical access to the thoracic cavity is the use of high frequency jet ventilation (HFJV). During HFJV the lungs are almost completely deflated as gas exchange does not rely on tidal ventilation.
- The most commonly encountered problem during one-lung ventilation is hypoxia, particularly in patients with bilateral lung disease. Measures that can be taken to improve oxygenation include (Kavanagh and Sandler, 1996):
  – increasing the inspired oxygen concentration
  – ensuring that the ventilated lung is clear of secretions and inflating adequately
  – applying PEEP to the ventilated lung
  – insufflating oxygen via a catheter to the non-ventilated lung
  – early clamping of the pulmonary artery to the non-ventilated lung during pneumonectomy

If hypoxia persists then re-ventilation of the collapsed lung may be essential.

3. General anaesthetic management of thoracotomy

The principles of management are the anticipation of a transient decline in respiratory status post-operatively, as many procedures are performed on patients with poor respiratory reserve. The potential for concurrent cardiovascular disease should also be considered. Anaesthetic aims are to avoid opioid-induced respiratory depression, to achieve a return to spontaneous ventilation in the immediate post-operative period, and to ensure adequate post-operative analgesia to facilitate deep breathing and coughing.

The pre-operative anaesthetic assessment and preparation should focus on (Coucher et al., 1997; Kavanagh and Sandler, 1996; Plummer et al., 1998; Zollinger and Pasch, 1998):

- The underlying thoracic pathology
- The degree of limitation of respiratory function
- Concomitant pathology, especially cardiovascular disease
- Drug therapy
- Laboratory investigations

Post-operative morbidity and mortality have been related to many indices of respiratory function but no one factor can be used exclusively.

Acknowledged risk factors include:

- FEV_1 <1 litre and FVC <2 litres are associated with secretion retention.
- FEV_1 <0.8 litre is generally considered a contraindication for lung resection.
- Maximum Breathing Capacity (MBC) 25–50 l/min (normal >60 l/min) is associated with severe respiratory impairment.
- Raised arterial carbon dioxide retention ($PaCO_2$ >6.0 kPa).
- Age over 70 years of age.

The more specialised tests of pulmonary artery pressure measurements to assess unilateral lung function and radionucleotide techniques to assess detailed quantification of regional ventilation and perfusion may be required for patients at the limit of acceptable operable risk. Calculation of predicted residual lung function after pulmonary resection should also be considered in-patients undergoing excision of lung tissue.

3.1. Premedication

The aim is to provide anxiolysis and sedation without respiratory depression. Many consider this best achieved with the avoidance of opioids and the use of benzodiazepines. Anti-sialogues (e.g. hyoscine) maybe used for their additional sedative effect; however, their use maybe associated with increased sputum retention. Bronchodilator therapy should be continued until surgery. Patients on steroids may require steroid supplementation to avoid development of secondary hypoadrenalism.

3.2. Monitoring for anaesthesia

The minimal standards of monitoring required for thoracic surgery include ECG, pulse oximetry, capnography, invasive arterial and central venous pressure measurement. Correct positioning of the catheter in the pulmonary artery to the non-operative lung can be difficult.

3.3. Choice of anaesthetic and conduct of anaesthesia

Choice of agent for intravenous induction is rarely critical, especially for longer procedures such as lung resection. Maintenance of anaesthesia is usually by inhalation of a volatile anaesthetic agent such as isoflurane or enflurane in a 50% oxygen:nitrous oxide or oxygen:air mix. 100% oxygen may be required during one-lung ventilation.

Muscle relaxation for endotracheal intubation is achieved by the administration of non-depolarising muscle relaxants such as atracurium, vecuronium and pancuronium according to the anticipated duration of the procedure.

4. Endobronchial intubation

One-lung anaesthesia is most commonly achieved with the use of a double lumen endobronchial tube inserted after induction of anaesthesia. There are two schools of thought as to the choice between right- or left-sided tubes. Some feel a left-sided tube should be used in all cases other then surgery involving the left main bronchus. This avoids the problem of accidental occlusion of the right upper lobe bronchus, resulting in upper lobe collapse. Others favour a routinely placed double lumen tube in the bronchus of the non-operative lung. In both situations, correct position should be confirmed by flexible bronchoscopy. Right endobronchial tubes have an additional orifice in the endobronchial limb for ventilation of the right upper lobe and this requires careful positioning (Simon et al., 1992).

Endobronchial tubes are bulky and may cause laryngeal and mucosal damage. Bronchial rupture can occur with overinflation of the distal cuff. Overinflation may also lead to the herniation of the bronchial cuff over the main bronchus of the lung to be operated on or may obstruct the lower trachea at the carinal level. (See Fig. 2.)

5. Lateral position and return to two-lung ventilation

Adoption of the lateral position for thoracotomy and institution of one-lung ventilation are associated with physiological changes in ventilation–perfusion matching.

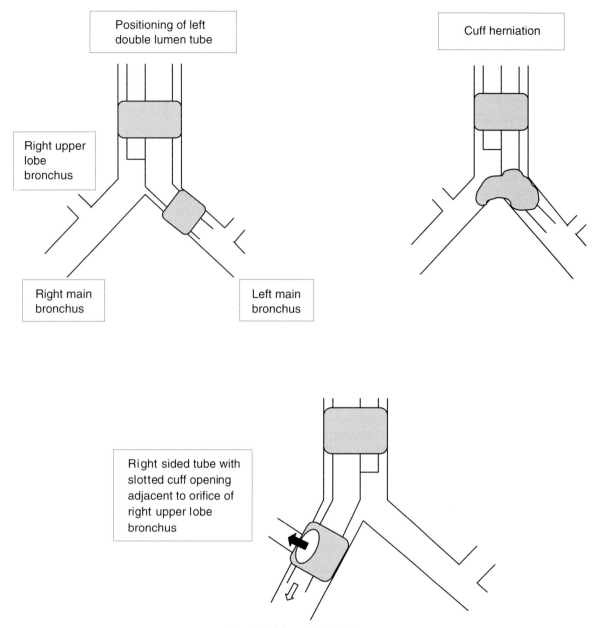

Fig. 2. Endobronchial intubation.

5.1. Lateral position

5.1.1. Ventilation–perfusion distribution

In the awake patient lying in the lateral position, blood flow increases by 60% to the lower (dependent) lung due to the effect of gravity. This is matched by an increase in ventilation as the lower lung is on the steep part of the pressure–volume loop.

In the spontaneous breathing patient under anaesthesia there is a reduction in FRC and both lungs decrease in volume due to the encroachment of abdominal contents on the diaphragm into the chest and the weight of the mediastinum. There is also loss of diaphragmatic tone. As a result, the upper lung now moves onto the steep portion of the pressure-volume curve such that it receives more ventilation than the dependent lung, whilst perfusion still preferentially flows to the lower lung resulting in ventilation–perfusion mismatch.

In the paralysed and ventilated patient for thoracotomy the situation remains the same, with preferential ventilation to the upper lung which may be accentuated by the open chest.

5.1.2. Venous admixture

Pulmonary blood flow continues to the upper lung, which is non-ventilated in one-lung anaesthesia, thereby creating a true shunt. This shunt is the major cause of hypoxaemia during one-lung ventilation. Venous admixture increases from a baseline value of approximately 20% during two-lung ventilation (due to the dependent related ventilation–perfusion ratios) to a level of 30–40% during one-lung ventilation. In the majority of cases adequate oxygenation can be maintained by using inspired oxygen at concentrations of 50–100%.

5.1.3. Hypoxic pulmonary vasoconstriction

In the normal state, the vasculature of poorly oxygenated alveoli will vasoconstrict; however, many factors during anaesthesia inhibit this mechanism: e.g. volatile anaesthetic agents, hypocapnia, and the use of vasodilator drugs. Intravenous anaesthetic agents do not seem to inhibit this response, but hypoxic pulmonary vasoconstriction itself does not appear to significantly reduce hypoxaemia during one-lung anaesthesia and, therefore, the benefits of total intravenous anaesthesia in comparison to inhaled agents are arguable.

5.2. Re-expansion of the collapsed lung and return to two lung ventilation

At the end of the procedure the lungs are re-inflated to 40 cm H_2O for 30–40 seconds several times to reverse any atelectasis and to enable leaks to be detected.

Re-inflation pulmonary oedema may develop due to inactivation of surfactant during the period of lung collapse, causing an increase in solute and water permeability of the alveolar–capillary barrier. This is compounded by the relatively increased blood flow through the remaining pulmonary vascular bed and reversal of hypoxic pulmonary vasoconstriction with reoxygenation of the alveoli.

6. Post-operative period

6.1. Cardiovascular complications

Following lung resection, the relative increased blood flow through the remaining pulmonary vascular bed may result in raised pulmonary vascular resistance and right ventricular failure, especially if the pulmonary artery pressure is elevated pre-operatively.

Supraventricular arrhythmias, common after lung resection are treated with digoxin or verapamil. Some centres prophylactically digitalise patients prior to pneumonectomy.

6.2. Respiratory complications

Pulmonary function changes following thoracotomy can result in more than 50% reduction from pre-operative values of FVC and FEV_1. This can lead to sputum retention and to respiratory failure. Pain limiting chest movement and lung expansion can compound this, whilst operative phrenic or laryngeal nerve damage will also result in increased risk of respiratory complications.

Chest physiotherapy and good analgesia are required to treat sputum retention. Mini tracheostomy should be considered to clear secretions and, if necessary, mechanical ventilation reinstituted, though this is associated with an increased incidence of airleak and is avoided where possible.

7. Analgesia

Good analgesia is essential to ensure optimal post-operative ventilatory effort, coughing and co-operation with physiotherapy.

7.1. Opioid use

Despite the potential respiratory depressant complications associated with their use, intravenous opioids by continuous infusion or patient-controlled pumps are widely used for post-operative analgesia. Intermittent intramuscular boluses on an 'as required' basis is generally a poor method of pain control due to relatively high dose requirements and periods of pain between doses.

7.2. Intercostal nerve blockade

If several nerves above and below the incision site are infiltrated under direct vision before closure of the chest, analgesia can be achieved for the immediate post-operative period. This can be prolonged by the use of a continuous infusion through an indwelling catheter left in the epi-pleural space.

7.3. Epidural analgesia

With this approach analgesia is achieved at the anterior and posterior spinal root and spinal cord level. Local anaesthetic (e.g. 10 ml 0.25% bupivacaine) is administered at a thoracic level T7–T9 by initial bolus. For post-operative analgesia a continuous infusion of e.g. 0.1% bupivacaine is commenced (Grant, 1999; Slinger, 1999).

The use of epidural opioids decreases local anaesthetic requirements, thereby reducing the extent of motor blockade caused, and increases the duration of block achieved. Lipophilicity of the opioid used determines the onset and duration of analgesia. Increased lipophilicity results in rapid distribution across the dura and penetration of the dorsal horn. Fentanyl 2 mcg/ml is commonly used in the local anaesthetic infusion solution. If opioids are used there is an increased risk of respiratory depression and observation in a High Dependency Unit is initially required.

7.3.1. Complications of epidural anaesthesia
- Hypotension due to sympathetic blockade resulting in loss of tone in resistance and capacitance vessels causing vasodilatation and decreased venous return.
- Bradycardia by cephalad spread to T2–T4 causing a block of cardioaccelerator fibres and preventing the ability to compensate for the circulatory changes.
- Respiratory impairment by cephalad spread may also result in reducing the ability to cough due to intercostal nerve blockade and, rarely, direct brain stem depression.
- Total spinal blockade through inadvertent dural puncture and large volume local anaesthetic administration into the CSF is recognised by rapid onset bradycardia, hypotension, respiratory arrest and loss of consciousness.
- Neural damage by direct trauma to spinal cord or nerve roots may occur. For this reason thoracic epidural placement is usually performed in the awake state to ensure early recognition of potential neurological impingement.
- Spinal abscess by the introduction of infection. Onset of fever and back pain over day 1–3 with

CSF leucocytosis should raise the suspicion of this and the risk of impending spinal cord compression.
- Spinal haematoma recognised by sharp back pain and features of nerve compression requires rapid decompression to avoid permanent neurological damage.
- Urinary retention.
- Shivering (reduced by the use of fentanyl with the local anaesthetic solution).
- Horner's syndrome, by cephalad tracking of local anaesthetic and sympathetic blockade.
- Puritis with opioid use.

References and further reading

Branson RD, et al. New modes of ventilatory support. Int Anaesthesiol Clin 1999 Summer; 37(3): 103–125.

Coucher I, et al. Anaesthesia for surgery of emphysema. Br J Anaesth 1997; 79: 530–538.

Engoren MC, et al. Propofol based versus fentanyl-isoflurane based anaesthesia in cardiac surgery. J Cardiothorac Vasc Anaesth 1998 Apr; 12(2): 177–181.

Grant RP. Con: every post-thoracotomy patient does not deserve thoracic epidural analgesia. J Cardiothorac Vasc Anaesth 1999 Jun; 13(3): 355–357.

Guarracino F, et al. Anaesthetic management is a major determinant of early extubation after elective cardiac surgery. Chest 1998 Jul; 114(1): 348.

Kavanagh BP, Sandler AN. Anaesthesia for thoracic surgery. Baillere's Clin Anaesthesiol 1996; 10(1): 77–98.

Michalopoulos A, et al. Effects of positive end expiratory pressure (PEEP) in cardiac surgery patients. Respir Med 1998 Jun; 92(6): 858–862.

O'Connor CJ. Pain relief and pulmonary morbidity after cardiac surgery. Crit Care Med 1999 Oct; 27(10): 2314–2316.

Plummer S, Hartley M, Vaughan RS. Anaesthesia for telescopic procedures in the thorax. Br J Anaesth 1998; 80: 223–234.

Price JA, et al. Post operative ventilatory management. Chest 1999 May; 115(5 supp): 1305–1375.

Radr MY, et al. Perioperative predictors of extubation failure and effects on clinical outcome after cardiac surgery. Crit Care Med 1999 Feb; 27(2): 340–347.

Simon BA, Hurford WE, Alfille PH et al. An aid to the diagnosis of malpositioned double lumen tubes. Anaesthesiology 1992; 76: 845–849.

Slinger PD. Pro: every post thoracotomy patient deserves thoracic epidural analgesia. J Cardiothorac Vasc Anaesth 1999 Jun; 13(3): 350–354.

Zaidi AM, et al. Good outcomes from cardiac surgery in the over 70s. Heart 1999 Aug; 82(2): 134–137.

Zollinger A, Pasch T. Anaesthesia for lung volume reduction surgery. Curr Opin Anesth 1998; 11: 45–49.

K. Moghissi, J.A.C. Thorpe and F. Ciulli (Eds.)
Moghissi's Essentials of Thoracic and Cardiac Surgery
© 2003 Elsevier Science B.V. All rights reserved

CHAPTER V.4

Surgery of congenital heart disease

V.T. Tsang and D.J. Penny

1. Introduction

Over the last 50 years, many palliative and reparative procedures have been developed for most congenital heart defects. The rapid progress in diagnosis, circulatory physiology, interventional cardiology, anaesthesia, cardiopulmonary bypass techniques and critical care have significantly improved the surgical outcome, even for very sick neonates and small infants. With the current philosophy of early reparative surgery to achieve as normal a development as possible, this may avoid the unfavourable influence of abnormal physiology and reoperations.

The content of this chapter is based on the curriculum for higher surgical training in cardiothoracic surgery. We try to cover some important aspects of the cardiac morphology, physiology of the neonatal, pulmonary and univentricular circulation, which are relevant to patients with congenital heart disease. Their appreciation, we believe, would help to understand the surgery of congenital heart disease. Should any specialist details be required, the trainees are encouraged to refer to several eloquently written major textbooks of congenital heart surgery. These are listed at the end of this chapter.

2. Classification of congenital heart disease

The classification of congenital heart disease remains one of the most contentious issues in paediatric cardiology. In most centres in this country, the sequential segmental approach pioneered by Anderson and colleagues (1987) is employed. The approach depends on a number of simple rules. First, diagnosis depends on observed anatomical facts and not on embryological speculation. Second, anomalies are described using a 'sequential' approach, in which the observer first describes the arrangement of the atriums, then the connections between the atrial and ventricular masses, then the connections between the ventricles and great arteries, and finally, considers any associated features. While this approach may appear to be like using a sledgehammer to crack a nut, in describing some of the simpler lesions, the advantage is that an unambiguous description of even the most complex anomalies is permitted.

2.1. Some aspects of cardiovascular physiology relevant to the patient with congenital heart disease

2.1.1. The fetal and neonatal circulation
Throughout development the cardiovascular system undergoes a series of profound changes in form and function. These changes are not merely of academic interest, but are fundamental to the understanding of congenital heart disease and its surgical management (Friedman and Fahey, 1993). In this respect, most patients with symptomatic congenital heart disease present at a time in their development when these fundamental changes are occurring in their circulatory physiology, while conversely, the normal developmental changes can be altered by some congenital heart lesions. Furthermore, the timing of operative intervention for some conditions is determined by the developmental stage of the patient's cardiovascular physiology.

An important feature of the fetal circulation is the presence of several intracardiac and extracardiac shunts, most importantly the oval foramen, the arterial duct and the ductus venosus. As a result of these shunts, *in utero*, unlike in the postnatal state, the perfusion of the systemic organs can be derived from both the left and right ventricles, operating in parallel. In general, under normal circumstances,

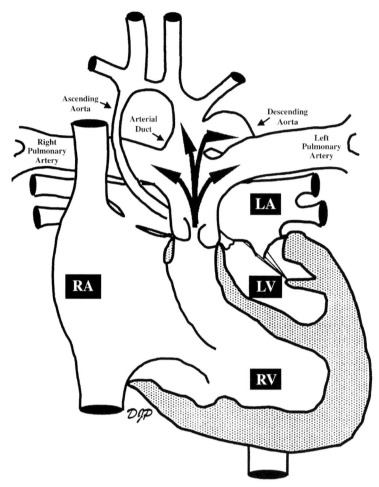

Fig. 1. Cartoon of the cardiac anatomy in aortic atresia with hypoplastic left heart syndrome. Right ventricular output is distributed between the pulmonary and systemic circulations according to the relative resistances of the pulmonary and systemic vascular beds.

3.1.1. Presentation

Closure of the ductus at birth produces the liga-mentum arteriosum. Persistent patency of the ductus, with the fall in pulmonary vascular resistance which naturally follows, is associated with a left-to-right shunt. The signs of excessive pulmonary blood flow and left ventricular volume overload may be present, depending on the size of the duct, the pulmonary vas-cular resistance, and associated anomalies. In infants with complex congenital heart disease, pulmonary or systemic blood flow may be dependent on the ductal patency, and decompensation occurs if the duct closes. Patients surviving into adulthood with a PDA may develop pulmonary hypertension and Eisenmenger syndrome.

3.1.2. Investigations

Two-dimensional echocardiography is the test to demonstrate the PDA and evaluate any associated anomalies. Cardiac catheterisation is indicated in older patients with suspected pulmonary vascular disease.

3.1.3. Management

In premature infants, pharmacological closure with indomethacin may be attempted. PDA is convention-ally closed via a left fourth space thoracotomy, either by ligation with silk or by Ligaclip in the very small infant (Fig. 3). Care must be taken to avoid damage to the recurrent nerve which loops around the ductus.

Thoracoscopic closure of PDA is routinely carried out in centres with the appropriate expertise. Non-sur-gical transcatheter closure of PDA with intravascular coils or an umbrella device has been established as a treatment of choice in the majority of patients, with very encouraging long-term follow-up data.

In some infants with obstructive right- or left-sided cardiac lesions, the ductus may need to be kept

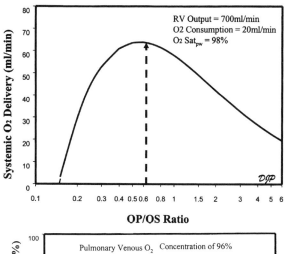

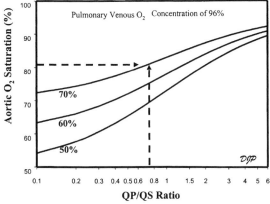

Fig. 2. Changes in systemic oxygen delivery with the pulmonary-to-systemic blood flow ratio (Qp/Qs) in the patient with hypoplastic left heart syndrome (top panel). Systemic oxygen delivery is optimised at a Qp/Qs ratio of slightly below 1. In the bottom panel, the aortic oxygen saturation is calculated, as Qp/Qs is altered, assuming a pulmonary venous oxygen saturation of 96% and mixed venous oxygen saturations of 50, 60 and 70%. With a mixed venous oxygen saturation of 70%, the appropriate aortic oxygen saturation for optimal systemic oxygen delivery is slightly greater than 80%. (Based on principles outlined in Barnea et al., 1998.)

open by prostaglandin to achieve a stable circulation (see above).

3.1.4. Outcome

Surgical closure of PDA carries an operative risk close to 0%. Hospital mortality is unlikely to be related to the procedure; it may instead be associated with the degree of prematurity or multisystem disease.

3.2. Coarctation of the aorta

Coarctation of the aorta is defined as a narrowing of the aortic lumen, usually around the aortic isthmus and arterial duct.

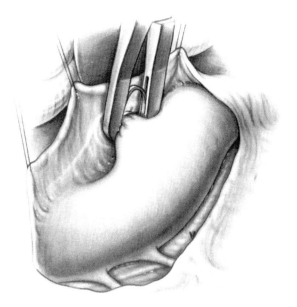

Fig. 3. Occlusion of PDA with a Ligaclip.

3.2.1. Presentation

The presentation of aortic coarctation can be quite complex. It may be determined by the degree of aortic flow obstruction, the presence of a patent arterial duct and other important cardiovascular lesions, such as left ventricular inflow or outflow obstruction and ventricular septal defect.

In infants, frequently the dominant feature is the hypoplastic arch and isthmus, with a large patent ductus arteriosus in continuity with the descending aorta. The coarctation is juxtaductal. Symptoms develop after ductal closure, which results in significant aortic obstruction compromising the blood supply to the distal organs. Renal failure and metabolic acidosis soon follow. In older children, coarctation may present with reduced femoral pulses and/or proximal systemic hypertension.

3.2.2. Investigations

The chest radiograph usually shows cardiomegaly and may have rib notching due to enlarged collateral arteries in the older children. The electrocardiogram may show left ventricular hypertrophy. Cross-sectional echocardiography allows the imaging of the coarctation with characteristic descending aortic flow velocity pattern. The long diastolic tail is due to the persistent gradient between the ascending and descending aorta throughout the cardiac cycle. Bicuspid aortic valve is commonly seen, and mitral valve anomalies may be present. Cardiac catheteri-

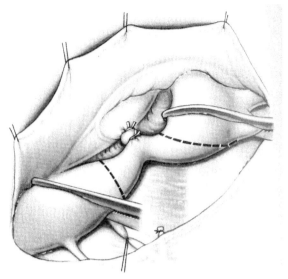

Fig. 4. Resection of coarctation and repair with an end-to-end anastomosis. Collaterals are preserved.

sation and/or magnetic resonance imaging may be indicated in cases of complex coarctation or recoarctation of the aorta.

3.2.3. Management
In neonates with coarctation, the ductal flow can be re-established with intravenous prostaglandin E1, an important component of resuscitation to support the lower body circulation by the right ventricle. Ventilatory and inotropic support may be required to improve the metabolic acidosis, and this allows early surgical repair to be done under optimal conditions.

The role of interventional catheterisation in the treatment of native coarctation is controversial. Resection and end-to-end anastomosis for discrete coarctation through a left fourth space thoracotomy is a very successful operation (Fig. 4).

The resection can be extended into the undersurface of the aortic arch when there is significant arch hypoplasia. Subclavian flap aortoplasty may be indicated if extensive circumferential mobilisation is undesirable (Fig. 5).

Prosthetic patch aortoplasty has been rarely performed because of the risk of subsequent aneurysm formation. Complications of coarctation repair include haemorrhage, chylothorax, recurrent nerve palsy, paraplegia and recoarctation.

Different from primary aortic coarctation, the treatment of choice for recoarctation is balloon dilation aortoplasty and/or stenting, with a small risk of aneurysm formation. Extra-anatomic conduit between the ascending and descending aorta is probably a last resort for complex recoarctation, placed via a median sternotomy.

3.2.4. Outcome
Surgical repair of coarctation carries a very low risk, and the operative mortality is probably associated with very small infants and the associated anomalies. Persistent hypertension may remain a long-term problem, even after a successful repair.

3.3. Atrial septal defect

Atrial septal defect (ASD) is defined as a deficiency of the atrial septum which allows shunting of blood

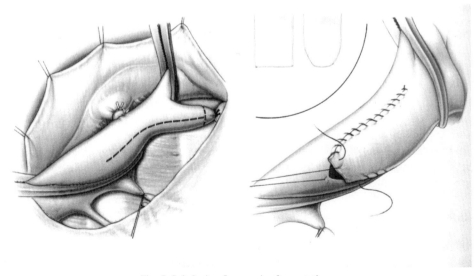

Fig. 5. Subclavian flap repair of coarctation.

between the two atrial chambers. The commonest defect is ostium secundum type, due to the absence of septal tissue in the oval fossa. It is different from the patent foramen ovale, which is a flap valve without true deficiency of the septum and usually closes after birth. Superior sinus venosus defect is located high in the atrial septum with an overriding superior vena cava. It is often associated with anomalous drainage of the right pulmonary veins. Ostium primum atrial septal defect, or partial atrioventricular septal defect, is caused by a deficiency in the atrioventricular septum and is always associated with abnormal atrioventricular valve anatomy. Most atrial septal defects do not close spontaneously.

3.3.1. Presentation

The degree of shunting across the atrial septal defect depends on the size of the defect and on the relative compliances of the left and right ventricles during diastole. The left-to-right shunt will increase the right heart volume load. Congestive heart failure may develop in early infancy, and this may indicate restriction of the mitral valve. However, despite the unrestrictive nature of the defect, most children remain asymptomatic. Pulmonary hypertension has been reported, but the incidence remains low.

3.3.2. Investigations

Transthoracic echocardiography identifies the precise defects in the majority of cases, the direction of shunting and other associated cardiac anomalies. Cardiac catheterisation is reserved for patients with associated abnormalities or suspected pulmonary hypertension.

3.3.3. Management

Closure of isolated secundum atrial septal defect is indicated if the pulmonary flow is more than 1.5 times the systemic flow, although in the current era, pulmonary blood flow is rarely measured. The operation is undertaken via a median sternotomy and cardiopulmonary bypass with bicaval cannulation is used. The heart is arrested with cardioplegia. Via a right atriotomy, the abnormal septal defect is demonstrated, and the pulmonary venous drainage is assessed. Primary suture is usually possible, but closure with a patch is more common for large defects to achieve no tension at the suture line (Fig. 6).

Repair of sinus venosus defect requires the placement of a patch to redirect the abnormal pulmonary venous drainage back to the left atrium. At the time of closure of the ostium primum defect, repair of

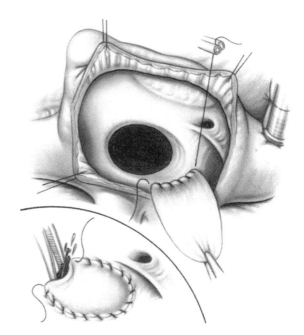

Fig. 6. Patch closure of ASD. De-airing prior to tying down the patch.

the left atrioventricular valve is often necessary. Care must be exercised to avoid the abnormally located conduction tissue in these patients.

In the majority of patients with small to moderate size secundum ASD, device closure at cardiac catheterisation has overtaken surgery as the treatment of choice.

3.3.4. Outcome

The risk of surgical closure of secundum septal defects for those without pulmonary hypertension should be less than 1% with no major long-term consequences. Symptomatic infants undergoing repair still have a considerable risk. In patients with ostium primum defect, the successful long term outcome depends on the competency of the left-sided atrioventricular valve repair.

3.4. Ventricular septal defects

Ventricular septal defects (VSDs) are defined as communications in the septum between the right and left ventricles. For simplicity, the ventricular septum is termed as having inlet, trabecular, and outlet portions, and VSDs can be described largely on this basis. The membraneous septum is located near the anterior septal commissure of the tricuspid valve. A VSD in the region of the membraneous septum is described as a perimembraneous defect. It is impor-

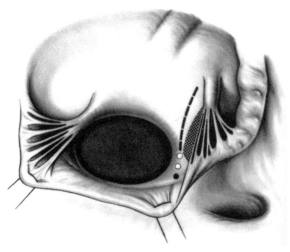

Fig. 7. Transatrial view of perimembraneous VSD with the conduction tissue closely related to its inferior margin. Stay sutures on the septal leaflet of the tricuspid valve.

tant to know that the bundle of His passes along the inferior margin of the defect (Fig. 7). Muscular VSDs are surrounded by a muscular margin, and can be single or multiple.

3.4.1. Presentation

The physiology of all VSDs is that of a left-to-right shunt. It is determined by the size of the defect and the relative resistance of the pulmonary and systemic circulations. Large and unrestrictive VSD may result in systemic levels of right ventricular pressure. If the VSD is restrictive with a pressure gradient across it, the right ventricular pressure is less elevated, but the pulmonary blood flow may still be significantly increased.

Small VSDs, particularly muscular type, may close without any intervention. Large VSDs present with congestive cardiac failure at an early age. Increased pulmonary blood flow may lead to pulmonary vascular disease, but it is uncommon to see severe changes before 2 years of age. High pulmonary vascular resistance may lead to bidirectional shunting across the VSD. Eisenmenger syndrome develops when there are irreversible pulmonary vascular changes with reverse shunting across the VSD. With subarterial VSD, closely related to both semilunar valves, there may be prolapse of the aortic valve cusp leading to aortic regurgitation. Other associated anomalies include coarctation and left ventricular outflow obstruction.

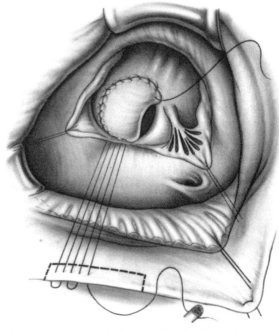

Fig. 8. Transatrial patch closure of VSD with continuous synthetic suture. Strip of autologous pericardium as pledget.

3.4.2. Investigations

Echocardiography with colour flow Doppler is the most useful diagnostic test in these patients, allowing the accurate definition of the location of the defect, the direction of shunting, and other associated anomalies. Cardiac catheterisation with oximetry to calculate the degree of shunting may be indicated in those with suspected pulmonary vascular changes.

3.4.3. Management

Patch closure for isolated significant VSD is the preferred treatment (Fig. 8). Most perimembraneous and some muscular defects can be closed via a right atrial approach. However, a right ventriculotomy may be necessary for some outlet and apical/anterior muscular defects. Subarterial defects are best approached via the pulmonary artery. Care must be taken to avoid the conduction tissue in the perimembraneous defects by suturing inferior to the bundle of His and along the tricuspid valve margin.

3.4.4. Pulmonary artery banding

Advances in neonatal cardiac surgery have made primary VSD closure the preferred technique, even in small infants. However, there is still a place for pulmonary artery banding to limit the pulmonary blood flow in small infants with multiple VSDs or non-committed VSD. Some very sick neonates, es-

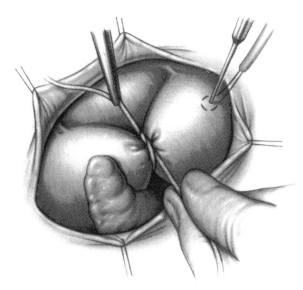

Fig. 9. Pulmonary artery banding with a distal pressure monitoring needle.

pecially those with an associated coarctation, can be safely treated by preliminary banding. For VSD, the constriction of the band is adjusted to a distal pulmonary artery pressure of about 30% of the systemic pressure (Fig. 9). Closure of the defect and removal of the band will be performed at a second operation.

3.4.5. Outcome
Closure of isolated VSD with no pulmonary hypertension carries a very low risk (less than 2%), even in the very young. In older patients, the presence of pulmonary vascular disease will increase the operative risk.

3.5. Atrioventricular septal defect (AVSD)

There is a wide spectrum of defects due to deficiency of atrioventricular septum and abnormal development of atrioventricular valve. The defect is characterised by an atrial septal defect of ostium primum type and a large inlet ventricular septal defect. There may be two separate valves or a common atrioventricular valve. When no VSD is present, the defect is termed partial AVSD. Patients with Trisomy 21 have a higher incidence of AVSD. Important associated defects include tetralogy of Fallot or coarctation of the aorta.

3.5.1. Presentation
Patients with AVSD usually present with heart failure in early infancy due to a large left-to-right shunt at ventricular level, sometimes with atrioventricular

valve regurgitation. Pulmonary vascular disease may develop early if left uncorrected.

3.5.2. Investigations
Two dimensional echocardiography is very useful in the diagnosis of AVSD and the atrioventricular valve function. If there is concern of elevated pulmonary vascular resistance and other anomalies, cardiac catheterisation may be necessary.

3.5.3. Management
Complete repair is usually undertaken at 3 to 6 months of age, using either a one-patch or two-patch technique. The latter consists of transatrial patch closure of VSD, recreation of two competent atrioventricular valves and another patch closure of the ostium primum ASD. The conduction tissue is situated in a more posterior and inferior position, towards the coronary sinus. The approach of preliminary pulmonary artery banding to limit the pulmonary blood flow has been abandoned, and early repair is preferred.

3.5.4. Outcome
Although these repairs can be difficult, the early mortality should be less than 5%. The long-term outcome depends on the competency of the left atriventricular valve.

3.6. Tetralogy of Fallot (TOF)

The key abnormality is the anterior deviation of the outlet septum. There is usually a large perimembraneous outlet VSD with the aorta overriding the crest of the ventricular septum, with a varying degree of right ventricular outflow tract obstruction (Fig. 10). The latter is due to hypertrophy of the infundibular septum and septoparietal trabeculations of the right ventricular outflow tract beneath a usually stenotic pulmonary valve. There may be branch pulmonary artery stenosis. Important associated defects include AVSD and anomalous left anterior descending artery from the right coronary artery.

3.6.1. Presentation
The initial presentation is dictated by the degree and the progression of the right ventricular outflow tract obstruction. If mild, there may be a left-to-right shunt across the VSD with pulmonary overflow (pink Fallot). If severe, the dominant lesion is right-to-left shunt across the VSD with progressive cyanosis. When pulmonary atresia is present, the pulmonary

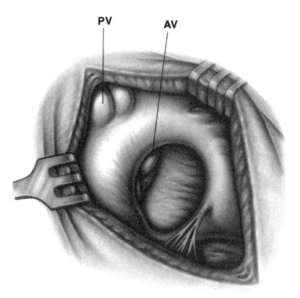

Fig. 10. Intracardiac anatomy of tetralogy of Fallot via a right ventriculotomy.

circulation is duct-dependent and its patency should be maintained with a prostaglandin infusion.

3.6.2. Investigations
Two-dimensional echocardiography can provide accurate assessment of the VSD, the right ventricular outflow tract, the proximal pulmonary artery and the proximal coronary artery. Cardiac catheterisation may be indicated if there is any doubt about distal pulmonary artery anatomy.

3.6.3. Management
Neonatal repair done at the time of diagnosis to avoid a systemic-to-pulmonary shunt operation and prolonged hypoxia has been advocated at some centres, but the operative risk and the reoperation rate is not insignificant. Conventionally, in small symptomatic infants with small pulmonary arteries, a modified Blalock-Taussig shunt is performed to increase pulmonary blood flow and promote growth of the pulmonary arteries. This is followed by definitive repair between the age of 6–12 months. The surgical repair consists of patch closure of the VSD and relief of right ventricular outflow obstruction, with or without a transannular patch.

The operation is performed via a median sternotomy, using hypothermic cardiopulmonary bypass and cardioplegic myocardial protection. Intraoperatively, the coronary anatomy is delineated. If indicated, the vertical incision in the pulmonary artery to examine the dysplastic pulmonary valve can be extended across the stenotic valve annulus (transannular incision) to adequately relieve the outflow tract obstruction. Obstructing muscle bundles may need to be resected. The VSD can be closed through the infundibular incision or a right atriotomy. Care must be taken to avoid the conduction tissue and the aortic valve. The infundibular and the pulmonary artery incision is patched with Gore-tex or autologous pericardium. The repair should aim to produce as normal a postoperative RV:LV pressure ratio as possible. A ratio of more than 0.75 is associated with increased early and late risk.

3.6.4. Modified Blalock–Taussig shunt
In patients with a left aortic arch, a right fourth space thoracotomy is used to expose the proximal right subclavian artery and the innominate artery. Care must be taken to avoid damaging the recurrent nerve. The right pulmonary artery is dissected out to confirm structural feasibility. An interposition graft (usually a 4 mm Gore-tex in neonates) between the proximal subclavian artery and the right pulmonary artery is carried out with systemic heparinisation.

3.6.5. Insertion of homograft valved conduit
In 1966, Ross and Somerville reported the use of aortic homograft in the repair of pulmonary atresia and VSD (Fallot type). The surgical concept has been applied extensively in the management of much complex congenital reconstructive surgery. To achieve good long term homograft function, it is essential to avoid any sternal compression by creating the appropriate accommodation for the conduit between the right ventricle and the distal pulmonary artery. The placement of the homograft valve close to the pulmonary bifurcation may minimise any distortion of the valve geometry, and the contour of the conduit can be optimised with the use of a Gore-tex graft extension onto the right ventriculotomy. In addition, any significant branch pulmonary artery stenosis should be dealt with at the time of homograft conduit insertion.

3.6.6. Outcome
The operative risk should be less than 3%. Reoperation for residual VSD or right ventricular outflow obstruction is not insignificant.

3.7. Transposition of the great arteries (TGA)

In this condition (discordant ventriculo-arterial connections), the anterior aorta arises from the right ventricle and the posterior pulmonary artery from the left ventricle. The pulmonary and systemic circulations are in parallel rather than in series, and there must be a connection between the two circuits to sustain life.

Most children with this lesion have an intact ventricular septum (IVS), or a VSD may be present. Left ventricular outflow tract obstruction may be present and is usually subvalvar.

3.7.1. Presentation
In infants with TGA/IVS, severe cyanosis occurs as soon as the duct is closed. With TGA/VSD there may be mixing at ventricular level with mild cyanosis. Without an ASD, VSD, or PDA, patients cannot survive.

3.7.2. Investigations
Echocardiography can demonstrate the abnormal origins of the great vessels, very importantly the coronary anatomy, the presence of PDA, ASD, VSD, and the left ventricular outflow tract. Cardiac catheterisation is rarely indicated.

3.7.3. Management
The use of prostaglandin infusion to reopen the duct, followed by urgent balloon atrial septostomy under echocardiographic control to create a good size ASD for better mixing, is our usual practice. In the past, atrial switch (Mustard or Senning procedures) was performed to obtain a physiological circulation using an intra-atrial baffle to direct systemic and pulmonary venous blood to the left and right ventricle respectively. The right ventricle remains as the systemic ventricle and there has been important long term morbidity and mortality with systemic ventricular dysfunction and arrhythmia.

At present, arterial switch is the treatment of choice for most forms of TGA by 'switching' the aorta back to the left ventricle and the pulmonary artery to the right ventricle, with reimplantation of the coronary arteries on to the neo-aorta (previously the proximal pulmonary artery) (Fig. 11). For TGA/IVS, the operation should be performed within the first few weeks of life, before the pulmonary vascular resistance falls to a lower postnatal level, thus the left ventricle becomes 'deconditioned' to cope with the systemic circulation. The operation is performed with deep hypothermic cardiopulmonary bypass and cardioplegic arrest. The aorta and the pulmonary artery are transected, followed by the transfer of the coronary buttons on to the neo-aorta. The pulmonary arteries are fully mobilised, and the

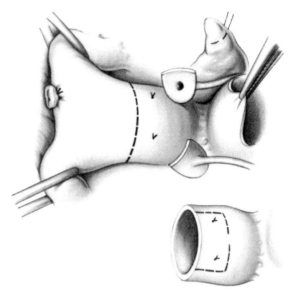

Fig. 11. Arterial switch: transfer of coronary arteries onto the neo-aorta (previously the main pulmonary artery).

aorta is usually positioned behind the pulmonary bifurcation (Lecompte manoeuvre).

In children with TGA/VSD, an arterial switch plus VSD closure can be performed during the first few months of life. In patients with an additional left ventricular outflow tract obstruction, it is usually possible to stage the repair with an initial systemic-to-pulmonary shunt to increase pulmonary blood flow. This is then followed by a 'Rastelli' type of repair by baffling the left ventricle to the anterior aorta, disconnecting and closing the proximal pulmonary artery, and finally reconnecting the right ventricle to the distal pulmonary artery with a homograft valved conduit.

3.7.4. Outcome
The overall operative mortality for simple TGA should be less than 5%. In the medium term, most children lead a normal life. Only with long-term follow-up would we be able to determine the real benefit of an arterial switch operation. Obstruction of the right ventricular outflow tract and occlusion of the transferred coronary arteries has been described.

3.8. Common arterial trunk

This malformation is characterised by a common arterial trunk with the branch pulmonary arteries coming off the posterior aspect of the trunk, and a large malalignment VSD. The truncal valve may be composed of more than 3 leaflets, and can be stenotic or regurgitant.

3.8.1. Presentation
The physiology is dictated by the unrestrictive communication between the pulmonary and systemic circulations. Most infants present with congestive cardiac failure with a high pulmonary blood flow.

3.8.2. Investigations
Echocardiography is the test to demonstrate the arterial trunk, the origins of the pulmonary arteries, the truncal valve status, the ventricular function, and other significant cardiac anomalies. Cardiac catheterisation may be indicated in older patients with suspected pulmonary vascular disease.

3.8.3. Management
Once the diagnosis is made, early corrective surgery is the most appropriate management. Cardiopulmonary bypass is instituted with distal ascending arterial cannulation and bicaval venous return. Pulmonary flow is occluded by placement of vascular slings on the branch pulmonary arteries during cooling. Cardioplegia can then be delivered into the truncal root after aortic cross-clamping.

The pulmonary arteries are detached from the arterial trunk. Caution must be exercised because of the close proximity of the left coronary artery. Via a right ventriculotomy, the VSD is patched so that the left ventricle is connected with the aorta. An extra-cardiac valved conduit, preferably a homograft, is inserted between the right ventricle and the disconnected pulmonary arteries.

3.8.4. Outcome
The hospital mortality ranges from 5–10%. The important factors are truncal valve regurgitation and other significant cardiac anomalies. The late issue is related to truncal valve dysfunction and the small homograft conduit inserted during early infancy, which would inevitably need to be replaced later on in life, with its associated risks.

3.9. Total anomalous pulmonary venous connection (TAPVC)

The most common type is 'supra-cardiac', in which the pulmonary venous drainage is via an ascending vertical vein behind the left atrium to the innominate vein and the right superior vena cava (Fig. 12a and 12b). A less common type is 'cardiac', in which the connection of pulmonary venous confluence is to the coronary sinus (Fig. 12c). This connection is only mildly stenotic. 'Infra-cardiac' type is via a descending vertical vein behind the left atrium into the portal system (Fig. 12d). A combination of pulmonary venous connections with the systemic veins is known as the 'mixed' type.

3.9.1. Presentation
Although the presentation depends on the degree of pulmonary venous obstruction, children with obstructive TAPVC always become very ill in early infancy with cyanosis and tachypnoea. In such cases, immediate resuscitation should be followed by surgery as soon as possible.

3.9.2. Investigations
Echocardiography is the most appropriate technique for diagnosis of TAPVC in sick neonates, and they should be distinguished from the newborns with persistent fetal circulation or lung disease.

3.9.3. Management
'Supra-cardiac' and 'infra-cardiac' TAPVC: The strategy of repair is to connect the pulmonary venous confluence with the left atrium, and ligate the abnormal connections to the systemic veins. Deep hypothermic circulatory arrest technique is commonly employed. Wide openings are made in the anterior wall of the pulmonary venous confluence and posterior wall of the left atrium, followed by direct anastomosis with continuous 7/0 Prolene.

'Cardiac' TAPVC: This is repaired by unroofing the coronary sinus into the left atrium, and the newly created ASD and the coronary sinus ostium is covered by a single patch.

3.9.4. Outcome
Hospital mortality is around 5% for obstructive TAPVC, and largely depends on the preoperative conditions. The use of nitric oxide has decreased the considerable risk of pulmonary hypertensive crises, which are still responsible for significant mortality and morbidity.

3.10. Functional single ventricle and the Fontan procedure

In some complex congenital heart conditions, including absent right atrioventricular connection (tricuspid atresia), double inlet ventricle and hypoplastic left heart syndrome, there is functionally a single ventricular chamber, with a small 'rudimentary' ventricle. Univentricular atrioventricular connection is a useful term in which the management strategy for

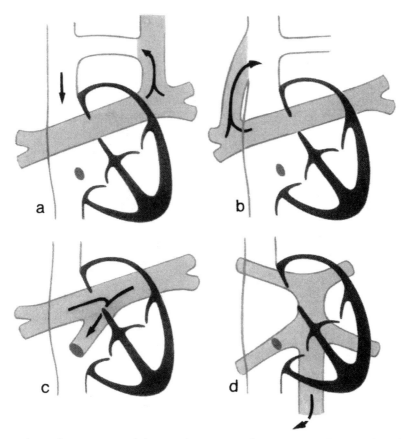

Fig. 12. Total anomalous pulmonary venous drainage (a, b = supra-cardiac type, c = cardiac type, d = infra-cardiac type).

these patients is directed towards a Fontan type of repair. This involves the 'pumpless' return of systemic venous blood directly to the pulmonary artery, and the dominant ventricle provides the systemic arterial output.

3.10.1. Presentation
For brevity, only the common forms of this type of lesion are considered. Their presentation depends on whether there is excessive or inadequate pulmonary blood flow, and any obstruction to the ventricular outflow. Systemic venous return may be abnormal.

3.10.2. Investigations
In the neonates, echocardiographic data should be sufficient, but in older children, detailed angiographic and haemodynamic assessment is essential.

3.10.3. Management
In the neonatal period, palliation is either by systemic-to-pulmonary shunt for inadequate pulmonary blood flow, or pulmonary artery banding if there is excessive pulmonary blood flow. Any obstruction to

the ventricular outflow should be avoided, and any abnormal pulmonary venous return should be dealt with. The aim is to achieve a balanced pulmonary and systemic circulation and optimise the patient's chances for a successful Fontan procedure.

3.10.4. Fontan procedure
Fontan and Baudet originally described the operation for tricuspid atresia in 1971, and the Fontan concept was subsequently applied to the management of other forms of functionally single ventricle. The circulation created depends entirely on the systemic ventricle for the production of forward blood flow through the lungs. The criteria for a well-functioning Fontan includes good ventricular function, no atrioventricular valve regurgitation and a low pulmonary vascular resistance.

Recently, major improvements and modifications of the Fontan operation have led to the introduction of total cavo-pulmonary connection (TCPC) with an intra-atrial tunnel. This provides better flow characteristics than the original Fontan (atrio-pulmonary connection). The creation of an inter-atrial fenestration allows the mixing of systemic and pulmonary venous blood, thus probably reduces post-operative effusions and generally contributes to a less complicating post-operative course. Since the mid-1990s, TCPC with an extra-cardiac conduit has become popularised, and it appears to provide better flow characteristics by avoiding over-distension of the right atrium.

3.10.5. Bidirectional cavo-pulmonary anastomosis

This right heart bypass operation diverts the superior vena caval blood to both the right and left pulmonary arteries. There is a tendency to undertake bidirectional cavo-pulmonary anastomosis as either a staging or part of a definitive palliation in cases that are less than optimal for a Fontan operation. The advantages of a systemic venous shunt over a systemic arterial shunt are more efficient oxygenation of venous blood and reduction of volume load on the heart. However, the efficiency of a bidirectional cavo-pulmonary anastomosis decreases with age, probably because the upper body venous return is proportionally greater in the young child.

3.11. Hypoplastic left heart syndrome (HLHS)

Hypoplastic left heart syndrome is a complex anomaly in which the left side of the heart is severely underdeveloped. In 1983, Norwood et al. suggested a series of operations to palliate this difficult condition. The first operation, Norwood stage 1, is performed soon after birth using cardiopulmonary bypass and deep hypothermic circulatory arrest to augment the aortic arch using the main pulmonary artery and the small ascending aorta and arch. A systemic-to-pulmonary shunt is created to provide pulmonary blood flow. For the stage 2 operation, bidirectional Glenn anastomosis, the systemic shunt is divided and the superior vena cava is anastomosed to the right pulmonary artery to provide pulmonary blood flow and reduce the volume load on the systemic ventricle. Finally, the third operation, Fontan/TCPC, is performed by creating an intra-atrial tunnel or extra-cardiac conduit to connect the inferior vena cava to the right pulmonary artery, thereby separating the systemic from the pulmonary circulation.

When introduced, this treatment carried a high mortality and a prolonged intensive care stay, but re-cent results from several major centres have demonstrated quite considerable improvements, at least in the medium term.

3.11.1. Outcome

Management of children with univentricular atrioventricular connection remains difficult, and the cardiac anatomy still dictates the short- as well as the long-term outcomes. The Fontan circulation itself carries its own late attrition, and atrio-pulmonary connection has several late problems, including pathway obstruction, arrhythmias, thromboembolism and congestive cardiac failure, with effusions and protein losing enteropathy. The Fontan modifications with intra-atrial tunnel and extra-cardiac conduit may minimise some of the problems, and only time will tell.

References and further reading

Anderson RH. Terminology. In: Anderson RH, Macartney FJ, Shinebourne EA, Tynan M (eds.), Paediatric Cardiology. UK: Churchill Livingstone, 1987; pp. 65–82.

Barnea O, Santamore WP, Rossi A, Salloum E, Chien S, Austin EH. Estimation of oxygen delivery in newborns with a univentricular circulation. Circulation 1998; 98: 1407–1413.

Castaneda AR, Jonas RA, Mayer JE, Hanley FL. Cardiac surgery of the neonate and infant. Philadelphia: WB Saunders, 1994.

Chang AC, Hanley FL, Wernovsky G, Wessel DL. Pediatric cardiac intensive care. Baltimore: Williams and Wilkins, 1998.

Fontan F, Baudet E. Surgical repair of tricuspid atresia. Thorax 1971; 26: 240–248.

Friedman AH, Fahey JT. The transition from fetal to neonatal circulation: normal responses and implications for infants with heart disease. Semin Perinatol 1993; 17: 106–121.

Jonas RA, Elliott MJ. Cardiopulmonary bypass in neonates, infants and young children. Oxford: Butterworth–Heinemann, 1994.

Kirklin JW, Barratt–Boyes BG. Cardiac surgery. New York: Churchill Livingstone, 1993.

Norwood WI, Lang P, Hansen DD. Physiologic repair of aortic atresia — hypoplastic left heart syndrome. N Eng J Med 1983; 308: 23–26.

Ross DN, Somerville J. Correction of pulmonary atresia with a homograft aortic valve. Lancet 1966; 2: 1446–1447.

Stark J, de Leval MR. Surgery for congenital heart defects. Philadelphia: WB Saunders, 1994.

Stark J, Pacifico AD. Reoperations in cardiac surgery. Berlin: Springer Verlag, 1989.

Wessel DL. Simple gases and complex single ventricles. J Thorac Cardiovasc Surg 1996; 112: 655–657.

CHAPTER V.5

Surgery of the aorta

D. Harrington and R.S. Bonser

1. Introduction

The aim of this chapter is to give an overview of the most important aspects of surgery of the aorta. A summary of the anatomy of the thoracic aorta is given first, followed by the important features of the most common congenital anomalies of the aortic arch. The next section covers infective problems of the aortic root including both native and prosthetic valve endocarditis. Aortic dissection is dealt with in some detail from incidence and classification, through to current management recommendations. This is followed by a similar section dealing with degenerative thoracic aortic aneurysms. The section on Marfan's syndrome describes its relevance to thoracic aortic surgery. The investigation and management principles of thoracic aortic trauma are then described. Operative techniques in thoracic aortic surgery include descriptions of aortic root replacement, total aortic arch replacement, descending thoracic aortic replacement and thoracoabdominal aortic replacement. The final section in this chapter then introduces the topic of neurological protection in aortic surgery and outlines the basic principles of widely used protective techniques.

2. Anatomy of the aorta

The aortic valve is tricuspid, consisting of three cup-like structures and the sinuses of Valsalva. These are dilated pockets of the aortic root whose walls are thinner than that of the normal aorta. The sinuses and cusps of the aortic valve are labelled right, left and non-coronary. The free edges of the cusps are tough, having a fibrous nodulus Aranti at the midpoint. The crescent shaped portion on either side is known as the lunula. The aortic valve mechanism is in continuity with the membranous interventricular septum and the anterior leaflet of the mitral valve (McMinn, 1994).

The ascending aorta is approximately 5 cm long and passes upwards and forwards towards the manubrium before the start of the arch. It gently spirals with the pulmonary trunk on its left. Both lie within the common sleeve of serous pericardium, and the fibrous pericardium blends with the aortic wall. The branches of the ascending aorta are the left and right coronary arteries.

The aortic arch begins at the level of the manubrio-sternal junction and passes backwards over the left main bronchus towards the body of T4 to the left of the midline. Its upper convexity reaches as high as the midpoint of the manubrium, where its branches are the brachiocephalic trunk, left common carotid artery and the left subclavian artery. The aortic arch is crossed on the left by the phrenic and vagus nerves and between them branches of the sympathetic and vagus nerves to the superficial cardiac plexus. The left superior intercostal vein passes forwards across the arch superficial to the vagus and deep to the phrenic nerve. The left recurrent laryngeal nerve hooks around the ligamentum arteriosum and passes upwards on the right of the aorta. The bifurcation of the pulmonary trunk is within the concavity of the arch of the aorta, the trachea and oesophagus are to the right. The adventitial layer of the aortic arch contains vagal baroreceptors, and the aortic bodies under the arch in the region of the ligamentum arteriosum are concerned with respiratory reflexes.

The descending aorta begins at the lower border of T4 to the left of the midline and leaves the posterior mediastinum in the midline at T12 where it passes behind the diaphragm between the crura. Its branches are nine posterior intercostals bilaterally, to be constructed as an open technique on the re-constituted non-instrumented aorta. During cooling, many surgeons clamp the ascending aorta while they effect a proximal repair. After opening the ascending aorta, the surgeon must first identify the presence of an intimal tear. Usually this lies transversely or obliquely approximately 2 cm distal to the left coronary ostium. If an intimal tear is not identified, then a detailed search of the aortic arch will be necessary during hypothermic circulatory arrest. Cold blood or crystalloid cardioplegia is next instilled directly via the coronary ostia to afford myocardial protection supplemented by topical cooling. Examination of the aortic root allows assessment of aortic valve competency and the integrity of the coronary ostia. Commonly coronary ostia have a degree of dissection, which can be repaired using appropriate adhesive. Some 80% of previously normal but disrupted aortic valves can be repaired by re-suspension of the prolapsing aortic commissures using Teflon buttressed 4'O' monofilament sutures. In certain instances, disruption of two or more commissures and extensive root dissection preclude safe repair and necessitate aortic root replacement. In others, root reconstruction is feasible allowing a supra-coronary graft to be used but aortic valve replacement is necessary for pre-existing valve pathology. Following valve re-suspension the dissected layers of the aortic root are re-affixed using gelatin–resorcinol-based surgical adhesive. It is important to warm the adhesive (but not the firing agent) prior to application. A firm adhesion takes 4 minutes and during this time the layers are compressed using forceps and soft clamps. The surrounding tissues must be carefully protected from the sclerosant effects of the glutaraldehyde/formaldehyde activator. Following satisfactory adhesion, the ascending aorta is completely transected just distal to the sino-tubular junction and at this juncture a buttressed over-sewing of the cut edge can be performed. An appropriately sized vascular graft is anastomosed to the transected aorta using a running monofilament suture. Teflon and pericardial buttressing is at the discretion of the surgeon. On completion of this anastomosis, its integrity and the competence of the aortic valve can be checked by pressurisation of the graft with cold cardioplegia. This check allows insertion of additional sutures as necessary with full surgical access to all areas of the anastomosis.

Attention is next directed to the aortic arch. At profound hypothermia, the aortic cross-clamp is removed, the ascending aorta is excised, including the clamp site and the interior of the aortic arch is inspected. An intimal tear within the arch, marked aneurysmal dilatation, rupture or extreme fragmentation are indications for a further resection and replacement of the aortic arch. Arch replacement is only necessary in the minority of cases. More commonly, reconstruction of the proximal aortic arch can be undertaken using gelatin-based adhesive with a Teflon collar buttress if necessary. A separate length of vascular graft is anastomosed to the distal aorta, and following this, the graft is pressurised by transferring the arterial return to the arch graft, and this simultaneously re-institutes orthograde flow via the true lumen. Inspection of this anastomosis under pressure at this stage allows insertion of further sutures as necessary. This open distal anastomosis appears to improve outcomes following type A dissection repair. Following rigorous arch air-drill and occlusion of the distal graft, cardiopulmonary bypass is re-established and the patient re-warmed. During re-warming the two lengths of graft are anastomosed together, the cross-clamped released and cardiac de-airing performed. During re-warming, super-heating of the brain should be avoided and once a nasopharyngeal temperature of 35°C is achieved, pump water temperatures should be set to 37°C. On completion of warming, cardiopulmonary bypass is discontinued in the normal manner.

Immediate post-operative management is similar to other open heart procedures but should include an early abdominal Doppler-ultrasound to confirm visceral and renal arterial flow signals. During convalescence, patients should be commenced on long-term beta-adrenergic antagonist therapy (Borst et al., 1996; Kirklin et al., 1993; Pretre et al., 1997).

5.6. Management of type B dissection

The early natural history of untreated type B dissection is superior to that of type A dissection, and for the majority of patients, medical therapy provides equivalent results to surgery (Glower et al., 1990). Rupture of the aorta is less likely than for type A and 70% of cases progress to a chronic form of dissection suitable for surveillance follow-up. Medical therapy is therefore indicated for those patients without complications and for those with significant co-morbidity. A complication-specific approach to surgery is usually adopted. Management is commenced by initiation of pain and blood pressure control. Both hypertension and left ventricular ejection velocity are related to dissection propagation and thus the mainstay of medical management includes the use of vasodilator agents and beta-adrenergic antagonists. Intravenous therapy is gradually shifted to oral anti-hypertensives as the patient stabilises. Indications for emergency surgery include haemothorax, unremitting pain, visceral, neurological or limb malperfusion and uncontrollable hypertension. A larger aortic size (>5 cm) at the site of the dissection may confer increased risk of early and late complications and is used by some as a primary indication for surgery (Borst et al., 1996; Kirklin et al., 1993; Pretre et al., 1997). Recently, various endovascular stenting devices have been used as a primary treatment of type B dissection and initial results are encouraging, although the patient with malperfusion phenomena remains at high risk. However, interventional radiological techniques to relieve malperfusion phenomena by true luminal stenting or percutaneous fenestration of the intimal flap may become important modalities of treatment in the future (Fann et al., 1999; Slonim et al., 1999).

Surgery for type B dissection is aimed at repair of aortic rupture, resection of the intimal tear, restoration of true luminal flow and obliteration of the false lumen. This will most commonly necessitate a short segment replacement of the distal aortic arch and proximal descending aorta. Re-affixation of the distal dissected layers is performed as in type A dissection. The conduct of the operation must include perfusion techniques to maintain distal perfusion or protect from spinal cord ischaemia during any period of aortic clamping. Such methods include the use of hypothermic circulatory arrest, partial cardiopulmonary bypass or left heart bypass techniques (e.g. left atrio–femoral bypass). The complications of surgery are common with other procedures on the descending and thoraco-abdominal aorta and include paraplegia (Elefteriades et al., 1999; Kitamura et al., 1995; Pretre et al., 1997).

5.7. Natural history

Untreated type A dissection carries a dismal prognosis with a 1-month survival of less than 5%. Although surgical treatment transforms survival rates, the operative mortality rate remains 5–30%. Deaths are due to haemorrhage, acute cardiac failure or the sequelae of malperfusion including stroke. Both the presence of an intimal tear within the aortic arch and the need for extended resection adversely affects survival. Medically treated type B dissection has a 1-month survival of 70–80%. Patients surviving the acute episode have a survival rate of approximately 80% and 40% at 5 and 10 years respectively. Two-thirds of late deaths are attributable to cardiovascular causes and of these, about half are due to progression of the aortic pathology. A persistently perfused false lumen increases the risk of subsequent aneurysmal expansion and aortic rupture. Regardless of initial treatment, patients with aortic dissection require continued out-patient surveillance with periodical imaging to monitor aneurysmal progression of the aorta. Some 15–30% patients potentially require late re-intervention for aneurysmal enlargement (Kirklin et al., 1993; Kitamura et al., 1995; Lansman et al., 1999; Pretre et al., 1997).

6. Degenerative aneurysms

Degenerative aneurysms of the aorta were previously thought to be atherosclerotic in aetiology. Although the processes of atherosclerosis and aneurysm formation may occur in parallel it is now recognised that aneurysm development is multi-factorial in origin with genetic and environmental components leading to a marked destruction of medial and adventitial lamellae and exaggerated connective tissue lysis. An understanding of the connective tissue matrix degradation may in future allow pharmacological strategies to prevent or retard aneurysm formation and growth. Degenerative aneurysm is primarily a disease of the elderly. Although the exact incidence of aneurysm formation is unknown, autopsy studies have suggested a prevalence in older patients of approximately 500 per 100,000 examinations with a marked increase in the eighth and ninth decade (Kouchoukos et al., 1997; Pitt et al., 1997). The incidence of ruptured thoracic aneurysm is approximately 5 per 100,000 population per annum. For degenerative aortic aneurysm, the descending aorta is at greatest rupture risk. The anatomical distribution of degenerative aneurysms is different to acute dissection with the majority affecting the descending aorta. Approximately 10% affect the thoraco-abdominal aorta. Thoraco-abdominal aneurysms are classified according to their anatomical extent. Crawford extent I aneurysms involve most of the descending aorta, but in the abdomen, terminate proximal to the renal artery ostia. Extent II aneurysms involve the renal arteries and extent III aneurysms involve the distal half of the descending aorta and the proximal abdominal aorta. Extent IV aneurysms involve the entire abdominal aorta and usually commence at the diaphragmatic hiatus (Safi et al., 1999).

6.1. Prognosis and presentation

Many degenerative aneurysms remain undetected during life. However, recognised aneurysms have a poor prognosis with >40% of deaths being secondary to aneurysm rupture. Aneurysms affecting the ascending aorta in association with aortic regurgitation have a dismal 2-year survival with almost all deaths secondary to rupture or cardiac failure. Although degenerative aneurysms of the descending and thoraco-abdominal aorta have a similar natural history to abdominal aortic aneurysms, a far greater fraction of deaths are due to rupture rather than other cardiovascular causes. The 5-year survival of patients with a large untreated thoracic aneurysm is less than 20%. Much recent work has been devoted to establishing the natural history of thoracic aortic aneurysms and the factors that impact upon prognosis. Aneurysm growth is exponential, with increasing rate of expansion with increasing size. Aneurysm growth appears to be accelerated in the presence of continued cigarette smoking and chronic obstructive lung disease. The risk of rupture is related to aneurysm size. Aneurysms less than 5.5 cm in diameter appear to have a low expansion rate and rupture risk while aneurysms >7 cm diameter carry a high risk. The decision to recommend operation is a careful balance between the potential risk of rupture and the attendant risks of surgery, which include death and permanent neurological disability (Coady et al., 1999; Griepp et al., 1999; Pitt et al., 1997; Shimada et al., 1999; Svensson, 1997).

Apart from fatal rupture, the most common presentation of thoracic aortic aneurysms is as an incidental finding on a chest X-ray whilst under investigation for another pathology. Hypertension is a common corollary and pain may occur due to either compression or erosion of vertebral bodies or due to a sudden increase in dimension. Pain may be chronic and very longstanding and difficult to clearly attribute to the aneurysms. Nevertheless, the presence of such chronic pain in the appropriate location appears to be a risk factor for rupture. Such aneurysms may also present due to compression or displacement phenomena. Hoarseness of voice due to stretching of the recurrent laryngeal nerve is a relatively common presenting symptom in distal arch aneurysms. Stridor and dysphagia can occur due to compression of the trachea and bronchi and oesophagus by descending aortic aneurysms while superior vena caval obstruction may complicate ascending aortic aneurysms (Coselli et al., 1997).

6.2. Investigation

Suspicion of the presence of an aneurysm is followed by a number of imaging investigations. Computed tomography is the most widely used investigation and provides information regarding site, size and extent, and serial investigations allow assessment of expansion rate. These data are also provided by magnetic resonance imaging, the use of which is primarily restricted by availability. MRI can additionally be used to assess the aortic valve, pericardium and left ventricular function. If an aneurysm is of sufficient size to warrant consideration of surgical intervention, further investigations are required to assess co-morbidity and to plan the operative approach. Such investigations usually include coronary angiography, carotid duplex scanning, spirometry, arterial blood gas analysis and renal function assessment. Aortography with selective arteriograms of the visceral arterial supplies is a common pre-requisite to repair of thoraco-abdominal aneurysms. Significant valvular heart disease, occlusive coronary and carotid disease should all be treated either before or contemporaneously with any repair of the aneurysm (Kouchoukos et al., 1997; Pitt et al., 1997; Safi et al., 1999).

6.3. Indications for and results of surgery

Although survival of untreated thoracic aneurysms is poor, the hazards of surgery remain substantial. Surgery of the aortic root for isolated annulo-aortic ectasia and Marfan's syndrome has the best reported results and in such circumstances can be recommended prophylactically in patients with aortic diameter >5.5 cm or less in the presence of a family history of sudden death or dissection (Bachet et al., 1997). Surgery of the ascending aorta and arch is more complex and requires strategies of brain protection to reduce cerebral injury. The risk of permanent neurological deficit for such procedures is 5–15% with a mortality of 5–30% (Wong et al., 1999). Because of the risks of aortic arch procedures, recommendation for surgery are restricted to those patients with symptoms attributable to the aneurysm or other features suggestive of imminent risk such as large size, rapid enlargement, pain or compression phenomena (Kouchoukos et al., 1997).

For patients with aneurysms affecting the descending and thoraco-abdominal aorta, surgery is advisable for those aneurysms of >6–7 cm diameter or if symptoms are present The decision to recommend surgery must be based upon local surgical results rather than the best published data in the literature. A few patients with descending and thoraco-abdominal aortic aneurysms may initially survive rupture when exsanguination is prevented by pleural containment. Following rupture, there is a brief time window during which emergency surgery can be contemplated. As in ruptured abdominal aortic aneurysm, the overall survival rate is low (Coady et al., 1999; Griepp et al., 1999; Kouchoukos et al., 1997; Svensson 1997).

The main complications of descending and thoraco-abdominal aortic aneurysm repair are myocardial failure, respiratory insufficiency, renal failure, bleeding and paraplegia or paraparesis. The occurrence of paraplegia is increased in association with bleeding and renal failure reflecting the vulnerability of spinal cord perfusion in the post-operative period. Two primary determinants of spinal cord injury relate to the duration of cord ischaemia and the extent of aortic dissection. In the descending aorta, complete replacement carries a higher risk than segmental replacement. Not surprisingly, resection of the distal descending aorta is more hazardous than a proximal resection. Thoraco-abdominal aneurysms carry a substantial risk (5–30%) of spinal cord injury. Again this is related to aneurysm extent. Crawford extent II aneurysms carry the greatest risk, followed by I, III and IV in that order (Kouchoukos et al., 1997; Safi et al., 1999; Svensson, 1999).

Survival rates following surgery are dependent upon site of resection and disease type. Isolated replacement of the aortic root for Marfan's syndrome and annulo-aortic ectasia are associated with a peri-operative mortality of 1–7% and five-year survival rates approaching 80% (Bachet et al., 1997; Baumgartner et al., 1999). Surgery of the descending aorta carries a mortality of 5–20% dependent on patient age, presentation and co-morbidity; but 5- and 10-year survival rates of 60% and 40% have been reported. Thoraco-abdominal surgery is confined to specialist centres and has similar short- and long-term results (Kouchoukos et al., 1999; Schepens et al., 1999).

7. Marfan's syndrome

This is an autosomal dominantly inherited disorder, the gene for which is located on chromosome 15q. It is a disorder of connective tissue causing abnormalities in the cardiovascular, skeletal and ocular systems. Mutant fibrillin is unable to bind calcium, causing elastic fibre degeneration. This results in

increased aortic wall stiffness, increased pulse pressure, increased wall stress and cardiac workload. Cardiovascular features include progressive dilatation of the proximal aorta causing aortic dissection and rupture. It may cause aortic valve incompetence and regurgitation (Baumgartner et al., 1999; LeMaire et al., 1997; Westaby, 1999).

Life expectancy in Marfan's syndrome is halved, with dissection being the commonest cause of death. Paramount is the prevention of dissection. There is compelling evidence that administration of beta-blockade therapy retards expansion of the aortic root. There is also evidence that prophylactic replacement of an excessively dilated root improves survival. Elective aortic root replacement should be considered when aortic root dimension exceeds 6 cm in the sinus portion or 5 cm beyond. Earlier repair is indicated in patients with chronic dissection, a positive family history of dissection or sudden death, and in females planning pregnancy. Surgical results are very satisfactory with operative mortality rates of <5%. Long term survival following root replacement appears excellent with 10-year survival exceeding 80%.

8. Trauma to the aorta

Penetrating trauma to the aorta is rare in the UK and most commonly the site of injury is within the abdomen. Motor vehicle accidents constitute the main source of blunt aortic trauma, and although injury is more common in young adults, it can also occur in the elderly, but rarely in children. By far the most common site of injury is the proximal descending aorta, just beyond the left subclavian artery at the level of the ligamentum arteriosum. During a rapid deceleration, the sudden arrest of forward motion of the heart, ascending aorta and arch results in a torsion effect at the distal arch-descending aortic junction. A shearing force develops, resulting in, most usually, a transverse tear in the medial aortic wall. Depending upon the interaction of these forces and the prior state of the aorta, the developing tear can affect a small arc of the aortic wall or the whole aortic circumference. Rarely, an ascending aortic transection can occur via the same traumatic mechanism. Many patients die immediately from exsanguination via a full thickness tear but a small number survive transfer to hospital allowing evaluation, investigation and treatment. In these cases, exsanguination has not occurred due to containment of blood loss by the aortic adventitia and mediastinal pleura (Demetiades, 1997; Kirklin et al., 1993; von Segesser et al., 1997).

8.1. Diagnosis and investigation

On occasion, clinical signs of a haemothorax may be present but most commonly there are no specific clinical signs. Aortic trauma should be suspected and excluded in any patient with a compatible mode of injury. The most sensitive chest X-ray finding is a widened mediastinum. Ancillary signs, including obliteration of the aortic knuckle contour, left 1st and 2nd rib fractures, haemothorax, apical pleural capping by haematoma and depression of the left main bronchus, may be present but are not diagnostic.

Although a high index of suspicion is justification for proceeding to aortography, this is often not immediately available and computed tomographic scanning of the aorta and other injured areas acts as a filter for further investigation. CT scanning is a coronal imaging method and cannot directly demonstrate a transverse tear, the detection of a peri-aortic haematoma at the classical site is an indication to proceed to aortography. Findings may include demonstration of an intimal tear manifest as a rosethorn arising from the inner curvature of the aorta or more florid changes including contrast extravasation pseudoaneurysm. Recently, trans-oesophageal echocardiography has been used in the diagnosis of traumatic aortic transection. In a typically sited lesion, this investigation appears to have satisfactory accuracy and may have a role in patients who are unable to withstand transfer to scanning facilities.

8.2. Management and results

Although there is controversy regarding the timing of surgery, the need for operation is generally agreed. Satisfactory results have been obtained in series of patients treated with hypotensives and beta-adrenergic antagonists, in whom aortic surgery has been delayed while other injuries are treated and stabilised but with this approach there remains a risk of unheralded exsanguination during the observation period. Therefore, in patients in whom the aortic injury is felt to be the main threat to life, immediate operation is the generally accepted option. Surgery is undertaken by a full left 4th space thoracotomy. The descending aorta is circumferentially mobilised just distal to the haematoma. Access to the proximal aorta is more difficult and it is essential to obtain a clamp position that maximises suture ac-

cess to the underside of the transverse aortic arch. After mobilisation of the phrenic nerve, the arch is mobilised between the innominate and left common carotid artery. Once this is done, dissection proceeds more distally to circumferentially mobilise the aorta between the left carotid and subclavian. Finally, if possible the arterial ligament is divided prior to aortic clamping. Approximately 50% of lesions can be repaired by direct suture, the remainder requiring a short interposition graft. The extent of repair needed cannot be predicted until the aorta is opened and for this reason it is advisable to utilise some form of bypass (most commonly left atrio-distal bypass) to maintain lower body perfusion during clamping. There is an escalating risk of paraplegia with durations of aortic clamping greater than 30 minutes. This risk can be attenuated by the use of shunting technique. The overall mortality of treated patients is approximately 30% with death due to the overall sequelae of polytrauma. Paraplegia rates of 5–15% are reported.

9. Operative techniques

9.1. Aortic root replacement

This is most frequently performed for annulo-aortic ectasia or an ascending aortic aneurysm with aortic valve incompetence (Fig. 2). Other indications include bacterial endocarditis of the aortic root with extensive abscess formation or acute/chronic aortic dissection with valvular incompetence and severe root disruption. In septic cases, allograft replacement of the aortic root is thought to provide resistance to recurrent infection.

If the aneurysm stops short of the innominate artery, the aorta may be cannulated in the usual fashion; if not, the common femoral artery may be used. The pulmonary artery needs to be cleanly separated from the back of the aorta to allow safe placement of the aortic cross clamp. Cardiopulmonary bypass is established and core cooling commenced. The chosen temperature is dependent upon the anticipated need to utilise hypothermic circulatory arrest to conduct arch repair or an open distal anastomosis. The cross clamp is applied proximal to the innominate artery and the ascending aorta is opened longitudinally and stay sutures applied. Cardioplegia can be administered either directly via the coronary ostia or retrogradely via the coronary sinus.

The replacement graft may either be an allograft aortic valve cylinder or a prosthetic valve cylin-

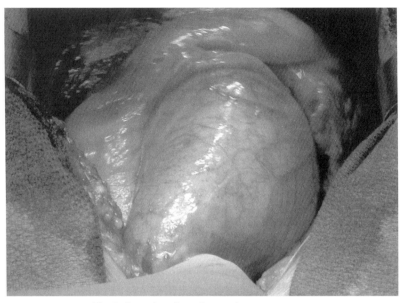

Fig. 2. Operative view of an aortic root aneurysm.

der. The native valve leaflets are excised and the proximal anastomosis performed using interrupted sutures, in the case of an allograft so that it lies orthotopically. For prosthetic aortic root replacement, the use of everting, buttressed mattress sutures of a strong multifilament suture is preferred. There remains debate regarding the ideal method of coronary re-implantation. The classical Bentall method utilised an in-situ technique in which the aortic wall around the coronary ostia was sutured to an ostium created in the graft wall. This technique appears to be associated with a significant incidence of coronary anastomotic leakage, perigraft haematoma and false aneurysm formation and in most centres a modified button technique is preferred. A circular incision then creates a button of native aortic wall around the coronary ostia, and the first part of the artery is mobilised. The ostia of the coronary arteries of the allograft are excised, or appropriate windows are cut in the prosthetic tube graft. The coronary buttons are then fitted and anastomosed with a continuous monofilament suture. The left anastomosis is performed first. Pressurisation of the graft with cardioplegia solution allows the integrity of these anastomoses to be checked. The right coronary implantation can be next performed but is sometimes deferred until the distal graft-aortic anastomosis is complete. This allows a more exact placement of the ostium within the graft. The distal aorta is transected in either an open or closed fashion, the graft being trimmed to an appropriate length and positioned to prevent torsion and folding of redundant material. The anastomosis is performed using a continuous suture technique.

In all aortic operations meticulous primary suture placement is essential as access to bleeding anastomoses following clamp release is particularly difficult. Isolated ascending aortic replacement is performed in a similar manner, the proximal anastomosis being constructed just distal to the sino-tubular junction (Borst et al., 1996; LeMaire et al., 1997).

9.2. Aortic arch replacement

Aortic arch replacement is occasionally required in cases of acute type A dissection but the most common indication is aneurysm due to either degenerative change or chronic dissection. Proximal aortic cannulation may be preferable during cooling to avoid the potential of embolism from a diseased descending aorta during perfusion using femoral arterial return. Although some centres use selective antegrade perfusion techniques for cerebral protection during aortic arch surgery, the majority utilises profound hypothermia with circulatory arrest often supplemented by retrograde cerebral perfusion via the superior vena cava. During cooling the aortic arch is mobilised avoiding excessive manipulation that could dislodge atheromatous material. Mobilisation includes the proximal portions of the epiaortic vessels, dissection of the plane posterior to the aorta and division of the ligamentum arteriosum. Such extensive mobilisation facilitates reconstruction and shortens the arrest period, a critical objective. Following a prolonged period of cooling to 15–18°C, the patient is placed in a steep Trendelenberg position and the extra-corporeal circulation arrested. Any cross clamp is removed and the aortic incision extended into the anterior aortic arch. Meticulous care is taken to prevent athero-embolism into the epi-aortic arteries. The innominate, left carotid and left subclavian artery ostia are usually mobilised as a single, elliptical Carrel patch with a full thickness excision. The distal arch is transected beyond the left subclavian and ligamentum. If the aneurysm is restricted to the transverse arch, the distal end of the graft is simply anastomosed end-to-end with the upper descending thoracic aorta. In cases where there is further aneurysmal dilatation of the proximal descending aorta, an elephant trunk technique can be used. To perform this, part of the arch of prosthetic graft is invaginated upon itself. The whole graft is passed into the upper descending aorta and an anastomosis constructed at the folding ring of the invagination. On completion, the graft is dis-invaginated leaving a trunk protruding into the descending aorta and a graft segment suitable for proximal reconstruction. An ellipse of graft tissue is excised opposite the epiaortic vessel patch, which is then re-implanted using a continuous suture technique. Following this the graft and aortic arch are de-aired meticulously and orthograde perfusion re-instituted. The proximal part of the procedure is then completed (Kirklin et al., 1993).

9.3. Descending thoracic aortic aneurysm repair

For this procedure the patient is placed in the right lateral decubitus position, with the left hip rolled back. The thorax is entered via a long postero-lateral incision through the 4th space. A second entrance through the 7th space may also be required. A limited dissection is performed around the aorta proximal and distal to the aneurysm. A prosthetic graft of matched size is selected and the proximal aortic clamp placed. The proximal anastomosis is performed, the distal clamp placed at an appropriate level and the aneurysm opened longitudinally. If possible, an oblique anastomosis is made to preserve intercostal arteries. Once both anastomoses are complete, the distal clamp is released and the proximal clamp gradually opened. In cases in which a proximal aortic clamp cannot be safely applied due to aortic fragility or extensive atheroma, core-cooling

techniques with open anastomoses under conditions of circulatory arrest are necessary. In cases in which clamping is possible there is increasing evidence that maintenance of distal perfusion using partial or left heart bypass techniques reduce the risk of paraplegia (Kirklin et al., 1993; Kouchoukos et al., 1999; Schepens et al., 1999).

9.4. Thoraco-abdominal aortic aneurysm repair

A thoraco-abdominal incision through the 9th intercostal space is made, extending obliquely across or down the abdomen vertically. A second intercostal incision may be needed. The diaphragm is opened via a peripheral incision, and the retroperitoneal space entered. A prosthetic graft is selected, the proximal clamp placed, the distal clamp placed if used and the aneurysm opened longitudinally. The proximal anastomosis is made within the aneurysm, an oval aperture created in the graft opposite the origin of the visceral arteries, and the graft sewn to the aorta around the origins. The distal anastomosis is made and both clamps are released. The aneurysm walls are wrapped around the graft. Replacement of the thoraco-abdominal aorta is a major undertaking and careful planning is necessary to maximise visceral and spinal cord protection to achieve satisfactory results (Kirklin et al., 1993).

10. Neurological protection

The brain is extremely sensitive to ischaemia, requiring protection for procedures involving an alteration of cerebral blood flow. A number of methods have been used during surgery on the aortic arch, to improve cerebral protection. The simplest method is that of profoundly hypothermic total circulatory arrest, using cardiopulmonary bypass for cooling and re-warming. This is based on the premise that reduced temperature will inhibit cerebral metabolism to allow a period of 'safe' circulatory standstill to be prolonged. The clinically safe duration of hypothermic circulatory arrest is thought to be approximately 40 minutes. Above this time there is a significantly higher incidence of permanent and temporary neurological deficit. Permanent neurological deficit rates of 7–15% are reported and the protection afforded by hypothermia alone remains limited (Svensson et al., 1993; Wong et al., 1999). Retrograde cerebral perfusion, whereby the brain is retrogradely perfused via the superior vena cava during the arrest period, has been used as a putative adjunct to cerebral protection during hypothermic circulatory arrest. Its theoretical advantages are substrate supply, catabolite removal, and maintenance of cooling and protection from gaseous and particulate embolism. Although popular and apparently safe, it has not been shown unequivocally to improve results (Wong et al., 1999).

Antegrade cerebral perfusion uses selective perfusion of the brachiocephalic arteries with cold blood to cool the brain independently. Cardiopulmonary bypass is discontinued and cerebral perfusion carried out during distal aortic repair. When this type of technique is used, body temperature may be advantageously maintained at moderate hypothermia during cold cerebral perfusion. However, results for stroke and mortality using these techniques are similar to those of hypothermic circulatory arrest and no controlled comparative studies have been undertaken (Bachet et al., 1991).

The key determinants of paraplegia during descending and thoraco-abdominal aneurysm repair would appear to be duration of ischaemia and non-reperfusion of critical important intercostal arteries that communicate with the anterior spinal artery. A number of techniques have been advocated in an attempt to reduce the risk. Detailed intercostal angiography in an effort to identify the artery of Adamkiewicz has been attempted by some groups while others have used evoked potential techniques both sensory and motor to predict which segmental arteries are critical to cord perfusion. Others have used techniques to improve the spinal cord's ischaemic tolerance such as whole body cooling or local cooling using epidural irrigation. Spinal fluid drainage, by reducing spinal venous pressure, may improve perfusion during aortic clamping or in the critical reperfusion period. At present no adjunct is universally utilised or of proven efficacy. Of obvious importance are expeditious surgery to minimise the ischaemic period and re-implantation of possible intercostal arteries in the critical T8–L1 segment (Connolly, 1998; Kouchoukos et al., 1999; Svensson, 1999).

References and further reading

Ala-Kulji K, Heikkinen L. Aneurysms after patch graft aortoplasty for coarctation of the aorta: long-term results of surgical management. Ann Thorac Surg 1989; 47: 853–856.

Aoyagi S, Akashi H, Tayama K, Fujino T. Aneurysm of aberrant right subclavian artery arising from diverticulum of Kommerell. Report of a case with tracheal compression. Eur J Cardiothorac Surg 1997; 12: 138–140.

Bachet J, Guilmet D, Goudot B et al. Cold cerebroplegia. A new technique of cerebral protection during operations on the transverse arch. J Thorac Cardiovasc Surg 1991; 102: 85–94.

Bachet J, Goudot B, Dreyfus G, et al. Current practice in Marfan's syndrome and annulo-aortic ectasia: aortic root replacement with a composite graft over a twenty-year period. J Card Surg 1997; 12: 157–166.

Baumgartner WA, Cameron DE, Redmond M, et al. Operative management of Marfan syndrome: the Johns Hopkins experience. Ann Thorac Surg 1999; 67: 1859–1860.

Borst HG, Heinemann MK, Stone CD. Surgical treatment of aortic dissection. New York: Churchill Livingstone, 1996.

Coady MA, Rizzo JA, Hammond GL, et al. Surgical intervention criteria for thoracic aortic aneurysms: a study of growth rates and complications. Ann Thorac Surg 1999; 67: 1922–1926.

Connolly JE. Prevention of spinal cord complications in aortic surgery. Am J Surg 1998; 176: 92–101.

Coselli JS, Poli de Figueiredo LF. Natural history of descending and thoracoabdominal aortic aneurysms. J Card Surg 1997; 12: 285–291.

David TE. Surgical management of aortic root abscess. J Card Surg 1997; 12: 262–269.

David TE, Komeda M, Brofman PR. Surgical treatment of aortic root abscess. Circulation 1989; 80(suppl I): I-269–I-274.

Davidian M, Kee ST, Kato N, et al. Aneurysm of an aberrant right subclavian artery: treatment with PTFE covered stentgraft. J Vasc Surg 1998; 28(2): 335–339.

Demetiades D. Penetrating injuries to the thoracic great vessels. J Card Surg 1997; 12: 173–180.

d'Udekem Y, David TE, Feindel CM, et al. Long-term results of operation for paravalvular abcess. Ann Thorac Surg 1996; 62: 48–53.

Elefteriades JA, Lovoulos CJ, Coady MA, et al. Management of descending aortic dissection. Ann Thorac Surg 1999; 67: 2002–2005.

Fann JI, Miller DC. Endovascular treatment of descending thoracic aortic aneurysms and dissections. Surg Clin North Am 1999; 79(3): 551–574.

Glower DD, Fann JI, Speier RH, et al. Comparison of medical and surgical therapy for uncomplicated descending aortic dissection. Circulation 1990; 82(suppl IV): IV-39–IV-46.

Griepp RB, Ergin A, Galla JD, et al. Natural history of descending thoracic and thoracoabdominal aneurysms. Ann Thorac Surg 1999; 67: 1927–1930.

Kirklin JW, Barratt-Boyes BG. Cardiac Surgery (2nd ed.). New York: Churchill Livingstone, 1993.

Kitamura M, Hashimoto A, Tagusari O, et al. Operation for type B aortic dissection: introduction of left heart bypass. Ann Thorac Surg 1995; 59: 1200–1203.

Kouchoukos NT, Dougenis D. Surgery of the thoracic aorta. N Engl J Med 1997; 336: 1876–1888.

Kouchoukos NT, Rokkas CK. Hypothermic cardiopulmonary bypass for spinal cord protection: rationale and clinical results. Ann Thorac Surg 1999; 67: 1940–1942.

Lansman SL, McCullough JN, Nguyen KH, et al. Subtypes of acute aortic dissection. Ann Thorac Surg 1999; 67: 1975–1978.

LeMaire SA, Coselli JS. Aortic root surgery in Marfan syndrome: current practice and evolving techniques. J Card Surg 1997; 12: 137–141.

McMinn RMH. Last's anatomy regional and applied (9th ed.). New York: Churchill Livingstone, 1994.

Miller DC (ed.). Thoracic aortic problems. Sem Thorac Cardiovasc Surg 1997; 3: 190–268.

Miller DC (ed.). New knowledge and treatments in thoracic aortic disease. Sem Thorac Cardiovasc Surg 1993; 1–99.

Owens WA, Tolan MJ, Cleland J. Late results of patch repair of coarctation of the aorta in adults using autogenous arterial wall. Ann Thorac Surg 1997; 64: 1072–1074.

Pitt MPI, Bonser RS. The natural history of thoracic aortic aneurysm disease: an overview. J Card Surg 1997; 12: 270–278.

Pretre R, von Segesser LK. Aortic dissection. Lancet 1997; 349: 1461–1464.

Sadler TW. Langman's medical embryology (5th ed.). Baltimore: Williams and Wilkins, 1985.

Safi HJ, Miller CC. Spinal cord protection in descending thoracic and thoracoabdominal aortic repair. Ann Thorac Surg 1999; 67: 1937–1939.

Schepens MAAM, Vermeulen FEE, Morshuis WJ et al. Impact of left heart bypass on the results of thoracoabdominal aortic aneurysm repair. Ann Thorac Surg 1999; 67: 1963–1967.

Shimada I, Rooney SJ, Pagano D, et al. Prediction of thoracic aortic aneurysm expansion: validation of formulae describing growth. Ann Thorac Surg 1999; 67: 1968–1970.

Slonim SM et al. Percutaneous balloon fenestration and stenting for life-threatening ischaemic complications in patients with acute aortic dissection. J Thorac Cardiovasc Surg 1999; 117: 1118–1127.

Svensson LG. An approach to spinal cord protection during descending or thoracoabdominal aortic repairs. Ann Thorac Surg 1999; 67: 1935–1936.

Svensson LG. Natural history of aneurysms of the descending and thoracoabdominal aorta. J Card Surg 1997; 12(Suppl): 279–284.

Svensson LG, Crawford ES. Cardiovascular and vascular disease of the aorta. Philadelphia: WB Saunders, 1997.

Svensson LG, Crawford ES, Hess KR et al. Deep hypothermia with circulatory arrest. Determinants of stroke and early mortality in 656 patients. J Thorac Cardiovasc Surg 1993; 106: 19–28.

von Segesser LK, Fischer A, Vogt P, Turina M. Diagnosis and management of blunt great vessel trauma. J Card Surg 1997; 12: 181–192.

Wells WJ, Prendergast TW, Berdjis F, et al. Repair of coarctation of the aorta in adults: the fate of systolic hypertension. Ann Thorac Surg 1996; 61: 1168–1171.

Westaby S. Aortic dissection in Marfan's syndrome. Ann Thorac Surg 1999; 67: 1861–1863.

Wong CH, Bonser RS. Retrograde cerebral perfusion: clinical and experimental aspects. Perfusion 1999; 14: 247–256.

Wong PH, Lee JW. Right aortic arch and Kommerell's diverticulum. Thorax 1983; 38: 553–555.

K. Moghissi, J.A.C. Thorpe and F. Ciulli (Eds.)
Moghissi's Essentials of Thoracic and Cardiac Surgery
© 2003 Elsevier Science B.V. All rights reserved

CHAPTER V.6

Coronary artery bypass surgery

M.J. Underwood and G.J. Cooper

1. Introduction

The syndrome of angina pectoris and its association with atherosclerotic coronary artery disease has been recognised for many centuries. Early surgical treatment attempted to lower the metabolic demands of the myocardium. The use of thoracocervical sympathectomy and thyroidectomy to achieve this were abandoned in favour of techniques aimed at increasing myocardial blood supply. A variety of techniques have been described (Vineberg, 1958) but it was not until the development of coronary angiography that direct myocardial revascularisation with bypass grafts became a reality. Saphenous vein bypass grafting was popularised by Favaloro at the Cleveland Clinic (Favaloro, 1968) and the first internal mammary artery graft was performed in 1964 (Kolessov, 1967). Since this time, the use of coronary artery bypass surgery for the treatment of patients with ischaemic heart disease has increased exponentially

Table 1

Indications for coronary artery bypass surgery

Clinical	Anatomical
(1) Stable angina on maximum medical therapy	(1) LMS stenosis >50%
(2) Unstable angina	(2) TVD with impaired LV
(3) Post MI angina	(3) TVD normal LV :inducible ischaemia
(4) Unsuccessful PTCA	(4) Two-vessel disease :proximal LAD stenosis
(5) Mechanical complications	(5) Severe LV impairment :reversible ischaemia
	(6) CAD prior to other surgery

LMS = Left main stenosis; TVD = Triple vessel disease; LV = Left ventricle; MI = Myocardial infarction; LAD = Left anterior descending coronary artery; CAD = Coronary artery disease.

and has become one of the commonest surgical procedures performed.

2. Indications for coronary artery surgery

The indications for coronary artery surgery can be divided into clinical (relief of symptoms) and anatomical (improved survival) (Table 1). It is important, however, to understand how these indications have been established and the limitations and controversies which exist when applied to current clinical practice.

2.1. Randomised trials of coronary bypass surgery

2.1.1. The trials
Randomised trials of medical therapy versus bypass surgery were advocated in the 1970s in an attempt to determine the place of surgery in the treatment of patients with ischaemic heart disease (Table 2). Three major studies were initiated which provided valuable information but each has limitations in study design and the conclusions must be applied with caution in the current era.

Veterans administration (VA) cooperative study. The VA study randomised 686 male patients who had stable angina for at least 6 months and evidence of ischaemia on resting or stress electrocardiography (Veterans Administration Coronary Artery Bypass Surgery Cooperative Study Group, 1984). Survival was improved for patients with left main disease who underwent surgery and also for patients in angiographic (triple vessel disease, EF <45%) or clinical (hypertension, and previous MI, Class III–IV symptoms, resting ST changes) 'high' risk groups. Relief of angina was better in the surgical group at

Table 2

Randomised trials of coronary artery surgery

	VA	ECSS	CASS
Year	1972–1974	1973–1976	1975–1979
No patients	686	768	780
Age	Any	<65 yrs	<65 yrs
Females	0	0	10%
Anginal Class %	3% I	58% I–II	15% I
	39% II	42% III	59% II
	55% III		22% post MI
	3% IV		:asymtomatic
EF %	>45% 74%	>50%	>50% 73%
	<45% 26%		<50% 21%

Table 3

Limitations of the randomised trials

- Intention to treat methodology
- Left Internal Mammary Artery not used
- Improvements in surgical techniques and myocardial protection
- No antiplatelet therapy in post-operative period
- Small number of female patients
- Small number of patients >65yrs
- Improvements in medical treatment of angina
- Advent of angioplasty and stenting

from: Kirklin et al., 1993, p. 1130.

7 years but this advantage was lost by 10 years. The operative mortality was 5.6% and the perioperative infarction rate nearly 10%.

European coronary surgery study. The European study randomised 768 men with preserved left ventricular function and stable angina (European Coronary Surgery Study Group, 1982). Surgery improved survival at 10 years in patients with left main stem disease, triple vessel disease and two vessel disease with proximal involvement of the left anterior descending coronary artery (LAD) and a positive exercise test. Relief of angina was also significantly improved at 5 years with surgery and the rate of fatal myocardial infarction lowered. The operative mortality was 3.3%.

Coronary artery surgery study. CASS randomised 780 patients to medical or surgical therapy (CASS Principle Investigators and their Associates, 1983). 90% were male and all were either asymptomatic or had Class I–II angina. Only patients with triple vessel disease and impaired ventricular function had a survival advantage at 10 years following surgery. Surgery reduced the incidence of fatal myocardial infarction at 5 years. The operative mortality was 1.4%.

2.1.2. Limitations

The main conclusions after analysis of all three studies were that surgery provides relief of angina, reduces the incidence of fatal myocardial infarction and improves survival in patients with left main stem disease or triple vessel disease with impairment of left ventricular function (Kaisser, 1986). These conclusions need to be applied with a knowledge of the study limitations (Table 3).

All trials were conducted on an 'intention to treat' basis which in essence means that the end results were correlated with the initial randomisation. Nearly 40% of patients in the medical arm crossed over to surgery by 10 years, a fact which may overestimate survival figures for the medical groups. This does suggest however that medical therapy can be safely continued until more advanced symptoms of angina are present. Only the VA study provided evidence of inducible angina in patients by exercise testing, and although all the studies correlated survival with severity of angina, extent of coronary disease, and degree of ventricular function, none of them examined the relationship between survival and the extent of ischaemia or myocardium 'at risk'. Patients with moderate to severe left ventricular impairment (EF <35%) represented only a small group in the VA study and were excluded in the other two. The application of the conclusions of these studies to women and patients over the age of 65 years are difficult since both the VA and ECSS excluded women (10% of study population in CASS) and both the ECSS and CASS studies excluded patients over 65 years.

A variety of other issues also need to be appreciated. The mortality (5.6%) in the VA study for patients with chronic stable angina would be considered unacceptable in current practice following improvements in anaesthesia, surgical technique and myocardial protection. The internal mammary artery was not used in any study and has since been shown to improve event-free and overall survival in surgical patients (Loop et al., 1986). Other arterial grafts are now being used and producing superior surgical outcomes for certain groups of patients (Lytle et al., 1999). Anti-platelet therapy has been shown to improve the early patency of vein grafts (Underwood et al., 1994) since these studies were conducted and all these factors suggest that the surgical results in the current era should be superior. The same can be said for medical therapies for angina which have also improved considerably.

3. Other indications

3.1. Unstable angina

Unstable angina is evidence of important myocardial ischaemia but urgent or emergency coronary surgery is only indicated when medical therapy fails to stabilise the patient. If the unstable angina subsides with medical therapy, the patient should be investigated further and recommendations based upon these results. However, the occurrence of unstable angina predisposes the patient to further events of this nature and also myocardial infarction and therefore the indications for surgery following an episode of unstable angina become stronger whichever symptomatic or anatomical group the patient falls into after investigation (Von Dohlen et al., 1989).

3.2. Following myocardial infarction

3.2.1. Uncomplicated Q wave
Surgery probably has little place in the management of these patients in the acute phase and only a few centres propose its use. Comparative benefits need to be assessed along with thrombolysis and angioplasty. A positive exercise test following successful medical treatment of these patients, however, may be predictive of a 15–20% one-year mortality and early angiography is indicated to determine which patients may benefit from revascularisation (Gibson, 1989).

3.2.2. Uncomplicated non-Q wave
These patients generally have the same indications as patients with unstable or post-infarction angina. However, the risk of re-infarction may be substantially higher than patients with a Q-wave infarct and this high incidence of recurrent ischaemic events may be an indication for early investigation and revascularisation as appropriate (Bosch et al., 1987).

3.2.3. Acute ischaemia following unsuccessful PTCA
When PTCA fails, resulting in vessel closure, the patient may develop angina, ECG changes, or haemodynamic insability. Several measures are now available to cardiologists to re-open the vessel and minimise myocardial damage, including the use of reperfusion catheters. Failure of these therapies, however, requires urgent surgery which must take into ac-

count general patient factors. Reperfusion catheters and insertion of an intra-aortic balloon pump may help stabilise the patient whilst surgery is organised (Greene et al., 1991).

3.2.4. Silent ischaemia
Patients with coronary artery disease but without angina, usually identified following myocardial infarction, may benefit from coronary artery bypass grafting.

The presence of silent ischaemia impairs prognosis (Weiner et al., 1988a; Weiner et al., 1995) and the magnitude of this impairment is related to the severity of the underlying coronary artery disease (Weiner et al., 1988a). In certain patients prognosis is improved by surgery. Surgically treated patients with three vessel disease and reduced ventricular function have a 7-year survival twice that of medically treated patients (Weiner et al., 1988b) and operation is indicated in patients with left main stem stenosis (Taylor et al., 1989).

3.2.5. Patients with heart failure
Coronary artery disease may not only present as heart failure but is also its commonest cause (SOLVD investigators, 1991). Data from the CASS registry suggests that coronary artery bypass is not beneficial in patients with predominant heart failure (Alderman et al., 1983) however the identification of the phenomenon of hibernating myocardium raises the possibility of improving ventricular function in these patients (Rahimtoola, 1989). Hibernating myocardium can be identified by dobutamine stress echocardiography, positron emission tomography, and thallium scintigraphy (Dilsizian et al., 1993). Revascularisation in these patients can improve left ventricular function (Vom Dahl et al., 1994; Dreyfus et al., 1994; Pagano et al., 1998) with an operative mortality of between 2% and 6% (Pagano et al., 1998). The long-term clinical benefit of this remains to be established, however.

4. Coronary bypass surgery versus angioplasty

Since the conduct of the randomised trials described above, interventional cardiology has expanded exponentially and the ability to perform angioplasty (PTCA) and stenting has also had an influence on the indications for coronary bypass surgery. Several randomised studies are in progress in an attempt to define the place of each in the management of patients with coronary artery disease. Early reports

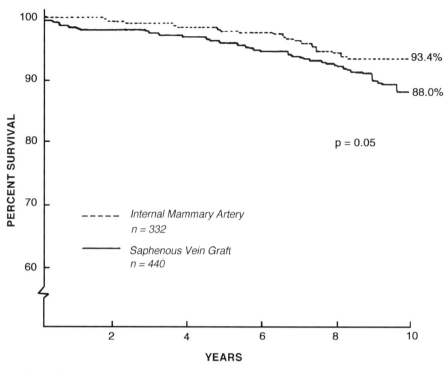

Fig. 1. Ten-year survival of patients with One-Vessel (Anterior Descending Artery) Disease.

Given the benefit of using one internal mammary artery, the expectation has been that using both would further improve outcome. This has been difficult to prove possibly because of the large number of possible combinations of graft and recipient coronary artery (Underwood et al., 1997). When the right internal mammary artery is placed to the right coronary artery, no benefit over a single internal mammary artery is found at 8 years (Carrel et al., 1996). However, in series where both mammary arteries have principally been placed to the left coronary artery, usually left-to-left anterior descending and right-to-circumflex coronary artery, survival advantages of 5% to 23% have been demonstrated at 10 years (Pick et al., 1997; Buxton et al., 1998; Schmidt et al., 1997). This survival advantage becomes apparent after 5 to 6 years (Pick et al., 1997) and may be greater in those with worse ventricular function, diabetes and peripheral vascular disease (Buxton et al., 1998).

To achieve a complete arterial revascularisation usually requires use of more than both internal mammary arteries. Reports of low patency with the inferior epigastric artery have reduced enthusiasm for its use (Perrault et al., 1993) and most surgeons prefer the radial or gastroepiploic arteries as the third conduit. Excellent five year results have been obtained with both radial (Borger et al. 1998) and gastroepiploic (Grandjean et al., 1996; Albertini et al., 1998) arteries.

5.3.3. Which conduits to use and when

Left internal mammary artery. The survival benefit of grafting the left anterior descending coronary artery with the left internal mammary artery is present in the elderly (Gardner et al., 1990), diabetics (Morris et al., 1991) and women (Cameron et al., 1988). Furthermore, its use may beneficially effect operative mortality (Grover et al., 1994). Concerns about inadequate flow through internal mammary artery grafts early after operation do not seem to have any great clinical significance (Cooper et al., 1995). The evidence supports using the left internal mammary artery whenever the left anterior descending coronary artery is to be grafted. The only exception is in the case of acute unrelieved ischaemia when a vein graft may provide speedier revascularisation. In patients with subclavian artery stenosis, the mammary artery should be used as a free graft.

Both internal mammary arteries. Use of both internal mammary arteries confers a substantial risk of sternal wound complications in diabetics (Cosgrove et al., 1988; Kouchoukos et al., 1990), the elderly

(Cosgrove et al., 1988) and the obese (Kouchoukos et al., 1990). Bilateral mammary artery grafting is indicated in patients in whom both internal mammary arteries can be placed to the left coronary artery, who are not at high risk for wound complications and in whom the expected survival advantage is judged to be important.

Total arterial revascularisation. A strategy of total arterial revascularisation has not been shown to be superior to one or two mammary arteries and supplementary vein grafts. It may be useful for selected younger patients and those in whom there is no venous conduit.

5.4. Operative mortality after coronary artery bypass

Despite a less favorable patient profile (Estafanous et al., 1998), during the past decade operative mortality for isolated coronary artery bypass has remained constant at around 3% in both the USA (Kirklin et al., 1991) and the UK (Keogh et al., 1999). In Europe, patients without any of the risk factors identified in the EuroSCORE have an operative mortality of 0.4% (Roques et al., 1999).

Many risk factors have been identified that increase the operative risk; these are summarised in Table 7.

6. Re-operative coronary surgery

6.1. Indications

Patients may re-present following coronary artery surgery with recurrent angina as a result of vein graft occlusion, native vessel disease or a combination of both. These patients require special consideration both in terms of the indications for operation and the appropriate surgical strategy.

The mortality following re-operation is significantly higher than that documented for first-time operations (Lytle et al., 1987). Only patients with a stenotic vein graft to the LAD have an improved survival with re-operative surgery (Lytle et al., 1992). Patients with a patent LIMA–LAD graft, minimal symptoms and who do not have large areas of myocardium placed at 'risk' due to diseased vein grafts have equivalent survival if managed medically and the presence of severe symptoms with good 'target' vessels are the only other indications for re-operation.

Table 7

Pre-operative and operative risk factors for increasing the probability of death early or late after a primary coronary bypass operation [a]

Risk factors
Demographic
– Age at coronary bypass operation (older)
– Body size (smaller)
– Gender (female)
Clinical status
– Angina (Canadian class 0 to IV) (more severe)
– Unstable angina
– Response to stress testing (more severe)
– Acute myocardial infarction
– Hemodynamic instability (grade 0 to 4) (more severe)
– NYHA functional class (I to IV) (higher)
Distribution and severity of coronary artery disease (greater)
Left ventricular dysfunction (grade 0 to 4) (more severe)
Aggressiveness of arteriosclerotic process
– Diffusely diseased coronary arteries
– Peripheral vascular disease
– Cerebrovascular disease
– Hyperlipidemia (more severe)
– Age at coronary bypass operation (younger)
Coexisting disease
– Diabetes
– Hypertension
– Pulmonary disease (more severe)
– Stroke
– Smoking
Surgical factors
– Date of operation (earlier)
– Non-use of IMA to LAD
– Incomplete revascularisation
– Peri-operative myocardial infarction (inadequate myocardial management)
– Surgeon
Institutional factors

IMA, internal mammary artery; LAD, left anterior descending coronary artery; NYHA, New York Heart Association.

[a] This table is not the result of a specific multivariable analysis, but is a composite depiction of data from many studies.

6.2. Operative techniques

Special attention has to be paid to a variety of issues (Table 8).

6.2.1. Patent LIMA–LAD grafts
A patent LIMA–LAD graft poses problems in terms of damage to the graft during sternotomy and mobilisation of the heart and also to the technique of myocardial protection. The graft is most at risk

Table 8

Technical considerations during re-operative coronary surgery

Consideration	Problem	Solution
Patent LIMA–LAD graft	Damage	Careful surgical technique
		Divide pericardium at first operation
	Myocardial protection	Add retrograde cardioplegia Occlude graft
Embolisation from vein grafts	Myocardial Infarction	Minimise mobilisation of grafts
		Add retrograde cardioplegia
		Replace grafts >5 yrs old
Replacing veins with arterial grafts	Hypoperfusion	Leave vein graft in-situ
Inadequate conduit	Incomplete revascularisation	'Recycle' existing arterial grafts

from damage if it lies high on the chest wall, an occurrence which should be prevented at the first operation by dividing the pericardium and allowing it to lie medial to the lung.

6.2.2. Myocardial protection

Antegrade cardioplegia alone may not be protective during re-operative coronary surgery. If the patient has a patent LIMA–LAD graft, this area of myocardium will not receive cardioplegia, and atherosclerosis in vein grafts may embolise, resulting in infarction. Additional infusion of cardioplegia via the retrograde route can minimise these problems, although there are concerns regarding protection of the right ventricle if it is used alone. The technique of cross-clamp fibrillation may also result in complications as a result of repeated clamping of the aorta, which is often calcified in these cases and it may also dislodge atherosclerotic debris in the proximal ends of diseased vein grafts. A combination of antegrade and retrograde cardioplegia seems the most sensible compromise.

6.2.3. Management of patent or stenotic vein grafts

Problems with patent or stenotic (as opposed to occluded) vein grafts include the potential for embolisation of atheromatous debris, and subsequent disease progression. It has been suggested that all grafts older than 5 years be replaced to avoid these complications (Marshall et al., 1986). However, this strategy also has to take into account the patient's age, the availability of suitable conduit and the quality of the distal coronary vessels and a sensible compromise reached.

6.2.4. Replacing vein grafts with pedicled arterial conduits

Patients with an occluded LAD and a stenosed vein grafts to this vessel who have the vein graft replaced

with the LIMA are at risk of hypoperfusion. A disadvantage to leaving the vein graft in situ is the potential for embolisation, but this appears to be small, and it appears this is the safest option for managing this situation unless a large diagonal vessel is also amenable to grafting and provides additional blood flow to the area of myocardium at risk of hypoperfusion (Cooper et al., 1995).

6.2.5. Re-operation following use of arterial grafts

This may be necessary because of progression of native vessel disease, technical problems during the primary operation or disease of additionally placed venous grafts. A variety of approaches have been described to minimise the potential for damaging patent arterial grafts at re-operation and techniques have also been described which allow 'recycling' of previously placed arterial grafts to circumvent the problems of inadequate conduit (Noirhomme et al., 1999).

7. Management of the patient following coronary artery surgery

Coronary bypass surgery is a palliative operation and should be considered only as a treatment incident in the overall management of the patient with coronary atherosclerosis. A variety of measures must be instigated post-operatively to ensure continued benefit for the patient (Table 9).

7.1. Smoking

Cessation of smoking is pivotal in prolonging the patency of venous bypass grafts and in reducing the incidence of progressive native vessel disease. A variety of studies and data from the CASS registry have shown that patients who continue to smoke following coronary revascularisation have a reduced survival, have more cardiac events and are readmitted to hos-

Table 9

Management of patients following coronary artery surgery

Proven benefit
- Stop smoking
- Aspirin for life
- Lipid lowering treatment if indicated
- Rehabilitation programmes

Anticipated Benefit
- Blood pressure control
- Control diabetes
- Dietary advice

pital more frequently than patients who have stopped smoking (Cavender et al., 1992). Many patients need help to achieve this and the use of rehabilitation programmes may be of great value.

7.2. Aspirin

Treatment with aspirin has clearly been demonstrated as being effective in improving early vein graft patency when given in the immediate post-operative period. This benefit has been shown to be present for at least a year post-operatively. Continued treatment should also be beneficial in these patients since they still have native vessel atherosclerosis and the benefits of secondary prevention demonstrated by meta-analysis may also be applicable to this cohort of patients although direct evidence is lacking (Underwood et al., 1994).

7.3. Lipid-lowering therapy

There is substantial evidence that lipid-lowering therapy promotes coronary plaque stabilisation by reducing the lipid content of the lesions, and regression of coronary atherosclerosis has also been demonstrated (Cashin-Hemphill et al., 1990). This may also be true for vein graft atherosclerosis and lipid levels should be monitored post-operatively and treatment initiated when indicated.

7.4. Other factors

Whilst there is no direct evidence of benefit in cohorts of patients following coronary bypass surgery, it seems sensible that other factors such as hypertension and diabetes should be monitored and treated accordingly following surgery. As stated, the use of rehabilitation programmes with education regarding diet and exercise allows all these factors to be

monitored and the success of the operation can be prolonged (Engblom et al., 1992).

7.5. Future considerations

Many areas of coronary surgery will change substantially in the next decade. With improvements in angioplasty and stent technology, these interventions may well become commonplace in multivessel disease whilst improved outcome in surgical patients undergoing multiple arterial revascularisation may challenge this. Minimally invasive coronary surgery is now established in some units and may be beneficial for certain subgroups of patients and indeed may be combined with angioplasty in certain situations (Izzat et al., 1997). Special retractors and stabilising devices have contributed to more widespread use of 'off-pump' revascularisation and its proponents will undoubtedly document superior results. Other innovative technologies using endoscopic techniques and CRT optics with robotic help will continue to develop and may gain a place in the armamentarium of the cardiac surgeon (Loop, 1998). Inhibition of vein graft disease using non-restrictive stents, gene therapy and even techniques to promote angiogenesis may improve outcome and may also be used in conjunction with angioplasty techniques (Jeremy et al., 1999). All these areas will develop over the next 10 years and provide unique tools to aid the surgeon managing patients with coronary atherosclerosis.

References and further reading

Acar C, Ramshey A, Pagny JY et al. The radial artery for coronary artery bypass grafting. Clinical and radiological results at five years. J Thorac Cardiovasc Surg 1998; 116: 981–989.

Albertini A, Lochegnies A, El Khoury G et al. Use of the right gastroepiploic artery as a coronary artery bypass graft in 307 patients. Cardiovasc Surg 1998; 6: 419–423.

Alderman E, Fisher L, Litwin P et al. Results of coronary artery surgery in patients with poor left ventricular function. Circulation 1983; 4: 785–795.

Borger MA, Cohen G, Buth KJ et al. Multiple arterial grafts. Radial versus right internal thoracic arteries. Circulation 1998; 98: II-7–II-14.

Bosch X, Theroux P, Waters DD et al. Early post-infarction ischaemia: clinical, angiographic and prognostic significance. Circulation 1987; 75: 988–995.

Buch M, Dion R. Current status of the inferior epigastric artery. Semin Thorac Surg Cardiovasc Surg 1996; 8: 10–14.

Buda AJ, Macdonald IL, Anderson MJ, Strauss HD, David TE, Berman ND. Long term results following coronary bypass operation: Importance of preoperative factors and complete revascularisation. J Thorac Cardiovasc Surg 1981; 82: 383–390.

Buxton BF, Komeda M, Fuller JA, Gordon I. Bilateral internal thoracic artery grafting may improve outcome of coronary artery surgery. Circulation 1998; 98: II-1–II-6.

Cameron A, Davis KB, Green G, Schaff HV. Coronary artery bypass surgery with internal thoracic artery grafts — effects on survival over a 15 year period. N Engl J Med 1996; 334: 216–219.

Cameron A, Davis KB, Green GE et al. Clinical implications of internal mammary artery grafting: The Coronary Artery Surgery Study experience. Circulation 1988; 77: 815–819.

Cameron A Kemp HG, Green GE. Bypass surgery with the internal mammary artery grafts: 15 year follow up. Circulation 1986; 74: III-30–III-36.

Carrel T, Horder P, Turina MI. Operation for 2-vessel coronary artery disease: Midterm results of bilateral ITA grafting versus unilateral ITA and saphenous vein grafting. Ann Thorac Surg 1996; 62: 1289–1294.

Cashin-Hemphill L, Mack WJ, Pogoda JM et al. Beneficial effects of combined colestipol–niacin therapy on coronary atherosclerosis: a 4 year follow up. JAMA 1990; 264: 3013–3017.

CASS principle investigators and their associates. Coronary Artery Surgery Study: a randomised trial of coronary artery bypass surgery. Survival data. Circulation 1983; 68: 939–950.

Cavender JB, Rogers WJ, Fisher LD et al. Effects of smoking on survival and morbidity in patients randomised to medical or surgical therapy in the CASS study: 10 year follow up. J Am Coll Cardiol 1992; 20: 287.

Cooper GJ, Angelini GD. Flow through arterial grafts. In: Angelini GD, Bryan AJ, Dion R (eds.), Arterial grafts in myocardial revascularisation. London: E Arnold, 1995: 46–54.

Cosgrove DM, Loop FD, Lytle BW et al. Determinants of 10 year survival after primary myocardial revascularisation. Ann Surg 1985; 202: 480–490.

Cosgrove DM, Lytle BW, Loop FD et al. Does bilateral internal mammary artery grafting increase surgical risk? J Thorac Cardiovasc Surg 1988; 95: 850–856.

Dilsizian V, Bonow RO. Current diagnostic techniques of assessing myocardial viability in patients with hibernating and stunned myocardium. Circulation 1993; 87: 1–20.

Dion R, Verhelst R, Fousseau M et al. Sequential mammary grafting. J Thorac Cardiovasc Surg 1989; 98: 80–89.

Donatelli F, Triggiani M, Benussi S, D'Ancona G. Inferior epigastric artery as a conduit for myocardial revascularisation: a two year clinical and angiographic follow up. Cardiovasc Surg 1998; 6: 52–54.

Dreyfus G, Duboc D, Blasco A et al. Myocardial viability assessment in ischaemic cardiomyopathy: benefits of coronary revascularisation. Ann Thorac Surg 1994; 57: 1402–1408.

Engblom E, Ronnemaa T, Hamalainen H et al. Coronary heart disease risk factors before and after bypass surgery: results of a controlled trial on multifactorial rehabilitation. Eur Heart J 1992; 13: 232–237.

Estafanous FG, Loop FD, Higgins TL et al. Increased risk and decreased morbidity of coronary artery bypass grafting between 1986 and 1994. Ann Thorac Surg 1998; 65: 383–389.

European Coronary Surgery Study Group. Long term results of prospective randomisation study of coronary artery bypass surgery in stable angina pectoris. Lancet 1982; 2: 1173–1180.

Favaloro RG. Saphenous vein autograft replacement of severe segmental coronary artery occlusion: operative technique. Ann Thorac Surg 1968; 5: 334–339.

Fitzgibbon GM, Leach AJ, Kafka HP, Keon WJ. Coronary bypass graft fate: long term angiographic study. J Am Coll Cardiol 1991; 17: 1075–1080.

Gardner TJ, Green PS, Rykil MF et al. Routine use of the left internal mammary artery graft in the elderly. Ann Thorac Surg 1990; 49: 188–194.

Gerola LR, Puig LB, Moreira LF et al. Right internal thoracic artery through the transverse sinus in myocardial revascularisation. Ann Thorac Surg 1996; 61: 1708–1712.

Gibson RS. Management of acute non-Q-wave myocardial infarction: role of prophylactic pharmacotherapy and indications for pre-discharge arteriography. Clin Cardiol 1989; 12: 26–32.

Grandjean JG, Voors AA, Boonstra PW, den Heyer P, Ebels T. Exclusive use of arterial grafts in coronary artery bypass operations for three vessel disease: use of both thoracic arteries and the gastroepiploic in 256 consecutive patients. J Thorac Cardiovasc Surg 1996; 112: 935–942.

Greene MA, Gray LA, Slater AD et al. Emergency aortocoronary bypass after failed angioplasty. Ann Thorac Surg 1991; 51: 194–199.

Grover FL, Johnson RR, Marshall G, Hammermeister KE. Impact of mammary artery grafts on coronary bypass operative mortality and morbidity. Ann Thorac Surg 1994; 57: 559–568.

Ivert T, Huttunen K, Landou C, Bjork VO. Angiographic studies of internal mammary artery grafts 11 years after coronary artery bypass grafting. J Thorac Cardiovasc Surg 1988; 96: 1–12.

Izzat MB, Yim APC, Mehta D et al. Staged minimally invasive coronary artery bypass and angioplasty for multivessel coronary disease. Int J Cardiol 1997; 62: 105–109.

Jeremy JY, Rowe D, Gadson P et al. Novel strategies in the treatment of late vein graft failure. Vasc Dis 1999; 2: 2–7.

Jones EL, Weintraub WS. The importance of completeness of revascularisation during long-term follow-up after coronary artery operations. J Thorac Cardiovasc Surg 1996; 112: 227–237.

Kaisser GC. CABG: lessons from the randomised trials. Ann Thorac Surg 1986; 42: 3–8.

Keogh BE, Kinsman R. National audit cardiac surgical database report. Society of Cardiothoracic Surgeons of Great Britain and Ireland. 1999.

Kirklin JW, Akins CW, Blackstone EH et al. ACC/AHA guidelines and indications for coronary artery bypass graft surgery. Circulation 1991; 83: 1125–1173.

Kolessov VI. Mammary artery-coronary artery anastomosis as method of treatment for angina pectoris. J Thorac Cardiovasc Surg 1967; 54: 535–544.

Kouchoukos NT, Wareing TH, Murphy SF, Pelate C, Marshall WG. Risks of bilateral internal mammary artery bypass grafting. Ann Thorac Surg 1990; 49: 210–217.

Loop FD. Coronary artery surgery: the end of the beginning. Eur J Cardiothorac Surg 1998; 14: 554–571.

Loop FD, Lytle BW, Cosgrove DM et al. Influence of the internal mammary artery on 10 year survival and other cardiac events. N Eng J Med 1986; 314: 1–6.

Lytle BW, Blackstone EH, Loop FD et al. Two internal thoracic artery grafts are better than one. J Thorac Cardiovasc Surg 1999; 117: 855–872.

Lytle BW, Loop FD, Cosgrove DM et al. Fifteen hundred coronary reoperations: results and determinants of early and late survival. J Thorac Cardiovasc Surg 1987; 93: 847–859.

Lytle BW, Loop FD, Taylor PC et al. Vein graft disease: the clinical impact of stenosis in saphenous vein bypass grafts to coronary arteries. J Thorac Cardiovasc Surg 1992; 103: 831–840.

Marshall WG, Saffitz J, Kouchoukos NT. Management during reoperation of aortocoronary saphenous grafts with minimal atherosclerosis by angiography. Ann Thorac Surg 1986; 42: 163–167.

Morris JJ, Smith LR, Jones RH et al. Influence of diabetes and mammary artery grafting on survival after coronary bypass. Circulation 1991; 84: III-275–III-284.

Navia D, Cosgrove DM, Lytle BE et al. Is the internal thoracic artery the conduit of choice to replace a stenotic vein graft? Ann Thorac Surg 1994; 57: 40–44.

Noirhomme PH, Underwood MJ, El Khoury G et al. Recycling arterial grafts during reoperative coronary operations. Ann Thorac Surg 1999; 67: 641–644.

Pagano D, Townend JN, Littler WA, Horton R, Camici PG, Bonser RS. Coronary artery bypass surgery as treatment for ischaemic heart failure: The predictive value of viability assessment with quantitative positron emission tomography for symptomatic and functional outcome. J Thorac Cardiovasc Surg 1998; 115: 791–799.

Perrault LP, Carrier M, Hebert Y, Cartier R, leclerc Y, Pelletier LC. Early experience with the inferior epigastric artery in coronary artery bypass grafting. A word of caution. J Thorac Cardiovasc Surg 1993; 106: 928–930.

Pick AW, Orszulak TA, Anderson BJ, Schaff HV. Single versus bilateral internal mammary artery grafts: 10 year outcome analysis. Ann Thorac Surg 1997; 64: 599–605.

Pym J, Brown P, Pearson M, Parker J. Right gastroepiploic to coronary artery bypass. The first decade of use. Circulation 1995; 92: II-45–II-49.

Rahimtoola SH. The hibernating myocardium. Am Heart J 1989; 117: 211–221.

Roques F, Nashef SAM, Michel P et al. Risk factors and outcome in European cardiac surgery: Analysis of the EuroSCORE multinational database of 19030 patients. Eur J Cardiothorac Surg 1999; 15: 816–823.

Schmidt SE, Jones JW, Thornby JI, Miller CC, Beal AC. Improved survival with multiple left sided bilateral internal thoracic artery grafts. Ann Thorac Surg 1997; 64: 9–15.

Sergeant P, Lesaffre E, Flameng W, Suy R. Internal mammary artery: Method of use and effect on survival. Eur J Cardiothorac Surg 1990; 4: 72–78.

Sergeant PT, Blackstone EH, Meyns BP. Does arterial revascularisation decrease the risk of infarction after coronary artery bypass grafting? Ann Thorac Surg 1998; 66: 1–11.

SOLVD investigators. Effect of enalapril on survival in patients with reduced left ventricular ejection fraction and congestive heart failure. N Engl J Med 1991; 325: 293–302.

Stoney WS, Alford WC, Burrus GR et al. The fate of arm veins used for aorta-coronary bypass grafts. J Thorac Cardiovasc Surg 1984; 88: 522–526.

Tatoulis J, Buxton BF, Fuller JA. Results of 1454 free right internal thoracic artery-to-coronary artery grafts. Ann Thorac Surg 1997; 64: 1263–1269.

Taylor HA, Deumite NJ, Chaitman BR et al. Asymptomatic left main coronary artery disease in the Coronary Artery Surgery Study registry. Circulation 1989; 79: 1171–1176.

Underwood MJ, Cooper GJ, Keogh B. Is one arterial graft enough? Total arterial revascularisation seems promising. BMJ 1997; 31: 1213–1214.

Underwood MJ, More RS. The aspirin papers. BMJ 1994; 308: 71–72.

The Veterans Administration Coronary Artery Bypass Surgery Cooperative Study Group. Eleven year survival in the Veterans Administration randomised trial of coronary bypass surgery for stable angina. N Eng J Med 1984; 311: 333–339.

Vineberg AM. Coronary vascular anastomosis by internal mammary artery implantation. Can Med Ass J 1958; 78: 871–879.

Vom Dahl J, Eitzman DT, al Aouar ZR et al. Relation of regional function, perfusion and metabolism in patients with advanced coronary artery disease undergoing surgical revascularisation. Circulation 1994; 90: 2356–2366.

Von Dohlen TW, Rogers WB, Frank MJ. Pathophysiology and management of unstable angina. Clin Cardiol 1989; 12: 363–369.

Voutilainen S, Verkkala K, Jarvinen A, Keto P. Angiographic 5 year follow-up study of right gastroepiploic artery grafts. Ann Thorac Surg 1996; 62: 501–505.

Weiner DA, Ryan TJ, McCabe CH et al. Comparison of coronary artery bypass surgery and medical therapy in patients with exercise-induced silent myocardial ischaemia: A report from the Coronary Artery Surgery Study registry. J Am Coll Cardiol 1988a; 12: 595–599.

Weiner DA, Ryan TJ, McCabe CH et al. Risk of developing an acute myocardial infarction or sudden coronary death in patients with exercise-induced silent myocardial ischaemia. A report from the Coronary Artery Surgery Study registry. Am J Cardiol 1988b; 62: 1155–1158.

Weiner DA, Ryan TJ, Parsons L et al. Significance of silent myocardial ischaemia during exercise testing in women: Report from the Coronary Artery Surgery study. Am Heart J 1995; 129: 465–470.

White HD. Angioplasty versus bypass surgery. Lancet 1995; 346: 1174–1175.

Zeff RH, Kangtahwom C, Iannone LA et al. Internal mammary artery versus saphenous vein to the left anterior descending coronary artery. Prospective randomised study with 10 year follow up. Ann Thorac Surg 1988; 45: 533–536.

K. Moghissi, J.A.C. Thorpe and F. Ciulli (Eds.)
Moghissi's Essentials of Thoracic and Cardiac Surgery
© 2003 Elsevier Science B.V. All rights reserved

CHAPTER V.7

Off-pump coronary artery bypass (OPCAB) surgery

R. Ascione, F. Ciulli and G.D. Angelini

1. Introduction

Off-pump coronary artery bypass (OPCAB) surgery has experienced a revival since the early 1990s due to the potential of reducing morbidity in coronary artery surgery and of allowing countries with scarce health resources access to a viable programme of coronary surgery at reduced cost (Kolesov, 1967; Benetti et al., 1991; Buffolo et al., 1996). A variety of enabling instruments have been developed since then to improve exposure and stabilisation of the target coronary site on the beating heart and to achieve a bloodless surgical field while minimising myocardial and coronary injury. Simultaneously, a large number of observational, case-matched, and prospective randomised studies have provided the evidence of the safety and efficacy of this technique.

2. Indications for OPCAB surgery

Theoretically, there are no limitations to the application of OPCAB surgery; however, in practice, its use varies from 0% to 100% depending on the phase of the learning curve and ethos of individual surgeons (Kolesov, 1967; Benetti et al., 1991; Buffolo et al., 1996; Watters et al., 2001; Tasdemir et al., 1998; Puskas et al., 2001; Cartier et al., 2000). In the absence of recognised guidelines, common sense suggests that a surgeon starting an OPCAB surgery programme should consider avoiding dilated or poor left ventricles, very small, intramyocardial, or diffusely diseased vessels, and haemodynamically unstable patients with recent myocardial infarction. The simultaneous presence of these factors, in fact, still remains a challenge even for the experienced surgeon.

3. Surgical technique of OPCAB surgery

3.1. Exposure and positioning of the beating heart

The chest is opened using median sternotomy. The primary aim of OPCAB surgery is to expose and position the three main coronary systems with minimal haemodynamic compromise while displacing anteriorly and rotating the beating heart anticlockwise. A combination of different manoeuvres has been proposed over time including the introduction of deep pericardial retraction sutures (Watters et al., 2001), the use of intracoronary shunt (Watters et al., 2001) and the redistribution of blood to prevent right ventricular dysfunction with a combination of the Trendelenburg manoeuvre and gauge rotation of the operating table towards the surgeon (Watters et al., 2001; Geskes et al., 1999; Grundeman et al., 1999). Tilting of the heart to reach the obtuse marginal branches and the distal branches of the right coronary artery caused significant impairment of right ventricular function due to inflow obstruction, disturbance of right ventricular contraction or development of tricuspid regurgitation, and a reduction of left ventricular output (Geskes et al., 1999). The rotation of the operating table toward the surgeon and the Trendelenburg manoeuvre facilitate blood redistribution and venous return, leading to a restoration of the coronary flow paralleled by recovery of cardiac output and mean arterial pressure (Watters et al., 2001; Geskes et al., 1999; Grundeman et al., 1999).

3.2. Snaring

Following appropriate exposure and positioning of the beating heart, the next step consists of approaching the coronary site to allow the construction of a

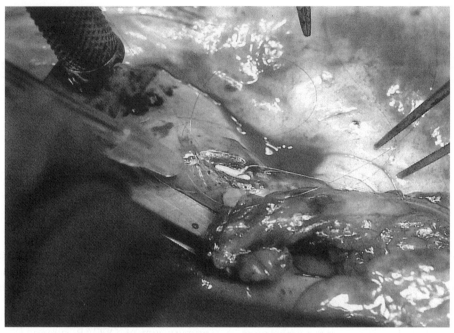

Fig. 1. Intracoronary shunt in place during the LIMA to LAD anastomosis.

precise anastomoses. The early approach consisted of a proximal and distal snare of the target coronary artery throughout the sewing of the anastomoses. Double snaring, however, raised many concerns because of the potential of iatrogenic coronary injury (Alessandrini et al., 1997).

3.3. Shunting

Intracoronary shunts are now used to prevent prolonged snaring of the coronary vessels and to allow distal myocardial perfusion avoiding myocardial ischaemia. This prevents the regional and global wall motion abnormalities and haemodynamic dysfunction described by Watters et al. (2001), Malkowski et al. (1998) and Lucchetti et al. (1999), while improving visibility of the coronary edges, minimising the use of a blower and preventing misplaced coronary sutures (Fig. 1).

3.4. Stabilisation

Excessive motion of the coronary target during the construction of the anastomosis might lead to a poor quality anastomosis (Cooley, 2000). During the early OPCAB experience, pharmacological agents like diltiazem, adenosine and esmolol were used to slow the heart rate to minimise this problem. The real breakthrough, however, was achieved with the introduc-

tion of either pressure or suction retractor-stabilisers (Watters et al., 2001; Pym, 1999; Grundeman et al., 1998). The use of the stabilisers in association with the preliminary manoeuvres of exposure and position of the beating heart described above, allowed surgeons to standardise the surgical technique for grafting of the three main coronary arteries.

4. Validation of OPCAB surgery

Over the last decade a number of prospective randomised trials, case-matched and observational reports have been published on OPCAB surgery. The Beating Heart Against Cardioplegic Arrest Studies (BHACAS 1 and 2) were two single-centre randomised trials carried out on a total population of 401 (200 off-pump) elective patients (Angelini et al., 2002). Completeness of revascularisation was similar in both groups, and in-hospital mortality did not differ (1% and 0% on- vs. off-pump). OPCAB surgery was associated with a significant reduction of chest infection, inotropic requirement, incidence of arrhythmias, total chest tube drainage and consequent transfusion requirement, intubation time, intensive care, hospital stay, and costs. The outcome of a multi-centre randomised trial in a cohort of 281 patients (142 off-pump) showed no difference in terms of in-hospital mortality and morbidity. The off-pump patients, however, had a shorter ventilation time, were discharged 1 day earlier and had a reduction of 41% release of CK–MB when compared to the on-pump patients (Van Dijk et al. 2001). In a multi-centre retrospective analysis of 118,140 CABG-only procedures (11,717 (9.9%) off-pump), a risk-adjusted analysis showed significant benefits associated with OPCAB surgery including operative mortality (from 2.9% to 2.3%), and major complication such as deep sternal infection, bleeding, renal failure, and prolonged ventilation (from 14.1% to 10.6%) (Cleveland et al., 2001). Others (Magee et al., 2001; Calafiore et al., 2001) have reported similar clinical outcomes.

The influence of OPCAB surgery on subsystem function also deserves mention. Several studies have reported minimal inflammatory activation (Diegeler et al., 2000a; Ascione et al., 2000a), and coagulation impairment (Angelini et al., 2002; Van Dijk et al., 2001; Calafiore et al., 2001; Ascione et al., 2001b) with OPCAB compared to conventional surgery. The lower release of troponin I during OPCAB surgery (Wan et al., 1999; Ascione et al., 1999a), suggests limited myocardial injury, a possible explanation for the reduced incidence of postoperative arrhythmias and inotropic support (Angelini et al., 2002; Ascione et al., 2000a). A protective effect of OPCAB surgery on renal function is suggested both by biochemical evaluation in elective patients (Ascione et al., 1999b), and by the post-operative incidence of acute renal failure in high-risk patients presenting either with diabetes (Magee et al., 2001), or with raised pre-operative serum creatinine (Ascione et al., 2001a). Although a lower release of S100 protein has been recorded soon after off-pump coronary surgery, the results regarding early and late cognitive dysfunction are controversial in the sense that they have been either better or similar when compared to conventional surgery (Diegeler et al., 2000b; Taggart et al., 1999).

Some data on mid-term clinical outcome are also available. The outcome of the two BHACAS trials (29.3 ± 7.4 and 15.7 ± 5.5 months for BHACAS 1 and 2 respectively) showed no differences in terms of mortality, cardiac-related events, and need for further coronary revascularisation procedure between groups (Angelini et al., 2002). These results are similar to those reported by Van Dijk et al. at 1 month of follow-up (2001), and are supported by the angiographic evidence reported by others (Cartier et al., 2000; Calafiore et al., 2001).

OPCAB surgery has evolved rapidly during the last decade and the use of specific stabilisation techniques, intracoronary shunts and blood flow redistribution techniques have made it a routine procedure. The available evidence suggests that OPCAB surgery is a safe and effective surgical technique of myocardial revascularisation with reduced early morbidity and organ dysfunction when compared with conventional CABG with CPB and cardioplegic arrest.

References and further reading

Alessandrini F, Gaudino M, Glieca F, Luciani N, Piancone FL, Zimarino M, Possati G. Lesions of the target vessel during minimally invasive myocardial revascularization. Ann Thorac Surg 1997; 64: 1349–1353.

Angelini GD, Taylor FC, Reeves BC, Ascione R. Early and midterm outcome after off-pump and on-pump surgery in Beating Heart Against Cardioplegic Arrest Studies (BHACAS 1 and 2): a pooled analysis of two randomised controlled trials. Lancet 2002; 359: 1194–1199.

Ascione R, Lloyd CT, Gomes WJ, Caputo M, Bryan AJ, Angelini GD. Beating versus arrested heart revascularization: evaluation of myocardial function in a prospective randomised study. Eur J Cardiothorac Surg 1999a; 15: 685–690.

Ascione R, Lloyd CT, MJ Underwood, WJ Gomes, GD Angelini. On pump versus off pump coronary revascularization: evaluation of renal function. Ann Thorac Surg 1999b; 68: 493–498.

Ascione R, Caputo M, Calori G, Lloyd CT, Underwood MJ, Angelini GD. Predictors of atrial fibrillation after conventional and beating heart coronary surgery: a prospective randomised study. Circulation 2000a; 102: 1530–1535.

Ascione R, Lloyd CT, Underwood MJ, Lotto AA, Pitsis AA, Angelini GD. Inflammatory response after coronary revascularisation with or without cardiopulmonary bypass. Ann Thorac Surg 2000b; 69: 1198–1204.

Ascione R, Nason G, Al-Ruzzeh S, Ko C, Ciulli F, Angelini GD. Coronary revascularisation with or without cardiopulmonary bypass in patients with preoperative nondialysis dependent renal insufficiency. Ann Thorac Surg 2001a; 72: 2020–2025.

Ascione R, Williams S, Lloyd CT, Sundaramoorthi T, Pitsis AA, Angelini GD. Reduced postoperative blood loss and transfusion requirement after beating-heart coronary operations: a prospective randomised study. J Thorac Cardiovasc Surg 2001b; 121: 689–696.

Benetti FJ, Naselli C, Wood M, Geffner L. Direct myocardial revascularization without extracorporeal circulation. Experience in 700 patients. Chest 1991; 100: 312–316.

Buffolo E, de Andrade CS, Branco JN, Teles CA, Aguiar LF, Gomes WJ. Coronary artery bypass grafting without cardiopulmonary bypass. Ann Thorac Surg 1996; 61: 63–66.

Calafiore AM, Di Mauro M, Contini M, Di Giammarco G, Pano M, Vitolla G, Bivona A, Carella R, D'Alessandro S. Myocardial revascularisation with and without cardiopulmonary bypass in multivessel desease: impact of the strategy on early outcome. Ann Thorac Surg 2001; 72: 456–463.

Cartier R, Brann S, Dagenais F, Martineau R, Couturier A. Systematic off-pump coronary artery revascularisation in multivessel disease: experience of three hundred cases. J Thorac Cardiovasc Surg 2000; 119: 221–229.

Cleveland JC, Shroyer LW, Chen AY, Peterson E, Grover FL. Off-pump coronary artery bypass grafting decreases risk-adjusted mortality and morbidity. Ann Thorac Surg 2001; 72: 1282–1289.

Cooley DA. Con: Beating-heart surgery for coronary revascularisation: is it the most important development since the introduction of the heart-lung machine? Ann Thorac Surg 2000; 70: 1779–1781.

Diegeler A, Doll N, Rauch T, Haberer D, Walther T, Falk V, Gummert J, Autschbach R, Mohr FW. Humoral immune response during coronary artery bypass grafting. A comparison of limited approach, 'off-pump' technique and conventional cardiopulmonary bypass. Circulation 2000a; 102(III): 95–100.

Diegeler A, Hirsch R, Schneider F, Schilling LO, Falk V, Rauch T, Mohr FW. Neuromonitoring and neurocognitive outcome in off-pump versus conventional coronary bypass operation. Ann Thorac Surg 2000b; 69: 1162–1166.

Geskes GG, Dekker AL, van der Veen FH, Cramers AA, Maessen JG, Shoshani D, Prenger KB. The enabler right ventricular circulatory support system for beating heart coronary artery bypass graft surgery. Ann Thorac Surg 1999; 68: 1558–1561.

Grundeman PF, Borst C, van Herwaarden JA, Verlaan CWJ, Jansen EWL. Vertical displacement of the beating heart by the Octopus stabilizer: influence on coronary flow. Ann Thorac Surg 1998; 65: 1348–1352.

Grundeman PF, Borst C, Verlaan CWJ, Meijburg H, Moues CM, Jansen EWL. Exposure of circumflex branches in the tilted, beating porcine heart: echocardiographic evidence of right ventricular deformation and the effect of right or left bypass. J Thorac Cardiovasc Surg 1999; 118: 316–323.

Gundry SR, Romano MA, Shattuck OH, Razzouk AJ, Bailey LL. Seven-year follow-up of coronary artery bypasses performed with and without cardiopulmonary bypass. J Thorac Cardiovasc Surg 1998 Jun; 115(6): 1273–1277.

Kolesov VI. Mammary artery–coronary artery anastomosis as method of treatment for angina pectoris. J Thorac Cardiovasc Surg 1967; 54: 535–544.

Lucchetti, V, Capasso F, Caputo M, Grimaldi G, Capece M, Brando G, Caprio S, Angelini GD. Intracoronary shunt prevents left ventricular function impairment during beating heart coronary revascularization. Eur J Cardiothorac Surg 1999; 15: 255–259.

Magee MJ, Dewey TM, Acuff T, Edgerton JR, Hebeler JF, Prince SL, Mack MJ. Influence of diabetes on mortality and morbidity: off-pump coronary artery bypass grafting versus coronary artery grafting with cardiopulmonary bypass. Ann Thorac Surg 2001; 72: 776–781.

Malkowski M, Kramer CM, Parvizi ST, Dianzumba S, Marquo J, Reichek N, Magovern JA. Transient ischemia does not limit subsequent ischemic regional dysfunction in humans: a transesophageal echocardiographic study during minimally invasive coronary artery bypass surgery. JACC 1998; 31: 1035–1039.

Puskas JD, Thourani VH, Marshall JJ, Dempsey SJ, Steiner MA, Sammons BH, Brown WM 3rd, Gott JP, Weintraub WS, Guyton RA. Clinical outcomes, angiographic patency, and resource utilization in 200 consecutive off-pump coronary bypass patients. Ann Thorac Surg 2001 May; 71(5): 1477–1483.

Pym J. Off pump arterial grafting: 125 cases using the Medtronic–Utrecht Octopus. Eur J Cardiothorac Surg 1999; 16: S88–S94.

Taggart DP, Browne SM, Halligan PW, Wade DT. Is CPB still the cause of cognitive dysfunction after cardiac operations? J Thorac Cardiovasc Surg 1999; 118: 414–420.

Tasdemir O, Vural KM, Karagoz H, Bayazit K. Coronary artery bypass grafting on the beating heart without the use of extracorporeal circulation: review of 2052 cases. J Thorac Cardiovasc Surg 1998; 116: 68–73.

Van Dijk D, Nierich AP, Jansen WL, Nathoe HM, Suyker WJ, Diephuis JC, van Boven WJ, Borst C, Buskens E, Grobbee DE, Robles De Medina EO, de Jaegere PP. Early outcome after off-pump versus on-pump coronary bypass surgery. Results from a randomised study. Circulation 2001; 104: 1761–1766.

Wan S, Izzat BM, Lee TW, Wan IY, Tang NL, Yim AP. Avoiding cardiopulmonary bypass reduces cytokine response and myocardial injury. Ann Thorac Surg 1999; 68: 52–57.

Watters MPR, Ascione R, Ryder IG, Ciulli F, Pitsis AA, Angelini GD. Haemodynamic changes during beating heart coronary surgery with the 'Bristol technique'. Eur J Cardiothorac Surg 2001; 19: 34–40.

Surgical treatment of acquired valvular disease

H. Huysmans

1. Introduction

Surgical treatment of diseases of the mitral valve was one of the earliest achievements in the history of heart surgery. Closed commissurotomy of the valve has been successfully performed by Cutler and Levine (1923) and by Souttar (1925). Their success was not really appreciated by their contemporaries and only twenty years later this procedure was done again simultaneously by Harken et al. (1948), Bailey (1949) and Baker et al. (1950).

The first heart valve prosthesis was successfully implanted only a few years later; in 1952 Hufnagel implanted his ball-valve heterotopically in the descending aorta in a case of aortic regurgitation (Hufnagel and Harvey, 1953). In 1956 Murray reported placement of an aortic homograft in the descending aorta (Murray, 1956).

The development of extracorporeal circulation in 1953 allowed orthotopic placement of heart valves. Many synthetic devises were tried, from materials like Silastic, Teflon, Mylar and polyurethane, all in the shape of valve cusps. The first successful prosthetic valves were placed in the aorta by Harken in 1960 (Harken et al., 1960) and in the mitral position by Starr in 1960 (Starr et al., 1961).

Tissue valves followed shortly afterwards. The aortic homograft was introduced by Ross (1962), the porcine aortic valve by Duran and Gunning (1965) and clinically implanted as a stentless valve by Binet et al. (1965). Ross (1967) then introduced the use of the pulmonary autograft. The reliability of the porcine tissue valves was enormously improved with the glutaraldehyde preservation proposed by Carpentier et al. (1969).

During the next decades valve surgery could be improved by the development of better valve prostheses and repair methods, but also by better knowledge of heart valve anatomy and function.

2. Aetiology

Rheumatic fever has for a long time been the most common cause of heart valve disease. But it has become far less common today, especially in the western world. In some other parts of the world it is still the main cause of valve dysfunction: stenosis and combined disease of the mitral valve, regurgitation and combined disease of the aortic valve and stenosis or regurgitation of the tricuspid valve.

Calcific degeneration is now the most common cause of aortic stenosis and sometimes of mitral regurgitation in elderly patients.

Degenerative disease like myxomatous degeneration, Marfan's syndrome, Ehlers-Danlos disease and others are responsible for many cases of mitral and aortic valve disease.

Endocarditis has increased as a reason for heart valve surgery. It causes regurgitation of aortic, mitral or tricuspid valve by destruction of parts of the valve apparatus.

Ischaemia caused by coronary artery disease can be the cause of mitral or tricuspid regurgitation.

Other causes of valve dysfunction are cardiomyopathy (dilated or restrictive) and conditions with elevated ventricular pressure.

3. Anatomy, function and pathology

Heart valves are part of a complicated structure. Understanding these structures and their relevance for valve function is essential when repairing or replacing valves. The aortic valve apparatus consists of a valve ring, three valve leaflets and three coronary

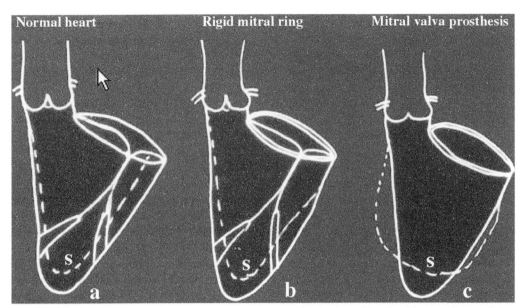

Fig. 1. Contraction patterns of the left ventricle. Left: in normal LV. Middle: after implantation of prosthesis in mitral annulus: no contraction of basic part of the LV-myocardium, abnormal contraction pattern. Right: after implantation of (semi-)rigid ring: no contraction of basic part of LV-myocardium, normal contraction of remaining part.

sinuses (Van Rijk-Zwikker et al., 1994a). The mitral valve consists of a valve ring, two asymmetric valve leaflets, three types of chordae and two papillary muscles (Van Rijk-Zwikker et al., 1994b; 1994c). The left ventricular myocardium is also an integral part of the aortic and mitral valve apparatus. Pulmonary and tricuspid valves have similar structures. In normal valves, all parts move in a well coordinated way, providing an optimal opening and closure pattern with low stresses and strains of the leaflets. Any change of anatomy by a pathological process in any of the contributing parts will cause dysfunction of the valve, either stenosis or regurgitation or a combination of the two.

The key properties of a normal natural valve are: undisturbed central flow, early closure, no disturbance of myocardial function, and a lifetime durability. When treating a diseased valve, one should always try to get back to these original properties as much as possible. Restoring the original geometry should be the goal in valve repair. Replacing a diseased valve with a mechanical or a stented bioprosthesis always leads to permanent loss of function of the myocardium (Fig. 1). Function of both natural and prosthetic heart valves is negatively influenced by disturbances of the heart rhythm (Van Rijk-Zwikker et al., 1994a, 1994c).

Pathology of diseased heart valves varies depending on the underlying process:

Leaflets can be thickened by fibrous scar tissue, calcified, torn or perforated and fused by inflammatory processes; they can prolapse due to tissue degeneration or chordal abnormalities.

The valve ring can be dilated, calcified or narrowed by scar tissue. Coronary sinuses can be dilated or calcified.

Chordae can be thickened, shortened, elongated or ruptured.

Papillary muscles can be shortened and scarred, elongated or ruptured.

Abnormalities of the myocardium caused by hypertrophy, ischaemia or myocardial infarction further contribute to disturbance of valve function.

4. Symptoms and Diagnosis

When the pathology has caused a stenosis of the valve opening, the signs and symptoms are related to pressure overload of atrium or ventricle. If the pathology has led to incomplete closure of the valve, the symptoms are caused by volume overload. In cases of combined disease (stenosis and regurgitation) there will be a combination of symptoms, mostly related to the dominating abnormality. Primary or secondary abnormalities of the myocardium will add further symptoms, like heart failure and cardiac arrhythmias (Bonow et al., 1998; Bonow et al., 1995).

The diagnosis of valve disease has to follow the classic pattern. History and physical examination with inspection, palpation, percussion and auscultation are still important and allow a good first diagnosis (Bonow et al., 1998).

A chest X-ray gives information about size and shape of the heart and the intrathoracic vessels; it also shows secondary abnormalities in the lungs. An ECG can show hypertrophy or damage of the myocardium or cardiac arrhythmias.

Today the most important tool for the diagnosis of valve disease is the echo-Doppler examination, both transthoracic (TTE) and transoesophageal (TEE). The M-mode echo allows evaluation of size and shape of heart chambers and intrathoracic vessels.

From the measurement of the peak flow velocity, valve area and mean transvalvular gradient can be calculated with the help of the Gorlin formula and the Bernoulli equation. Regurgitation can be demonstrated, located and quantified by Doppler colour flow mapping and analysis of the velocity curves (Cheitlin et al., 1997; Otto 1997).

CT scan or MRI can give important information, especially in cases were the aortic root is also involved (Hundley et al., 1995).

Additional information can be obtained from catheterisation and angiography. These investigations are not, however, always necessary (Tribouilloy et al., 1996).

5. Different types of valve disease

5.1. Aortic valve disease

5.1.1. Aortic stenosis (AS)

Degenerative calcific AS is the most common valve lesion today in the western world. It is also caused by rheumatic fever in some patients. Both causes can be responsible for AS in patients with a congenital bicuspid aortic valve.

The disease usually develops slowly over a long period of time. The pressure overload of the LV leads to LV-hypertrophy. This in turn may cause increased wall stress and ischaemia of the wall, leading to decrease of LV-diastolic function with elevated LVedp and also to LV-arrhythmias. Left heart failure with pulmonary edema develops at a late stage.

Complaints and symptoms frequently appear after a considerable time and sudden death is a well known danger. Rarely however sudden death is not preceded by some symptoms.

The diagnosis is made based on the typical systolic murmur, LV-hypertrophy on ECG and the findings of the echo-Doppler.

AS is diagnosed with TTE according to the following criteria for valve area: normal 3.0 to 4.0 cm^2, mild >1.5 cm^2, moderate 1.0 to 1.5 cm^2, and severe <1.0 cm^2. These values are not reliable in patients with a very large or very small body surface area, in which case the indexed area is more reliable. The diagnostic criteria are: 0.9 cm^2/m^2 for mild, 0.6 to 0.9 cm^2/m^2 for moderate, and 0.6 cm^2/m^2 for severe stenosis. In cases of severe stenosis the mean transvalvular gradient is usually >50 mmHg (Bonow et al., 1998; Burwash et al., 1993).

Cardiac catheterisation is only recommended if there is a distinct discrepancy between clinical and echocardiographic findings. Angiography or coronary angiography is recommended in patients over 35 years of age.

5.1.2. Aortic regurgitation (AR)

The most common causes for aortic regurgitation are aortic dilatation (idiopathic, myxomatous, Marfan's syndrome, etc.), rheumatic fever, calcific degeneration, infective endocarditis and type I dissection of the aorta.

Depending on the cause the regurgitation is acute or chronic. Acute regurgitation as caused by endocarditis or aortic dissection, causes massive LV-volume overload with increased LVedp and acute left heart failure and pulmonary edema. Usually there is rapid forward failure too with cardiogenic shock. Chronic regurgitation is much better tolerated. By development of LV-dilatation and LV-hypertrophy the stroke volume will be increased and the overload can be compensated for. Eventually the increase in afterload will cause decrease of systolic function.

Symptoms develop when the systolic LV-function starts to decrease, usually starting with early fatigue and later symptoms of left heart failure (Bonow et al., 1983; Borer et al., 1998).

Examination will show a diastolic murmur, LV-hypertrophy and an enlarged LV on chest X-ray.

Echo-Doppler shows reverse flow on colour flow mapping. The ratio of colour flow jet area to left ventricular outflow tract area or the ratio of jet height to outflow tract height can give an indication for the severity of regurgitation. Different cut-off values are given; an area ratio below 20% is considered non-important regurgitation. Height ratios are usually interpreted as follows: <20% means unimportant, 20 to 30% mild, 30 to 45% moderate, and >45% means severe.

Another method to express the severity of regurgitation is the pressure half-time, calculated from the slope of the continuous wave Doppler regurgitant jet. Pressure half-time of <400 ms are considered a sign of severe regurgitation.

On aortic root angiography the opacification of the LV is a measure of severity of regurgitation.

5.1.3. Combined aortic disease

Some degree of regurgitation is rather common in AS. Signs and symptoms are depending on the dominance of stenosis or regurgitation. The development of symptoms is usually faster than in isolated disease.

Both a systolic and diastolic murmur are present. Diagnostic methods are the same as described for AS and AR.

5.1.4. Aortic root disease

Aortic regurgitation can be secondary to diseases of the aortic root. Medial degeneration like in Marfan's syndrome or Ehlers-Danlos' disease can lead to dilatation of the aortic root and annulus. Type I aortic dissection can cause severe regurgitation without any disease of the valve leaflets. Endocarditis can destruct annulus, leaflets and parts of the aortic root. Exact diagnosis is important to be able to make the right choice of surgical treatment.

CT-scan and MRI will usually give a better picture of the pathologic anatomy than echo-Doppler studies alone. To define associated lesions like fistulae the use of all diagnostic modalities is important in these cases.

5.2. Mitral valve disease

5.2.1. Mitral stenosis (MS)

Mitral stenosis is caused by rheumatic fever and less frequently by degenerative calcific disease. In rheumatic disease, thickening and fusion of the mitral leaflets along their free edges is the first cause of stenosis, but frequently thickening and fusion of chordae cause a subvalvular stenosis also. Calcification of these structures leads to further limitation of movement and increases the degree of stenosis.

Mitral stenosis is a slowly progressive disease; there can be a long period between the original rheumatic fever and the development of symptomatic stenosis. After onset of symptoms the condition remains good for quite a long period and survival is good for the first 10 years. After that time progression becomes more rapid.

Complaints are primarily shortness of breath and early fatigue. Elevated left atrial pressure and atrial dilatation induce atrial fibrillation. Later symptoms of left heart failure and pulmonary hypertension and finally right heart failure, with symptoms of congested liver, peripheral edema and ascites, can occur.

On auscultation, an accentuated mitral closure sound, an opening snap and a rumbling mid-diastolic murmur can be heard.

Chest X-ray shows an enlarged left atrium and later enlargement of pulmonary arteries and right ventricle. Calcification of leaflets and/or annulus can also be diagnosed on X-ray. Kerley-lines in the lower lobes indicate chronic slow lymphatic drainage.

Echo-Doppler shows a diminished mitral valve opening area (MVA). Normally it is 4.0 to 5.0 cm^2, in mild stenosis from 1.5 to 2.5 cm^2, moderate between 1.0 and 1.5 cm^2 and severe <1.0 cm^2. Mitral transvalvular gradient can be calculated from the continuous wave Doppler signal and is considered to be moderate if it remains <5 mmHg at rest. Pulmonary artery pressure (PAP) can be calculated from the continuous wave Doppler of tricuspid valve regurgitation. For a complete diagnosis, TEE is the best method (Bonow et al., 1998).

Catheterisation and angiography are usually not needed for the diagnosis of mitral stenosis.

5.2.2. Mitral regurgitation (MR)

There are many causes for mitral regurgitation, e.g. myxomatous degeneration, rheumatic fever, calcific degenerative disease, Marfan's syndrome, endocarditis, and myocardial ischaemia or infarction.

The regurgitation can be acute or chronic, depending on the cause. Acute volume overload, as seen in endocarditis or myocardial infarction with chordal rupture, is poorly tolerated and leads to severe symptoms of pulmonary oedema and forward failure. Chronic regurgitation develops slower and allows for compensatory dilatation and hypertrophy of LA and LV. It is not as well tolerated as mitral stenosis, and severe symptoms of congestive heart failure, caused by progressive loss of contractile function, develop within ten years in almost all patients. Ischaemic mitral regurgitation, due to ischaemic damage or to ischaemic dysfunction, has a worse prognosis.

Mitral regurgitation causes a harsh holosystolic murmur. The ECG shows LV-hypertrophy and often at a later stage atrial fibrillation. Chest X-ray shows enlarged LA and LV.

Echocardiography (preferably TEE) can assess the degree of regurgitation by the length of the colour jet into the left atrium. More precise estimates can be made with the proximal isovelocity surface area (PISA) method, based on calculation of volumetric flow proximal to the mitral valve from the colour images. Calculation should be made very carefully, because of the asymmetric regurgitant jet and its varying location in the atrium. Severe regurgitation is defined as 60 ml regurgitant volume per beat or as 50% regurgitant fraction (Carabello, 1998).

Catheterisation and angiography are not needed for the diagnosis of mitral regurgitation.

5.2.3. Combined mitral disease
Mixed stenosis and regurgitation is usually of rheumatic or degenerative calcific origin. MS is frequently the dominating disease.

Signs and symptoms are a combination of those of MS and MR, depending on the dominating lesion.

A reliable diagnosis can be made with echo-Doppler examination (TEE).

5.3. Tricuspid valve disease

5.3.1. Tricuspid stenosis (TS)
Tricuspid stenosis is caused by rheumatic fever. It is very rarely an isolated disease: it usually is combined with mitral or aortic valve disease. Thickening and fusion of leaflets is the common pathology. Calcification and chordal abnormalities are less frequent than in mitral valve disease.

Symptoms develop slowly. A mid-diastolic murmur is present; raised central venous pressure is an early sign. Later an enlarged liver and peripheral edema will develop. Chest X-ray shows an enlarged right atrium.

A complete diagnosis can be made by echo-Doppler study, using the methods already described for the mitral valve.

5.3.2. Tricuspid regurgitation (TR)
Tricuspid regurgitation is much more common than tricuspid stenosis. It has many potential causes. Rheumatic fever, endocarditis, degenerative disease, ischaemia and pulmonary hypertension (of all origins) are among the more frequent ones.

When tricuspid regurgitation develops slowly, compensatory dilatation and hypertrophy of right atrium and right ventricle will make the disease tolerable for a long period of time. Acute regurgitation, as in endocarditis or ischaemic chordal or papillary muscle rupture is usually not so well tolerated.

Signs and symptoms are a holosystolic murmur, a raised central venous pressure, an enlarged, pulsating liver, and peripheral edema and ascites. In case of combined mitral or aortic valve disease the clinical picture can be dominated by the former disease.

A complete diagnosis and an estimate of the severity of regurgitation can be made by echo-Doppler studies (Child, 1989).

5.3.3. Combined tricuspid disease
Combined TS and TR is common, when rheumatic fever is the cause.

Signs and symptoms are as described before, with a holosystolic- and a diastolic murmur, and depend on the dominating lesion.

Diagnosis can also be completely made by echo-Doppler examination.

6. Indications and timing for surgery

An indication for surgical treatment of heart valve disease exists, when a patient has serious complaints (NYHA class III or IV) or when symptoms have reached a certain level. A balance should be found between the mortality risk without surgery, the risk of surgery and the prognosis after surgery. The prognosis is related to the pre-operative condition (especially irreversible damage to the heart), age, concomitant disease and the type of surgery to be performed. Repair of a heart valve has a lower post-operative risk of complications than replacement; different types of valve prostheses have different post-operative complication rates.

In asymptomatic patients with AS, surgery is indicated when the AS is severe or when signs of failing LV-function are present. Surgery for coronary disease can be an indication to treat even moderate AS (Bonow et al., 1998; Carabello, 1997).

Surgery for AR is indicated when it is severe or when signs of failing LV-function develop. Extreme LV-dilatation (end-systolic >55 mm, end-diastolic >70 mm) is also an indication.

Acute AR usually presents an urgent/emergency indication, because of LV-dysfunction.

In aortic root disease an indication is present for the same reasons as in AR, but dilatation of the root of >50 mm is also an indication.

Surgery for MS is indicated when a patient reaches NYHA class III or IV. In patients with class I or II symptoms and moderate or severe MS, repeated emboli under anticoagulant treatment or newly developed atrial fibrillation surgical treatment is also indicated.

In MR, surgery is indicated for NYHA class III and IV patients. In other patients surgical treatment can be advised as soon as LV-function shows deterioration. Ejection fraction <60% or end-systolic diameter >45 mm are an indication for surgery. Recently developed atrial fibrillation, pulmonary hypertension and ventricular arrhythmias are also indications for surgery (Acar et al., 1991).

Acute MR is usually an indication for surgery, because of the disturbed LV-function. It is important to treat atrial fibrillation by surgery (Maze procedure) or cryo-ablation simultaneously (Cox et al., 1995a; Cox et al., 1995b).

Tricuspid disease should be treated surgically when the symptoms are severe (class II or IV) or in less severe cases, when there is an indication for mitral or aortic surgery.

Concomitant disease, especially coronary artery disease, can give an independent indication for surgery. Moderate valve lesions can then be treated simultaneously (Lytle et al., 1988; Ashraf et al., 1994).

Indications for surgery are not essentially different in elderly patients (Olsson et al., 1992; Freeman et al., 1991) or pregnant women (Oakley, 1994; Oakley, 1996).

7. Surgery

7.1. Surgical approach

Incisions for valve surgery are variable. A midsternal approach offers good access to all valves. The mitral valve and the tricuspid valve can also be approached through a right anterior thoracotomy. A left anterior thoracotomy can be used to approach the mitral valve.

Other alternatives are a proximal mini-sternotomy for the aortic (and mitral?) valve and a small right anterior thoracotomy at the second intercostal space for mitral (and aortic) surgery (Loulmet et al., 1998).

Thoracoscopic surgery for valve repair is still in a development phase.

7.2. Valve repair

All valve repair should be aimed at reconstructing the original geometry as precisely as possible. But even when complete reconstruction is impossible, a repaired valve is often better than a replaced valve, because it will allow more normal movement and has fewer post-operative complications associated with it.

Valve stenosis can be repaired by commissuro-tomy, either blunt or sharp. To obtain a satisfactory result it is important that the pliability of the leaflets can be maintained or restored.

Valve repair by commissurotomy has been reasonably successful in mitral stenosis, where the effect may last for several decades. In aortic stenosis the effect has been less durable. The mitral procedure can be performed as a closed commissurotomy, through a left thoracotomy and left auricular incision, or as an open procedure, whereby a more accurate opening of the fused commissures can be done. Closed balloon commissurotomy can be an option for elderly patients, pregnant patients, or patients in very poor condition (Dean et al., 1996).

Valve regurgitation can be repaired most successfully in mitral and tricuspid valves; a careful choice has to be made between repair and replacement (Akins et al., 1994; Cohn et al., 1988; Cohn et al., 1995; Grossi et al., 1998).

Aortic regurgitation can be successfully be repaired, but long term results are uncertain (Duran et al., 1991; David et al., 1995). Good techniques for these repairs are described by Carpentier (1983), Duran et al. (1991), de Vega and several others (David et al., 1995; Cosgrove, 1989).

Leaflets can be repaired by excision in case of redundant tissue, by patch reconstruction in case of insufficient leaflet material and by closure of tears or perforations. Shrunken (aortic) leaflets can be extended by patches (Duran et al., 1991).

A dilated valve annulus can be reduced by simple sutures — especially in the tricuspid valve (Duran, 1994) — or by a properly sized prosthetic ring, semi-rigid or flexible. A flexible ring might be better, because it reduces myocardial mobility around the annulus only minimally (Van Rijk-Zwikker et al., 1990; Rivera et al., 1985). Simple suturing of the free edges of the mitral leaflets can also repair the regurgitation in certain cases (Fucci et al., 1995; Maisano et al., 1998).

Repair of fused, thickened, shortened or elongated chordae is more difficult, but can be done with great success. Chordae and papillary muscles can be divided, lengthened or shortened. In case of ruptured chordae there are several options for repair: quadrangular (posterior mitral leaflet, Fig. 2) or triangular (anterior mitral leaflet) resection, 'flap-over' plasty from a part of the posterior mitral leaflet with its chordae to the anterior leaflet, or replacement of the chordae by synthetic material (David et al., 1991; Smedira et al., 1996). Often a combination of several of these techniques is necessary.

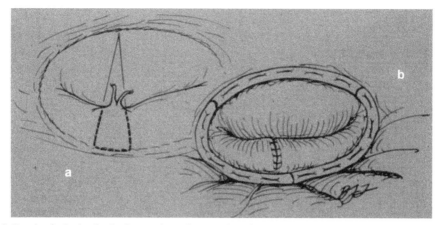

Fig. 2. Repair of mitral valve leaflet: quadrangular resection of the posterior leaflet in case of ruptured chordae.

As a basic rule, as little material as possible should be used for reconstruction. If material is needed, it should preferably be autologous, porcine or bovine pericardium. Synthetic material should be as inert as possible and only be used in small quantities (e.g. Gore-Tex chorda replacement).

Peri-operative evaluation of the repair by transoesophageal or epicardial echo is needed, to prevent early reoperation in case of an unsatisfactory result (Practical guidelines for peri-operative transesophageal echocardiography, 1996; Griffin, 1997; Stewart et al., 1990).

7.3. Valve replacement

7.3.1. Mechanical valves

All mechanical valves do have an abnormal flow pattern, due to the presence of an occluder in the bloodstream (Paulsen et al., 1988; Kleine et al., 1998; Van Rijk-Zwikker et al., 1996). As there is no longer a well-coordinated valve system after valve replacement, opening and closure are later and less complete than in the natural valve. All mechanical valves do interfere with myocardial function, because of the immobilisation of the myocardium around the rigid prosthesis ring (Fig. 3). In mitral valves a loss of 25 to 30% of LV-function has been measured in experiments (Van Rijk-Zwikker et al., 1989). Preservation of the (mural) chordae can reduce this effect with approximately 50% (Van Rijk-Zwikker et al., 1989; David et al., 1984; Horstkotte et al., 1993). Due to these abnormalities there is a tendency for valve thrombosis and thrombo-embolic complications, necessitating lifelong anticoagulant therapy. Other disadvantages are haemolysis, susceptibility for endocarditis and noise.

Basically there are three types of mechanical valves: caged ball valves, tilting disc valves and bileaflet valves (Fig. 4). There are some differences in flow patterns, thrombogenicity and noise, but a

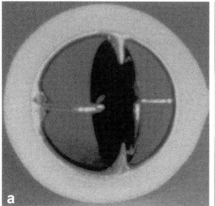
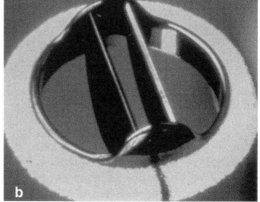

Fig. 3. Two of the most widely used types of mechanical valve prostheses. (a) Tilting disc valve (Medtronic-Hall). (b) Bileaflet valve (St. Jude Medical).

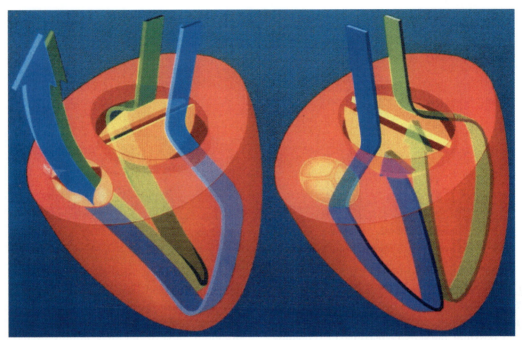

Fig. 4. Importance of orientation of a bileaflet prosthesis. (a) When oriented perpendicular to the ventricular septum, the flow through all openings of the prosthesis goes towards the aortic valve. (b) When oriented parallel to the ventricular septum, the flow is turned back to the prosthesis, causing early closure.

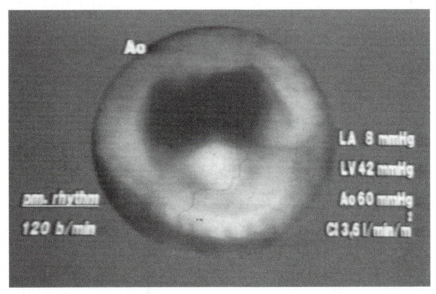

Fig. 5. Typical incomplete opening (the leaflet opposite of the aorta does not open) of a stented bioprosthesis, when implanted in the mitral position (picture from intra-cardiac video).

clear superiority of any one of the three types has never been demonstrated (Akins, 1995). Tilting disc valves and bileaflet valves need to be implanted in the proper orientation, to avoid unfavourable flows and incomplete opening and closing of the disc or leaflets (Van Rijk-Zwikker et al., 1996 — Fig. 5).

7.3.2. Biological/tissue valves
Tissue valves have the advantage of an unobstructed central flow, giving less tendency towards thrombo-embolic problems. These valves, if stented, are no longer part of a well-coordinated structure anymore and therefore show abnormal opening and clos-

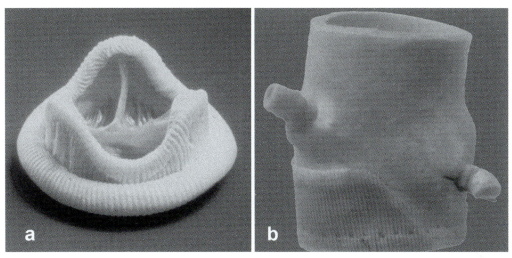

Fig. 6. Two common types of biological valve prostheses. (a) Porcine aortic stented valve (Hancock II). (b) Stentless porcine aortic root (Medtronic Freestyle).

ing patterns. The use of an aortic (model of) tissue valve in the mitral position enhances this shortcoming (Fig. 6). Stented tissue valves also interfere with myocardial function in the same way as mechanical prostheses. Due to the imperfect design, especially in stented valves, and to biochemical surface processes, the durability of tissue valves is limited (Christie, 1992; Thrubikar et al., 1983; Rousseau, 1985). Patient factors play an important role, too (Jamieson et al., 1999a; Jamieson et al., 1997). In homografts, rejection is probably a factor reducing durability.

There are three types of tissue valves: autografts from the patient's own valves or pericardium, homografts (or allografts) from other humans, and xenografts (or heterografts) from animal valves or pericardium.

Autografts are used for aortic valve replacement (Ross procedure), whereby the patient's own pulmonary valve is used to replace the aortic valve, as root replacement (Fig. 7), root inclusion or subcoronary replacement.

Parts of the tricuspid valve have been used to replace the mitral valve (Hvass et al., 1996). The

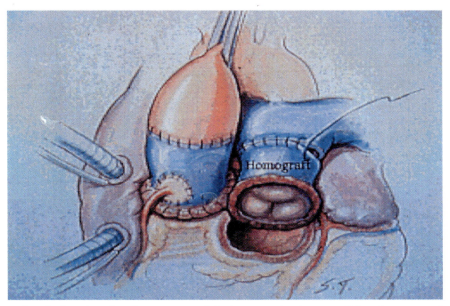

Fig. 7. Ross procedure: implantation of a pulmonary autograft in the aorta and replacement of the pulmonary root by a homograft.

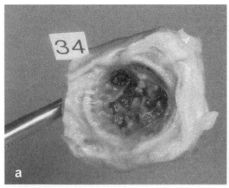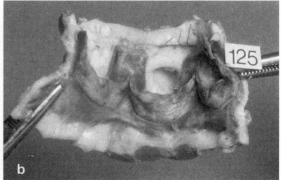

Fig. 8. Better durability by stentless design (animal experiment, 6 months implantation). (a) Stented porcine valve: severe calcification, leaflet tears. (b) Stentless porcine valve: no macroscopic abnormalities.

disadvantage of these techniques is that the autograft has to be replaced by a homograft, making a one-valve operation into a two-valve procedure (Oury et al., 1999).

Stented tissue valves, made from the patient's own pericardium during surgery, have not yet been fully evaluated.

Homografts can be used for aortic replacement mainly, with any of the three techniques mentioned above for the autograft (Langley et al., 1999; Lund et al., 1999). Mitral homograft replacement is still not completely successful (Edmunds, 1987; Cannegieter et al., 1995). The disadvantage of homografts is the limited availability, the potential problem of rejection and the limited durability, maybe related to the method of preservation (fresh, antibiotics or cryopreserved).

Xenografts are made from porcine aortic valves or constructed with bovine pericardium. They can be suspended in a frame (Fig. 8) or used without external support. All xenografts have a limited durability. Most xenografts are fixed and preserved by glutaraldehyde solution. Factors influencing the post-operative calcification and durability are the concentration of the glutaraldehyde solution and the pressure under which the valves have been fixed; low pressure fixation gives better function and durability. Better methods of fixation and preservation are being investigated.

Stentless valves (autografts, homografts, xenografts) allow preservation of the original geometry of the donor valve, especially when used as a root replacement (Butchart, 1992a). These valves have (almost) normal flow patterns, no negative influence on myocardial function (Cannegieter et al., 1994) and normal flows, creating the potential for return to a completely normal situation after valve replacement

(Acar et al., 1996; Kumar et al., 2000; Durack et al., 1994; David et al., 1990; Joyce et al., 1995). Because of their natural design, stentless prostheses are probably more durable (Lytle et al., 1996 — Fig. 8).

7.3.3. Sizing and suture techniques

The size of a valve prosthesis should be the same or somewhat larger than the size of the natural valve ring. Height and weight of the patient play a role. A parameter for the optimal size is the relationship between effective orifice area (EOA) of the prosthesis and the body surface area (BSA). In aortic valve replacement, this relationship, the body surface area index (BSAI), should be not less than $0.85 \text{ cm}^2/\text{m}^2$ (patient–prosthesis mismatch). In mitral valve replacement there is usually no problem if the EOA of the prosthesis is $>2.5 \text{ cm}^2$.

Sizing of a stentless valve should be as precise as possible; in case of doubt a slightly larger size is preferred.

Implanting a valve prosthesis can be done using running sutures or interrupted single or mattress sutures. Interrupted sutures can be reinforced by felt pledgets, especially in cases with frail annulus tissue after decalcification. The superiority of any method has never been proven; the suturing method is a choice of the surgeon primarily.

Valves can be implanted annular or supra-annular. The latter method may allow the use of a bigger sized prosthesis.

Dangers to be aware of when implanting a valve prosthesis are dehiscence and impingement. Dehiscence, leading to paravalvular leakage, can be avoided by taking sufficiently large bites of the annulus tissue and equally spacing them. Impingement, interference of tissue or a suture end between the prosthesis ring and the occluder, can be avoided by careful inspection of the disc or leaflet movement before closure and by tying the sutures well away from the prosthesis. Impingement can be a lethal complication.

7.3.4. Complications

All replacement valves can have potential complications. Valve thrombosis, thrombo-embolic complications, anticoagulant related bleeding, haemolysis, endocarditis, structural degeneration, non-structural dysfunction, paravalvular leak and reoperation are the well-known complications, which have to be reported when evaluating the performance of replacement devices. Reporting has to be done in a standard way, following the guidelines and criteria published a few years ago (Hazekamp et al., 1993).

In mechanical prostheses thrombosis, thromboembolic complications and bleeding are the most common problems (Del Rizzo et al., 1999) Valve thrombosis is relatively rare; it can in some cases be treated by thrombolysis and aggressive anticoagulant therapy (Walter et al., 1999). There are some differences in the frequency of these complications between the different types of prosthesis and also between different makes (Akins, 1995). The yearly mortality rate after replacement with a mechanical valve is 1–3% for aortic and 3–5% for mitral valves. Structural failure of mechanical valves is very rare nowadays.

The main problem in tissue valves is structural degeneration. All valves fail after a period of time that is defined by type of valve, mode of fixation and preservation, mode of implantation, age of patient and some other patient-related factors (Christie, 1992; Thrubikar et al., 1983; Rousseau, 1985; Jamieson et al., 1999b; Jamieson et al., 1997). The still limited experience with stentless devices shows a lower complication rate and mortality rate (Acar et al., 1996).

7.3.5. Post-operative care

Apart from the usual post-operative care, prevention of infection and of thrombosis needs extra attention in valve replacement patients.

Usually routine antibiotic prophylaxis for 24 hours is sufficient to protect the patient against early endocarditis. Only in cases of active endocarditis or in the presence of other infections should a therapeutic antibiotic regimen be used.

Anticoagulant therapy with coumadines (some centres prefer to start with heparin) should be started immediately after surgery in all valve-replacement patients. In tissue valves it can be stopped after 6 to 12 weeks; in mechanical valves it should be maintained lifelong. There are different opinions about the level of anticoagulation. It should be somewhat higher after mitral valve replacement than after aortic valve replacement: 2.5–3.0 INR for aortic and 3.0–3.5 INR for mitral valves (Jin et al., 1997; Westaby et al., 1998; Vogt et al., 2000; Genomi et al., 2000; Cobanoglu et al.; 1987).

Echo-Doppler evaluation of prosthesis function before dismissal from the hospital is advisable.

7.3.6. Choice of prosthesis

Factors influencing the choice of prosthesis are type and rate of complications, durability, ease of implant, skills and preference of the surgeon and finally the patient's choice.

Long-term results (Lund et al., 1999; Edmunds et al., 1996; Jamieson et al.; 1998; Jin et al., 1995; O'Brien et al., 1995; Sintek et al., 1995; Bach and Boling, 1996) will have to support the choice of prosthesis. As the available data on valve prostheses can be interpreted in different ways, it is hard to give clear advice on the choice of prosthesis. General practice is not to implant stented tissue valves in younger patients (<65 years), because these valves will fail in a relatively short period of time (7 to 10 years). In patients over 65 years of age the same valves may last much longer.

All stentless valves have a lower complication rate than other valve types and allow a normal life, because they do not need anticoagulants and frequently have a totally normal heart function. Even when their durability is still limited, these advantages might compensate the additional risk of reoperation at the time of failure.

At present, if repair is impossible, a mechanical prosthesis is probably the best choice for mitral valve replacement, because tissue valves, both stented and stentless, have a very limited durability. In elderly patients and in the presence of contra-indications for anticoagulation, a stented bioprosthesis is an acceptable choice.

For aortic valve replacement there is a wider choice. In very young patients an autograft offers the advantage of growth potential. In patients below the age of 65 to 70 years, a mechanical prosthesis is still the usual choice, but stentless devices (homograft, xenograft) can be considered as an alternative. Elderly patients should have a tissue valve.

7.3.7. Redo valve-prosthesis surgery

Structural degeneration, paravalvular leak and endocarditis are the most common cause for reoperation after valve replacement. The indications for surgery are in essence the same as for primary valve replacement. The operative risk and the post-operative complication rate are somewhat higher than in primary valve surgery, but have today come down to very acceptable values (Horstkotte et al., 1995; Horstkotte et al., 1994; Butchart, 1992b). Early reoperation, when clear signs of dysfunction are present, is advocated (Kon et al., 1995).

8. Infective endocarditis

Bacterial endocarditis is a relatively common disease, caused by a wide range of microorganisms. Most notorious are *Staphylococcus aureus*, *S. epidermidis*, *E. coli*, *Pseudomonas sp.* and different types of fungi and yeasts.

Criteria for diagnosis are well defined (Tyers et al., 1995). A positive blood culture confirms the diagnosis. Echo-Doppler studies can give complete information about the extent and anatomical details of the disease. When only the leaflets are diseased it is called simple endocarditis; all others are complex.

Indication for surgery is given when the disease does not immediately react to antibiotic treatment, when the disease is progressive on serial TTE, when the disease is complex, when the causing microorganism is very aggressive and when there are signs of progressive heart failure or dangerous arrhythmias. In case of prosthetic endocarditis early operation is indicated (Gillinov et al., 1997). Timely operation is decisive for the post-operative outcome.

The basic principle for surgery is to remove all infected tissue completely. After that a repair is rarely possible. Replacement should be done by autograft or homograft preferably in aortic endocarditis (Scully et al., 1995). A Ross procedure is another option (Nitter–Hauge et al., 1996). In mitral endocarditis it is probably best to follow the usual choice of prosthesis. Additional repair for other lost structures can best be done with autologous or other pericardium.

9. Summary

Valve surgery demands a profound knowledge of anatomy and function of the heart valves. The surgeon has to be familiar with physical examination and the diagnostic methods of cardiology, especially echo–Doppler studies.

The aim of surgical treatment should always be to reconstruct the original geometry as well as possible. Repair is therefore preferable if that can be done.

Valve prostheses are still being further developed. It is wise to follow these developments closely, but not to decide to use a new valve until there is sufficient proof of its safety.

Complicated procedures, like the Ross procedure and the treatment of complex endocarditis, require great surgical skills and experience. To get optimal results for the patient, it might be wise to concentrate these procedures in the hands of experienced surgeons.

References and further reading

Acar C, Tolan M, Berrebi A, et al. Homograft replacement of the mitral valve. Graft selection, technique of implantation and results in forty-three patients. J Thorac Cardiovasc Surg 1996; 111: 367–378.

Acar J, Michel PL, Luxereau P, et al. Indications for surgery in mitral regurgitation. Eur Heart J 1991; 12(b): 52–54.

Akins C, Hilgenberg A, Buckley M. Mitral valve reconstruction versus replacement for degenerative or ischemic mitral regurgitation. Ann Thorac Surg 1994; 58: 668–676.

Akins C. Results with mechanical cardiac valvular prostheses. Ann Thorac Surg 1995; 60: 1836–1844.

Ashraf SS, Shaukata N, Odom N, et al. Early and late results following combined coronary bypass surgery and mitral valve replacement. Eur J Cardiothorac Surg 1994; 8: 57–62.

Bach DS, Boling SF. Improvement following correction of secondary mitral regurgitation in end-stage cardiomyopathy. Am J Cardiol 1996; 78: 966–999.

Bailey CP. The surgical treatment of mitral stenosis (mitral commissurotomy). Dis Chest 1949; 15: 377.

Baker C, Brock RC, Campbell M. Valvulotomy for mitral stenosis: report of six successful cases. BMJ 1950; 1: 283.

Binet, JP, Duran CG, Carpentier A, et al. Heterologous aortic valve transplantation. Lancet 1965; 2: 1275.

Bonow RO, Carabello B, de Leon AC, et al. ACC/AHA Guidelines for the management of patients with valvular heart disease. A report of the American College of Cardiology/American Heart Association Task Force on practical guidelines (Committee on Management of Patients with Valvular Heart Disease). J Am Coll Cardiol 1998; 32: 1486–1488, Circulation 1998; 98(18): 1949–1984.

Bonow RO, Nikas D, Elefteriades JA. Valve replacement for regurgitant lesions of the aortic or mitral valve in advanced left ventricular dysfunction. Cardiol Clin 1995; 13: 73–83.

Bonow RO, Rosing DR, McIntosh CL, et al. The natural history of asymptomatic patients with aortic regurgitation and normal left ventricular function. Circulation 1983; 68: 509–517.

Borer JS, Hochreiter C, Herrold EM, et al. Prediction of indications for valve replacement among asymptomatic or minimally symptomatic patients with chronic aortic regurgitation and normal left ventricular performance. Circulation 1998; 97: 525–534.

Burwash IG, Forbes AD, Sadahiro M, et al. Echocardiographic

volume flow and stenosis severity measures with changing flow rate in aortic stenosis. Am J Physiol 1993; 265(H1): 734–1743.

Butchart EG. Prosthesis-specific and patient-specific anticoagulation. In: Butchart EG, Bodnar E (eds.). Current Issues in Heart Valve Disease, Thrombosis, Embolism and Bleeding. London: ICR publishers, 1992a; p. 293.

Butchart EG. Thrombogenicity, thrombosis and embolism. In: Butchart EG, Bodnar E (eds.). Current issues in heart valve disease: thromosis, embolism and bleeding (1st ed.). London: ICR Publishers, 1992b; pp. 172–205.

Cannegieter SC, Rosendaal FR, Briët E. Thromboembolic and bleeding complications in patients with mechanical heart valve prostheses. Circulation 1994; 89: 635–641.

Cannegieter SC, Rosendaal FR, Wintzen AR, et al. Optimal oral anticoagulant therapy in patients with mechanical heart valves. N Engl J Med 1995; 333: 11–17.

Carabello BA. Timing of valve replacement in aortic stenosis: moving closer to perfection. Circulation 1997; 95: 2241–2243.

Carabello RA. Mitral valve regurgitation. Curr Probl Cardiol 1998; 202–241.

Carpentier A. Cardiac valve surgery: The 'French connection'. J Thorac Cardiovasc Surg 1983; 86: 323–337.

Carpentier A, Lamaigre CG, Robert L, et al. Biological factors affecting long-term results of valvular heterografts. J Thorac Cardiovasc Surg 1969; 58: 467.

Cheitlin MD, Alpert JS, Armstrong WF, et al. ACC/AHA Guidelines for the Clinical Application of Echocardiography. A report of the American College of Cardiology/American Heart Association Task Force on Practice Guidelines (Committee on Clinical Application of Echocardiography). Developed in collaboration with the American Society of Echocardiography. Circulation 1997; 95: 1686–1744.

Child JS. Improved guides to tricuspid valve repair: 2-D echocardiographic analysis of tricuspid anulus function and color flow imaging of severity of tricuspid regurgitation. J Am Coll Cardiol 1989; 14: 1275.

Christie GW. The anatomy of aortic heart valve leaflets: The influence of glutaraldehyde fixation. Eur J Cardiothorac Surg 1992; 6(Suppl 1): S25–S33.

Cobanoglu A, Jamieson WRE, Miller DC, et al. A tri-institutional comparison of tissue and mechanical valves using a patient oriented definition of 'treatment failure'. Ann Thorac Surg 1987; 43: 245.

Cohn LH, Kowalker W, Bhatia S, et al. Comparative morbidity of mitral valve repair versus replacement for mitral regurgitation with and without coronary artery disease. Ann Thorac Surg 1988; 45: 284–290.

Cohn LH, Rizzo RJ, Adams DH, et al. The effect of pathophysiology on surgical treatment of iscemic mitral regurgitation: operative and late risks of repair versus replacement. Eur J Cardiothorac Surg 1995; 9: 568–574.

Cosgrove DM. Surgery for degenerative mitral valve disease. Semin Thorac Cardiovasc Surg 1989; 1: 183.

Cox JL, Boineau JP, Schuessler RB, et al. Modification of the maze procedure for atrial flutter and atrial fibrillation. I. Rationale and surgical results. J Thorac Cardiovasc Surg 1995a; 110: 473–484.

Cox JL, Jaquiss RD, Schuessler RB, et al. Modification of the maze procedure for atrial flutter and atrial fibrillation. II. Surgical technique of the maze III procedure. J Thorac Cardiovasc Surg 1995b; 110: 485–495.

Cutler EC, Levine SA. Cardiotomy and valvotomy for mitral stenosis: experimental observations and clinical notes concerning an operated case with recovery. Boston Med Surg J 1923; 188: 1023.

David T, Bos J, Rakowski H. Mitral valve repair by replacement of chordae tendineae with polytetrafluoroethylene sutures. J Thorac Cardiovasc Surg 1991; 101: 495.

David TE, Bos J, Christakis GT, et al. Heart valve operations in patients with active infective endocarditis. Ann Thorac Surg 1990; 49: 701–705.

David TE, Burns RJ, Bacchus CM, et al. Mitral valve replacement for mitral regurgitation with and without preservation of chordae tendineae. J Thorac Cardiovasc Surg 1984; 88: 718–725.

David TE, Feindel CM, Bos J. Repair of the aortic valve in patients with aortic insufficiency and aortic root aneurysm. J Thorac Cardiovasc Surg 1995; 109: 345–351.

Dean L, Mickel M, Bonan R, et al. Four year follow-up of patients undergoing percutaneous balloon commissurotomy: A report from the National Heart Lung and Blood Institute Balloon Valvuloplasty Registry. J Am Coll Cardiol 1996; 28: 1452–1457.

Del Rizzo D, Abdoh A, Cartier P, et al. The effect of prosthetic valve type on survival after aortic valve surgery. Semin Thorac Cardiovasc Surg 1999; 11(Suppl 1): 1–8.

Durack DT, Lukes AS, Bright DK. New criteria for diagnosis of infective endocarditis: utilization of specific echocardiographic findings. Am J Med 1994; 96: 200–209.

Duran CG, Gunning AJ. Heterologous aortic-valve transplantation in the dog. Lancet 1965; 2: 114.

Duran CG, Kumar N, Gometza B, et al. Indications and limitations of aortic valve reconstruction. Ann Thorac Surg 1991; 52: 447–453.

Duran CG. Tricuspid valve surgery revisited. J Card Surg 1994; 9: 242–247.

Edmunds LH Jr, Clark RE, Cohn LH, et al. Guidelines for reporting morbidity and mortality after cardiac valvularoperations: the American Association for Thoracic Surgery, ad hoc Liaison Committee for Standardizing Definitions of Prosthetic Heart Valve morbidity. Ann Thorac Surg 1996; 62: 932–935, J Thorac Cardiovasc Surg 1996; 112: 708–711.

Edmunds LH Jr. Thrombotic and bleeding complications of prosthetic heart valves. Ann Thorac Surg 1987; 44: 430–445.

Freeman WK, Schaff HV, O'Brien PC, et al. Cardiac surgery in the octogenarian: Perioperative outcome and clinical follow-up. J Am Coll Cardiol 1991; 18: 29–35.

Fucci C, Sandrelli L, Pardini A, et al. Improved results with mitral valve repair using new surgical techniques. Eur J Cardiothorac Surg 1995; 9: 621–626.

Genomi M, Frantzen D, Vogt P, et al. Paravalvular leakage after mitral valve replacement: improved long-term survival with aggressive surgery? Eur J Cardiothorac Surg 2000; 17:14–19.

Gillinov AM, Cosgrove DM, Lytle BW, et al. Reoperation for failed mitral valve repair. J Thorac Cardiovasc Surg 1997; 113: 467–475.

Griffin B. Echocardiography in patient selection, operative planning and intraoperative evaluation of mitral valve repair. In: Otto CM (ed.): The Practice of Clinical Echocardiography. Philadelphia: WB Saunders, 1997.

K. Moghissi, J.A.C. Thorpe and F. Ciulli (Eds.)
Moghissi's Essentials of Thoracic and Cardiac Surgery
© 2003 Elsevier Science B.V. All rights reserved

CHAPTER V.9

Thoracic organ transplantation

K. McNeill, M. Yeatman and F. Ciulli

1. Introduction

Thoracic organ transplantation involves heart, lung, bilateral lung, or heart-lung block transplantation for the treatment of end-stage and irreversible congenital or acquired disease. The International Society for Heart and Lung Transplantation (ISHLT) has been compiling an International Registry of thoracic organs transplanted since 1982 (Fig. 1). The registry now comprises over 57,000 heart transplants from 321 centres, 2861 heart-lung transplants from 126 centres, 7204 single lung transplants from 161 centres, and 5420 bilateral lung transplants from 148 centres worldwide (Hosenpud et al., 2001).

Heart transplantation is currently the treatment of choice for selected patients with irreversible and otherwise not treatable cardiac disease where quality of life and longevity are severely compromised. The ISHLT Registry database shows the 1-, 5-, 10- and 15-year actuarial survival figures of over 52,000 cases (Fig. 2a and b) (Hosenpud et al., 2001). The success of cardiac transplantation is the result of careful pre-operative evaluation and management of arrhythmia and heart failure (Hunt et al., 2001), surgical and post-operative care, modern immunosuppressive regimes, and the management of post-operative infections. There is still a need to address issues such as chronic shortage of organ donors (20–40% of

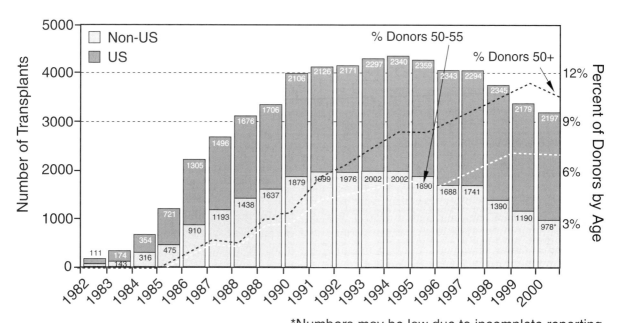

*Numbers may be low due to incomplete reporting

Fig. 1. Thoracic organs transplanted since 1982 (ISHLT Registry).

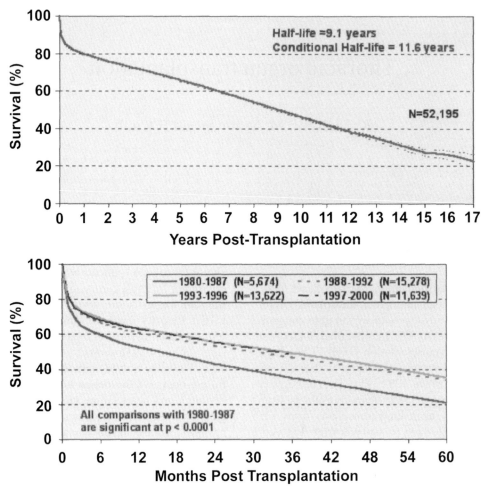

Fig. 2 (a and b). Heart transplantation survival rates (ISHLT Registry).

patients listed for cardiac transplantation die before a suitable organ can be found) (Carrier et al., 1992), the lack of specific, non-toxic immunosuppression, and late allograft failure from graft atherosclerosis.

2. Cardiac transplantation

2.1. History of cardiac transplantation

The first experimental heart transplant was performed in 1905 by Carrel and Guthrie (1905). Between 1940 and 1956, Demikhov (1962), working in the Soviet Union, developed a canine intrathoracic heterotopic heart model with survival of up to 32 days. Developments in cardioplegia and cardiopulmonary bypass facilitated the development of orthotopic techniques. Lower and Shumway (1960) described the use of separate right and left atrial anastomoses instead of multiple caval and pul-

monary venous anastomoses and this is one of the techniques still in use today. Azathioprine and prednisolone were shown to be effective following experimental heart transplantation in dogs (Reemtsma et al., 1962; Blumenstock et al., 1963). Hardy et al. (1964) performed the first chimpanzee-to-human orthotopic heart xenotransplant. The transplanted heart was however unable to support the recipient circulation and bypass was discontinued after one hour. In late December 1967, Christiaan Barnard (1967) performed the first allogenic human heart transplant but the recipient succumbed to *Pseudomonas pneumonitis* on the 18th post-operative day. During the following 12 months, 102 transplants were performed in 17 countries by 64 surgical teams. The results were so discouraging that by the end of 1969, only a few groups persisted with active cardiac transplant programmes (Stanford, USA; Cape Town, South Africa; and La Pitie Hospital, Paris).

Table 1

Indications for cardiac transplantations (ISHLT Registry data, 2000)

Cardiomyopathy	43.7%
Coronary artery disease	44.3%
Valvular heart disease	3.6%
Retransplantation	2.0%
Congenital heart disease	1.5%
Miscellaneous conditions	4.9%

Cyclosporin A was first isolated in 1970 (Dreyfuss et al., 1976). Calne and colleagues demonstrated its efficacy in preventing organ graft rejection in experimental models (Kostakis et al., 1977). The introduction of cyclosporin by Oyer and colleagues (1983) into cardiac transplant programmes ushered in the era of modern cardiac transplant surgery.

2.2. Indications, recipient selection and contraindications for cardiac transplantation

The indications for heart transplantation as reported to the ISHLT Registry (Hosenpud et al., 2001) are shown in Table 1. Absolute and relative contraindications to cardiac transplantation are shown in Table 2. The upper age limit for transplantation has gradually increased over the years, and for many centres 55 years is now the limit for patients with ischaemic heart disease, and 60 years for those with cardiomyopathy. Age is considered 'biological' which thus leaves a way open for otherwise good candidates to be accepted onto the waiting list. Orthotopic transplantation is contraindicated in the presence of an elevated transpulmonary gradient (≥ 15 Wood units) but heterotopic transplantation is a possible alternative for these patients. The timing of heart trans-

Table 2

Contraindications to orthotopic cardiac transplantation

1. *Absolute Contraindications*
Active infection
Untreated malignancy
Coexisting systemic illness likely to limit survival
Severe and irreversible other major organ dysfunction
Fixed elevated pulmonary vascular resistance

2. *Relative Contraindications*
Advanced age (over 55 for IHD; over 60 for CM)
Recent or unresolved pulmonary infarction
Active peptic ulceration
Marked peripheral or cerebrovascular disease
Psychological instability, substance abuse, mental illness

plantation in the treatment of end-stage heart failure is now less clear (Radovancevic et al., 1999) due to improvements in the medical treatment of heart failure (Bristow et al., 1994; Hunt et al., 2001) and to evolving technologies such as ventricular assist devices and implantable defibrillators (Frazier et al., 1992). Absolute indications for heart transplantation however have become more scientific with the introduction of peak VO_2 measurements. Achievement of anaerobic metabolism with VO_2 max of 10 ml/kg/min is an absolute indication; 14 ml/kg/min is a relative indication.

2.3. Evaluation of candidates for transplantation

A thorough assessment prior to listing for cardiac transplantation is necessary in order to determine whether conventional modalities of treatment are feasible and whether the candidate will tolerate the inevitable involvement of the medical teams peri- and post-operatively. Some groups have found that up to 20% of potential recipients may be suitable for other forms of treatment (Griepp et al., 1971; Ciulli et al., 1992). Unfortunately donor organs have always been a scarce resource and recipient selection must be stringent and multidisciplinary in order to make the best use of these organs and attain the best results in terms of longevity and quality of life.

All patients undergo systematic medical screening including cardiac catheterisation, glucose tolerance test, respiratory function tests, bacteriological screening, and dental examination. Serological tests for previous exposure to Hepatitis B, Hepatitis C, HIV, VDRL, Epstien Barr Virus (EBV), and Cytomegalovirus (CMV) are also carried out. Donor–recipient matching is based on ABO compatibility as well as height and weight. The routine use of HLA typing is not conducted because of limited time between the donor organ becoming available and transplantation. Some teams include a psychosocial evaluation to screen possible problems with compliance with medication and levels of support following discharge.

2.4. Evaluation and management of the cardiac donor

The acceptance of the medico-legal definition of brain-stem death in the 1970s since Harvard Medical School published its landmark criteria regarding the clinical definition of 'brain death' in 1968 (The Ad Hoc Committee of the Harvard Medical School to

Examine the Definition of Brain Death, 1968) and distant procurement programmes have both played a role in increasing the availability of donor organs. There is still however a significant discrepancy between supply and demand worldwide. The majority of organs offered for donation follow death related to road traffic accidents, intracranial haemorrhage, suicide, and primary intracranial malignancy. The establishment of brain-stem death requires that two clinicians, unrelated to the transplant team, perform brain-stem function tests twice during a twelve-hour period (Working Group of Conference of Medical Colleges and their Faculties in the United Kingdom, 1995).

Review of medical records excludes the presence or history of cardiovascular disease, chest trauma, prolonged periods of hypotension, or cardiac arrest. Active infection or extra-cranial malignancy is a contraindication to donation. A chest radiograph, 12 lead ECG, and routine blood tests are performed. Serological testing for HBSAg, VDRL, HIV, and CMV is mandatory to avoid transmission of donor infections. Donor and recipient are matched for ABO compatibility, height, and weight. Potential recipients with pre-formed lymphocytotoxic antibodies must have a negative crossmatch with the donor prior to transplantation.

Once accepted for donation, continuing intensive care treatment of the donor is critical. The Cushing response, due to increased sympathetic outflow, may lead to catecholamine-induced subendocardial ischaemia and myocardial injury. Hypotension may also be exacerbated by intense vasodilatation combined with hypovolemia. Initial vasopressor support is normally good practice using low-dose Aramine or Noradrenaline infusion. Subsequently inotropic support with Dopamine (up to 10 mcg/kg/min) may be commenced. A Swan–Ganz catheter should be in use by this stage to avoid unnecessary over-use of catecholamines which will deplete myocardial energy stores essential for survival of the myocardium during the period of ischaemia prior to and during transplantation. Brain stem-death is also associated with depletion of myocyte high-energy phosphate stores and a decrease in serum free thyroxine, free tri-iodothyronine, thyroid-stimulating hormone, cortisol, insulin, and antidiuretic hormone. These endocrine responses potentiate haemodynamic collapse and are associated with myocardial instability due to electrolyte disturbance. Novitzky has demonstrated the improvement in myocardial function of brain-stem dead pigs following the use

of tri-iodothyronine, insulin and cortisol (Novitzky et al., 1987). Many centres now administer both tri-iodothyronine and antidiuretic hormone to the donor prior to organ procurement and to monitor haemodynamic parameters and cardiac output with a pulmonary artery cardiac output catheter (MacLean and Dunning, 1997).

2.5. Techniques of donor cardiectomy and orthotopic transplantation

Multiple organ retrieval requires communication and cooperation between operating teams, donor hospitals and the recipient centres. Transplant coordinators play a fundamental role in organising the multi-disciplinary donor organ harvesting teams. They are specifically trained in approaching grieving relatives to obtain consent for organ donation. There can be more than 3 teams involved in the donor organ harvest procedure.

Once the donor operation has started, the heart is approached through a median sternotomy incision and a thorough macroscopic examination is performed, including palpation of the coronary arteries for signs of disease and presence of thrills over the heart valves. Once the heart is considered suitable for transplantation, the recipient hospital is informed so that the appropriate timings can be set for the recipient operation to be started, depending on the estimated operating time of the abdominal organ retrieval teams and the travel time to the recipient centre. In coordination with the other donor surgical teams (liver, kidney, pancreas), the heart is arrested using cold cardioplegia generally crystalloid and infused into the aortic root, taking care to vent the left and right side of the heart through the pulmonary veins and vena cavae respectively. The donor cardiectomy is performed leaving as much cuff on the pulmonary veins, pulmonary artery and aorta as possible. Many teams worldwide have been performing bi-caval anastomoses instead of the original Shumway right atrial anastomosis (Aziz et al., 1999). This consequently has led to the harvest of longer segments of superior vena cava. The excised organ is stored in Ringer's lactate at 4°C for transport to the recipient hospital. The upper limit ischaemic time has not been determined, but 4 hours is accepted as a safe limit and allows retrieval from distances of up to 1250 miles. Longer times of up to 6 hours have been achieved successfully; however, the organs must be from young donors on little or, better yet, no inotropic support pre-donation (Aziz et al., 1999).

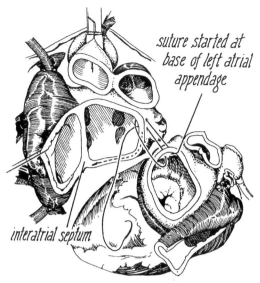

suture started at base of left atrial appendage

interatrial septum

Fig. 3. Left atrial anastomosis.

The recipient operation is timed to coincide with the arrival of the donor heart. Immunosuppression and broad spectrum antibiotic prophylaxis is commenced. The native heart is excised, taking care to leave a suitable cuff of aorta, pulmonary artery, left atrium and atrium (or SVC/IVC separately). Transplantation of the donor heart can then commence in orthotopic position starting from the left atrial anastomosis (Fig. 3). Generally the right atrial, pulmonary artery and aortic anastomoses are performed in order. Following transplantation, the recipient is weaned from cardiopulmonary bypass with an isoprenaline infusion to encourage intrinsic sinus rhythm and facilitate the lowest pulmonary artery pressure. Atrial and ventricular pacing wires are placed routinely so that weaning off isoprenaline can be done safely after the first 24–48 hours. The patient is returned to the intensive care unit and extubated once able to maintain a satisfactory airway with normal arterial blood gases, has re-warmed to 36.5°C and is not bleeding. Prophylactic antibiotics are discontinued after 24 hours. A–V sequential pacing should be established to maintain a resting heart rate of 90–100/min for the first 3–5 days.

2.6. Immunosuppression

Allograft rejection remains an important cause of morbidity and mortality amongst recipients of cardiac transplants; current regimens — although they prolong survival — lack specificity, do not reduce

Table 3

Mechanism of action of commonly-used immunosuppressive agents

Agent	Major mechanism of action
Cyclosporin	Inhibits interleukin-2 synthesis
Aziathioprine	Inhibits purine synthesis
Corticosteroids	Inhibits interleukin-1 and prostaglandin synthesis
Antithymocyte globulin	Depletes circulatory T-lymphocytes
OKT3	Depletes circulatory T-lymphocytes Prevents antigen recognition
Cyclophosphamide	Alkylates DNA
Methotrexate	Inhibits purine synthesis

allograft vasculopathy, are toxic, and predispose to the development of opportunistic infections and malignancy. Significant milestones in the development of immunosuppressive therapy and the evaluation of its effectiveness include the development of endomyocardial biopsy techniques (Caves et al., 1973), a system of grading rejection (Billingham, 1979), the clinical use of RATG (Rabbit Antithymocyte Globulin) (Hiestand et al., 1992), and the introduction of cyclosporin (Oyer et al., 1983). The mechanism of action of commonly-used immunosuppressive agents is shown in Table 3. A balance must be achieved between suppressing the immune response thus avoiding rejection of the graft, and the development of opportunistic infections. There are three phases of immunotherapy:

2.6.1. Induction
Induction commences peri-operatively and continues for one to two months post-operatively. Acute rejection episodes are more frequent during this phase, and drug doses are correspondingly higher. Some centres employ an anti T-cell immunoglobulin (either ATG or OKT3) during induction; however more frequently high dose i.v. steroid (methyl-prednisolone) is used. Cyclosporin and azathioprine are also introduced during this phase.

2.6.2. Maintenance phase
Maintenance is characterised by lower levels of immuno-suppressant therapy as the risk of rejection diminishes with time. Generally oral steroids (prednisolone) are weaned or stopped altogether. Maintenance immunosuppression therefore consists of oral Cyclosporin and Azathioprine with or without Prednisolone.

2.6.3. Treatment of acute rejection episodes

The treatment of acute rejection episodes is usually with intravenous methyl-prednisolone. RATG, OKT3 or total lymphoid irradiation may be used for recurrent episodes of acute rejection.

Unfortunately, these drugs are all associated with considerable side effects and morbidity; therefore, new immuno-suppressants are continually under clinical investigation.

2.7. The diagnosis and treatment of acute allograft rejection

Acute allograft rejection and infection are the two most frequent causes of death during the first 12 months following cardiac transplantation. Endomyocardial biopsy (EMB) developed by Phillip Caves while working at Stanford is still the gold standard for screening and diagnosing rejection (Caves et al., 1973). Rejection may be asymptomatic and so a regular surveillance protocol is essential during the first 12 months. The EMB screening protocols vary from centre to centre; however, weekly biopsies are taken for the first 4 weeks and then generally monthly for the first 6 months according to how many rejection episodes there have been. Diagnostic EMBs are also obtained when rejection is suspected clinically. Signs are generally quite aspecific and may start with general chest discomfort leading to retrosternal pain. Dyspnea and signs of heart failure constitute an emergency and the patient should be hospitalised and treated with IV steroids. Arrythmia such as atrial fibrillation (AF) or flutter may also be a sign and an EMB should be performed as soon as possible. Treatment of acute rejection is dependent upon the grade of rejection and time since transplantation. The presence of haemodynamic compromise, symptoms and incidence of previous rejection episodes will also help determine the timing and course of action. Rejection occurring during the first three months following transplantation is generally treated aggressively using IV steroids. Mild rejection is treated by increasing Cyclosporin dosage and performing serial biopsies to assess progression; this may occur in approximately one third of cases requiring enhanced steroid treatment. Moderate rejection following the first three months is treated with an oral taper of Prednisolone over 2 weeks starting with 1 mg/kg. Cytolytic therapy should be used for recurrent or steroid-resistant episodes of rejection. Polyclonal antilymphocytic globulins have been shown to be effective in reversing acute cardiac rejection and have been in use for some time (O'Connell et al., 1989).

2.8. Infectious complications following cardiac transplantation

Infection remains a major cause of morbidity and mortality following heart transplantation and alongside rejection and primary graft failure still represents a major risk of death in the first postoperative year (Hosenpud et al., 2000). The majority of patients experience at least one infection episode during the post-transplant period and those occurring within the first month are usually due to nosocomial bacteria, including staphylococci and Gram-negative bacilli. Thereafter, opportunistic infections such as Cytomegalovirus, *Toxoplasma gondii*, *Pneumocystis carinii*, Herpes Simplex, and fungi (*Aspergillus*/*Candida*) predominate. Every effort is made to reduce the possibility of infection in the transplant recipient. Donor-transmitted infections are rare given the careful screening of the donor before transplantation. Perioperative antimicrobial prophylaxis is commenced at induction of anaesthesia and continued for up to 48 hours post-operatively. Strict aseptic techniques are observed in all invasive procedures, although recipients are no longer barrier-nursed in isolation. Any pyrexia exceeding 37.5°C should be investigated thoroughly with a careful review of symptoms, physical examination, and the taking of appropriate culture specimens. Unless the sepsis is causing grave problems, antibiotic therapy should only be commenced after identification of a pathogen and sensitivity testing has become available. Collaboration with the microbiology department is therefore essential. Prophylaxis with Trimethoprim-sulphamethoxazole is given to reduce the incidence of Pneumocystis and toxoplasmosis infections. CMV can be a major problem following transplantation whether it is a primary infection (CMV mismatch: donor positive /recipient negative) or reactivation (CMV positive recipient). Various methods have been used to reduce the incidence of post-transplant infection with CMV; however, the incidence of clinical disease remains high especially in the mismatch group (50–75%). Some strategies used are: avoidance of mismatching recipients and donors for CMV, the use of CMV-negative blood products, CMV hyperimmune globulin, active immunisation with an attenuated vaccine, and the prophylactic administration of gancyclovir (Rubin, 2000).

2.9. Post-transplant malignancy

The development of malignancy following heart transplantation is a well-recognised long-term complication of immunosuppression with the reported incidence of *de novo* malignant tumours in cardiac transplant recipients from 1% to 16%, an incidence 100 times greater than that of the matched general population (Penn, 1984). The most common neoplasms in cyclosporin-treated patients are cutaneous malignant lesions, non-Hodgkin's lymphomata, carcinoma of the lung, and Kaposi's sarcoma. The development of lymphoproliferative disease in cyclosporin-treated patients seems to be associated with Epstein-Barr infection following cardiac transplantation (Armitage et al., 1990). Treatment involves conventional techniques and consideration must be given to reducing the level of immunosuppression as much as possible, particularly Cyclosporin. Lymphoma continues to play an important role as a post-transplant cause of death particularly after 12 months from transplantation (Hosenpud et al., 2000; Hosenpud et al., 2001).

2.10. Coronary artery vasculopathy

Together with malignancy, coronary artery vasculopathy (CAV) affects long-term survival following transplantation of the heart. Serial coronary angiography of cardiac transplant recipients has shown an annual incidence of coronary vasculopathy of 10% (Costanzo et al., 1998). Reports demonstrate the presence of cardiac allograft vasculopathy as early as 3 months post-transplant and in patients as young as 4 years. Afferent denervation of the cardiac graft prevents the development of typical angina pectoris in the early years following transplantation; therefore most patients with this condition suddenly develop congestive cardiac failure, myocardial infarction or sudden death. A diagnosis can be made by coronary angiography which demonstrates diffuse obliteration of the distal vessels. A variety of non-invasive methods have been investigated to diagnose CAV, including echocardiography, radio-isotope scanning (oral dipyridamole thallium-201 scanning and single photon emission computed tomographic imaging) and Holter monitoring. The results are imprecise and the role of non-invasive methods remain uncertain. Intra-coronary ultrasonography has been shown to be more sensitive than angiography in detecting and quantifying the coronary artery disease and Doppler angiographic catheters have recently been used to measure coronary flow reserve.

Currently CAV is irreversible, unpreventable and the definitive treatment is retransplantation, the results of which are inferior to primary transplantation.

2.11. Results of heart transplantation (Figs. 2a and b)

Since the Registry of the International Society for Heart and Lung Transplantation commenced in 1982, 57,818 cardiac transplants have been reported. The overall 1-year survival is 80%, the patient half-life (time to 50% survival) is 9.1 years and the annual mortality rate from years 1 to 14 is constant (4% per year). The 1-, 5-, 10- and 15-year survival figures now approach 80%, 65%, 50% and 35% respectively.

The registry data from 1994 to 2000 show that there is remarkably good rehabilitation amongst the cardiac transplant population. Of patients surviving the first transplant year, 90% have no activity limitations. Less than 10% require some form of assistance and 1% require total assistance or hospitalisation (Hosenpud et al., 2001).

2.12. Cardiac retransplantation

Controversy exists as to the appropriateness of retransplantation given the limited supply of donor organs. There are two principal indications for retransplantation: the first is acute rejection or 'non-specific' primary graft failure, and the second is chronic allograft coronary artery vasculopathy. Actuarial survival at 1 year after retransplantation is 6–12% lower than for patients undergoing primary cardiac transplantation. These relatively poor survival figures have dissuaded many from recommending retransplantation on the basis of severe limitation of a precious resource and the belief that organs should only be used to promote maximal possible gain. The Stanford group has reported the results of 63 cardiac retransplantions (Smith et al., 1994). For those patients undergoing retransplantation after 1981 and, therefore, benefiting from cyclosporin-based immunosuppression, the actuarial survival rates at 1, 5, and 10 years were 55%, 33%, and 22% respectively. They concluded that, despite these results, they maintain a firm commitment to retransplanting a highly select group of patients in whom a reasonable longevity and quality of life could be expected. The individual clinician must balance the therapeutic obligation to the transplant recipient with the current limitation of organs.

2.13. Alternatives to cardiac transplantation

The discrepancy between donor organ availability and supply severely limits the extent of cardiac transplantation. The shortfall in supply has caused a decline in the number of transplant operations performed since 1995. Unfortunately, measures such as presumed consent, educational programmes, and domino transplantation would not significantly affect this mismatch. As a consequence, considerable effort is being applied to alternatives to allograft cardiac transplantation and these include the development of ventricular assist devices and xenotransplantation.

The use of a skeletal muscle wrap to augment cardiac function has been thought to be an alternative to transplantation for many years. Since first described by Carpentier and Chachques in 1985, 112 patients have been entered into the phase 1 multi-centre trial. Skeletal muscle, acting as an auto graft, is chronically electrically stimulated to induce morphological, biochemical and physiological changes to prevent the development of fatigue. After a period of conditioning the muscle is wrapped around the ventricles in an effort to improve ventricular function. The early results were disappointing: early mortality was 22.3%, and there was only a small improvement in ejection fraction and symptomatic status. At present it has not gained the favour of the surgical community and is not recommended by the American Heart Association Guidelines (Hunt et al., 2001).

Ventricular assist devices have been used as a bridge to transplantation during the period prior to the isolation of a suitable donor organ. At the present time, the Novacor system (LVAS) (Baxter Healthcare Corporation, Novacor Left Ventricular Assist System, Oakland, California) and the Heart-Mate LVAD (Thermo Cardiosystems, Woburn, Michigan, USA) devices have been evaluated in multi-centre trials (Constanzo-Nordin et al., 1993). A reported 226 patients have received ventricular assist devices (132 Novacor, 94 TCI Heart-Mate) with 61% subsequently receiving a heart transplant. The maximal implantation period to date is 460 days. The hospital survival following transplantation was 89% and 85% respectively. Technical advances continue, and despite the high cost of such devices, the aim is for a permanent implantable device. At present the clinical use has been orientated towards a 'bridge to transplantation' rather than instead of transplantation due to durability and reliability of biocompatible material. Long-term use still only relates to 2–3 years experience. Thromboembolism and infection still re-main the major limiting factors as they were nearly twenty years ago when the first Jarvik was implanted into Barney Clarke in Salt Lake City (Kasirajan, 2000).

Xenotransplantation refers to the grafting of tissue or organs from different species. The degree of genetic similarity determines whether such grafts are concordant or discordant. Although the use of non-human primates is an attractive prospect immunologically, with the potential for less aggressive rejection, moral, ethical and practical issues have led investigators to examine the possibilities of utilising farm animals for transplantation into humans. Pigs expressing regulators of complement activity on endothelial surfaces (transgenic) have been engineered and may allow successful clinical transplant programmes to become established. However, the world experience so far of xenotransplantation is extremely limited and much preliminary work has still to be conducted. There have been eight attempts at cardiac xenotransplantation (five using non-human primate hearts), the most recent by Czaplicki in 1992, but maximum survival was only 20 days.

2.14. Summary

Cardiac transplantation has developed into a highly successful treatment for selected patients with end-stage cardiac failure. Expected 1-year survival is 80–90%, with 90% of survivors living with no limitations to activity. The 5-year survival is around 70–75%. The long-term results are limited by the development of coronary artery vasculopathy, infection and malignancy. The activity of transplantation programmes worldwide is severely limited by the availability of donor organs. Further refinements of immunosuppressive agents could result in improved prevention of both acute and chronic rejection. Every effort is being made to extend the donor pool; however, it is unlikely to change significantly enough to address the shortfall in organ supply. Alternative methods to allograft transplantation need further investigation to increase the number of therapeutic options available for those patients with end-stage heart failure.

3. Lung transplantation

3.1. Introduction

For many patients with end-stage lung disease, the only prospect for better survival and quality of life is through a successful lung transplant. Since the first heart-lung transplant in 1981 there have been over 11,000 pulmonary transplants reported to the international registry. This falls considerably short of the number of patients with advanced lung disease and indeed one of the major challenges facing lung transplantation is the critical shortage of donor organs.

The lung allograft is unique within solid organ transplantation as it is in direct contact with the external environment. This exposes the allograft directly to potential infections and allergens, which predispose to many of the numerous problems encountered immediately post-transplant and in the longer term.

The transplant process involves recipient selection, donor selection, donor/recipient matching, the surgical procedure, immediate post-operative care, and long-term follow-up.

3.2. Recipient selection

Most end-stage pulmonary diseases can be treated with transplantation. The most common disease indications are emphysema/COPD, cystic fibrosis, pulmonary fibrosis, and pulmonary vascular disease (primary pulmonary hypertension and Eisenmenger's syndrome). Disease should be confined to the thorax, although in carefully selected patients, certain systemic diseases with pulmonary manifestations (scleroderma, sarcoidosis, etc.) can be transplanted successfully. Most patients are listed when their survival is estimated to be less than 2 years. The prognosis of cystic fibrosis, primary pulmonary hypertension and cryptogenic fibrosing alveolitis can now be reliably estimated. In patients with Eisenmenger's syndrome and emphysema, however, survival on the waiting list can be as good or better than following transplantation. In this setting, transplantation is performed primarily for quality of life issues. Table 4 summarises referral recommendations based on guidelines recently published by the International Society for Heart and Lung Transplantation.

Contraindications are well defined. Most are relative and are considered in the context of the patient's overall status. Selected patients with significant co-existing kidney or liver disease can be considered for combined thoracic and abdominal organ transplantation. 'Absolute' exclusion criteria are confined to active malignancy (excluding localised cutaneous malignancies), major psychosis, active extra-pulmonary infection and significant extra-thoracic organ dysfunction with the exceptions noted above.

Table 4

Disease-specific indications for lung transplantation

Patients with the following characteristics should be referred for a transplant assessment.

1. Obstructive Lung Disease/Non CF Bronchiectasis
   FEV_1 <25% predicted without reversibility
   Respiratory failure
   Cor pulmonale
   Severely limited quality of life (NYHA class III–IV dyspnoea)

2. Cystic Fibrosis
The following parameters are associated with a 2-year survival on the waiting list of 20%:
   FEV_1 <25% predicted
   Respiratory failure
   Severely reduced exercise capacity: ≤500 metres on a 12 minute walk
   Compromised nutrition: BMI ≤17
In addition, adolescent females with rapidly declining lung function should be referred early.

3. Primary Pulmonary Hypertension
The following parameters are associated with a median survival of only 12 months, and an overall survival of <20% at 3 years. Patients requiring increasing doses of prostacycline should also be referred for assessment.
   Mean right atrial pressure >15 mmHg
   Mixed venous oxygen saturation <60%
   Cardiac index <2.0 l/min/m²
Eisenmenger's Syndrome
   Severely compromised quality of life
   Refractory right heart failure
   Frequent pre-syncopal or syncopal events
   Poorly controlled dysrhythmia

4. Cryptogenic Fibrosing Alveolitis
These patients often deteriorate rapidly, with up to a 50% death rate on the waiting list after only 12 months. Consequently, they should be referred early. Gas transfer values <60% predicted are indicative of advanced disease.
   Progressive disease/failure of immunosuppression
   Respiratory failure
   NYHA Class III dyspnoea

3.3. Donor selection

Most donors are brain-stem-dead. However, select cardiopulmonary transplant centres around the world perform living-related lobar donations. Generally the recipients of these organs are children with cystic fibrosis. The allograft is assessed on the basis of function (gas exchange and compliance) and appearance (macroscopic, bronchoscopic and radiographic). In heart-lung transplantation, cardiac function is assessed via haemodynamic performance and the macroscopic appearance of the coronary arteries (angiography and echocardiography are not routinely available at every donor hospital).

Lung donors are generally under 55 years of age, although because of the organ shortage, there is an increasing trend to accept organs from donors older than this with acceptable results.

Matching the donor organ with a suitable recipient is simply on the basis of ABO blood group, and size (based on total lung capacity). Perfect size matching is rarely achieved. Oversizing should be avoided because the resultant lung compression and atelectasis predisposes to infection post-operatively.

3.4. Surgery

There are three basic options when replacing diseased lung tissue: single lung transplantation (SLT), bilateral sequential single (double lung) transplantation (BLT), and heart-lung transplantation (HLT). The choice of procedure is determined by the recipient's underlying disease and surgical preference. Diseases involving the heart and lungs such as Eisenmenger's syndrome mandate HLT. Septic lung diseases such as cystic fibrosis and bronchiectasis require replacement of both lungs (either BLT or HLT). SLT can usually be applied to most other diseases.

Bilateral lung transplantation is performed as two sequential single lung transplants. This can be done via a sternotomy or bilateral thoracotomy, with or without cardiopulmonary bypass. Heart-lung transplantation mandates cardiopulmonary bypass and is performed via a sternotomy.

There are 2 surgical principles essential for a successful outcome: careful and unhurried dissection minimises bleeding complications and damage to mediastinal (phrenic, vagus and recurrent laryngeal) nerves; and careful implantation reduces the chances of vascular or airway anastamotic complications post-transplant. Ideally implantation and reperfusion is achieved within 6 hours. Shorter ischaemic times are generally associated with better immediate and longer term results, especially when older donors are utilised.

3.5. Post-operative care

The first 24–48 hours post-transplantation are critical. Immediate post-operative care is aimed specifically at reducing the effects of the endothelial injury resulting from ischaemia and reperfusion. This injury results in a breakdown of the normal capillary endothelial barrier with resultant leakage of fluid into alveoli causing impaired gas exchange. Severe injury may necessitate prolonged mechanical ventilatory support with an increased risk of infection and barotrauma and irreversible damage to the allograft.

3.5.1. Early extubation
Early extubation permits active coughing and clearance of secretions, the institution of enteral nutrition, and the early commencement of rehabilitation. In the majority of patients, extubation is possible within 12 hours of the procedure (in many cases much less than this).

3.5.2. Fluid (crystalloid) restriction and diuresis
Fluid (crystalloid) restriction and diuresis minimises the development of the pulmonary oedema characteristic of ischaemia-reperfusion injury. Colloid solutions are used for haemodynamic requirements.

3.5.3. Early mobilisation
Early mobilisation prevents complications such as basal atelectasis and deep venous thrombosis, improves appetite and promotes sleep.

Patients with end-stage lung disease are usually debilitated and it is vitally important they are mobilised as early as possible. Most patients are able to sit out of bed within 24 hours and can participate in a gymnasium program by day 3. Adequate analgaesia is imperative for effective rehabilitation at this early stage.

3.5.4. Nutrition
Patients with end-stage lung disease are usually nutritionally compromised and an adequate calorie intake is necessary to overcome the severe catabolism stimulated by surgery. Enteral feeding can usually be started within 24 hours (either orally or via a nasogastric tube). If the gut is not functioning, parenteral nutrition should be used.

3.5.5. Prevention of infection
Bacterial infection remains the most significant problem encountered in the peri-operative period and is responsible for most deaths during this time. The organism is usually recipient-derived. Antibiotic prophylaxis is administered until the patient is mobile, all drains have been removed and respiratory secretions are clear. The choice of agent is dictated by the underlying disease and/or pre-transplant microbiology results. In cystic fibrosis and other septic lung diseases, antibiotics are chosen to cover *Pseudomonas aeruginosa* and *Staphylococcus aureus*. In other patients, community-acquired respiratory pathogens (*Pneumococcus*, *Haemophilus*, etc.) and *Staphylococcus aureus* are targeted.

Oropharyngeal candidiasis is common post-transplant and is effectively controlled with topical nystatin or amphotericin. Routine systemic prophylaxis against candida is not generally necessary. Aspergillus is the commonest cause of invasive fungal disease in this period. In SLT and BLT, nebulised amphotericin prophylaxis (5 mg tds) given for the first month post-transplant is effective in reducing aspergillus-related problems. Routine use of itraconazole prophylaxis is dependent on local policy and experience. It is very uncommon for HLT recipients to have problems with aspergillus in this period as the tracheal anastamosis is not ischaemic and all diseased lung tissue is removed. Routine prophylactic strategies are therefore not required in this setting.

Viral infections (specifically herpes viruses) tend to occur later in the recovery period but prophylaxis must be administered from the early stages to be effective. Ganciclovir is very effective in reducing both the incidence and severity of CMV-related illness. There is no consensus on the optimal prophylaxis regimen, but most units opt for a combination of intravenous followed by oral therapy for 1–3 months. Herpes simplex virus (HSV) most commonly causes muco-cutaneous infection. It is effectively covered by ganciclovir. In the occasional CMV negative donor/recipient match (where ganciclovir is unnecessary), acyclovir is used.

Co-trimoxazole prophylaxis is effective in preventing both pneumocystis infection and toxoplasma reactivation. Standard therapy is 480 mg daily or 960 mg three times a week. Therapy is usually continued for a minimum of 12 months or until corticosteroid doses have been reduced to physiological replacement doses. If cotimoxazole is not tolerated, nebulised pentamidine (300 mg per month) is an effective alternative for pneumocystis prophylaxis.

3.5.6. Prevention of rejection

In lung transplantation there are 3 phases of immunosuppression (induction, consolidation, and maintenance), and although the details of the exact combinations and doses of agents used vary from unit to unit, the principles are similar. A typical regimen is shown in Table 5. Most regimens employ a combination of 2 or more agents and are based on calcineurin inhibitors.

Anti-thymocyte globulin (ATG) is a polyclonal immunoglobulin directed at T lymphocytes. Increasingly, monoclonal antibodies directed at the IL-2 receptor are being used for induction although formal trial results are lacking.

Cyclosporin is a calcineurin inhibitor and works by preventing IL-2 production by activated T-cells. Tacrolimus is a widely used alternative.

These agents are usually combined with a bone marrow suppressive agent such as azathioprine. Mycophenolate mofetil works in a similar fashion via its acion as a purine analogue interfering with *de novo* DNA synthesis. Corticosteroids have a lympholytic action and are commonly employed in the standard 'triple immunosuppression' regimens.

Table 5

Immunosuppression regimen based on protocol from Papworth Hospital

Arrival:	azathioprine	2 mg/kg orally or IV
Induction of anaesthesia:	methylprednisolone	500 mg IV infusion over 30 minutes
Commencement of cardio-pulmonary bypass:	rabbit anti-thymocyte globulin (RATG)	1–2 mg/kg. Dilute in 250 ml 0.9% saline. Run over 10 hours. Pre medicate with 10 mg IV chlorpheniramine.
Reperfusion:	methylprednisolone	500 mg IV infusion over 30 minutes
Immediate post-op period:	methylprednisolone, 3 doses given 8, 16 and 24 hours post-op	125 mg IV bolus
	RATG days 1 and 2 (pre-med. with paracetamol and chlorpheniramine)	1–2 mg/kg aiming for T-cells <20% lymphocyte count
Maintenance therapy:	Prednisolone	1 mg/kg/day in 2 divided doses, reducing by 5 mg/day to 0.2 mg/kg/day
	Azathioprine	1–2 mg/kg single daily dose. Titrate to WCC $4–6 \times 10^9$/l
	Cyclosporin	First dose day 3. Commence 50 mg, increase 50 mg per dose to total 10 mg/kg/day in 2 divided doses (tds regimen for CF patients). Aim for cyclosporin level of ≥ 400 ng/l (EMIT assay) by day 7.

Newer agents such as rapamycin and its derivatives are still undergoing trials in pulmonary transplantation and their use is not widespread in this population.

3.6. Follow-up

The incidences of acute rejection and infection are highest in the first 3 months. Baseline lung function is usually established by 6–9 months post-transplant. This baseline is used to define the Bronchiolitis Obliterans Syndrome (BOS). This is discussed in detail below. As time from the transplant increases, out-patient visits occur less frequently, usually 3–6 monthly. The thrust of management in the longer term is to maintain allograft function, and to minimise the side effects of immunosuppression. Immunosuppression can be slowly reduced aiming to stop prednisolone after 12 months and reduce cyclosporin levels. Immunosuppression must however be tailored to individual requirements, and prevention of acute rejection must be the primary goal.

Monitoring of symptoms, chest X-ray and spirometry are the basis of allograft surveillance. Small hand-held spirometers enable daily home monitoring of lung function. A 10% or greater fall in the forced expiratory volume in 1 second (FEV_1) prompts review and investigation of the cause.

In the event of allograft dysfunction, transbronchial biopsies (TBBx) are performed. Acute rejection and infection cannot be distinguished clinically, and may occur simultaneously. Histopathological diagnosis of the cause of dysfunction is therefore mandatory. Some units perform regular surveillance TBBx. There is no evidence, however, that this influences long-term outcomes.

3.7. Specific complications

Many of the complications experienced by lung transplant recipients are common to all forms of solid organ transplantation and relate to drug side effects (hypertension, renal dysfunction, osteoporosis, hypercholesterolaemia etc.). The following problems relate specifically to lung transplantation.

3.7.1. Rejection

Lung allograft rejection is defined by immunological events and histological changes. Acute and chronic rejection are not defined by the timing of occurrence after transplant. Acute rejection can occur at any time post-transplant, and so-called 'chronic rejection' can occur within 3–6 months. In addition, the 2 processes can co-exist and probably have distinct immunopathological aetiologies. Histopathological criteria, standardised by the International Society of Heart and Lung Transplantation are listed in Table 6.

Acute rejection is treated conventionally with intravenous methyprednisolone (typically 0.5–1 g daily for 3 days). This is effective in the majority of cases. Steroid resistant rejection is usually treated with either a polyclonal (ATG) or monoclonal (OKT3) anti-lymphocytic agent. In addition, it is now usual to also change the background immunosuppression by substituting either tacrolimus for cyclosporin, or mycophenolate for azathioprine (or both).

Table 6

Working formulation for the classification and grading of pulmonary allograft rejection (adapted from International Society of Heart and Lung Transplantation Guidelines)

A: Acute Rejection — diagnosed on transbronchial lung biopsy. At least 5 alveolated pieces of lung are required for confident diagnosis.

Grade 0   none

Grade 1   minimal – scattered perivascular mononuclear cell infiltrates, not obvious at low magnification.

Grade 2   mild – frequent perivascular mononuclear cell infiltrates recognisable at low magnification.

Grade 3   moderate – dense perivascular mononuclear cell infiltrates usually associated with endothelialitis. Extension of inflammation into surrounding tissue.

Grade 4   severe – diffuse lymphocytic, eosinophilic and nuetrophil infiltrates with pneumocyte damage, hyaline membranes and haemorrhage.

B: Airway inflammation — deleted in this revised classification.

C: Chronic airway rejection — obliterative bronchiolitis

a. active

b. inactive

D: Chronic vascular rejection — accelerated graft vascular sclerosis

---

3.7.2. Chronic rejection

In lung transplantation, the term 'chronic rejection' is used to denote the presence of obliterative bronchiolitis (OB). Chronic rejection is defined histologically (airway fibrosis and/or vascular sclerosis), not by the time of occurrence after transplant. The aetiology, natural history and treatment are discussed in the following section.

3.7.3. Obliterative bronchiolitis (OB)

This term describes the pathological entity that represents 'chronic rejection' in lung transplantation. The term 'chronic rejection' is however a misnomer in this setting, as there are many processes (both allo-immune and non-allo-immune) which may result in fibrotic obliteration of the airway lumen. The term 'chronic allograft dysfunction' is therefore preferred.

The histopathology of OB is a fibro-proliferative scarring leading to either total or subtotal obliteration of the affected airway. This translates into fixed airflow obstruction, and this has enabled a non-invasive marker of the presence and severity of OB to be developed. The Bronchiolitis Obliterans Syndrome (BOS) is defined by a fall in the forced expiratory volume in one second (FEV_1), as measured from a baseline defined as the average of the 2 best FEV_1 measurements achieved post-transplant, taken at least 1 month apart. No reversible cause of the fall in lung function should be present. Table 7 summarises the BOS grading system. It has been confirmed in a number of large series that BOS accurately reflects the presence and severity of OB, and it is widely used in clinical practice for this purpose.

OB is the major cause of death in longer-term survivors of lung transplantation, with infection complicating OB the most common terminal event.

3.7.4. Treatment

There are no controlled trials to guide treatment of this condition. In some cases the disease arrests spontaneously. Augmented immunosuppression is rarely effective (although usually tried) and increases the risk of infection. Most experienced centres change immunosuppression early in the disease, substituting tacrolimus for cyclosporin, or mycophenolate for azathioprine. If the disease progresses despite the above changes, it is now common practice to reduce immunosuppression in an attempt to minimise the impact of infections.

3.7.5. Malignancy

Solid organ and lymphoid malignancies occur at an increased frequency in lung transplantation, affecting up to 4% of recipients. Lymphoproliferative disorders (LPD) are Epstein-Barr driven and related to the intensity of immunosuppression. In lung transplantation most cases are focused in the allograft and the majority occur in the first 12–18 months post-transplant. Patients are usually given a 1–2 month trial of aciclovir and reduced immunosuppression, with either non-response or progression of disease indicating the need for chemotherapy.

Reduction of immunosuppression involves cutting cyclosporin levels by 30–50%, stopping azathioprine and reducing prednisolone to less than 10 mg per day. There are no evidence-based data to support these recommendations, which are based on clinical experience only. The prognosis of these disorders is surprisingly good, especially if confined to a single organ system; however, patients diagnosed with advanced disease invariably have a poor outcome.

The most common solid organ malignancy seen is cutaneous malignancy (squamous or basal cell carcinoma). Provided these are diagnosed early and treated appropriately, they carry a very good prognosis. In contrast, other solid organ malignancy (lung, gastrointestinal tract etc.) carries a very poor prognosis and usually result in death within 12 months of diagnosis.

3.7.6. Airway complications

The bronchial anastamosis is devoid of its normal bronchial arterial supply and therefore prone to the development of problems. Most units experience an airway complication rate of around 10%. Complications range from asymptomatic narrowing, to severe narrowing requiring surgical intervention, to dehiscence and death. Bronchial artery revascularisation procedures are time consuming, technically

Table 7

Classification of Bronchiolitis Obliterans Syndrome (BOS)

Baseline:	Average of 2 best FEV_1 measurements achieved post-transplant, taken at least 1 month apart.	
BOS grade 0	FEV_1 >80%	baseline
BOS grade 1	FEV_1 66–79%	baseline
BOS grade 2	FEV_1 51–65%	baseline
BOS grade 3	FEV_1 <50%	baseline

Histopathology

a = no obliterative bronchiolitis or no biopsy

b = obliterative bronchiolitis demonstrated

demanding, and are therefore not widely performed. Bronchial stenosis can be treated with dilatation or stenting.

The situation in heart-lung transplantation is completely different. The tracheal anastamosis has a collateral blood supply derived from the coronary arteries. The airway is well vascularised and therefore serious airway/anastamotic problems are rare.

3.8. Outcome

Many studies have shown that lung transplantation confers significant survival and quality of life benefits to the majority of those patients lucky enough to receive a transplant. Survival figures of better than 80% at 1 year and 50% at 5 years are now achieved for all types of transplant and underlying disease category.

The main cause of death in the first 12 months is infection (predominantly bacterial). Acute rejection rarely causes death directly. OB is the major factor determining long-term survival in the majority of lung transplant recipients. Coronary occlusive disease affecting the cardiac allograft in a heart-lung transplant occurs predominantly in the setting of OB and it is the airway disease that dominates the clinical picture.

Survival is usually associated with markedly improved lung function and this translates into an improved functional capacity. As long as lung function is maintained (implying an absence of BOS) quality and quantity of life are maintained. Many patients are able to return to work and live a near normal life. Several female recipients have undergone normal pregnancies without specific transplant-related complications.

3.9. Conclusion

Lung and heart-lung transplantation offers the only therapeutic option for many patients with a variety of end-stage pulmonary and cardio-pulmonary diseases. With increasing experience and the development of more effective immunosuppression, survival figures continue to improve. The effectiveness of this process overall, however, continues to be limited, firstly by the critical shortage of donor organs (which limits the opportunity for transplantation to a select few), and secondly the occurrence of OB which limits the long term outcome in those fortunate to have been transplanted.

References and further reading

The Ad Hoc Committee of the Harvard Medical School to Examine the Definition of Brain Death. A definition of irreversible coma. JAMA 1968; 205(6): 337–340.

Armitage JM, Griffith BP, Hardesty RL, Kormos RL, Dummer JS. Lymphoproliferative disease in heart and lung transplant recipients: the University of Pittsburgh experience. J Heart Transplant 1990; 9: 60.

Aziz TM, Burgess MI, El-Gamel A, Campbell C, Rahman AN, Deiraniya AK, Yonan NA. Orthotopic cardiac transplantation technique: a survey of current practice. Ann Thorac Surg 1999 Oct; 68: 1242–1246.

Barnard CN. A human cardiac transplant: An interim report of a successful operation performed at Groote Schurr Hospital, Capetown. S Afr Med J 1967; 4: 1271–1274.

Barr ML, et al. Recipient and donor outcomes in living related and unrelated lobar transplantation. Transplant Proc 1998; 30, 915–922.

Bieber CP, Griepp RB, Oyer PE et al. Use of rabbit antithymocyte globulin in cardiac transplantation. Transplantation 1976; 22: 478–488.

Billingham ME. Diagnosis of cardiac rejection by endomyocardial biopsy. J Heart Transplant 1979; 1: 25.

Blumenstock DA, Hechtman HB, Collins JA, et al. Prolonged survival of orthotopic homotransplants of the heart in animals treated with methotrexate. J Thorac Cardiovasc Surg 1963; 46: 616.

Bristow MR, O'Connell JB, Gilbert EM et al. Dose-response of chronic beta-blocker treatment in heart failure from either idiopathic dilated or ischaemic cardiomyopathy. Circulation 1994; 89: 1632–1642.

Carpentier A, Chachques JC. Myocardial substitution with a stimulated skeletal muscle: first successful clinical case. Lancet 1985; 1: 126 (letter).

Carrel A, Guthrie CC. The transplantation of veins and organs. Am Med 1905; 10: 1101–1102.

Carrier M, Emery RW, Riley JE, et al. Cardiac transplantation in patients over 50 years of age. J Am Coll Cardiol 1992; 8: 285.

Caves PK, Stinson EB, Billingham ME Shumway ME. Percutaneous endomyocardial biopsy in human heart recipients. Ann Thorac Surg 1973; 16(4) 325–336.

Ciulli F, English TAH, Caine N, Mullins P, Biocina B, Schofield P, Wallwork J, Large S. Management of end-stage heart disease: conventional surgery or transplantation. Eur Heart J 1992; 13: 230.

Constanzo–Nordin MR, Cooper DKC, Jessup M, Renlund DG, Robinson JA, Rose EA. Task force 6: future developments. J Am Coll Cardiol 1993; 22: 54–64.

Costanzo MR, Naftel DC, Pritzker MR et al. Heart transplant coronary artery disease detected by coronary angiography: a multi-institutional study of preoperative donor and recipient risk factors. J Heart Lung Transplant 1998; 17: 744–753.

Czaplicki J, Blonska B, Religa Z. The lack of hyperactive xenogeneic heart transplant rejection in a human. J Heart Lung Transplant 1992; 11: 393–398 (letter).

Demikhov VP. Experimental transplantation of vital organs. Haigh B (transl), Consultants' Bureau, New York, 1962.

Dennis CM, et al. Heart-lung transplantation for end-stage respiratory disease in patients with cystic fibrosis at Papworth

Hospital. J Heart Lung Transplant 1993; 12: 893–902.

Dennis CM, et al. Heart-lung-liver transplantation. J Heart Lung Transplant 1996; 15: 536–538.

Dreyfuss M, Harri E, Hoffman H, Kobel H, Pache W, Tscherter H. Cyclosporin A and C, new metabolites from *Trichoderma polysporum*. Eur J Appl Microbiol 1976; 3: 125.

Frazier OH, Rose EA, Macmanus Q, et al. Multicenter clinical evaluation of the Heart-Mate 1000 IP left ventricular assist device. Ann Thorac Surg 1992; 53: 1080–1090.

Griepp RB, Stinson EB, Dong E, et al. Determinants of operative risk factors in human heart transplantation. Am J Surg, 1971; 122: 192.

Gross CR, et al. Long-term health status and quality of life outcomes of lung transplant recipients. Chest 1995; 108, 1587–1593.

Hardy JD, Chavez CM, Kurrus FD, et al. Heart transplantation in man. JAMA 1964; 188: 114–119.

Heng D, et al. Bronchiolitis obliterans syndrome: incidence, natural history, prognosis, and risk factors. J Heart Lung Transplant 1998; 17: 1255–1263.

Hiestand PC, Graber M, Hurtenbach U, et al. The new cyclosporine derivative, SDZ IMM 125: in vitro and in vivo pharmacological effects. Transplant Proc 1992; 24: 31–38.

Higgins R, et al. Airway stenosis after lung transplantation: management with expanding metal stents. J Heart Lung Transplant 1994; 13: 774–778.

Hosenpud JD, et al. The registry of the International Society for Heart and Lung Transplantation: sixteenth official report, 1999. J Heart Lung Transplant 1999; 18: 611–626.

Hosenpud JD, Bennett LE, Berkeley M, Keck MK, Boucek MM, Boucek M, Novick RJ. The registry of the International Society for Heart and Lung Transplantation: seventeenth official report, 2000. J Heart Lung Transplant 2000; 19(10): 909–931.

Hosenpud JD, Bennett LE, Keck MK, Boucek MM, Novick RJ. The registry of the International Society for Heart and Lung Transplantation: eighteenth official report, 2001. J Heart Lung Transplant 2001; 20(8): 805–815.

Hunt SA, Baker DW, Chin MH, Cinquegrani MP, Feldman AM, Francis GS, Ganiats TG, Goldstein S, Gregoratos G, Jessup ML, Noble R, Packer M, Silver MA, Stevenson LW. ACC/AHA guidelines for the evaluation and management of chronic heart failure in the adult: executive summary: a report of the American College of Cardiology/American Heart Association Task Force on Practice Guidelines. J Am Coll Cardiol 2001; 38: 2101–2113.

Joint Statement of the American Society for Transplant Physicians / American Thoracic Society / European Respiratory Society / International Society for Heart and Lung Transplantation. International guidelines for the selection of lung transplant candidates. Am J Respir Crit Care Med 1998; 158: 335–339.

Jonas M, Oduro A. Management of the multi-organ donor. In: Higgins RSD et al. (eds.), The Multi-Organ Donor. Selection and Management. Cambridge, MA, USA: Blackwell Scientific Publications, 1997; pp. 123–129.

Kasirajan V, McCarthy PM, Hoercher KJ, Starling RC, Young JB, Banbury MK, Smedira NG. Clinical experience with long-term use of implantable left ventricular assist devices: indications, implantation, and outcomes. Semin Thorac Cardiovasc Surg 2000 Jul; 12(3): 229–237.

Kostakis AJ, White DJG, Calne RY. Prolongation of rat heart allograft survival by cyclosporin A. IRCS Med Sci 1977; 5: 280.

Lower RR, Shumway NE. Studies on orthotopic homotransplantation of the canine heart. Surg Forum 1960; 11: 18–19.

MacLean A, Dunning J. The retrieval of thoracic organs: donor assessment and management. Br Med Bull 1997; 53(4): 829–843.

McNeil K, Dennis CM. Heart-lung transplantation: intensive care. In: Klinck JR, Lindop MJ (eds.), Anaesthesia and intensive care for organ transplantation. London: Chapman and Hall, 1998; 115–120.

McNeil K, Wallwork J. Principles of lung allocation. In: Collins GM, et al. (eds.), Procurement, preservation and allocation of vascularised organs. Dordrecht, the Netherlands: Kluwer Academic Publishers, 1997; 223–226.

Meester JD, et al. Lung transplant waiting list: differential outcome of type of end-stage lung disease, one year after registration. J Heart Lung Transplant 1999; 18: 563–571.

Novitzky D, Wicomb WN, Cooper DKC, et al. Improved cardiac function following hormonal therapy in brain dead pigs: Relevance to organ donation. Cryobiology, 1987; 24: 1.

O'Connell JB, Renlund DG, Gay WA et al. Efficacy of OKT3 re-treatment for refractory cardiac allograft rejection. Transplantation 1989; 47: 788–792.

Oyer PE, Stinson EB, Jamieson SA, et al. Cyclosporin A in cardiac allografting: A preliminary experience. Transplant Proc, 1983; 15: 1247–1252.

Penn I. Neoplastic consequences of immunosuppression. In: Dean JH, Munson AE, Luster M (eds.), Toxicology of the immune system. New York: Raven Press, 1984.

Radovancevic B, Frazier OH. Heart transplantation. Texas Heart Inst J 1999; 26(1): 60–70.

Reemtsma K, Williamson WE, Inglesias F, et al. Studies in homologous canine heart transplantation: Prolongation of survival with a folic acid antagonist. Surgery 1962; 52: 127.

Rubin RH. Prevention and treatment of cytomegalovirus disease in heart transplant patients. J Heart Transplant 2000; 19(8): 731–735.

Smith JA, Ribakove GH, Hunt SA et al. Cardiac retransplantation (CRTX): the 25 year experience at a single institution. J Heart Lung Transplant 1994; 13: S557.

Working Group of Conference of Medical Colleges and their Faculties in the United Kingdom. Criteria for the diagnosis of brain stem death. J R Coll Phys (Lond) 1995; 29: 281–282.

Yeatman M, et al. Lung transplantation in patients with systemic diseases: an eleven year experience at Papworth Hospital. J Heart Lung Transplant 1996; 15: 144–149.

Yousem SA, et al. Revision of the 1990 working formulation for the classification of pulmonary allograft rejection: lung rejection study group. J Heart Lung Transplant 1996; 15: 1–15.

The rehabilitation of cardiothoracic patients

L. Boruta and K. Pearson

1. Introduction

This chapter aims to provide an overview of the role of rehabilitation within the holistic package of care for cardiac and thoracic patients. Detailed discussion is beyond the scope of this chapter and references are provided for more in-depth reading. Best practice is emphasised, but it is acknowledged that services will vary according to available resources.

2. The rehabilitation of cardiac surgery patients

Participation in a comprehensive cardiac rehabilitation programme has the potential to reduce overall and cardiovascular mortality by 25% in MI (myocardial infarction) patients. This information was determined by two meta-analyses of 32 randomised control trials (RCTs) and almost 9000 patients (Oldridge et al., 1988; O'Connor et al., 1989). Although these seminal studies focused upon MI patients, there is evidence that the benefits of cardiac rehabilitation also apply to other cardiac populations (Julian, 1995; McCleod et al., 1995; Broustet et al., 1995; Banner, 1992; Noy, 1998) such as:

- cardiac surgery
- heart failure
- interventional cardiology
- angina
- transplantation

Cardiac rehabilitation can offer other benefits (Chartered Society of Physiotherapy, 1999) besides a reduction in mortality, namely:

- a reduction in frequency and severity of angina
- normalisation of blood pressure
- improved lipid profiles
- improved exercise tolerance, participation in leisure pursuits and daily activities
- reduced anxiety and depression
- improved compliance with risk factor modification
- improvement rates of return to work
- increased confidence and well-being
- improved understanding of condition by family and friends.

The economic justification for cardiac rehabilitation has been described by the British Cardiac Society working party report in 1992 on cardiac rehabilitation (Horgan et al., 1992). They suggested that approximate running costs per patient session were between £4 and £15 and that capital costs for setting up a programme were small. Pre-existing facilities were utilised and little in the way of extra equipment is required. More recent data (Gray et al., 1997) suggest the median cost per patient per session to be £26. An American study in 1993 (Oldridge et al., 1993) attempted to cost cardiac rehabilitation per quality adjusted life year (QALY). In 1997 this was recalculated at £6,900 to reflect costs within the UK (Cardiac Rehabilitation, 1998). Much of this work examined the service delivery to MI patients, but it is reasonable to presume that costs for other groups of cardiac patients would be similar. The heterogeneity of cardiac rehabilitation services and the range of different factors that can affect calculations of cost effectiveness make it difficult to conclude that all cardiac rehabilitation programmes are cost-effective. They are more likely to be so when patients receive only the specific interventions they require. This is the 'menu-based' approach which will be discussed below (Cardiac Rehabilitation, 1998).

2.1. Current service provision

The World Health Organisation (World Health Organisation, 1993) provides a comprehensive definition of cardiac rehabilitation:

"The rehabilitation of cardiac patients is the sum of activities required to influence favourably the underlying cause of the disease, as well as to ensure the patients the best possible physical, social and mental conditions so that they may, by their own efforts, preserve, or resume when lost, as normal a place as possible in the life of the community."

The gold standard for a comprehensive programme requires a service delivered by expert practitioners, to patients (and family members), when and where they need it, and in a way that allows the individual to take appropriate action for life-long benefits.

The working party report (Horgan et al., 1992) concluded that every major district hospital that treats patients with heart disease should provide a cardiac rehabilitation service. It is vital that these services are developed as an integral part and incorporated into service contracts from the outset rather than as an 'add-on' service. Sufficient funding should be included to allow services to develop in line with evidence-based national guidelines (Chartered Society of Physiotherapy, 1999; Thompson et al., 1996; Lewin et al., 1998; Thompson et al., 1997; Stokes et al., 1998) and research findings.

The needs of patients should drive rehabilitation programmes and flexibility is essential. The 'menu-based' approach (Thompson et al., 1996) allows patients to identify, with guidance, the appropriate aspects of a programme and access them accordingly. This way programmes are tailored to meet the needs of individual patients and not vice versa. As previously noted this should also make the programme more cost-effective.

Flexibility of staffing is a feature of many rehabilitation programmes, and an expert, interdisciplinary team represents the ideal (Horgan et al., 1992). The team may include (Lewin et al., 1998):

- physiotherapists
- nurses
- occupational therapists (OT)
- social workers
- pharmacists
- dieticians
- medical staff
- primary care team members
- exercise physiologists
- community-based exercise instructors
- vocational advisers
- psychologists/counsellors
- health promotion officers

Ward staff also play a vital role and are in a unique position to work with patients during an important stage in their rehabilitation. Patients and their families are less well acknowledged key members of the rehabilitation team.

Each team member offers specialist knowledge and skills and there may be areas where these overlap. Regardless of membership, however, the service should offer:

- risk factor management
- lifestyle and behavioural change
- health promotion
- counselling
- medical information

All team members have a responsibility to ensure that their knowledge and skills are evidence-based and remain in line with national and clinical guidelines. The service they provide must be clearly presented and in a format and language that is easily understood. Good intentions are wasted, however unless the team assesses whether patients and families *really* understand what is said to them!

2.2. Programme structure

Cardiac rehabilitation is usually divided into four phases which followed the recovery of patients post-MI. Stokes et al. (1995) describe this structure as helping to clarify "what should be done, when, where, to whom and by whom."

It is clear that with a planned event such as surgery, the opportunity exists for rehabilitation to commence as soon as a decision for surgery is made. It is useful, therefore to consider a further phase, namely the pre-operative phase (Table 1).

2.2.1. Pre-operative phase

This phase extends from the decision for surgery through to the operation. The focus is upon preparation for surgery and introduction to risk factor modification and the rehabilitation process.

It has been recognised that one of the most powerful predictors of cardiac rehabilitation uptake is the strength of medical recommendation (Ades et al., 1992). The initial consultation provides an excellent opportunity to enrol patients and their partners in the rehabilitation process and this enhances postoperative recovery. It provides an ideal opportunity to work with patients to minimise deterioration in cardiac function and physical ability, establish rapport, harness motivation and decrease fears and anxieties.

Table 1

The phases of cardiac rehabilitation for surgical patients.

	Hospital			
Community		**Community**		
Pre-op phase	Phase I *In-patient period*	Phase II *Early post-discharge*	Phase III *Intermediate post-discharge*	Phase IV *Long-term maintenance and independence*

The benefits of providing pre-operative information have been widely acknowledged (Haywood, 1975; Boore, 1978; Wilson-Barnett, 1986; Devine et al., 1983) and topics included are:
- identification of general and individual risk factors and guidance in their management
- correct use of medication to minimise symptoms and maximise compliance
- guidance in maintaining activity levels to maximise pre-operative fitness and minimise post-operative complications
- practical information about the hospital stay, including visits to the ward and intensive care areas for patients and/or families
- setting short- and long-term goals with professional guidance
- physiotherapy advice regarding respiratory care and the importance of early ambulation
- individual concerns of patients and families
- the role patients play in their own recovery

Problems travelling to a hospital-based programme, dislike of group settings and language or communication difficulties require that information be delivered in a variety of ways. Strategies used must consider the needs of group members and where possible several methods of presenting information should be available. These may include:
- written information
- video tapes
- audio tapes
- individual face-to-face discussion
- group discussion
- telephone contact
- other agencies such as national cardiac organisations and patient support groups
- information targeted at groups with specific needs such as religious and cultural groups, women and the elderly.

However the information is delivered, access to team members should be available to address issues arising during the sometimes lengthy waiting period.

2.2.2. The post-operative phases
The post-operative phases focus upon recovery and secondary prevention and encourage patients to pursue the ultimate goal of informed independence.

2.2.3. Phase I: the in-patient period
This phase lasts approximately 3–10 days as patients move from recovery from anaesthetic, through increasing independence to discharge home.

Rehabilitation usually begins on the intensive care unit on the first post-operative day and the physiotherapist plays a key role in this. Respiratory care and the prevention of musculo-skeletal complications are the key issues (Kieran et al., 1993). Positioning and early mobilisation play a vital role in both of these (Hough, 1984; Dean, 1985; Jenkins et al., 1989). Ambulation commences as soon as patients are cardiovascularly stable and is progressed daily. This is undoubtedly the most important rehabilitation intervention at this stage (Dean, 1994), and allows patients to take the first steps towards independence and resuming their role in their recovery. As recovery progresses, individuals learn to measure the amount of exertion they experience and how they should modify it. One tool used to facilitate this is the Borg Rated Perceived Exertion (RPE) scale (Borg, 1982).

The emphasis shifts quickly towards preparation for discharge. This should be inter-disciplinary and encompass progressive independence and education. Information to facilitate progress at home should be discussed prior to discharge and should include the family. Patients may lack confidence or have short-term memory problems associated with cardio-pulmonary bypass and may require further support and advice when at home. To this end, relevant contact numbers should be provided for use by patients and family members. Domiciliary visits, where available, are provided by primary or secondary care teams.

From experience, more intensive input may be required during this phase if surgery was performed as an emergency. There will have been no time for

tation will highlight the requirements specific to the needs of thoracic surgery patients.

Each thoracic procedure has its own requirements for rehabilitation, ranging from minimal to comprehensive. The aims of rehabilitation will differ depending on whether surgery is curative or palliative. A palliative procedure should not exclude a patient from receiving rehabilitation.

Thoracic surgery patients have little in the way of formalised rehabilitation programmes. Many centres, however, offer pulmonary rehabilitation programmes for those with chronic lung conditions and appropriate sections of this could be offered to those who have undergone surgery. Surgery-specific services would then be provided separately.

3.1. Key issues in rehabilitation programmes

The following topics are key issues in a rehabilitation programme for thoracic surgery patients and will be discussed below.
- Pain management
- Improving/maintaining lung function
- Exercise conditioning
- Musculo-skeletal and postural exercise
- Psychological/emotional support
- Activities of daily living (ADL)
- Education
- Nutrition
- Medication

3.1.1. Education
Although identified here as a separate issue, education is inherent within all of the following topics. Team members, topics, methods of delivery and timing of information mirror those of cardiac rehabilitation. Patients and their families place great store by the information provided by the team and this calls for precise, clear, consistent and accurate communication.

3.1.2. Pain management
Good pain management is fundamental to recovery and rehabilitation and is usually the primary concern of patients. It should begin pre-operatively with an assessment encompassing the patient's anxieties and preferences. Different types of pain may be present for the individual, notably:
- Surgical — acute and chronic
- Malignant
- Postural — due to joint stiffness and lack of movement

- Pre-existing pain relating to the presenting condition
- Pre-existing non-related pain

Obviously more than one type of pain may exist at any one time and a good pain management strategy will address this. Pain management techniques include:
- Pertinent choice of drugs and method of delivery
- Correct movement and handling
- Counselling
- Explanation and patient education including relaxation
- Posture correction and exercise
- Transcutaneous Electrical Nerve Stimulator (TENS)
- Acupuncture
- Hypnosis

The key team members here are the surgeon, pharmacist, physiotherapist, and nurses.

3.1.3. Improving/maintaining lung function
Potential problems associated with the presenting condition and/or the procedure include:
- atelectasis
- reduction in functional residual capacity and tidal volume
- impaired thoracic expansion
- retention of secretions
- ventilation/perfusion mismatches

These problems may occur before and/or after any thoracic operation and are due to the presenting condition, the effects of anaesthetic, pain (and fear of pain) and alteration in the normal mechanics of ventilation resulting from the surgery.

Patients who are at high risk of developing pulmonary complications or require active interventions, such as stopping smoking, should be identified prior to surgery. They should have access to this support before admission.

Key team members are the primary care team, physiotherapists and specialist nursing staff.

3.1.4. Exercise conditioning
Poor exercise tolerance is frequently a problem pre-operatively and much may be gained by attempting to stabilise or maximise it prior to surgery. Participation in an existing pulmonary rehabilitation programme or individual sessions with a physiotherapist or respiratory nurse may address this. However the intervention is delivered, the pre-operative aims remain the same. Hough (1991) describes them as being to:
- alleviate symptoms and fear of breathlessness

- teach energy conserving techniques
- decrease the number and frequency of acute episodes and resulting loss of function
- allow the patient to regain some control over their symptoms
- improve the capacity to perform activities of daily living (ADL)
- teach the judicious use of oxygen therapy during activity.

Pulmonary rehabilitation programmes are also used prior to lung volume reduction surgery (LVRS) (Harden, 1997; Grant, 1997; Nanheim et al., 1996; ACCP/AACVPR Pulmonary Rehabilitation Guidelines Panel, 1997) and lung transplantation (Downs, 1996). These patients benefit by maximising exercise tolerance and preparing for the intensive rehabilitation that follows these procedures. Lack of resources, however, remains an insurmountable obstacle to this ideal in many centres.

Post-operatively an appropriate cardiovascular exercise regime should be developed, aimed at maximising physical potential. The patient may initially require supervision, but then be encouraged to continue independently using a suitable self-assessment tool, such as the Borg RPE scale (Borg, 1982).

3.1.5. Musculo-skeletal and postural exercise

Post-operative problems will be affected by pre-existing musculo-skeletal problems. These include (Vibekk, 1991; Anderson et al., 1993):

- increased thoracic kyphosis
- reduced thoracic expansion, either due to stiff joints or underlying restrictive lung disease or both
- over-developed accessory muscles resulting in muscle imbalance and adaptive shortening.

Musculo-skeletal complications developing post-operatively include:

- reduced movement around the neck and thorax due to incisional pain and fear of pain.
- changes in the mechanics of ventilation and restriction of movement due to disruption of the thoracic cage.

Physiotherapists and nursing staff are best placed to address these issues by prescribing and encouraging good posture, appropriate exercise and stretching routines for use in the hospital and continuation at home.

3.1.6. Psychological/emotional support

Emotional and environmental factors and the patient's prognosis affect the perception of symptoms such as pain and breathlessness (Holland, 1991).

Help is needed in acknowledging these issues and identifying coping strategies such as relaxation techniques. Some patients and their families also require assistance with adaptation from illness to health.

Hospital-based and/or domiciliary services may be available, offering pre- and post-operative support. Key members for providing this are the OT, counsellor and psychologist.

Palliative care needs and cancer services should be provided by specialists in this field. In the UK this would be via hospice staff and charitably funded nurses (e.g. MacMillan nurses).

3.1.7. Activities of daily living

These issues need to be addressed at the pre-operative stage. This will prevent delay in discharge and promote early independence.

Issues to consider include:

- the inability to perform ADL due to any of the problems previously discussed
- unsuitable home environment; the need for aids, adaptations or re-housing
- review of the level of care/assistance required
- review of the need for financial assistance, e.g. state benefits or insurance claims
- return to work/re-training

The social worker and OT are key players at this stage.

3.1.8. Nutrition

Some patients require considerable input from the dietician/nutritionist; for others it will be minimal.

Interventions include:

- pre-operative improvement in nutritional status
- healthy eating advice
- modified diets
- parenteral nutrition
- dietary supplements
- high-calorie or reducing diets
- education about portion size and frequency of meals.

Partnership between primary and secondary care is once again invaluable.

3.1.9. Medication

The patient needs to understand the effects, side effects and method of delivery of all appropriate medications in order to maximise compliance. The consequences of non-compliance should be made clear. Advice regarding the possible effects of taking non-prescribed drugs such as herbal remedies, tobacco and alcohol also needs to be emphasised.

Pharmacists, medical and nursing staff are best placed to address these issues.

3.2. Summary

Clearly, the content and delivery of a rehabilitation service for thoracic surgery patients is very dependent upon many factors:

- pre-operative health status of the patient
- surgery performed
- prognosis
- recovery pathway
- resources

In order to address these effectively, a menu-based rehabilitation programme is required, which follows national guidelines and standards. Regular audit is essential to ensure the continuing development of the service.

4. Chapter summary

Ideally rehabilitation is interdisciplinary and multi-faceted in its approach. It takes place in both hospital and community and the two must work in harmony to best meet the needs of the individual patient. The approach should be consistent, be accessible to the majority and ensure efficient use of scarce resources. Funding issues must be addressed if rehabilitation programmes are to even begin to achieve this ideal.

References and further reading

ACCP/AACVPR Pulmonary Rehabilitation Guidelines Panel. Pulmonary rehabilitation: Joint ACCP/AACVPR evidence-based guidelines. Chest 1997; 112(5): 1363–1396.

Ades PA, Waldemann ML, McCann WJ, Weaver SO. Predictors of cardiac rehabilitation participation in older coronary patients. Arch Intern Med 1992; 152: 1033–1035.

American Association of Cardiovascular and Pulmonary Rehabilitation. Guidelines for cardiac rehabilitation programmes. Champaign, Illinois: Human Kinetics Books, 1991.

Anderson J, Jenkins SC. Physiotherapy problems and their management. In: Webber B and Pryor J (eds.), Physiotherapy for respiratory and cardiac problems. Edinburgh: Churchill Livingstone, 1993; pp. 199–233.

Banner N. Exercise physiology and rehabilitation after heart transplant. J Heart Lung Transplant 1992; 11(4 pt 2): S237–S240.

Bell J, Coats AJS, Hardman AE. Exercise testing and prescription. In: Coats A, McGee H, Stokes H, Thompson D (eds.), BACR guidelines for cardiac rehabilitation. Oxford: Blackwell Science, 1995; pp. 56–91.

Bethell HJN. Community based cardiac rehabilitation. In: Jones D, West R (eds.), Cardiac rehabilitation. London: BMJ Publishing Group, 1995; pp. 167–183.

Boore J. Prescription for recovery. London: Royal College of Nursing, 1978.

Borg G. Psycho-physical bases of perceived exertion. Med Sci Sports Exerc 1982; 14: 377–379.

Bowman GS, Bryar RM, Thompson DR. Is the place for cardiac rehabilitation in the community? Soc Sci Health 1998; 4(4): 243–254.

Broustet J-P, Douard H. Rehabilitation after cardiac surgery. In: Jones D, West R (eds.), Cardiac rehabilitation. London: BMJ Publishing Group, 1995; pp. 128–143.

Buckley J, Holmes J, Mapp G. Exercise on prescription: Cardiovascular activity for health. Oxford: Butterworth Heinemann, 1999.

Cardiac Rehabilitation. Effective Health Care 1998; 4(4).

Channer KS, Barrow D, Barrow R, Osborne M, Ives G. Changes in haemodynamic parameters following Tai Chi Chuan and aerobic exercise in patients recovering from acute myocardial infarction. Postgrad Med J 1996; 72: 349–351.

The Chartered Society of Physiotherapy. Standards for the exercise component of phase III cardiac rehabilitation. London, June 1999.

Coats A, McGee H, Stokes H, Thompson D (eds.). BACR guidelines for cardiac rehabilitation. Oxford: Blackwell Science, 1995.

Curfman GD. Is exercise beneficial — or hazardous — to your heart? N Engl J Med 1993; 329(23): 1730–1731.

Dean E. Effect of body position on pulmonary function. Phys Ther 1985; 65(5): 613–618.

Dean E. Oxygen transport: a physiologically based conceptual framework for the practice of cardiopulmonary physiotherapy. Physiother 1994; 80(6): 347–355.

De Bono D. Models of cardiac rehabilitation. BMJ 1998; 316: 1329–1330.

Department of Health National Service Framework for Coronary Heart Disease (Emerging Findings). UK Department of Health, Nov 1998 (HSC 1998/218).

Devine E, Cook R. A meta analytical analysis of psychoeducational interventions on length of post surgical stay. Nurs Res 1983; 32(5): 267–274.

Downs AM. Physical therapy in lung transplantation. Phys Ther 1996; 76(6): 626–642.

Gohlke H, Gohlke-Bärwolf C. Cardiac rehabilitation: Where are we going? Eur Heart J 1998; 19(suppl O): O5–O12.

Grant A. Lung volume reduction surgery. Clarification of the controversy. Physiother 1997; 83(9): 491–494.

Gray AM, Bowman GS, Thompson DR. The cost of cardiac rehabilitation services in England and Wales. J R Coll Physicians Lond 1997; 31: 57–61.

Harden B. Lung volume reduction surgery for emphysema: Cure or controversy. Physiother 1997; 83(3): 136–140.

Haywood J. Information: a prescription against pain. London: Royal College of Nursing, 1975.

Holland L. Breathlessness. In: Pryor J (ed.), Respiratory care. Edinburgh: Churchill Livingstone, 1991; pp. 5–26.

Horgan J, Bethell H, Carson P, Davidson C, Julian D, Mayou RA, Nagle R. Working party report on cardiac rehabilitation. Br Heart J 1992; 67: 412–418.

Hough A. Effects of posture on lung function. Physiother 1984; 70: 3: 101–104.

Hough A. Physiotherapy in respiratory care: A problem-solving approach. London: Chapman and Hall, 1991.

Jenkins SC, Soutar SA, Loukota JM, Johnson LC, Moxham J. Physiotherapy after coronary artery surgery — are breathing exercises necessary? Thorax 1989; 44: 634–639.

Jones D, West R (eds.). Cardiac rehabilitation. London: BMJ Publishing Group, 1995.

Julian DG. Medical background to cardiac rehabilitation. In: Jones D, West R (eds.), Cardiac rehabilitation. London: BMJ Publishing Group, 1995; pp. 4–30.

Kavanagh T. The role of exercise training in cardiac rehabilitation. In: Jones D, West R (eds.), Cardiac rehabilitation. London: BMJ Publishing Group, 1995; pp. 54–82.

Kieran M, McCoy P, Webber BA, Pryor J. Surgical patients and patients requiring intensive care. In: Webber B, Pryor J (eds.). Physiotherapy for respiratory and cardiac problems. Edinburgh: Churchill Livingstone, 1993; pp. 237–279.

Lan C, Chen SY, Lai JS, Wong MK. The effect of Tai Chi on cardiorespiratory function in patients with coronary artery bypass surgery. Med Sci Sports Exerc 1999 May; 31(5): 634–638.

Lewin RJP, Ingleton R, Newens AJ, Thompson DR. Adherence to cardiac rehabilitation guidelines: a survey of rehabilitation programmes in the UK. BMJ 1998; 316: 1354–1355.

McCleod A, Coats AJS. Medical aspects of cardiac rehabilitation. In: Coats A, McGee H, Stokes H, Thompson D (eds.), BACR guidelines for cardiac rehabilitation. Oxford: Blackwell Science, 1995; pp. 40–55.

Nanheim KS, Ferguson MK. The current status of lung volume reduction operations for emphysema. Ann Thorac Surg 1996; 62: 601–612.

Noy K. Cardiac Rehabilitation: structure, effectiveness and the future. Br J Nurs 1998; 7(17): 1033–1040.

O'Connor GT, Buring JE, Yusuf S, Goldhaber SZ, Olmstead EM, Paffenbarger RS, Hennekens CH. An overview of randomised controlled trials of rehabilitation with exercise after myocardial infarction. Circulation 1989; 80: 234–244.

Oldridge NB, Furlong W, Seeny D, Torrance G, Guyatt G, Crowe J, Jones N. Economic evaluation of cardiac rehabilitation soon after acute myocardial infarction. Am J Cardiol 1993; 72: 154–161.

Oldridge NB, Guyatt GH, Fischer ME, Rimm AA. Cardiac rehabilitation after myocardial infarction: combined experience of randomised clinical trials. JAMA 1988; 260: 945–950.

Outreach phase III cardiac rehabilitation programme for CABG patients (information pack and video, 1996). *From:* Cardiac Rehabilitation, Papworth Hospital, Papworth Everard, Cambridge CB3 8RE, UK.

Stokes HC, Thompson DR, Seers K. The implementation of multiprofessional guidelines for cardiac rehabilitation: a pilot study. Coronary Health Care 1998; 2: 60–71.

Stokes H, Turner S, Farr A. Cardiac rehabilitation: programme structure, content, management and administration. In: Coats A, McGee H, Stokes H, Thompson D (eds.), BACR guidelines for cardiac rehabilitation. Oxford: Blackwell Science, 1995; pp. 12–39.

Thompson DR, Bowman GS, de Bono DP, Hopkins A. The development and testing of a cardiac rehabilitation audit tool. J R Coll Physicians Lond 1997; 31: 317–320.

Thompson DR, Bowman GS, Kitson AL, de Bono DP, Hopkins A. Cardiac rehabilitation in the United Kingdom: guidelines and audit standards. Heart 1996; 75: 89–93.

Tod AM, Pearson K, McCabe M. Cardiac rehabilitation: Integrating primary and secondary care. Coronary Health Care 1998; 2: 150–155.

Vibekk P. Chest mobilisation and respiratory function. In: Pryor J (ed.), Respiratory care. Edinburgh: Churchill Livingstone, 1991; pp. 103–120.

Wilson–Barnett J. The prevention and alleviation of stress in patients. Nursing 1986; 10: 432–436.

World Health Organisation. Needs and action priorities in cardiac rehabilitation and secondary prevention in patients with coronary heart disease. Geneva: WHO Technical Report Service, WHO Regional Office for Europe, 1993; p. 831.

Subject Index